The Year in Metabolism

1977

The Year in Metabolism

The Year in Metabolism

1977

Edited by

Norbert Freinkel, M. D.

Kettering Professor of Medicine,
Professor of Biochemistry,
Director, Center for Endocrinology, Metabolism, and Nutrition,
Northwestern University Medical School,
Chicago, Illinois

PLENUM MEDICAL BOOK COMPANY
NEW YORK AND LONDON

The Library of Congress cataloged the first volume of this work as follows:

Main entry under title:

The year in metabolism, 1976.

Includes bibliographies and index.
1 Metabolism, Disorders of. 2. Metabolism.
I. Freinkel, Norbert. [DNLM: 1. Metabolism–Period. W1 YE41]
RC627.54.Y4 616.3'9 76-44885

ISBN 978-1-4684-2501-7 ISBN 978-1-4684-2499-7 (eBook)
DOI 10.1007/978-1-4684-2499-7

Library of Congress Catalog Card Number 76-44885

Softcover reprint of the hardcover 1st edition 1978
227 West 17th Street, New York, N. Y. 10011

Plenum Medical Book Company is an imprint of Plenum Publishing Corporation

Contributors

Gerald D. Aurbach, M.D. • Chief, Metabolic Diseases Branch, National Institute of Arthritis, Metabolism, and Digestive Diseases, National Institutes of Health, Bethesda, Maryland 20014

Jack W. Coburn, M.D. • Chief, Nephrology Section, Medical Services, Veterans Administration Wadsworth Hospital Center; Professor of Medicine, University of California Los Angeles School of Medicine, Los Angeles, California 90073

Stefan S. Fajans, M.D. • Professor of Internal Medicine; Head, Division of Endocrinology and Metabolism; Director, Metabolism Research Unit, The University of Michigan, Ann Arbor, Michigan 48109

Philip Felig, M.D. • Professor and Vice Chairman, Department of Internal Medicine; Chief, Section of Endocrinology, Yale University School of Medicine, New Haven, Connecticut 06510

DeWitt S. Goodman, M.D. • Tilden-Weger-Bieler Professor, Department of Medicine, College of Physicians and Surgeons of Columbia University, New York, New York 10032

David L. Hartenbower, M.D. • Clinical Investigator, Medical and Research Services, Veterans Administration Wadsworth Hospital Center, Los Angeles, California 90073

Jules Hirsch, M.D. • Professor and Senior Physician; Chairman, Department of Human Behavior and Metabolism, The Rockefeller University, New York, New York 10021

Charles R. Kleeman, M.D. • Professor of Medicine; Chief, Division of Nephrology, Department of Medicine, University of California Los Angeles School of Medicine, Los Angeles, California 90073

Veikko Koivisto, M.D. • Visiting Research Fellow, Section of Endocrinology, Department of Internal Medicine, Yale University School of Medicine, New Haven, Connecticut 06510

Charles S. Lieber, M.D. • Director, Alcohol Research Center; Chief, Section and Laboratory of Liver Disease and Nutrition, Veterans Administration Hospital, Bronx, New York 10468; Professor of Medicine and Pathology, Mount Sinai School of Medicine of the City University of New York, New York, New York 10029

Ferid Murad, M.D., Ph.D. • Professor, Departments of Internal Medicine and Pharmacology; Director, Division of Clinical Pharmacology; Director, Clinical Research Center, University of Virginia, Charlottesville, Virginia 22903

Leon E. Rosenberg, M.D. • Professor and Chairman, Department of Human Genetics, Yale University School of Medicine, New Haven, Connecticut 06510

J. Edwin Seegmiller, M.D. • Professor of Medicine; Head, Division of Rheumatology, The University of California San Diego, La Jolla, California 92093

Kay Tanaka, M.D. • Senior Research Scientist, Department of Human Genetics, Yale University School of Medicine, New Haven, Connecticut 06510

Roger H. Unger, M.D. • Staff Physician, Veterans Administration Hospital, Dallas, Texas 75216; Professor of Internal Medicine, University of Texas Southwestern Medical School, Dallas, Texas 75235

Hibbard E. Williams, M.D. • Chief, Medical Service, San Francisco General Hospital Medical Center; Professor and Vice Chairman, Department of Medicine, University of California, San Francisco, California 94110

Myron Winick, M.D. • R. R. Williams Professor of Nutrition; Professor of Pediatrics; Director, Institute of Human Nutrition, College of Physicians and Surgeons of Columbia University, New York, New York 10032

Preface

In the words of Disraeli, "To be conscious that you are ignorant of the facts is a great step to knowledge." For most of us, the conscious awareness of relative ignorance is an uncomfortable aspect of daily life. New data appear in such inexorable profusion that the necessity for continuous retooling has joined death and taxes as an inescapable component of our destinies. Perhaps it is this "consciousness of ignorance" that accounts for the success of the preceding volumes of this new series. *The Year in Metabolism* and *The Year in Endocrinology* series were introduced with the avowed intention of "providing an efficient and enjoyable bridge between those who are creating new knowledge at the bedside and the professional consciousness of those for whom such knowledge is ultimately intended." That objective seems particularly appropriate at a time when the award of the 1977 Nobel Prize in Medicine or Physiology to Guillemin, Schally, and Yalow has served to emphasize the epoch-making advances that have characterized the recent course of endocrinology and metabolism. For the 1977 volume of *The Year in Metabolism,* the previous formula has been preserved. The same internationally recognized authorities again have contributed commentaries about the progress in their areas of expertise. They have been joined by Drs. Jack W. Coburn, David L. Hartenbower, and Charles R. Kleeman, who have provided a new section on Divalent Ion Metabolism. All the authors have again combined erudition with lucidity and informality. The Editor hopes that the readers will find in the

1977 edition a series of profitable encounters with a remarkable group of teachers. If so, "great steps to knowledge" will have been taken and "ignorance of the facts" diminished.

Norbert Freinkel, M.D.

Contents

Chapter 1
Cyclic GMP in Metabolism: Interrelationships of Biogenic Amines, Hormones, and Other Agents
Ferid Murad and Gerald D. Aurbach

1.1. Introduction 1
1.2. Formation and Degradation of Cyclic GMP 3
1.2.1. Guanylate Cyclases 3
1.2.2. Cyclic Nucleotide Phosphodiesterases and Other Mechanisms of Cyclic Nucleotide Disposal 8
1.2.3. Cyclic Nucleotide Protein Kinases 10
1.3. Regulation of Cyclic GMP in Tissues 11
1.3.1. Effects of Hypophysectomy and Adrenalectomy 11
1.3.2. Effects of Choline Esters 12
1.3.3. Effects of α-Adrenergic Agonists 13
1.3.4. Effects of Prostaglandins 13
1.3.5. Effects of Calcium 14

1.3.6. Effects of Azide, Hydroxylamine, and Various Nitro Compounds 15
1.3.7. Effects of Other Agents 16
1.4. Some Physiologic Effects That May Correlate with Cyclic GMP 17
1.4.1. Smooth-Muscle Contraction 17
1.4.2. Heart 18
1.4.3. Secretion and Transport 18
1.4.4. Histamine Release 18
1.4.5. Cell Growth and Proliferation 19
1.4.6. Platelet Aggregation 19
1.4.7. Other Processes 20
1.5. Clinical Studies with Cyclic Nucleotides 20
1.5.1. Cyclic Nucleotides in Tissues 20
1.5.1.1. Psoriasis 20
1.5.1.2. Tumors 20
1.5.2. Cyclic Nucleotides in Extracellular Fluids 21
1.5.2.1. Parathyroid Disorders 21
1.5.2.2. Cystic Fibrosis 22
1.5.2.3. Cushing's Disease 22
References 23

Chapter 2
Diabetes Mellitus
Stefan S. Fajans

2.1. Heterogeneity of Diabetes Mellitus 33
2.1.1. Genetic Heterogeneity 33
2.1.1.1. The Histocompatability System *(HLA)* and Genetic Susceptibility to Diabetes Mellitus 34
2.1.1.2. Inheritance of (Genetic Susceptibility to) Virus-Induced Diabetes Mellitus 36
2.1.1.3. Autoimmunity in Diabetes Mellitus 38
2.1.1.4. Environmental Factors—Viruses and Other Infectious or Chemical Agents 42
2.1.2. Insulin Secretion 43
2.1.2.1. Prognostic Significance of Heterogeneity of Insulin Responses to Glucose in Mild Diabetes 43
2.1.2.2. Mechanism of Insulin Secretion Relevant to Clinical Diabetes Mellitus 44

2.1.2.3. Measurement of Beta-Cell Secretory Products—Connecting Peptide 48
2.1.3. Insulin Resistance 49
2.1.3.1. Evidence for Insulin Resistance 49
2.1.3.2. Mechanism for Insulin Resistance: Decreased Insulin Binding to Insulin Receptors 52
2.2. Relationship of Fuels to Hormonal Release and Fuel Economy 54
2.3. Glucagon Secretion—Somatostatin 54
2.4. Epidemiological Findings 54
2.5. Control of Diabetes 59
2.5.1. General Considerations 59
2.5.2. Glycosylated Hemoglobin and Diabetic Control 60
2.6. Long-Term Complications 62
2.6.1. Diabetic Microangiopathy 62
2.6.1.1. Changes in Plasma Proteins 62
2.6.1.2. Changes in Microvascular Permeability 63
2.6.1.3. Biochemical Studies 64
2.6.1.4. Muscle Capillary Basement Membrane Thickening 64
2.6.1.5. Diabetic Retinopathy 66
2.6.1.6. Diabetic Nephropathy 69
2.6.2. Diabetic Macroangiopathy 73
2.6.2.1. Prevalence 73
2.6.2.2. Pathogenetic Factors 74
2.6.3. Diabetic Neuropathy 75
2.6.3.1. Clinical Aspects 75
2.6.3.2. Pathogenetic Factors 77
2.6.4. Disturbance of Growth and Accelerated Aging in Diabetes Mellitus 77
2.6.5. Prevention and Treatment—Islet and Pancreas Transplantation 78
2.7. Diabetes in Pregnancy 78
2.8. Treatment of Diabetes Mellitus 79
2.8.1. Dietary Treatment 79
2.8.2. Insulin Treatment 82
2.8.2.1. Ketoacidosis 82
2.8.2.2. Chronic Therapy 85
2.8.3. Oral Hypoglycemic Therapy 86
2.8.3.1. Sulfonylureas 86
2.8.3.2. Phenformin 87
References 89

Chapter 3
Glucagon and Somatostatin
Roger H. Unger

3.1. Immunoreactive Glucagons in Tissues and Plasma 101
3.1.1. Primary Structure of Glucagon 101
3.1.2. "Glucagonlike Immunoreactivity" 102
3.1.3. Glucagon Biosynthesis 102
3.1.4. Tissue Immunoreactive Glucagon 103
3.1.5. Plasma Immunoreactive Glucagon 103
3.2. Structure–Function Relationships of Glucagon 104
3.2.1. Biological 104
3.2.2. Immunologic 105
3.3. Molecular Basis for Glucagon Actions 106
3.4. Glucagon Metabolism, Clearance, and Degradation 106
3.5. Physiologic Actions of Glucagon 107
3.5.1. Hepatic Glycogenolysis 107
3.5.2. Gluconeogenesis 108
3.5.2.1. Molecular 108
3.5.2.2. Physiologic 108
3.5.3. Ketogenesis 109
3.6. Physiologic Roles of Glucagon in Fuel Homeostasis 109
3.6.1. Maintenance of Basal Hepatic Glucose Production .. 109
3.6.2. Increase in Hepatic Glucose Production during Protein Meals 109
3.6.3. Increase in Hepatic Glucose Production during Exercise 110
3.6.4. Effects of Glucagon on Lipids and Ketones 110
3.7. Concept of the Bihormonal Unit 110
3.8. Control of Glucagon Secretion 111
3.8.1. Glucose 111
3.8.2. Amino Acids 113
3.8.3. Free Fatty Acids 113
3.8.4. Calcium 113
3.8.5. Cyclic 3′,5′-Adenosine Monophosphate 114
3.8.6. Adrenergic Stimulation—Stress and Exercise 114
3.8.7. Hormones 114
3.8.7.1. Gastrointestinal Hormones 114
3.8.7.2. Growth Hormone 115
3.8.7.3. Neurotensin and Substance P 115
3.8.7.4. Glucocorticoids 115
3.8.7.5. Prostaglandins 115

3.9. Extrapancreatic Glucagon 116
3.10. Somatostatin 117
3.10.1. Pancreatic Somatostatin 118
3.10.1.1. Paracrine Actions of Somatostatin 118
3.10.1.2. Endocrine Actions of Somatostatin 118
3.10.1.3. Mechanism of Action on Islet Cells 120
3.11. Morphofunctional Interrelationships of the Endocrine Pancreas: Microanatomic Organization of the Islets of Langerhans 120
3.11.1. Organization of Islet Cells 121
3.11.2. Subcellular Specialization of Islet Cells 121
3.12. Importance of Glucagon in Clinical Medicine—Diabetes Mellitus 123
3.12.1. A-Cell Function in Human Diabetes 123
3.12.2. The Bihormonal Abnormality Hypothesis 124
3.12.3. Glucagon Suppression as a Therapeutic Adjunct in Juvenile Diabetes 126
3.12.4. Glucagonoma 127
References 129

Chapter 4
Body Fuel Metabolism
Philip Felig and Veikko Koivisto

4.1. Introduction 143
4.2. Glucose Metabolism 143
4.2.1. Glucose Absorption: Effects of Somatostatin 143
4.2.2. Glucose Production 145
4.2.2.1. Protein Ingestion 145
4.2.2.2. Starvation 146
4.2.2.3. Evanescent Effects of Hyperglucagonemia . 148
4.2.2.4. Evanescent Effects of Hypoglucagonemia: Prolonged Infusion of Somatostatin 149
4.2.3. Insulin and Hepatic Glucose Output 151
4.2.4. Counterregulation during Insulin Hypoglycemia 152
4.2.5. Neonatal Hypoglycemia 153
4.3. Amino Acid Metabolism 153
4.3.1. Alanine Synthesis in Muscle 153
4.3.2. Metabolism of Branched-Chain Amino Acids in Normal and Diabetic Subjects 156
4.4. Ketone and Fatty Acid Metabolism 157

4.4.1. Hormonal Regulation of Ketogenesis 157
4.4.2. Substrate Regulation of Ketogenesis 158
4.4.3. Role of Ketone Disposal in Hyperketonemia 158
4.5. Fuel Metabolism in Exercise 160
4.5.1. Influence of Glucose Ingestion 160
4.5.2. Glucose-Sparing Effect of Free Fatty Acids 160
4.5.3. Interaction of Exercise and Insulin in Diabetes 161
References 163

Chapter 5
What's New in the Treatment of Obesity?
Jules Hirsch

5.1. Introduction 169
5.2. The Core Problem of Treatment 170
5.3. Hypothetical Defended Variables in Obesity 170
5.3.1. Hyperphagia 170
5.3.2. Symbolic Meaning of Obesity 171
5.3.3. A Life Style 172
5.3.4. Adipose Mass 173
5.4. Implications for Treatment 173
5.5. Current New Approaches in Treatment 174
5.5.1. The Protein-Sparing Modified Fast 174
5.5.2. Behavior Modification 176
5.5.3. Jejunoileal Shunt 179
5.6. Conclusion 180
References 181

Chapter 6
Disorders of Lipid and Lipoprotein Metabolism
DeWitt S. Goodman

6.1. Introduction 183
6.2. Lipoprotein Structure and Metabolism 184
6.2.1. General Review 184
6.2.2. The Lp(a) Lipoprotein 185
6.2.3. Lipoprotein-X and Liver Disease 187
6.3. Hyperlipidemias 187
6.3.1. Definition and Classification 187

6.3.2. Epidemiology 188
6.4. High-Density-Lipoprotein Levels and Coronary Heart Disease 189
6.4.1. Epidemiologic Studies 189
6.4.2. Familial Hyperalpha and Familial Hypobeta Lipoproteinemia 191
6.4.3. Possible Mechanisms 192
6.4.4. Implications 193
6.5. Type III Hyperlipoproteinemia 193
6.6. Cholesterol Metabolism and Its Regulation 194
6.6.1. In Intact Humans 194
6.6.2. In Cultured Cells 196
6.7. Familial Hypercholesterolemia 199
6.7.1. Genetics 199
6.7.2. Pathogenesis 199
6.7.3. Therapy 201
6.8. β-Sitosterolemia and Cerebrotendinous Xanthomatosis 203
6.9. Hypertriglyceridemia 204
6.9.1. Pathophysiology and Other Features 204
6.9.2. Hypertriglyceridemia and Coronary Heart Disease .. 206
6.10. Chronic Renal Failure and Hyperlipidemia 207
6.11. Treatment of Hyperlipidemia 208
6.11.1. Diet 208
6.11.2. Drugs 210
6.11.3. Partial Ileal Bypass Surgery 211
6.11.4. Primary Prevention of Ischemic Heart Disease 211
References 212

Chapter 7
Metabolism of Amino Acids and Organic Acids
Leon E. Rosenberg and Kay Tanaka

7.1. Introduction 219
7.2. Phenylketonuria and Its Variants 220
7.2.1. Phenylalanine Hydroxylation: Enzymes and Coenzymes 221
7.2.1.1. The Hydroxylation System 221
7.2.1.2. The Defect in Classic Phenylketonuria 222
7.2.1.3. "Benign" Hyperphenylalaninemia 223
7.2.1.4. Dihydropteridine Reductase Deficiency 224
7.2.2. Clinical Phenylketonuria: Incidence and Outcome .. 226

7.2.2.1 Phenylketonuria as a Balanced Polymorphism 226
7.2.2.2 Dietary Treatment of Phenylketonuria 227
7.2.2.3 Maternal Phenylketonuria 229
7.3. The γ-Glutamyl Cycle and 5-Oxoprolinuria 229
7.3.1. 5-Oxoprolinuria 229
7.3.2. The γ-Glutamyl Cycle 231
7.3.3. Biochemical Basis of 5-Oxoprolinuria 232
7.3.4. Evidence For and Against the Role of the γ-Glutamyl Cycle in Amino Acid Transport 235
7.4. Jamaican Vomiting Sickness and Glutaric Aciduria Type II: Similar Organic Acidurias with Different Etiologies 238
7.4.1. Jamaican Vomiting Sickness 238
7.4.1.1. Metabolic Effects of Hypoglycin 239
7.4.1.2. Inhibition of Acyl-CoA Dehydrogenases by Methylenecyclopropylacetic Acid 241
7.4.1.3. Recent Studies on Jamaican Vomiting Sickness 244
7.4.2. Glutaric Aciduria Type II 245
References 246

Chapter 8
Disorders of Purine and Pyrimidine Metabolism

J. Edwin Seegmiller

8.1. Introduction 253
8.2. Purine Metabolism 257
8.2.1. Role of Liver in Processing Purines of the Bloodstream 257
8.2.2. Purines as a Source of Ammonia Production 258
8.2.3. Regulation of Purine Synthesis 260
8.2.4. Effects of Purine Compounds on the Immune System 263
8.2.5. Changes in Adenosine Metabolism with Mitogenic Stimulation 266
8.2.6. Possible Role of Cyclic AMP in Immunosuppression 267
8.2.7. Role of Adenosine Deaminase in Metabolism or Action of Drugs 268
8.3. Adenosine Deaminase (ADA) Deficiency Associated with Severe Combined Immunodeficiency Disease 269
8.3.1. Frequency 270

8.3.2. Metabolic Studies of ADA-Deficient Patients 270
8.3.3. New Approach to Treatment of ADA Deficiency ... 271
8.3.4. Metabolic Consequences of ADA Deficiency 272
8.3.5. Tissue Distribution of ADA 274
8.3.6. Tissue Forms of ADA 274
8.3.7. Genetic Heterogeneity of Residual ADA Activity 275
8.3.8. Possible Pathogenetic Mechanism of ADA Deficiency 275
8.4. Increased Activity of ADA in Red Cells Associated with Hereditary Hemolytic Anemia 277
8.5. Purine Nucleoside Phosphorylase (PNP) Deficiency 278
8.5.1. Clinical Presentation 278
8.5.2. Metabolites in Urine 280
8.5.3. Metabolites in Blood and Serum 282
8.5.4. PNP Enzyme Activity and Metabolism of Erythrocytes and Fibroblasts 283
8.5.5. Purine Production in Cultured Fibroblasts 284
8.5.6. Possible Pathogenetic Mechanisms of PNP Deficiency 284
8.5.7. Properties of Purified PNP 286
8.6. Purine 5′-Nucleotidase Deficiency in Primary Hypogamma-globulinemia 286
8.6.1. Clinical Presentation 287
8.7. Hereditary Xanthinuria 288
8.8. Hypoxanthine-Guanine Phosphoribosyl transferase (HPRT) Deficiency 289
8.8.1. Clinical Correlations with HPRT Activity 290
8.8.2. Biochemical Mechanism of the Neurological Defect . 291
8.8.3. Nature of the Enzyme Abnormality 292
8.8.4. Mechanism of Purine Overproduction 293
8.8.5. Genetics of HPRT Deficiency 293
8.8.6. Other Conditions Associated with HPRT Deficiency . 294
8.9. Increased Activity of Phosphoribosylpyrophosphate Synthetase 294
8.9.1. Inheritance 295
8.10. Adenine Phosphoribosyltransferase (APRT) Deficiency 295
8.10.1. Clinical Presentation 295
8.10.2. Chemical Composition of Calculi 296
8.10.3. Therapy 297
8.10.4. APRT Activity in Erythrocytes 297
8.10.5. Adenine and Other Purine Metabolites in Urine 297
8.10.6. Genetics 298
8.10.7. APRT Deficiency in Cell Culture 298
8.11. Nucleoside Triphosphate Pyrophosphohydrolase Deficiency . 298
8.12. Gouty Arthritis 299

8.12.1. Metabolic Abnormalities Associated with Gout 299
8.12.2. Clinical Features of Gouty Arthritis 301
8.12.3. Local Conditions That Favor Urate Deposition 301
8.12.4. Characteristics of the Monosodium Urate Crystal ... 302
8.12.5. Uric Acid and the Kidney 303
8.12.6. Treatment of Gout 303
8.13. Abnormalities of Pyrimidine Metabolism 304
8.13.1. Pyrimidine 5′-Nucleotidase Deficiency 304
8.13.2. Hyperammonemia with Orotic Aciduria 305
8.13.3. Drug and Nutritional Factors That Affect Pyrimidine Metabolism 305
8.13.4. Orotic Aciduria Accompanying Other Errors of Metabolism 306
8.14. Chemotherapy of Malignancies and Viral Diseases 306
References 307

Chapter 9
Divalent Ion Metabolism

Jack W. Coburn, David L. Hartenbower, and Charles R. Kleeman

9.1. Regulation of Calcium Homeostasis 327
9.1.1. Parathyroid Hormone 328
9.1.1.1. Divalent Ion Control of Parathyroid Hormone Secretion 328
9.1.1.2. Actions of Parathyroid Hormone on Bone 330
9.1.1.3. Actions of Parathyroid Hormone on the Kidney 331
9.1.1.4. Immunoassay for Parathyroid Hormone .. 332
9.1.2. Vitamin D 333
9.1.2.1. Chemistry and Metabolism of Vitamin D .. 334
9.1.2.2. Actions of Vitamin D 337
9.1.2.3. Plasma Transport of Vitamin D 342
9.1.2.4. Assays for 25(OH)D, $1,25(OH)_2D$, and Other Vitamin D Sterols 342
9.1.2.5. Vitamin D Toxicity 343
9.1.2.6. Absence of Vitamin D Action 344
9.1.3. Other Factors That Affect Calcium Homeostasis 355
9.1.3.1. Calcium-Handling by the Kidney 355
9.2. Phosphate Metabolism 356
9.2.1. Regulation by the Kidney 356
9.2.1.1. Effects of Dietary Intake of Phosphorus ... 356

9.2.1.2. Effects of Parathyroid Hormone 357
9.2.1.3. Effects of Serum Calcium Level 358
9.2.1.4. Actions of Vitamin D 358
9.2.1.5. Other Factors That Affect Renal Phosphate-Handling 359
9.2.2. Phosphate Depletion 360
9.3. Magnesium Metabolism 364
9.3.1. The Kidney in Magnesium Homeostasis 364
9.3.2. Magnesium Depletion 365
References 367

Chapter 10
Nutrition, Growth, and Development
Myron Winick

10.1. Introduction 379
10.2. Malnutrition and the Mechanisms of Cellular Growth 379
10.3. Genetic Obesity 386
10.3.1. Changes in Adipose Tissue during Normal Growth . 386
10.3.2. Animal Models of Genetic Obesity 387
10.3.3. Human Studies 388
10.4. Nutrition and Pregnancy 389
References 392

Chapter 11
Metabolic Aspects of Renal Stone Disease
Hibbard E. Williams

11.1. Introduction 399
11.2. Incidence of Renal Stone Disease 400
11.3. Classification of Renal Stone Disease 400
11.4. Renal Stone Disease Secondary to Increased Crystalloid Excretion 401
11.4.1. Hypercalciuria 401
11.4.2. Hyperoxaluria 402
11.4.3. Hyperuricosuria 403
11.4.4. Cystine and Xanthine Stones 403
11.5. Renal Stone Disease Secondary to Physicochemical Changes in Urine Composition 404

11.6. Idiopathic Renal Stone Disease 405
11.7. Treatment of Renal Stone Disease 406
References 408

Chapter 12
Metabolism and Metabolic Actions of Ethanol
Charles S. Lieber

12.1. Metabolism of Ethanol 411
12.1.1. Role of Alcohol Dehydrogenase and Interaction of Dietary Factors with Ethanol and Acetaldehyde Metabolism 411
12.1.2. Role, Nature, and Metabolic Consequences of Non-ADH Pathways for Ethanol Oxidation 413
12.1.3. Effects of Chronic Ethanol Consumption on Ethanol Metabolism 415
12.1.4. Influence of Liver Disease, Ethnic Background, Circadian Rhythm, and Other Factors on Ethanol Metabolism 418
12.2. Interaction of Ethanol with Androgen Metabolism 420
12.3. Interaction of Ethanol with Amino Acid Metabolism 423
12.4. Effects of Ethanol on the Gastrointestinal Tract 424
12.4.1. Metabolic Consequences of Gastric Alterations Induced by Alcohol 424
12.4.2. Metabolic Consequences of Intestinal Changes Produced by Alcohol 425
References 428

Index 435

1

Cyclic GMP in Metabolism: Interrelationship of Biogenic Amines, Hormones, and Other Agents

Ferid Murad and Gerald D. Aurbach

1.1. Introduction

Many hormones, neurohormones, autacoids, drugs, and bacterial toxins produce their effects in various tissues by modifying the accumulation of cyclic AMP (cAMP) (Robison *et al.*, 1971). While many agents enhance adenylate cyclase activity and cAMP synthesis, some agents can decrease its synthesis and accumulation or alter its degradation by cyclic nucleotide phosphodiesterase. Presumably, cAMP levels in tissue could also be modi-

FERID MURAD • Professor of Internal Medicine and Pharmacology; Director, Division of Clinical Pharmacology; Director, Clinical Research Center; University of Virginia, Charlottesville, Virginia 22903. GERALD D. AURBACH • Chief, Metabolic Diseases Branch, National Institute of Arthritis, Metabolism, and Digestive Diseases, National Institutes of Health, Bethesda, Maryland 20014.

fied by agents that alter its release into interstitial fluid and plasma. Hormone–receptor interactions, formation of cAMP, and processes regulated by this cyclic nucleotide were topics covered in the preceding volume of *The Year in Metabolism* (Aurbach, 1976). In this chapter, we wish to emphasize in particular interactions of cyclic GMP (cGMP), the other naturally occurring cyclic nucleotide. In addition, we have continued the review begun last year of clinical aspects of cyclic nucleotides in extracellular fluids. Future chapters of this continuing annual series will focus on these as well as other aspects of cyclic nucleotides and their roles in metabolism.

cGMP was first found in urine (Ashman *et al.*, 1963). This discovery led to a search for (1) enzymes involved in its formation (Hardman and Sutherland, 1969; White and Aurbach, 1969; Ishikawa *et al.*, 1969; Schultz *et al.*, 1969) and hydrolysis (Brooker *et al.*, 1968); (2) hormone and drug regulation of its accumulation in tissues (Hardman *et al.*, 1969; Goldberg *et al.*, 1969, 1973); and (3) a physiologic role for this cyclic nucleotide. Our knowledge regarding the regulation of cGMP accumulation and its function is quite meager compared with that of cAMP. This is in part related to the methods by which the two nucleotides were discovered. cAMP was isolated as an intermediate of hormone-induced changes in liver phosphorylase activity and glycogenolysis (Sutherland and Rall, 1958). Thus, in the course of the examination of a hormone-induced function, cAMP was found to be an intermediate. cGMP was not discovered in the course of examining a physiologic process (Ashman *et al.*, 1963). The lower concentrations of cGMP in tissues (generally about 5–10% of that of cAMP) and the lag in the development of some cGMP and guanylate cyclase methodologies also account for less understanding of cGMP.

An assumption has been made that the presence of cGMP in essentially all tissues and extracellular fluids examined and its altered concentrations with some agents and processes indicate that this cyclic nucleotide should also have important physiologic roles that remain to be defined. With the appropriate agent, one can observe in some tissues an increase in one cyclic nucleotide with a concomitant decrease in the other (Goldberg *et al.*, 1973). This tends to be the exception, however, since usually a perturbation or the addition of a hormone or drug to a tissue alters the accumulation of one cyclic nucleotide without changing the other. Clearly, the accumulation of each cyclic nucleotide occurs independently of the other (Kimura *et al.*, 1974). There has been speculation that the two systems could be directly or indirectly coupled under some conditions. If coupling of the two systems does occur, a positive or negative interaction might take place to alter the accumulation or effect or both of the other cyclic nucleotide. This is an intriguing hypothesis that would obviously add greater complexity to cyclic nucleotide metabolism and effects. However, there is little direct evidence to support this view.

1.2. Formation and Degradation of Cyclic GMP

1.2.1. Guanylate Cyclases

The formation and degradation of cGMP and cAMP have many similarities, as summarized in Fig. 1. There are, however, some very distinct differences in the two systems. In mammalian tissues, adenylate cyclase catalyzes the conversion of ATP to cAMP and pyrophosphate, and is located exclusively in particulate fractions of tissue homogenates (Rall and Sutherland, 1962). While the enzyme is found predominantly in plasma membranes (Davoren and Sutherland, 1963), it has also been described in other fractions such as endoplasmic reticulum and Golgi from several tissues (Entman *et al.*, 1969; Katz *et al.*, 1974; McKeel and Jarret, 1974; Kimura and Murad, 1975a). With few exceptions, hormones that alter cAMP accumulation in intact tissues also alter adenylate cyclase activity assayed in cell-free systems. The specificity of hormone effects on

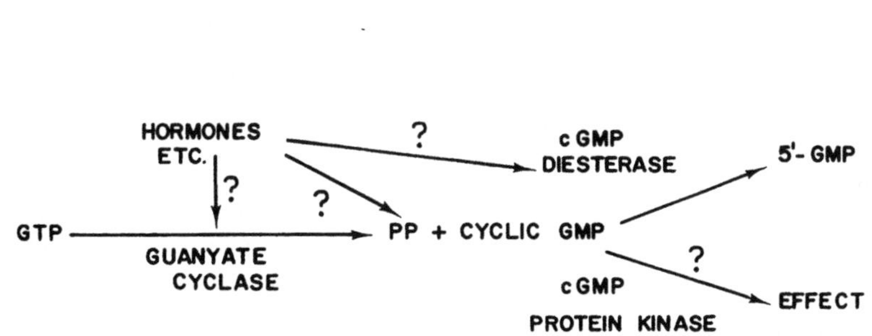

Fig. 1. Comparisons of cAMP and cGMP metabolism. The analogies in the two systems for synthesis, metabolism, and probable mechanism of action are apparent. The question marks designate possible areas for control or effects or both in which data are lacking or inconclusive.

cAMP formation in both intact tissues and cell-free systems invariably correlates with the agents expected to produce physiologic effects in a given tissue; i.e., generally, only the hormones known to have effects in a specific tissue are able to alter cAMP metabolism. Adenylate cyclase activity in preparations of liver plasma membranes, endoplasmic reticulum, and Golgi (Kimura and Murad, 1975a) can be increased with glucagon, fluoride ion, and other agents (Murad and Kimura, unpublished). The significance of activation of adenylate cyclase in these different particulate locations is not known.

In many of the early studies with guanylate cyclase, the enzyme was thought to reside predominantly in soluble fractions of tissue homogenates (Hardman and Sutherland, 1969; White and Aurbach, 1969; Schultz *et al.,* 1969). In subsequent studies, however, both soluble and particulate activities have been described in all mammalian tissues examined (Table I) (Kimura and Murad, 1974b; Chrisman *et al.,* 1975; Kimura and Murad, 1975a,b). The relative distribution of soluble and particulate activity is a function of the tissue and species examined. Much of the particulate activity in tissues is also latent and activated three- to ten-fold by detergents such as Triton X-100 or Lubrol PX (Hardman *et al.,* 1973; Kimura and Murad, 1974b, 1975a). Thus, in most tissues, guanylate cyclase is in fact predominantly particulate when distribution of detergent-activated enzyme is examined. Unfortunately, most studies have neglected the particulate enzyme, since it was not thought to represent a significant portion of homogenate activities. In rat liver, the particulate enzyme is found in purified preparations of plasma membranes, Golgi, endoplasmic reticulum (Kimura and Murad, 1975a,c), and nuclei (Earp *et*

Table I. Guanylate Cyclase Activity in Various Rat Tissues

	cGMP formed (nmol/min per g tissue)		
Tissue	Homogenate	Supernatant[a]	Particulate[a]
Lung	20.5	16.1 (79)	3.2 (16)
Intestinal mucosa	15.1	0.40 (3)	11.2 (74)
Intestinal smooth muscle	5.7	3.8 (67)	1.5 (26)
Liver	3.0	2.2 (73)	0.87 (29)
Kidney	3.0	2.0 (67)	1.0 (33)
Spleen	2.9	3.2 (110)	0.65 (22)
Cerebral cortex	2.6	1.7 (65)	1.4 (54)
Cerebellum	2.3	0.70 (30)	1.5 (65)
Pancreas	1.4	1.1 (79)	0.30 (21)
Epididymal fat pad	0.27	0.15 (56)	0.14 (52)
Skeletal muscle	0.21	0.16 (76)	0.10 (48)

[a]The values in parentheses are the percentages of homogenate activity.

Table II. Some Properties of Soluble and Particulate Guanylate Cyclase from Rat Heart, Lung, and Liver

Property	Soluble	Particulate
Molecular weight	150,000–200,000	300,000–400,000
K_m for GTP	12–65 μM	50–100 μM
Nucleotide sites	1	2 or more
K_a for free Mn^{2+}	≈0.2 mM	≈0.2 mM
Effect of Ca^{2+}	Generally stimulates	Generally inhibits
Effect of detergents	Stimulates 30–100%	Stimulates >300%
50% inhibition of ATP	≈0.4 mM	>1 mM

al., 1977). Guanylate cyclase has also been reported in sarcoplasmic reticulum preparations from heart (White, 1975) and nuclear preparations from calf uterus (Siegel *et al.*, 1976). Reports of some guanylate cyclase activity in crude mitochondrial preparations may be due to some contamination. Additional studies with the subcellular localization of guanylate cyclase and adenylate cyclase are needed.

The diverse subcellular location of guanylate cyclase suggests that multiple factors and small as well as large hormones and peptides could influence guanylate cyclase activity and cGMP formation in these different compartments. In contrast to the cAMP system, however, no hormones have been found to reproducibly increase guanylate cyclase activity in cell-free systems. The few instances in which agents such as secretin, pancreozymin (Thompson *et al.*, 1973), or acetylcholine (George *et al.*, 1975) seemed to increase guanylate cyclase activity are attributable to bile salt contaminants (Ichihara *et al.*, 1977) or other probable artifactual effects (Kimura and Murad, 1974a), and have not been confirmed by a number of laboratories. The agents that have been tested include choline esters, histamine, serotonin, prostaglandins, insulin, and many others that have been reported to increase cGMP levels in various intact-tissue preparations. The dearth of direct hormone effects on guanylate cyclase activity has obviously hindered research in this area and prevented formulations of potential physiologic roles for this cyclic nucleotide.

Guanylate cyclase activities in various tissue fractions have different kinetic properties and molecular sizes (Kimura and Murad, 1974b, 1975a,b; Chrisman *et al.*, 1975). Properties of the soluble and particulate forms of guanylate cyclase from rat heart, lung, and liver are summarized in Table II. The soluble enzyme from mammalian tissues is about 150,000 daltons, about one-half the apparent size of the particulate enzyme (Neer, 1976). The enzyme from *Escherichia coli* is considerably smaller, about 30,000 (Macchia *et al.*, 1975). Generally, Mg^{2+} is about 5–10% as effective as a cofactor as Mn^{2+}. In the presence of low Mn^{2+}, some but not all preparations of native enzyme will effectively utilize Mg^{2+} (Kimura and

Murad, 1975a,b). When guanylate cyclase is activated with sodium azide, sodium nitroprusside, and other nucleophilic agents, the enzyme can effectively utilize Mg^{2+} or Mn^{2+} (Kimura *et al.*, 1976; Katsuki *et al.*, 1977). The ability of the inactive and active forms of the enzyme to utilize Mg^{2+} as cofactor may be very important in view of the normally low concentrations of Mn^{2+} in tissues (Thiers and Vallee, 1957). Most soluble fractions of guanylate cyclase are activated by high concentrations of Ca^{2+} (1–4 mM), while the particulate form of the enzyme is generally inhibited with Ca^{2+} (Kimura and Murad, 1974b; Chrisman *et al.*, 1975). There are some exceptions, however, to this general rule; e.g., Ca^{2+} increases particulate activity from rat intestinal mucosa and increases or decreases particulate activity from rat lung depending on the Mn^{2+} concentration in incubations (Murad *et al.*, 1976). The potential role of Ca^{2+} in the regulation of cGMP accumulation in tissues is discussed in Section 1.3.5. The activation of guanylate cyclase with detergents is probably due in part to solubilization of enzyme and increased availability of substrate and cofactors (Hardman *et al.*, 1973). Detergents also activate soluble guanylate cyclase 30–100%, however, which suggests that activation is not exclusively a solubilization phenomenon (Hardman *et al.*, 1973; Kimura and Murad, 1974b). Therefore, the mechanisms of detergent activation are not totally understood. Activation of guanylate cyclase with bile salts is probably an effect similar to that of detergents (Ichihara *et al.*, 1977). Activation with low concentrations of arachidonic acid and other fatty acids is probably due to another mechanism (Wallach and Pastan, 1976). The soluble form of the enzyme is also more sensitive to inhibition by ATP at concentrations present in tissues (Kimura and Murad, 1974b; Criss *et al.*, 1976). This suggests that the soluble enzyme may be relatively inactive in tissues, and that the particulate form of the enzyme takes on greater significance in regulating tissue levels of cGMP (Kimura and Murad, 1975b–d).

Some minor differences in the properties of guanylate cyclase in preparations of plasma membranes, Golgi, endoplasmic reticulum, and nuclei have also been noted (Kimura and Murad, 1975a,c; Siegel *et al.*, 1976). These observations indicate that several different kinetic forms of the enzyme may exist in particulate fractions of tissues. The multiple forms of guanylate cyclase in tissues with different kinetic properties and subcellular location suggest that the different forms could be regulated independently of one another. This hypothesis has been supported with several studies in which the activities of the soluble and particulate forms were apparently altered independently in regenerating liver, fetal liver, and some tumors (Kimura and Murad, 1975d; Goridis and Reutter, 1975; Criss *et al.*, 1976).

Kinetic studies with crude preparations of particulate guanylate cyclase and GTP demonstrate cooperativity with curved double-reciprocal plots (Kimura and Murad, 1974b; Chrisman *et al.*, 1975). In contrast, typical Michaelis–Menten kinetics are seen with soluble guanylate cyclase preparations that imply a single nucleotide site on the enzyme. Highly purified particulate guanylate cyclase from sea urchin sperm gives linear double-reciprocal plots with GTP, while cooperativity is observed with crude preparations (Garbers, 1976). These observations indicate that both soluble and particulate enzyme have a single nucleotide site. The different properties of soluble and particulate enzymes in crude systems could result from different enzyme forms or similar proteins with different kinetic properties due to their particulate or soluble environment. The kinetic properties of particulate guanylate cyclase are not altered with detergent solubilization (Kimura and Murad, 1974b). Thus, the question whether there is a single enzyme with different properties due to environment or truly multiple enzyme forms has not been resolved. Perhaps a single particulate form exists in tissues, and the soluble activity is due to homogenization and stripping or releasing some activity from particles. Altered distribution of particulate and soluble activities in proliferating tissues supports the hypothesis of multiple forms (Kimura and Murad, 1975d; Criss *et al.*, 1976). Detailed studies with purified preparations are needed to resolve this question.

The different forms and pools of guanylate cyclase imply that there could be different pools of cGMP in tissues with perhaps different functions. While these questions are significant to assign possible functions to cGMP, current methods unfortunately are not adequate to test such hypotheses meaningfully.

Properties of the enzyme are markedly altered after activation of guanylate cyclase with azide, hydroxylamine, nitrite, nitroprusside, nitric oxide, and other nucleophilic agents (Kimura *et al.*, 1975a, 1976; Katsuki *et al.*, 1977; Arnold *et al.*, 1977a,b). Some properties of enzyme activated with sodium azide, summarized in Table III, indicate that inactive, latent, and active forms of the enzyme may exist in tissues. This has resulted in a

Table III. Alteration in the Properties of Guanylate Cyclase with Activation with NaN_3 and Other Agents

Property	Remarks
Apparent molecular size	Unaltered
K_m for GTP	Increased or unchanged
Requirement for free Mn^{2+}	Markedly decreased
Ability to utilize Mg^{2+}	As effective as Mn^{2+}
Heat stability	More labile
ATP inhibition	Unaltered
Ability to catalyze cAMP formation	Markedly increased
Calcium activation	Absent

great deal of complexity in examining guanylate cyclase in tissues. However, knowledge of the mechanisms and conditions required for interconversion of these forms in tissues should permit us to design more meaningful experiments and models in which the effects of hormones and drugs can be tested.

An interesting alteration in the properties of guanylate cyclase that occurs with activation is its ability to catalyze the conversion of ATP to cAMP (Mittal and Murad, 1977). Thus, another pathway for cAMP synthesis can exist in tissues. The significance of this alternate synthetic pathway for cAMP formation is not known, nor it is known what role it may play in various hormone- and drug-induced effects in tissues that were assumed to be due to adenylate cyclase activation.

1.2.2. Cyclic Nucleotide Phosphodiesterases and Other Mechanisms of Cyclic Nucleotide Disposal

Reduction of tissue content of cAMP and cGMP could be accomplished by (1) degradation with cyclic nucleotide phosphodiesterases, (2) release or extrusion into interstitial fluid and plasma, or (3) sequestration or binding within compartments in tissue. The latter two phenomena have received little attention. Both cAMP and cGMP are found in essentially all extracellular fluids (for reviews, see Broadus *et al.*, 1971; Murad, 1973). Also, both cyclic nucleotides are released into incubation media to varying degrees with many different kinds of tissues. Since tissue concentrations of the cyclic nucleotides are generally several orders of magnitude greater than in incubation media and plasma, an active transport mechanism does not need to be involved. This is not to say that an energy requirement is not involved or that the process is not important in regulating tissue levels of cyclic nucleotides.

Recent studies with rat atria incubations have shown free and bound compartments of cAMP (Terasaki and Brooker, 1977). Addition of catecholamines effected increases in total cAMP that were reflected in increases in both compartments, but greater increases in free cAMP. With the low concentrations of cGMP in tissues, analogous studies with this cyclic nucleotide are not currently feasible. The immunohistochemical technique (Steiner *et al.*, 1976) shows specific differences in localization of bound cAMP and cGMP in several tissues. The method does not detect free cyclic nucleotides, but further application in conjunction with analyses of total cyclic nucleotides in tissues in response to hormones or drugs could yield important information.

The only enzymatic degradation of cyclic nucleotides known at present is via cyclic nucleotide phosphodiesterase (Butcher, R. W., and Sutherland, 1962; Appleman and Terasaki, 1975). This pathway is obviously functional and important in maintaining or altering concentrations of cyclic nucleotides. This has been demonstrated in numerous studies in which methylxanthine inhibitors such as theophylline, caffeine, 1-methyl-3-isobutylxanthine (MIX), and others increase cyclic nucleotide accumulation in many tissues. These phosphodiesterase inhibitors frequently mimic or potentiate, or both, hormone responses (Robison *et al.*, 1971).

Chromatographic separation of tissue extracts usually reveals two or three forms of cyclic nucleotide phosphodiesterase (for a review, see Appleman and Terasaki, 1975). One form specifically hydrolizes cGMP. A second form hydrolizes either cGMP or cAMP, and a third form specifically hydrolizes cAMP. The number of forms and their kinetic properties vary with different tissues. As with guanylate cyclase, the kinetic behavior of these multiple forms is quite complex. With some forms, cAMP and cGMP may compete with one another for hydrolysis (Murad *et al.*, 1970), or low concentrations of cGMP may increase cAMP hydrolysis (Beavo *et al.*, 1971). Studies such as these have suggested that interactions of the cAMP and cGMP systems could occur in tissues. Addition of cGMP to some tissues results in cAMP accumulation, probably by decreasing endogenous cAMP hydrolysis (Murad *et al.*, 1969). High concentrations of either cyclic nucleotide can also activate both cAMP-dependent and cGMP-dependent protein kinases (Beavo *et al.*, 1975). Interactions such as these also make it extremely difficult to evaluate effects of adding exogenous cyclic nucleotide to tissues. Calcium ion or endogenous protein factors or both can increase activity of some phosphodiesterase forms (Cheung, 1971; Wang *et al.*, 1975; Kakiuchi *et al.*, 1975). The functions of these activating factors and calcium are not known.

In general, particulate fractions from tissue homogenates possess a phosphodiesterase with a low K_m for cAMP, and soluble fractions, a high-K_m form for cAMP and a low-K_m form for cGMP (Appleman and Terasaki, 1975). Various agents including methylxanthines (Butcher, R. W., and Sutherland, 1962), insulin (Loten and Sneyd, 1970), prostaglandins, steroids (Manganiello and Vaughan, 1972a,b), and cAMP (Manganiello *et al.*, 1971; Bourne *et al.*, 1973) can influence synthesis or activity of phosphodiesterase and cAMP hydrolysis. With retinal preparations, light increases phosphodiesterase activity and the hydrolysis of both cAMP and cGMP (Bitensky *et al.*, 1975). Effects with many agents are generally on the low-K_m activity in particulate fractions.

When hormones are added to tissue incubations, cAMP concentrations usually reach a peak in several minutes and then decline even though the hormone is continuously present. The term "refractoriness" or "desensitization" was introduced to describe this phenomenon (Manganiello *et al.*, 1971). Refractoriness probably occurs through a variety of mechanisms. The mechanisms may include alterations in receptor numbers and affinity (Mukherjee *et al.*, 1975), inhibition of adenylate cyclase and cAMP synthesis by one or more factors (Ho and Sutherland, 1975), and increased degradation by phosphodiesterase (Manganiello *et al.*, 1971). In some tissues, the accumulation of cAMP clearly leads to increased phosphodiesterase activity (Manganiello and Vaughan, 1972a,b; Bourne *et al.*, 1973). Thus, through mechanisms that are poorly understood, cAMP can influence its own accumulation. Analogous studies with cGMP hydrolysis are not available.

1.2.3. Cyclic Nucleotide Protein Kinases

Probably all or most effects of cAMP in mammalian tissues are due to the activation of cAMP-dependent protein kinase (Greengard, 1971). The holoenzyme has a molecular weight of 160,000, consists of four subunits, and is inactive (Beavo *et al.*, 1975). Binding of two molecules of cAMP to two receptor subunits results in dissociation of the enzyme to yield two active catalytic units and the receptor dimer bound to cAMP as summarized in Fig. 2 (Beavo *et al.*, 1975). The active unit (C-unit) catalyzes the transfer of gamma phosphate of ATP to a variety of protein substrates including phosphorylase kinase, glycogen synthase, hormone-sensitive lipase, histone, casein, protamine, and others. Phosphorylation of specific serine residues on these enzymes markedly alters activity. In some instances, membranous or structural proteins or both are phosphorylated with possible regulatory changes in transport or other processes (Rudolph and Greengard, 1974). The physiological significance and consequence of these phosphorylation mechanisms are not totally understood for membrane proteins.

The effects of cAMP on messenger RNA (mRNA) formation and enzyme induction in bacterial systems appear to have no requirement for protein kinase activation (Pastan and Perlman, 1972). In these systems, cAMP binds to another receptor protein that leads to mRNA synthesis and ultimately protein synthesis. However, most of all cAMP effects in mammalian tissues are consistent with the model of protein kinase activation (Greengard, 1971). Some tissues contain two forms of cAMP-depen-

$$\underset{\text{(INACTIVE)}}{R_2C_2} + 2\,\text{cAMP} \rightleftharpoons \underset{\text{(ACTIVE)}}{R_2\text{cAMP}_2 + 2\text{C}}$$

$$C_2 + 2\,\text{cGMP} \rightleftharpoons C_2\,\text{cGMP}_2$$

Fig. 2. Activation of protein kinases with cAMP or cGMP binding. Adapted from Beavo *et al.* (1975) and Gill *et al.* (1976).

dent protein kinase (Corbin *et al.*, 1975; Beavo *et al.*, 1975). These enzymes are separable, similar in size, and possess identical catalytic subunits but different receptor subunits. One form is capable of autophosphorylation (Rosen *et al.*, 1975). Whether or not there are functional differences in these kinases is not known.

The many similarities of the cAMP and the cGMP systems led to a search for a cGMP-dependent protein kinase. This enzyme was first described in arthropods (Kuo, J. F., *et al.*, 1971) and recently in mammalian tissues (Kuo, J. F., *et al.*, 1976; Gill *et al.*, 1976; Lincoln *et al.*, 1976). Very recent studies indicate that the enzyme is quite different from cAMP-dependent protein kinase. cGMP-dependent protein kinase from lung and silkworm has a molecular weight of 150,000 daltons and consists of two similar subunits (Gill *et al.*, 1976; Takai *et al.*, 1976; Lincoln *et al.*, 1976). Binding of cGMP results in activation of the enzyme without its dissociation (Fig. 2). It should be pointed out that some investigators believe that cGMP-dependent protein kinase also dissociates into subunits after binding to cGMP (Kuo, J. F., *et al.*, 1976). Disappointingly in preliminary studies, the protein substrates for both cAMP-dependent and cGMP-dependent protein kinases have been similar. If differences in substrate specificity exist, some clues regarding physiologic effects of cGMP might be provided if one assumes that most cGMP-induced effects are due to this mechanism. A heat-stable protein inhibitor of cAMP-dependent protein kinase (Appleman *et al.*, 1966) and a heat-stable protein activator of cGMP-dependent protein kinase (Kuo, W. N., *et al.*, 1976) have been described. While these materials have been useful as research tools, their physiological significance is not known. cGMP increases phosphorylation of endogenous proteins in smooth muscle preparations (Casnellie and Greengard, 1974), but the function of these proteins is not known. Nor is it known whether effects of cGMP require a phosphorylation mechanism.

1.3. Regulation of Cyclic GMP in Tissues

1.3.1. Effects of Hypophysectomy and Adrenalectomy

After the finding of cGMP in urine (Ashman *et al.*, 1963), it was reported that urinary excretion of cGMP in rats was decreased with either hypophysectomy, adrenalectomy, or thyroparathyroidectomy (Hardman *et al.*, 1969). The reduced excretion with hypophysectomy was reversed with large doses of thyroxine and hydrocortisone or a mixture of anterior pituitary hormones. The effects of adrenalectomy and thyroparathyroidectomy were reversed with hydrocortisone and thyroxine, respectively (Hardman *et al.*, 1969). These early studies suggest that hormones might regulate cGMP metabolism, as has been observed in studies with other agents. Recent clinical studies have extended these observations to alterations of cGMP excretion in Cushing's disease (Wray *et al.*, 1975).

Adrenalectomy of rats increased the cGMP content of skeletal muscle (Steiner *et al.*, 1972), and decreased it in liver (Thompson and Williams, 1974). Alterations of guanylate cyclase activity in these and other tissues were also observed, but did not completely parallel cGMP concentrations; i.e., adrenalectomy increased liver guanylate cyclase activity (Thompson and Williams, 1974). Some of these effects were prevented with cortisone administration. Administration of estrogens in intact animals increases cGMP levels in uterus (Kuehl *et al.*, 1974: Flandroy and Galand, 1975). Since effects of steroids and thyroid hormone on cGMP content or guanylate cyclase activity are usually not observed in *in vitro* systems, it has not been possible to determine which of these effects on cGMP metabolism are direct or indirect.

1.3.2. Effects of Choline Esters

The first report of a specific humoral agent influencing cGMP *in vitro* was reported (George *et al.*, 1970) for acetylcholine and rat heart. There have followed many reports of choline esters causing increased cGMP concentrations in diverse tissues. Acetylcholine and the cholinesterase-resistant analogue, carbachol, increase cGMP levels in preparations of heart, brain (Lee *et al.*, 1972), smooth muscle (Lee *et al.*, 1972; Schultz *et al.*, 1973), adipose tissue (Illiano *et al.*, 1973), lung (Kimura *et al.*, 1974; Stoner *et al.*, 1974), pancreas (Christophe *et al.*, 1976), thyroid (Yamashita and Field, 1972), sympathetic ganglia (Weight *et al.*, 1974), leukocytes (Ignarro and Cech, 1975; Sandler *et al.*, 1975), and other tissues. Many of these effects are time- and dose-dependent and are invariably blocked with atropine, indicating specifically the muscarinic effects of acetylcholine. The effects on cGMP accumulation are increased in many tissues with phosphodiesterase inhibitors, as would be predicted. Although it has been reported that choline esters increase guanylate cyclase activity in cell-free systems of heart (George *et al.*, 1975), these effects have not been confirmed by a number of laboratories working with the same tissue and conditions as well as other systems.

The effects of choline esters (and many other agents) on cGMP accumulation in intact tissues require calcium ion in the incubation media (Schultz *et al.*, 1973). Since many of the agents that increase cGMP levels in tissues also alter calcium uptake and release, effects of acetylcholine and other agents on cGMP accumulation may be mediated indirectly through calcium. If this hypothesis is correct, hormone activation of guanylate cyclase in broken-cell systems would be extremely difficult to demonstrate. Carbachol and other agents increase cGMP in pancreatic acinar cell preparations, and this effect is observed in the absence of added Ca^{2+} (Christophe *et al.*, 1976). This observation is one of the few exceptions of the general trend in which external Ca^{2+} is required for hormone-induced changes in cGMP levels. Choline esters also decrease cAMP formation in some tissues, and this effect is demonstrable in some cell-free preparations (Murad *et al.*, 1962). Although cGMP increases or cAMP decreases, or both, in tissues treated with choline esters in some instances correlate with effects of these agents, it is not established that these are direct or indirect effects on cyclic nucleotides or that changes in concentration of either nucleotide mediate the effects of acetylcholine.

1.3.3. Effects of α-Adrenergic Agonists

There is a great deal of evidence to support the view that β-adrenergic agents produce their diverse effects through activation of adenylate cyclase and increased accumulation of cAMP. Since α-adrenergic agents can decrease cAMP levels in some tissues, it was proposed that these agents could produce their effects through such a mechanism (Robison *et al.*, 1967). Because numerous effects of α-adrenergic agents are not accompanied by alterations in cAMP levels, this hypothesis has received little support. These agents can increase the cGMP content of ductus deferens (Schultz *et al.*, 1973), parotid (Butcher, F. R., 1975), and liver (Pointer *et al.*, 1976). Effects on cGMP in these tissues are usually prevented with α-adrenergic blockers such as phenoxybenzamine or phentolamine, but not β-adrenergic blockers such as propranolol. In a recent report with glioma cell cultures, however, β-adrenergic agonists increased cGMP accumulation (Schwartz, 1976).

1.3.4. Effects of Prostaglandins

Many of the diverse effects of prostaglandins can be attributed to increased adenylate cyclase activity and cAMP formation in tissues. In a few tissues such as adipose tissue, these agents decrease cGMP accumulation (Butcher, R. W., *et al.*, 1968). Whether prostaglandins decrease cAMP synthesis or increase its hydrolysis in this tissue is not known. A significant complexity in understanding the mechanism of action of prostaglandins is the altered activity and even opposite effects of prostaglandins possessing minor structural differences, such as the prostaglandins of the E and F series. This has suggested that their mechanisms of action are different. Prostaglandin E_2 increases cAMP accumulation in isolated veins and is associated with relaxation. Prostaglandin $F_2\alpha$, however, increases cGMP accumulation and produces contraction (Dunham *et al.,* 1974).

Prostaglandin synthetase (cyclooxygenase) catalyzes the conversion of arachidonic acid to an endopetroxide that is the immediate precursor of either prostaglandins or thromboxanes (Kolata, 1975; Anderson and Ramwell, 1974). The effects of prostaglandin synthetase inhibitors such as indomethacin on cAMP accumulation and some processes were inconsistent with the known effects of prostaglandins. An example is platelets, in which prostaglandins increase cAMP levels and inhibit aggregation (Haslam, 1975). The inhibitory effects of indomethacin and salicylates on platelet aggregation are probably due to decreased formation of endoperoxides and thromboxanes. These latter agents increase cGMP accumulation in platelets and increase aggregation (Davies *et al.,* 1976). A recent report described stimulation of guanylate cyclase activity with arachidonic acid in preparations of fibroblast cultures (Wallach and Pastan, 1976). It is not known whether this serves as a precursor for thromboxanes or prostaglandins in this system or has some other effect.

1.3.5. Effects of Calcium

Most agents that increase cGMP levels in tissues require Ca^{2+} in the incubation medium (Schultz *et al.,* 1973; Katsuki and Murad, 1977). This has been frequently observed with choline esters, α-adrenergic agents, histamine, phosphodiesterase inhibitors, the ionophore A23187, and other agents in several different tissues. An exception with pancreas preparations and pancreozymin was noted above (Christophe *et al.,* 1976).

With appropriate conditions, Ca^{2+} can stimulate soluble guanylate cyclase activity in many tissues. Thus, the question has been introduced whether these agents alter cGMP synthesis and accumulation because of their effects on Ca^{2+} transport or distribution or both in tissues, or whether their effects on cGMP are mediated in some other manner. More specifically, is Ca^{2+} relocation a more primary effect of these agents that leads to cGMP accumulation? The changes in cGMP may occur parallel or coincident with changes in Ca^{2+}, or could occur subsequent to Ca^{2+} and merely be "tracking" changes in this ion, as illustrated in Fig. 3 (for a review, see Berridge, 1975).

Serotonin can induce increases in cGMP in umbilical artery segments and does not require Ca^{2+} in the external medium, unlike the effects of choline esters and other agents (Clyman *et al.,* 1975). Similarly, sodium azide, hydroxylamine, sodium nitroprusside, nitroglycerin, or nitric oxide increases cGMP levels in either cerebral cortex, tracheal smooth muscle, liver, or other tissues, and does not require Ca^{2+} in the medium (Kimura

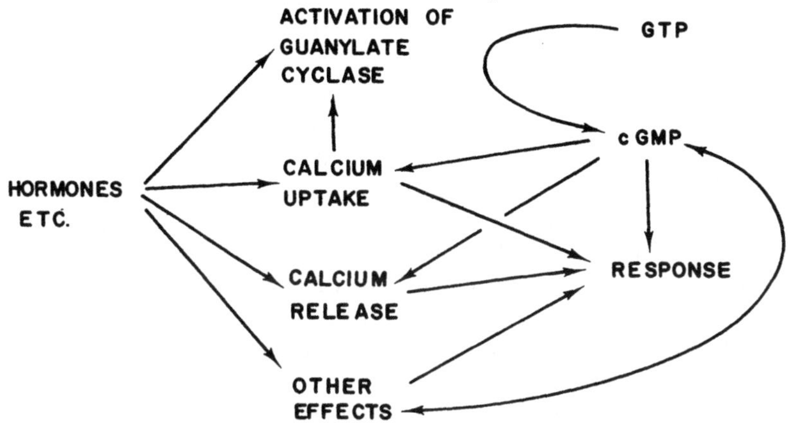

Fig. 3. A scheme designating possible interactions of cGMP and Ca^{2+}. Most of these potential interactions are hypothetical, and in some instances may be bidirectional.

et al., 1975b; Katsuki and Murad, 1977; Arnold *et al.,* 1977). Increases in cGMP in some of these tissues with choline esters, histamine, A23187, or depolorizing concentrations of K^+ require Ca^{2+}. These studies indicate that cGMP increases in tissues can occur through at least two mechanisms, one dependent on external calcium and another independent of external calcium. Agents that increase cGMP in the absence of Ca^{2+} are usually capable of activating guanylate cyclase in cell-free systems. Agents that require Ca^{2+} have not been convincingly shown to alter guanylate cyclase activity directly. The effects of the latter group of agents may lead to increased cGMP levels as a result of their effects on calcium distribution. If such is the case, effects of these agents on guanylate cyclase activity in cell-free systems would be extremely difficult to demonstrate, and could account for the numerous published and unpublished negative studies.

cGMP accumulation may also alter calcium intracellular distribution or its release or both. Thus, in some situations, calcium may influence cGMP accumulation, or cGMP could effect Ca^{2+}, or both effects could occur.

1.3.6. Effects of Azide, Hydroxylamine, and Various Nitro Compounds

In the process of examining the kinetic properties of various forms of guanylate cyclase, sodium azide was added to incubations to inhibit GTP hydrolysis (Kimura *et al.,* 1975a). This agent had small effects on substrate preservation, but markedly increased guanylate cyclase activity (Kimura *et al.,* 1975a). No effects on cyclic nucleotide phosphodiesterase were observed. The stimulatory effect of azide was tissue-specific, and in many tissues was also seen with hydroxylamine, NO_2^-, phenylhydrazine, nitroglycerin, nitroprusside, and nitric oxide (Kimura *et al.*, 1975a; Katsuki *et al.*, 1977; Arnold *et al.*, 1977a,b). The tissue specifity of these effects is attributable to protein activator factors such as catalase that are required for the stimulation and other proteins that can inhibit these effects (Kimura *et al.*, 1975a; Mittal *et al.*, 1975, 1977). The stimulatory effects of these agents can be observed in almost all guanylate cyclase preparations at different degrees of purification from various tissues if the conditions of incubation are carefully selected and protein activator preparations are added. These stimulatory agents can directly or indirectly give rise to reactive nitro groups such as nitric oxide (NO), which also activates guanylate cyclase preparations (Katsuki *et al.*, 1977; Arnold *et al.*, 1977a,b). With activation of guanylate cyclase by these agents, the properties of the enzyme are markedly altered, as discussed earlier.

These activators of guanylate cyclase also increase cGMP levels in a variety of intact tissue preparations such as cerebral cortex, cerebellum, liver, tracheal smooth muscle, and others (Kimura *et al.*, 1975b; Katsuki and Murad, 1977; Arnold *et al.*, 1977a,b). As mentioned above, increases in cGMP levels in tissues with these agents do not require Ca^{2+} in the incubation medium. Similar effects were also observed with nitrosoamines (DeRubertis and Craven, 1976). These latter agents probably also produce their effects by the formation of NO in tissues. These nucleophilic agents and NO donors have become extremely interesting probes with which to examine cGMP synthesis and accumulation in tissues. They should also prove to be very useful in defining the physiologic role(s) of cGMP and its effects in tissues in the presence and absence of calcium.

1.3.7. Effects of Other Agents

A number of other agents have been reported to increase cGMP levels in tissues or extracellular fluids. These agents include histamine (Murad and Kimura, 1974), pancreozymin (Christophe *et al.*, 1976), erythropoeitin (Rodgers *et al.*, 1976), parathyroid hormone (Kaminsky *et al.*, 1970a,b; Murad, 1973), and others. The mechanism or mechanisms by which cGMP is increased with these agents is not known, since the agents do not alter guanylate cyclase or phosphodiesterase activity in broken-cell preparations. Activation of guanylate cyclase with crude preparations of secretin and pancreozymin is due to bile salt contaminants that have effects analogous to detergents (Ichihara *et al.*, 1977). The biologically active octapeptide fragment of pancreozymin increases cGMP content in preparations of pancreas (Christophe *et al.*, 1976).

Administration of parathyroid hormone increases urine and plasma cGMP (Kaminsky *et al.,* 1970 a,b; Murad, 1973) as well as cAMP levels (Chase *et al.,* 1969; Kaminsky *et al.,* 1970a,b). The effects on cGMP require large doses of parathyroid hormone and are thought to be indirect, perhaps due to altered calcium. Intravenous infusions of calcium decrease parathyroid hormone secretion and cAMP excretion (Chase and Aurbach, 1967; Kaminsky *et al.,* 1970a,b), and increase urinary excretion of cGMP (Kaminsky *et al.,* 1970a,b). Administration of calcitonin increases urinary cAMP and cGMP. These latter effects are probably secondary to parathyroid hormone secretion, however, since they are not observed in thyroparathyroidectomized patients (Murad and Pak, 1972) and rats (Chase and Aurbach, 1967).

Administration of pressor agents such as catecholamines and angiotensin increases urinary cGMP (Ball *et al.,* 1972; Rosman *et al.,* 1976). These effects are probably secondary to reflex increases in parasympathetic activity and should be prevented with atropine.

1.4. Some Physiologic Effects That May Correlate with Cyclic GMP

1.4.1. Smooth-Muscle Contraction

The first suggestion of a physiologic role for cGMP came from studies with several smooth-muscle models. With ductus deferens (Schultz *et al.,* 1973), veins (Dunham *et al.,* 1974), tracheal rings (Murad and Kimura, 1974), intestinal smooth muscle (Lee *et al.,* 1972), umbilical artery (Clyman *et al.,* 1975), and uterus (Kuehl *et al.,* 1974), a number of agents that contract these smooth-muscle preparations increased cGMP accumulation. These agents included choline esters, α-adrenergic agents, histamine, bradykinin, serotonin, and prostaglandin $F_2\alpha$ (for a review, see Hardman *et al.,* 1975). On further examination with uterus (Diamond and Holmes, 1975), arterial segments (Diamond and Blisard 1976), and tracheal smooth muscle (Katsuki and Murad, 1977), the correlation of cGMP accumulation and contraction of these preparations does not hold up. Contraction usually precedes significant increases in cGMP. Also, with dose–response curves, low concentrations of choline esters produce some contraction without accompanying changes in cGMP. Furthermore, azide, nitroglycerin, nitroprusside, and other nitro compounds relax smooth-muscle preparations and increase cGMP concentration (Katsuki and Murad, 1977). Phosphodiesterase inhibitors relax these preparations and increase both cAMP and cGMP (Schultz *et al.,* 1973; Murad and Kimura,

1974). β-Adrenergic agonists relax and increase cAMP without altering cGMP. If cGMP is involved in smooth-muscle contraction or relaxation, several compartments or pools of cGMP with different physiologic functions must exist in this tissue.

1.4.2. Heart

Choline esters decrease contractility of various heart preparations. This tissue was the first in which humoral agents produced increased cGMP levels in *in vitro* preparations (George *et al.*, 1970). These observations have since been confirmed by many laboratories. In functioning-heart preparations, the negative inotropic effect may occur at the same time as the increase in cGMP. Choline esters also decrease adenylate cyclase activity in cell-free preparations (Murad *et al.*, 1962) and decrease cAMP levels in intact-cell preparations of heart (George *et al.*, 1970). Studies are not sufficiently complete to allow one to conclude that the effects of choline esters or perhaps other negative inotropic agents are due to increases in cGMP, decreases in cAMP, or both.

1.4.3. Secretion and Transport

Increased secretion of amylase from parotid preparations with choline esters or α-adrenergic agonists (Durham and Butcher, 1974; Wojcik *et al.*, 1975) and pancreatic preparations with choline esters or pancreozymin (Christophe *et al.*, 1976; Albano *et al.*, 1976) may be mediated by increased accumulation of cGMP. These agents influence calcium uptake or release or both in these preparations. It is difficult to conclude (see Fig. 3) at present what the roles of Ca^{2+} or cGMP or both are in these phenomena. It has also been suggested that cGMP accumulation in intestinal mucosa influences ion transport (Brasitus *et al.*, 1976). A variety of agents increase cGMP levels in leukocytes (Sandler *et al.*, 1975). Lysosomal enzyme secretion from neutrophils is also associated with increases in cGMP (Ignarro and Cech, 1975).

1.4.4. Histamine Release

It was first noted that antigen-induced histamine release from leukocyte preparations was inhibited by agents that increased cAMP accumulation, such as β-adrenergic agonists and phosphodiesterase inhibitors (Lichtenstein and Margolis, 1968). A similar phenomenon has been reported with lung preparations. Choline esters increase cGMP content in this tissue and increase the release of histamine and slow-reacting substance of anaphylaxis (Kaliner *et al.*, 1972). Addition of a phosphodiesterase-resistant cGMP analogue, 8-bromo cGMP, also increased histamine release (Austen, 1974). Thus, Austen and co-workers suggested that cGMP accumulation is associated with increased histamine release and cAMP accumulation with decreased release. It is not known, however, that these effects are clearly mediated by cyclic nucleotides.

1.4.5. Cell Growth and Proliferation

From cell culture studies, it has been observed that in many cell lines, there is a reciprocal relationship of cAMP levels and growth rates (Pastan *et al.,* 1975; Friedman, 1976). In some cell lines, cAMP accumulation or addition inhibits growth and increases differentiated functions. It should be pointed out, however, that there are exceptions to these phenomena and some disagreement about the role of cAMP in cell growth and differentiation (for reviews, see Chlapowski *et al.,* 1975; Friedman, 1976). A concern has been the increased levels of cAMP observed in a variety of solid transplantable tumors (Thomas *et al.,* 1973; Murad, 1976).

It has also been reported that lymphocyte proliferation with various mitogens is associated with cGMP accumulation (Hadden, 1975; Weinstein *et al.,* 1975). Fibroblast growth factor also increases proliferation of fibroblasts and increases cGMP (Rudland *et al.,* 1974). cGMP is found in increased concentration in a variety of transplantable Morris hepatomas, renal tumors (Thomas *et al.,* 1973; Murad, 1976), and colon carcinomas (DeRubertis *et al.,* 1976).

At present, it is extremely difficult to assess the roles, if any, of cAMP and cGMP in cell growth and differentiation. Until many additional studies are performed, one cannot and should not extrapolate from present observations to the development of clinical chemotherapeutic protocols.

1.4.6. Platelet Aggregation

As noted earlier, agents that increase cAMP in platelets such as prostaglandins and β-adrenergic agonists inhibit their aggregation induced by various mechanisms (for a review, see Haslam, 1975). Until recently, no explanation of the mechanism of the inhibitory effects of salicylates and indomethacin on platelet aggregation could be offered. These agents inhibit cyclooxygenase and prostaglandin synthesis, with decreased conversion of arachidonic acid to prostaglandins (for a review, see Anderson and Ramwell, 1974). Thus, one would have predicted increased platelet aggregation with these agents. Inhibition of this enzyme, however, also leads to decreased formation of prostaglandin endoperoxide and thromboxanes (Hamberg *et al.,* 1975). Some of these precursors and products increase cGMP accumulation in platelets and increase their aggregation (Davies *et al.*, 1976; Miller and Gorman, 1976). Agents that induce platelet aggregation such as ADP, collagen, serotonin, and arachidonic acid increase cGMP accumulation.

1.4.7. Other Processes

It has been suggested that cGMP could mediate some of the effects of insulin (Illiano *et al.*, 1973), mitogens (Hadden *et al.*, 1972), and some other agents, and is important in neuronal function (Ferrendelli *et al.*, 1972) and other processes (Goldberg *et al.*, 1973). In many instances, the data are usually less supportive of a role of cGMP than the processes discussed earlier.

1.5. Clinical Studies with Cyclic Nucleotides

1.5.1. Cyclic Nucleotides in Tissues

1.5.1.1. Psoriasis

Voorhees *et al.* (1976) reported that psoriatic skin possesses lower concentrations of cAMP and higher concentrations of cGMP than normal tissue. Since psoriasis can be viewed as a process of accelerated skin growth, these observations parallel and support the studies with cyclic nucleotides in many proliferating cell culture systems. As with solid tumor studies, the cellular heterogeneity and necrosis make it extremely difficult to utilize appropriate control tissues and normalize cyclic nucleotide levels for tissue weight, protein, DNA, or analagous parameters.

1.5.1.2. Tumors

As discussed above, a variety of transplantable solid tumors contain high concentrations of cGMP (Thomas *et al.*, 1973; Criss and Murad, 1976). In rats, some of these hepatomas and renal tumors are associated with increased urinary cGMP with normal cAMP concentrations (Murad *et al.*, 1975a; Criss and Murad, 1976). With some tumors, urine cGMP correlates with tumor size. Irradiation of these tumors, administration of 5-fluorouracil, or surgical removal causes reduction of urinary cGMP to normal. These studies have suggested that perhaps some tumors in patients will show increased urinary cGMP. This hypothesis, if borne out, could have significant implications for diagnosis and treatment of some tumors. A recent preliminary report described increased urinary cGMP in several patients with hepatomas (Neethling and Shanley, 1976). Additional studies are obviously needed for further evaluation of the potential clinical significance of these findings.

1.5.2. Cyclic Nucleotides in Extracellular Fluids

1.5.2.1. Parathyroid Disorders

The administration of parathyroid hormone increases urinary cAMP (Chase and Aurbach, 1967; Chase *et al.*, 1969). Parathyroid extract at a dose of 200 U intravenously also increases plasma cAMP and cGMP and urinary cGMP (Kaminsky *et al.*, 1970a,b; Murad, 1973). Urinary cAMP and cGMP are significantly elevated in patients with hyperparathyroidism, whether this is due to parathyroid hyperplasia, adenomas, or "ectopic PTH-producing tumors" (for a review, see Murad, 1973). Excretion of both cyclic nucleotides returns to normal with correction of the hyperparathyroidism. Patients with non-parathyroid-mediated osteoporosis, nephrolithiasis, or hypercalcemia generally show normal or reduced urinary excretion of cAMP or cGMP. Urinary cAMP has been quite helpful as a diagnostic acid for hyperparathyroidism, and is more useful than cGMP, which is increased less frequently (Murad and Pak, 1972; Murad, 1973). The specificity and utility of urinary cAMP for diagnosis of hyperparathyroidism can be improved if one determines the nephrogenous portion of cAMP in urine, rather than total urinary cAMP, which represents that cleared from plasma plus that contributed by the kidney (A. E. Broadus, personal communication).

A deficient or defective urinary cAMP response to parathyroid hormone has become the diagnostic test of choice in pseudohypoparathyroidism (Chase *et al.*, 1969). Smaller changes in urinary cGMP or plasma cAMP with parathyroid hormone in this disorder might also be used. However, the larger percentage changes in urinary cAMP in normal patients make this an easier analysis and test. Tomlinson *et al.* (1976) showed that the plasma cAMP response to parathyroid hormone can be used to rapidly separate pseudohypoparathyroid subjects (nonresponders) from normal subjects or those with surgical hypoparathyroidism. Shaw *et al.* (1977) further examined the diagnostic utility of the urinary cAMP/creatinine ratio in differentiating between primary hyperparathyroidism or ectopic hyperparathyroidism, on the one hand, and non-parathyroid-hormone-related hypercalcemia on the other. As shown originally by Dohan *et al.* (1972), patients with malignancy and hypercalcemia (non-parathyroid-related) show low urinary cAMP excretion, reflecting suppressed secretion of parathyroid hormone.

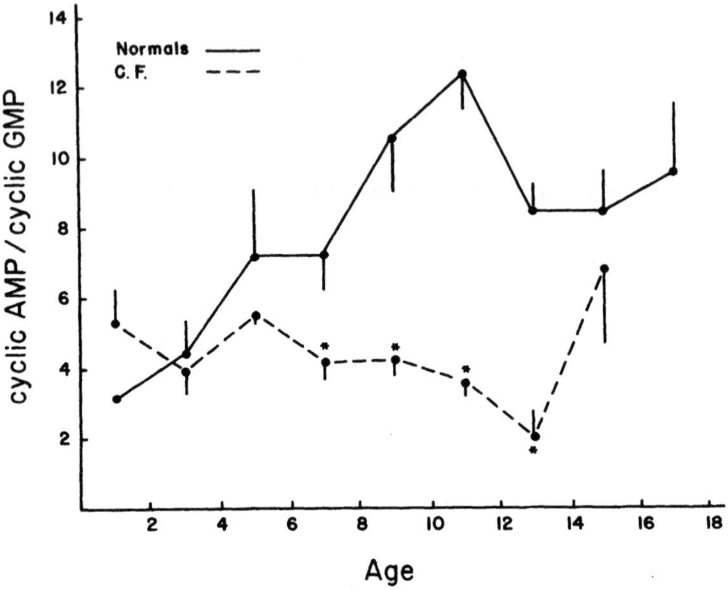

Fig. 4. Ratio of cAMP to cGMP excreted daily in urine in normal children and those with cystic fibrosis. Values are means ± S.E. for the age groups designated. Asterisks designate values that are significantly different from normals. From Murad *et al.* (1975b).

1.5.2.2. Cystic Fibrosis

Patients with cystic fibrosis have lower urinary excretion of cAMP and greater excretion of cGMP (Murad *et al.,* 1975b). This is best illustrated by the ratio of cAMP to cGMP excreted in normal children and those with cystic fibrosis (Fig. 4). The significance of these observations is not known. Lung and intestinal mucosa are rich sources of guanylate cyclase with high levels of cGMP (Ishikawa *et al.,* 1969; Chrisman *et al.,* 1975). Perhaps the increased urinary cGMP in these patients reflects their pulmonary injury and malabsorption with pancreatic insufficiency.

1.5.2.3. Cushing's Disease

Hypophysectomy or adrenalectomy decreases urinary cGMP in rats (Hardman *et al.,* 1969). Excretion of cGMP is increased with pitituary hormones, thyroxine, and steroids. A recent preliminary report described increased urinary cGMP in patients with adrenal hyperplasia, adenomas, and carcinoma with hypercorticism (Wray *et al.,* 1975).

References

Albano, J., Bhoola, K. D., Croker, M., Harvey, R. F., and Heap, R. F., 1976, Stimulation–secretion coupling in the pancreas: role of cyclic GMP in modulating enzyme secretion produced by acetylcholine and cholecystokinin-pancreozymin, *J. Biol.* **258**:87.

Anderson, N. H., and Ramwell, P. W., 1974, Biological aspects of prostaglandins, *Arch. Intern. Med.* **133**:30.

Appleman, M. M., and Terasaki, W. L., 1975, Regulation of cyclic nucleotide phosphodiesterase, *Adv. Cyclic Nucleotide Res.* **5**:153.

Appleman, M. M., Birnbaumer, L., and Torres, H. N., 1966, Factors affecting the activity of muscle glycogen synthetase. III. The reaction with adenosine triphosphate, Mg^{++}, cyclic 3′,5′-adenosine monophosphate, *Arch Biochem. Biophys.* **116**:39.

Arnold, W. P., Katsuki, S., Mittal, C. K., and Murad, F., 1977a, Stimulation of guanylate cyclase by nitric oxide gas, in: Proceedings of the Third International Conference on Cyclic Nucleotides, *Adv. Cyclic Nucleotide Res.* **9**: (in press).

Arnold, W. P., Mittal, C. K., Katsuki, S., and Murad, F., 1977b, Nitric oxide activates guanylate cyclase and increases guanosine 3′,5′-cyclic monophosphate levels in various tissue preparations, *Proc. Natl. Acad. Sci. U.S.A.* **74**:3203.

Ashman, D. F., Lipton, R., Melicow, M. M., and Price, T. D., 1963, Isolation of adenosine 3′,5′-monophosphate and guanosine 3′,5′-monophosphate from rat urine, *Biochem. Biophys. Res. Commun.* **11**:330.

Aurbach, G. D., 1976, Hormone receptors, cyclic nucleotides, and control of cell function, in: *The Year in Metabolism 1975–1976* (N. Freinkel, ed.), pp. 1–43, Plenum Press, New York.

Austen, K. F., 1974, Reaction mechanisms in the release of mediators of immediate hypersensitivity from human lung tissues, *Fed. Proc. Fed. Amer. Soc. Exp. Biol.* **33**:2256.

Ball, J. H., Kaminsky, N. I., Hardman, J. G., Broadus, A. E., Sutherland, E. W., and Liddle, G. W., 1972, Effects of catecholamines and adrenergic-blocking agents on plasma and urinary cyclic nucleotides in man, *J. Clin. Invest.* **51**:2124.

Beavo, J. A., Hardman, J. G., and Sutherland, E. W., 1971, Stimulation of adenosine 3′,5′-monophosphate hydrolysis by guanosine 3′,5′-monophosphate, *J. Biol. Chem.* **246**:3841.

Beavo, J. A., Bechtel, P. J., and Krebs, E. G., 1975, Mechanism of control for cyclic AMP dependent protein kinase from skeletal muscle, *Adv. Cyclic Nucleotide Res.* **5**:241.

Berridge, M. J., 1975, The interaction of cyclic nucleotides and calcium in the control of cellular activity, *Adv. Cyclic Nucleotide Res.* **6**:1.

Bitensky, M. W., Miki, N., Keirns, J. J., Keirns, M., Barabon, J. M., Freeman, J., Wheeler, M. A., Lacy, J., and Marcus, F. R., 1975,Activation of photoreceptor disk membrane phosphodiesterase by light and ATP, *Adv. Cyclic Nucleotide Res.* **5**:213.

Bourne, H. R., Tompkins, G. M., and Dion, S., 1973, Regulation of phosphodiesterase synthesis: Requirement for cyclic adenosine monophosphate-dependent protein kinase, *Science* **181**:952.

Brasitus, T. A., Field, M., and Kimberg, D. V., 1976, Intestinal mucosal cyclic GMP: regulation and relation to ion transport, *Amer. J. Physiol.* **231**:275.

Broadus, A. E., Hardman, J. G., Kaminsky, N. I., Ball, J. H., Sutherland, E. W., and Liddle, G. W., 1971, Extracellular cyclic nucleotides, *Ann. N.Y. Acad. Sci.* **185**:50.

Brooker, G., Thomas, L. J., and Appleman, M. M., 1968, The assay of adenosine 3′,5′-cyclic monophosphate and guanosine 3′,5′-monophosphate in biological materials by enzymatic radioisotopic displacement, *Biochemistry* **7**:4177.

Butcher, F. R., 1975, The role of calcium and cylcic nucleotides in α-amylase release from slices of rat parotid: Studies with the divalent cation ionophore A-23187, *Metabolism* **24**:409.

Butcher, R. W., and Sutherland, E. W., 1962. Adenosine 3′,5′-phosphate in biological materials. Purification and properties of cyclic 3′,5′-nucleotide phosphodiesterase and use of this enzyme to characterize adenosine 3′,5′-phosphate in human urine, *J. Biol. Chem.* **237**:1244.

Butcher, R. W., and Baird, C. E., 1968, Effects of prostaglandins on adenosine 3′,5′-monophosphate levels in fat and other tissues, *J. Biol. Chem.* **243**:1713.

Casnellie, J. E., and Greengard, P., 1974, Guanosine 3′,5′-monophosphate dependent phosphorylation of endogenous substrate proteins in membranes of mammalian smooth muscle, *Proc. Natl. Acad. Sci. U.S.A.* **71**:1891.

Chase, L. R., and Aurbach, G. D., 1967, Parathyroid function and the renal excretion of 3′,5′-adenylic acid, *Proc. Natl. Acad. Sci. U.S.A.* **58**:518.

Chase, L. R., Melson, G. L., and Aurbach, G. D., 1969, Pseudohypoparathyroidism: Defective excretion of 3′,5′-AMP in response to parathyroid hormone, *J. Clin. Invest.* **48**:1832.

Cheung, W. Y., 1971, Cyclic 3′,5′-nucleotide phosphodiesterase. Evidence for and properties of a protein activator, *J. Biol. Chem.* **246**:2859.

Chlapowski, F. J., Kelly, L. A., and Butcher, R. W., 1975, Cyclic nucleotides in cultured cells, *Adv. Cyclic Nucleotide Res.* **6**:245.

Chrisman, T. D., Garbers, D. L., Parks, M. A., and Hardman, J. G., 1975, Characterization of particulate and soluble guanylate cyclases from rat lung, *J. Biol. Chem.* **250**:374.

Christophe, J. P., Frandsen, E. K., Conlon, T. P., Krishna, G., and Gardner, J. D., 1976, Action of cholecystokinin, cholinergic agents and A-23187 on accumulation of guanosine 3′,5′-monophosphate in dispersed guinea pig pancreatic acinar cells, *J. Biol. Chem.* **251**:4640.

Clyman, R. I., Blacksin, A. S., Sandler, J. A., Manganiello, V. C., and Vaughan, M., 1975, The role of calcium in regulation of cyclic nucleotide content in human umbilical artery, *J. Biol. Chem.* **250**:4718.

Corbin, J. D., Keely, S. L., Soderling, T. R., and Park, C. R., 1975, Hormonal regulation of adenosine 3′,5′-monophosphate-dependent protein kinase, *Adv. Cyclic Nucleotide Res.* **5**:265.

Criss, W. E., and Murad, F., 1976, Urinary excretion of cyclic guanosine 3′,5′-

monophosphate and cyclic adenosine 3′,5′-monophosphate in rats bearing transplantable liver and kidney tumors, *Cancer Res.* **36**:1714.

Criss, W. E., Murad, F., Kimura, H., and Morris, H. P., 1976, Properties of guanylate cyclase in adult rat liver and several Morris hepatomas, *Biochem. Biophys. Acta* **445**:500.

Davies, T., Davidson, M. M., McClenaghan, M. D., Say, A., and Haslam, R. J., 1976, Factors affecting platelet cyclic GMP levels during aggregation induced by collagen and by arachidonic acid, *Thromb. Res.* **9**:387.

Davoren, P., and Sutherland, E. W., 1963, The effects of L-epinephrine and other agents on the synthesis and release of adenosine 3′,5′-phosphate of whole pigeon erythrocytes, *J. Biol. Chem.* **238**:3009.

DeRubertis, F. R., and Craven, P. A., 1976, Calcium-independent modulation of cyclic GMP and activation of guanylate cyclase by nitrosamines, *Science* **193**:897.

DeRubertis, F. R., Chayoth, R., and Field, J. B., 1976, The content and metabolism of cyclic adenosine 3′,5′-monophosphate and cyclic guanosine 3′,5′-monophosphate in adenocarcinoma of the human colon. *J. Clin. Invest.* **57**:641.

Diamond, J., and Blisard, K. S., 1976, Effects of stimulant and relaxant drugs on tension and cyclic nucleotide levels in canine femoral artery, *Mol. Pharmacol.* **12**:668.

Diamond, J., and Holmes, T. G., 1975, Effects of potassium chloride and smooth muscle relaxants on tension and cyclic nucleotide levels in rat myometrium, *Can. J. Physiol. Pharmacol.* **53**:1099.

Dohan, P. H., Yamashita, K., Larsen, P. R., Davis, B., Deftos, L., and Field, J. B., 1972, Evaluation of urinary cyclic 3′,5′-adenosine monophosphate excretion in the differential diagnosis of hypercalcemia, *J. Clin. Endocrinol. Metab.* **35**:775.

Dunham, E. W., Haddox, M. K., and Goldberg, N. D., 1974, Alteration of vein cyclic 3′,5′-nucleotide concentrations during changes in contractility, *Proc. Natl. Acad. Sci. U.S.A.* **71**:815.

Durham, J. P., and Butcher, F. R., 1974, The effect of catecholamine analogues upon amylase secretion from the mouse parotid gland in vivo: Relationship to changes in cyclic AMP and cyclic GMP levels, *FEBS Lett.* **47**:218.

Earp, H. S., Smith, P., Ong, S. H., and Steiner, A. L., 1977, Regulation of hepatic nuclear guanylate cyclase, *Proc. Natl. Acad. Sci. U.S.A.* **74**:946.

Entman, M. L., Levey, G. S., and Epstein, S. E., 1969, Demonstration of adenyl cyclase activity in canine cardiac sarcoplasmic reticulum, *Biochem. Biophys. Res. Commun.* **35**:728.

Ferrendelli, J. A., Kinscherf, D. A., and Kipnis, D. M., 1972, Effects of amphetamine, chlorpromazine, and reserpine on cyclic GMP and cyclic AMP levels in mouse cerebellum, *Biochem. Biophys. Res. Commun.* **46**:2114.

Flandroy, L., and Galand, P., 1975, Oestrogen-related changes in uterine and vaginal cAMP and cGMP, *Arch. Int. Physiol. Biochim.* **83**:965.

Friedman, D. L., 1976, Role of cyclic nucleotides in cell growth and differentiation, *Physiol. Rev.* **56**:652.

Garbers, D. L., 1976, Sea urchin sperm guanylate cyclase, purification and loss of cooperativity, *J. Biol. Chem.* **251**:4071.

George, W. J., Polson, J. B., O'Toole, A. G., and Goldberg, N. D., 1970, Elevation of guanosine 3',5'-cyclic phosphate in rat heart after perfusion with acetylcholine, *Proc. Natl. Acad. Sci. U.S.A.* **66**:398.

George, W. J., Ignarro, L. J., and White, L. E., 1975, Muscarinic stimulation of cardiac guanylate cyclase, *Recent Adv. Stud. Cardiac Struct. Metab.* **7**:381.

Gill, G., Holdy, K. E., Walton, G. M., and Kanstein, C. B., 1976, Purification and characterization of 3',5'-cyclic GMP-dependent protein kinase, *Proc. Natl. Acad. Sci. U.S.A.* **73**:3918.

Goldberg, N. D., Dietz, S. B., and O'Toole, A. G., 1969, Cyclic guanosine 3',5'-monophosphate in mammalian tissues and urine, *J. Biol. Chem.* **244**:4458.

Goldberg, N. D., O'Dea, R. F., and Haddox, M. F., 1973, Cyclic GMP, *Adv. Cyclic Nucleotide Res.* **3**:155.

Goridis, C., and Reutter, W., 1975, Plasma membrane-associated increase in guanylate cyclase activity in regenerating rat liver, *Nature (London)* **257**:698.

Greengard, P., 1971, On the reactivity and mechanism of action of cyclic nucleotides, *Ann. N.Y. Acad. Sci.* **185**:18.

Hadden, J. W., 1975, Cyclic nucleotides in lymphocyte function, *Ann. N.Y. Acad. Sci.* **256**:352.

Hadden, J. W., Hadden, E. M., Haddox, M. K., and Goldberg, N. D., 1972, Guanosine 3',5'-cyclic monophosphate: A possible intracellular mediator of mitogenic influences in lymphocytes, *Proc. Nat. Acad. Sci. U.S.A.* **69**:3024.

Hamberg, M., Svensson, J., and Samuelsson, B., 1975, Thromboxanes: A new group of biologically active compounds derived from prostaglandin endoperoxides, *Proc. Natl. Acad. Sci. U.S.A.* **72**:2994.

Hardman, J. G., and Sutherland, E. W., 1969, Guanyl cyclase an enzyme catalyzing the formation of guanosine 3',5'-monophosphate from guanosine triphosphate, *J. Biol. Chem.* **244**:6363.

Hardman, J. G., Davis, J. W., and Sutherland, E. W., 1969, Effects of some hormonal and other factors on the excretion of guanosine 3',5'-monophosphate and adenosine 3',5'-monophosphate in rat urine, *J. Biol. Chem.* **244**:6354.

Hardman, J. G., Chrisman, T. D., Gray, J. P., Suddath, J. L., and Sutherland, E. W., 1973, Guanylate cyclase: Alteration of apparent subcellular distribution and activity of detergents and cations, in: *Pharmacology and the Future of Man,* Vol. 5, pp. 134–145, Karger, Basel.

Hardman, J. G., Garbers, D. L., Wells, J. N., and Chrisman, T. D., 1975, The biosynthesis and degradation of cyclic GMP in smooth muscle and other tissues, in: *Smooth Muscle Pharmacology and Physiology* (M. Worcel and G. Vassort, eds.), pp. 73–82, Inserm, Paris.

Haslam, R. J., 1975, Roles of cyclic nucleotides in platelet function, *Ciba Found. Symp.* **35**:121.

Ho, R. J., and Sutherland, E. W., 1975, cAMP-mediated feedback regulation in target cells, *Adv. Cyclic Nucleotide Res.* **5**:533.

Ichihara, K., Larner, J., Kimura, H., and Murad, F., 1977, Activation of liver guanylate cyclase of bile salts and contaminants in crude secretion and pancreozymine preparations, *Biochim. Biophys. Acta* **481**:734.

Ignarro, L. J., and Cech, S. Y., 1975, Lysosomal enzyme secretion from human neutrophils mediated by cyclic GMP: Inhibition of cyclic GMP accumulation and neutrophil function by glucocorticoids, *J. Cyclic Nucleotide Res.* **1**:283.

Illiano, G., Tell, G. P., Siegel, M. I., and Cuatrecasas, P., 1973, Guanosine 3',5'-cyclic monophosphate and the action of insulin and acetylcholine, *Proc. Natl. Acad. Sci. U.S.A.* **70**:2443.

Ishikawa, E., Ishikawa, S., Davis, J. W., and Sutherland, E. W., 1969, Determination of guanosine 3',5'-monophosphate in tissues and of guanyl cyclase in rat intestine, *J. Biol. Chem.* **244**:6371.

Kakiuchi, S., Yamazaki, R., Teshima, Y., Uenishi, K., and Miyamoto, E., 1975, Ca^{2+}/Mg^{2+}-dependent cyclic nucleotide phosphodiesterase and its activator protein, *Adv. Cyclic Nucleotide Res.* **5**:163.

Kaliner, M., Orange, R. P., and Austen, K. F., 1972, Immunologic release of histamine and slow reacting substance of anaphylaxis from human lung. IV. Enhancement of cholinergic and alpha adrenergic stimulation, *J. Exp. Med.* **136**:556.

Kaminsky, N. I., Ball, J. H., Broadus, A. E., Hardman, J. G., Sutherland, E. W., and Liddle, G. W., 1970a, Hormonal effects on extracellular cyclic nucleotides in man, *Trans. Assoc. Amer. Phys.* **83**:235.

Kaminsky, N. I., Broadus, A. E., Hardman, J. G., Jones, D. J., Ball, J. H., Sutherland, E. W., and Liddle, G. W., 1970b, Effects of parathyroid hormone on plasma and urinary adenosine 3',5'-monophosphate in man, *J. Clin. Invest.* **49**:2387.

Katsuki, S., and Murad, F., 1977, Regulation of adenosine 3',5'-cyclic monophosphate and guanosine 3',5'-cyclic monophosphate levels and contractility in bovine tracheal smooth muscle, *Mol. Pharmacol.* **13**:330.

Katsuki, S., Arnold, A. P., Mittal, C. K., and Murad, F., 1977, Stimulation of guanylate cyclase by sodium nitroprusside, nitroglycerin and nitric oxide in various tissue preparations and comparison to the effects of sodium azide and hydroxylamine, *J. Cyclic Nucleotide Res.* **3**:23.

Katz, A. M., Tada, M., Repke, D. I., Iorio, J. M., and Kirchberger, M. A., 1974, Adenylate cyclase: Its probable localization in sarcoplasmic reticulum as well as sarcolemma of the canine heart, *J. Mol. Cell. Cardiol.* **6**:73.

Kimura, H., and Murad, F., 1974a, Nonenzymatic formation of guanosine 3',5'-monophosphate from guanosine triphosphate, *J. Biol. Chem.* **249**:329.

Kimura, H., and Murad, F., 1974b, Evidence for two different forms of guanylate cyclase in rat heart, *J. Biol. Chem.* **249**:6910.

Kimura, H., and Murad, F., 1975a, Localization of particulate guanylate cyclase in plasma membranes and microsomes of rat liver, *J. Biol. Chem.* **250**:4810.

Kimura, H., and Murad, F., 1975b, Two forms of guanylate cyclase in mammalian tissues and possible mechanisms for their regulation, *Metabolism* **24**:439.

Kimura, H., and Murad, F., 1975c, Subcellular localization of guanylate cyclase, *Life Sci.* **17**:837.

Kimura, H., and Murad, F., 1975d, Increased particulate and decreased soluble guanylate cyclase activity in regenerating liver, fetal liver, and hepatoma, *Proc. Natl. Acad. Sci. U.S.A.* **72**:1965.

Kimura, H., Thomas, E., and Murad, F., 1974, Effects of decapitation, ether and pentobarbital on guanosine 3′,5′-phosphate and adenosine 3′,5′-phosphate levels in rat tissues, *Biochim. Biophys. Acta* **343**:519.

Kimura, H., Mittal, C. K., and Murad, F., 1975a, Activation of guanylate cyclase from rat liver and other tissues by sodium azide, *J. Biol. Chem.* **250**: 8016.

Kimura, H., Mittal, C. K., and Murad, F., 1975b, Increases in cyclic GMP levels in brain and liver with sodium azide, an activator of guanylate cyclase, *Nature (London)* **257**:700.

Kimura, H., Mittal, C. K., and Murad, F., 1976, Appearance of magnesium guanylate cyclase activity in rat liver with sodium azide activation, *J. Biol. Chem.* **251**:7769.

Kolata, G. B., 1975, Thromboxanes: The power behind the prostaglandins, *Science* **190**:770.

Kuehl, F. A., Ham, E. A., Zanetti, M. E., Sanford, C. H., Nicol, S. E., and Goldberg, N. D., 1974, Estrogen-related increases in uterine guanosine 3′,5′-cyclic monophosphate levels, *Proc. Natl. Acad. Sci. U.S.A.* **71**:1866.

Kuo, J. F., Wyatt, G. R., and Greengard, P., 1971, Cyclic nucleotide-dependent protein kinases. IX. Partial purification and some properties of guanosine 3′,5′-monophosphate dependent and adenosine 3′,5′-monophosphate-dependent protein kinases from various tissues and species of Arthropoda, *J. Biol. Chem.* **246**:7159.

Kuo, J. F., Patrick, J. G., and Seery, V. L., 1976, Subunit structure of cyclic GMP-dependent protein kinase from guinea pig fetal lung: Dissociation of holoenzyme by cyclic GMP and histone, *Biochem. Biophys. Res. Commun.* **72**:996.

Kuo, W. N., Shoji, M., and Kuo, J. F., 1976, Stimulatory modulator of guanosine-3′,5′-monophosphate-dependent protein kinase from mammalian tissues, *Biochim. Biophys. Acta* **437**:142.

Lee, T. P., Kuo, J. F., and Greengard, P., 1972, Role of muscarinic cholinergic receptors in regulation of guanosine 3′,5′-cyclic monophosphate content in mammaliam brain, heart muscle, and intestinal smooth muscle, *Proc. Natl. Acad. Sci. U.S.A.* **69**:3287.

Lichtenstein, M., and Margolis, S., 1968, Histamine release *in vitro:* Inhibition of catecholamines and methylxanthines, *Science* **161**:902.

Lincoln, T. M., Hall, C. L., Park, C. R., and Corbin, J. D., 1976, Guanosine 3′,5′-cyclic monophosphate binding proteins in rat tissues, *Proc. Natl. Acad. Sci. U.S.A.* **73**:2559.

Loten, E. G., and Sneyd, J. G. T., 1970, An effect of insulin on adipose tissue adenosine 3′,5′-cyclic nucleotide phosphodiesterase, *Biochem. J.* **120**:187.

Macchia, V., Varrone, S., Weissbach, H., Miller, D. L., and Pastan, I., 1975, Guanylate cyclase in *Escherichia coli:* Purification and properties, *J. Biol. Chem.* **250**:6214.

Manganiello, V., and Vaughan, M., 1972a, Prostaglandin E_1 effects on adenosine 3′,5′-cyclic monophosphate concentration and phosphodiesterase activity in fibroblasts, *Proc. Natl. Acad. Sci. U.S.A.* **69**:269.

Manganiello, V., and Vaughan, M., 1972b, An effect of dexamethasone on adenosine 3′,5′-monophosphate content and adenosine 3′,5′-monophosphate phosphodiesterase activity of cultured hepatoma cells, *J. Clin. Invest.* **51**:2763.

Manganiello, V. C., Murad, F., and Vaughan, M., 1971, Effects of lipolytic and antilipolytic agents on cyclic 3′,5′-adenosine monophosphate in fat cells, *J. Biol. Chem.* **246**:2195.

McKeel, D. W., and Jarrett, L., 1974, The enrichment of adenylate cyclase in the plasma membrane and Golgi subcellular fractions of porcine adenohypophysis, *J. Cell Biol.* **62**:231.

Miller, O. V., and Gorman, R. R., 1976, Modulation of platelet cyclic nucleotide content by PGE_1 and the prostaglandin endoperoxide PGG_2, *J. Cyclic Nucleotide Res.* **2**:79.

Mittal, C. K., and Murad, F., 1977, Formation of adenosine 3′,5′-monophosphate by preparations of guanylate cyclase from rat liver and other tissues, *J. Biol. Chem.* **252**:3136.

Mittal, C. K., Kimura, H., and Murad, F., 1975, Requirement for a macromolecular factor for sodium azide activation of guanylate cyclase, *J. Cyclic Nucleotide Res.* **1**:261.

Mittal, C. K., Kimura, H. K., and Murad, F., 1977, Purification and properties of a protein required for sodium azide activation of guanylate cyclase, *J. Biol. Chem.* **252**:4384.

Mukherjee, C., Caron, M. G., and Lefkowitz, R. J., 1975, Catecholamine-induced subsensitivity of adenylate cyclase associated with loss of β-adrenergic receptor binding sites, *Proc. Natl. Acad. Sci. U.S.A.* **72**:1945.

Murad, F., 1973, Clinical studies and application of cyclic nucleotides, *Adv. Cyclic Nucleotide Res.* **3**:355.

Murad, F., 1976, Cyclic GMP metabolism in transplantable tumors, in: *Cyclic Nucleotides and the Regulation of Cell Growth* (M. Abou-Sabe', ed.) Dowden, Hutchinson and Ross, Stroudsburg, Pa., pp. 191–206.

Murad, F., and Kimura, H., 1974, Cyclic nucleotide levels in incubations of guinea pig trachea, *Biochim. Biophys. Acta* **343**:275.

Murad, F., and Pak, C. Y., 1972, Urinary excretion of adenosine 3′,5′-monophosphate and guanosine 3′,5′-monophosphate, *N. Engl. J. Med.* **286**:1382.

Murad, F., Chi, Y. M., Rall, T. W., and Sutherland, E. W., 1962, Adenyl cyclase III. The effects of catecholamines and choline esters on the formation of adenosine 3′,5′-phosphate by preparations from cardiac muscle and liver, *J. Biol. Chem.* **237**:1233.

Murad, F., Manganiello, V., and Vaughan, M., 1970, Effects of guanosine 3′,5′-monophosphate on glycerol production and accumulation of adenosine 3′,5′-monophosphate by fat cells, *J. Biol. Chem.* **245**:3352.

Murad, F., Kimura, H., Hopkins, H. A., Looney, W. B., and Kovacs, C. J., 1975a, Increased urinary excretion of cyclic guanosine monophosphate in rats bearing Morris hepatoma 3924a, *Science* **190**:58.

Murad, F., Moss, W. W., Johanson, A. J., and Selden, R. F., 1975b, Urinary excretion of adenosine 3′,5′-monophosphate and guanosine 3′,5′monophosphate in normal children and those with cystic fibrosis, *J. Clin. Endocrinol. Metab.* **40**:552.

Murad, F., Kimura, H., Mittal, C. K., and Arnold, W. P., 1976, Guanylate cyclase:

Properties and regulation, in: *Proceedings of the Vth International Congress of Endocrinology,* Excerpta Medica, Amsterdam.

Neer, E. J., 1976, The size of adenylate cyclase and guanylate cyclase from the rat renal medulla, *J. Supramol. Struct.* **4**:51.

Neethling, A. C., and Shanley, B. C., 1976, Cyclic GMP excretion and hepatoma, *Lancet* **2**:578.

Pastan, I., and Perlman, R. L., 1972, Regulation of gene transcription in *E. coli* of cyclic AMP, *Adv. Cyclic Nucleotide Res.* **1**:11.

Pastan, I. H., Johnson, G. S., and Anderson, W. B., 1975, Role of cyclic nucleotides in growth control, *Annu. Rev. Biochem.* **44**:491.

Pointer, R. H., Butcher, F. R., and Fain, J. N., 1976, Studies on the role of cyclic guanosine 3′,5′-monophosphate and extracellular Ca^{2+} in the regulation of glycogenolysis in rat liver cells, *J. Biol. Chem.* **251**:2987.

Rall, T. W., and Sutherland, E. W., 1962, Adenyl cyclase II. The enzymatically catalyzed formation of adenosine 3′,5′-phosphate and inorganic pyrophosphate from adenosine triphosphate, *J. Biol. Chem.* **237**:1228.

Robison, G. A., Butcher, R. W., and Sutherland, E. W., 1967, Adenyl cyclase as an adrenergic receptor, *Ann. N.Y. Acad. Sci.* **139**:703.

Robison, G. A., Butcher, R. W., and Sutherland, E. W., 1971, *Cyclic AMP,* Academic Press, New York, 531 pp.

Rodgers, G. M., Fisher, J. W., and George, W. J., 1976, Elevated cyclic GMP concentrations in rabbit bone marrow culture and mouse spleen following erythropoietic stimulation, *Biochem. Biophys. Res. Commun.* **70**:287.

Rosen, O. M., Erlichman, J., and Rubin, C. S., 1975, Molecular structure and characterization of bovine heart protein kinase, *Adv. Cyclic Nucleotide Res.* **5**:253.

Rosman, P. M., Agrawal, R., Goodman, A. D., and Steiner, A. L., 1976, Effect of angiotensin II on cyclic guanosine monophosphate and cyclic adenosine monophosphate in human plasma, *J. Clin. Endocrinol. Metab.* **42**:531.

Rudland, P. S., Gospodarowicz, D., and Seifert, W., 1974, Activation of guanyl cyclase and intracellular cyclic GMP by fibroblast growth factor, *Nature (London)* **250**:741.

Rudolph, S. A., and Greengard, P., 1974, Regulation of protein phosphorylation and membrane permeability of β-adrenergic agents and cyclic adenosine 3′,5′-monophosphate in the avian erythrocyte, *J. Biol. Chem.* **249**:5684.

Sandler, J. A., Gallin, J. I., and Vaughan, M., 1975, Effects of serotonin, carbamylcholine, and ascorbic acid on leukocyte cyclic GMP and chemotaxis, *J. Cell. Biol.* **67**:480.

Schultz, G., Böhme, E., and Munske, K., 1969, Guanyl cyclase: Determination of enzyme activity, *Life Sci. Part II Biochem. Gen. Mol. Biol.* **8**:1323.

Schultz, G., Hardman, J. G., Schultz, K., Baird, C. E., and Sutherland, E. W., 1973, The importance of calcium ions for the regulation of guanosine 3′,5′-cyclic monophosphate levels, *Proc. Natl. Acad. Sci. U.S.A.* **70**:3889.

Schwartz, J. P., 1976, Catecholamine-mediated elevation of cyclic GMP in the rat C-6 glioma cell line, *J. Cyclic Nucleotide Res.* **2**:287.

Shaw, J. W., Oldham, S. B., Rosoff, L., Bethune, J. E., and Fichman, M. P., 1977, Urinary cyclic AMP analyzed as a function of the serum calcium and parathy-

roid hormone in the differential diagnosis of hypercalcemia, *J. Clin. Invest.* **59**:14.
Siegel, M. I., Puca, G. A., and Cuatrecasas, P., 1976, Guanylate cyclase: Existence of different forms and their regulation of nucleotides in calf uterus, *Biochem. Biophys. Acta* **438**:310.
Steiner, A. L., Pagliara, A. S., Chase, L. R., and Kipnis, D. M., 1972, Radioimmunoassay for cyclic nucleotides. II. Adenosine 3′,5′-monophosphate and guanosine 3′,5′-monophosphate in mammalian tissues and body fluids, *J. Biol. Chem.* **247**:1114.
Steiner, A. L., Ong, S., and Wedner, H. J., 1976, Cyclic nucleotide immunocytochemistry, *Adv. Cyclic Nucleotide Res.* **7**:115.
Stoner, J. S., Manganiello, V., and Vaughan, M., 1974, Guanosine cyclic 3′,5′-monophosphate and guanylate cyclase activity in guinea pig lung: Effects of acetylcholine and cholinesterase inhibitors, *Mol. Pharmacol.* **10**:155.
Sutherland, E. W., and Rall, T. W., 1958, Fractionation and characterization of a cyclic adenine ribonucleotide formed by tissue particles, *J. Biol. Chem.* **232**:1077.
Takai, Y., Nakaya, S., Inoue, M., Kishimoto, A., Nishiyama, K., Yamamura, H., and Nishizuka, Y., 1976, Comparison of mode of activation of guanosine 3′:5′-monophosphate-dependent and adenosine 3′:5′-monophosphate-dependent protein kinases from silkworm, *J. Biol. Chem.* **251**:1481.
Terasaki, W. L., and Brooker, G., 1977, Cardiac adenosine 3′,5′-monophosphate: Free and bound forms in the isolated rat atrium, *J. Biol. Chem.* **252**:1041.
Thiers, R. E., and Vallee, B. L., 1957, Distribution of metals in subcellular fractions of rat liver, *J. Biol. Chem.* **226**:911.
Thomas, E. W., Murad, F., Looney, W. P., and Morris, H. P., 1973, Adenosine 3′,5′-monophosphate and guanosine 3′,5′-monophosphate concentrations in Morris hepatomas of different growth rates, *Biochim. Biophys. Acta* **297**:564.
Thompson, W. J., and Williams, R. H., 1974, Effect of adrenalectomy on cyclic 3′,5′-guanosine monophosphate metabolism of rat liver and other tissues, *Arch. Biochem. Biophys.* **165**:468.
Thompson, W. J., Williams, R. H., and Little, S. A., 1973, Activation of guanyl cyclase and adenyl cyclase by secretin, *Biochim. Biophys. Acta* **302**:329.
Tomlinson, S., Hendy, G. N., and O'Riordan, J. L. H., 1976, A simplified assessment of response to parathyroid hormone in hypoparathyroid patients, *Lancet* **1**:62.
Voorhees, J. J., Duell, E. A., Creehan, P., Staiviski, M., and Harrell, E. R., 1976, Cyclic AMP and cyclic GMP in epidermal physiology and pathophysiology, *Curr. Prob. Dermatol.* **6**:107.
Wallach, D., and Pastan, I., 1976, Stimulation of guanylate cyclase of fibroblasts by free fatty acids, *J. Biol. Chem.* **251**:5802.
Wang, J. H., Teo, T. S., Ho, H. C., and Stevens, F. C., 1975, Bovine heart protein activator of cyclic nucleotide phosphodiesterase, *Adv. Cyclic Nucleotide Res.* **5**:179.
Weight, F. F., Petzold, G., and Greengard, P., 1974, Guanosine 3′,4′-monophosphate in sympathetic ganglia: Increase associated with synaptic transmission, *Science* **186**:942.

Weinstein, Y., Segal, S., and Melmon, K. L., 1975, Specific mitogenic activity of 8-Br-guanosine 3′,5-monophosphate on B lymphocytes, *J. Immunol.* **115**:112.

White, A. A., 1975, Guanylate cyclase activity in heart and lung, *Adv. Cyclic Nucleotide Res.* **5**:353.

White, A. A., and Aurbach, G. D., 1969, Detection of guanyl cyclase in mammalian tissues, *Biochim. Biophys. Acta* **191**:686.

Wojcik, J. D., Grand, R. J., and Kimberg, D. V., 1975, Amylase secretion by rabbit parotid gland. Role of cyclic AMP and cyclic GMP, *Biochim. Biophys. Acta* **411**:250.

Wray, H. L., Corrigan, D. F., Burton, J., Schaaf, M., and Earle, J. M., 1975, Elevated urinary cyclic GMP in patients with Cushing's syndrome, in: *Proceedings of the 57th Annual Meeting of the Endocrine Society,* p. 362.

Yamashita, K., and Field, J. B., 1972, Elevation of cyclic guanosine 3′,5′-monophosphate levels in dog thyroid slices caused by acetylcholine and sodium fluoride, *J. Biol. Chem.* **247**:7062.

2

Diabetes Mellitus

Stefan S. Fajans

2.1. Heterogeneity of Diabetes Mellitus

2.1.1. Genetic Heterogeneity

Evidence has accumulated that primary or idiopathic diabetes mellitus is a heterogenous group of disorders that share hyperglycemia and, in part, the complications of diabetes mellitus. As such, it is a syndrome, not a single specific disease. In primary diabetes mellitus, genetic as well as environmental factors appear to be involved. Various environmental factors, superimposed on differences in genetic susceptibility, may be important in the pathogenesis of different forms of the disease. Evidence supporting the hypothesis of genetic heterogeneity was reviewed in Chapter 2 of *The Year in Metabolism 1975–1976* (Fajans, 1976), at an international workshop on the genetics of diabetes mellitus (Creutzfeldt *et al.*, 1976), and by Zonana and Rimoin (1976). To recapitulate briefly, at least five different lines of evidence have emerged to support the concept of

Stefan S. Fajans • Department of Internal Medicine, Division of Endocrinology and Metabolism and the Metabolism Research Unit, The University of Michigan, Ann Arbor, Michigan 48109.

genetic heterogeneity in diabetes: (1) histocompatibility (HLA) studies; (2) analysis of prevalence of diabetes and HLA types in identical twins; (3) pedigree analysis of two forms of diabetes in young people; (4) evidence of autoimmune phenomenon as expressed in the finding of circulating pancreatic islet-cell antibodies; and (5) evidence of autoimmune abnormalities as expressed by the finding of cell-mediated immunity.

This concept of genetic heterogeneity has been challenged solely on the basis of some recalculations and criticisms of the twin data of Tattersall and Pyke (Rosenthal *et al.*, 1976a–c). The latter authors adhere to older views that diabetes mellitus is inherited as a single genetic disorder. The multiple lines of evidence for genetic heterogeneity reviewed imply that different mechanisms of genetic susceptibility operate in the two major clinical forms of diabetes (Pyke *et al.*, 1976a, b; Cudworth and Woodrow, 1976a; Rimoin and Rotter, 1976; Burch, 1976).

2.1.1.1. The Histocompatibility System (HLA) and Genetic Susceptibility to Diabetes Mellitus

Following the recent studies of the major histocompatibility (HLA) system in man, it was found that in classic juvenile-onset-type diabetes (JOD), the major genetic susceptibility is HLA-linked. Looking for an association between the HLA system and a particular disease is more likely to be productive when there is familial aggregation and where virus and autoimmunity seem to be involved. As reviewed last year, and as will be expanded on in this chapter, in JOD there is evidence for the existence of all these possible pathogenetic factors. The HLA system probably contains the so-called "immune response" (Ir) genes or determinants (Svejgaard, 1976). If this is true, the associations observed with four types of cell surface antigens, HLA-A, -B, -C, and -D of chromosome 6 must be considered secondary to primary associations with Ir determinants in linkage disequilibrium with unknown HLA markers. Ir determinants may confer susceptibility to autoimmune disorders. The triggering of autoimmunity could be due to an infecting virus-carrying antigen resembling host antigens causing the release of self-constituents from infected organs. It has also been suggested that some HLA factors may serve as receptors for virus, or perhaps they could interfere with the interaction between the virus and its receptor.

The previously reported association between the increased prevalence of certain second-series HLA antigens and JOD was confirmed in a larger series of patients (Cudworth and Woodrow, 1976b). In 280 patients with insulin-dependent diabetes who were age 30 or under at onset, there was a significant positive association with HLA-B8 and BW15, as well as with B18, as previously reported from Montpelier (Seignalet *et al.*, 1975). In subjects who possess two of these antigens, the risk appears to be additive, suggesting that these antigens may be operating through different pathogenetic mechanisms (Cudworth and Woodrow, 1976b; Nerup *et al.,* 1976).

In 50 insulin-dependent diabetics with an age at onset greater than 30 years, there was evidence of significant association with HLA-B8 (Cudworth and Woodrow, 1976b). This suggests that an HLA-linked diabetogenic gene or genes have a major role in all cases of insulin-dependent JOD. On the other hand, in late-onset non-insulin-dependent diabetics (maturity-onset-type diabetics, MOD), there was no significant departure from normal frequency of any of the HLA antigens in 100 patients. This again provides strong evidence for the existence of genetic heterogeneity and further evidence for the existence of different pathogenetic mechanisms in the two major clinical forms of diabetes mellitus.

HLA-B8 and -BW15 can be demonstrated in 65% of patients with JOD as compared with 39% in the background population. The finding of HLA-B8 and -BW15 in a subject can be demonstrated to give an increased likelihood of developing JOD of about 2.5 times that of the subject not carrying these antigens (Nerup *et al.,* 1976). Another group (Ludwig *et al.,* 1976b) noted in JODs a close association with HLA-B8, HLA-BW15, and HLA-CW3, but a decrease in HLA-B7 frequency. This was also found when the data were combined with those of various other centers. The combined data give a 13.2% positivity in patients with JOD and a 26.8% positivity in control subjects. Thus, B7 may be a marker for a protective effect of the B7 antigen (Cudworth and Woodrow, 1976b; Van De Putte *et al.,* 1976). The protective effect was not absolute, but a B7-positive person had 14.5 times less chance of developing JOD than his B7-negative sib (Van De Putte *et al.,* 1976).

An even stronger association was demonstrated between JOD and HLA-DW3 and -DW4 antigens of the D series of the HLA system (Nerup *et al.,* 1976). In subjects possessing these antigens, the increased likelihood of developing JOD is 6.4 and 3.7 times greater, respectively. The antigens of this fourth locus of the major human histocompatibility region on chromosome 6 can at present be typed for only by means of unidirectional mixed lymphocyte cultures and thus differ from the other histocompatibility antigens. DW3 and DW4 were found to occur in 80% of JOD patients compared with 24% of the control population.

Another report describes the results of complete HLA typing of 10 families with one or more children with JOD (Rubinstein *et al.,* 1976). In all the patients, the age of onset was 16 years or less. A statistically significant association was found between JOD and HLA-D (DW3) antigen (mixed lymphocyte or *D*-locus antigens. No such association was detectable with the seriologically defined (SD) antigens of the HLA-A, HLA-B, or HLA-C series. These studies suggested to Rubinstein *et al.* (1976) that the HLA system is not directly involved in JOD, but that it maintains linkage disequilibrium (LD) with nearby genes that are so involved. HLA disease association was previously postulated to be due to a linkage disequilibrium in the *HLA* locus as a possible mechanism to explain the association between a serological antigen and the clinical disease. The risk of developing JOD is significantly increased in the sibs of patients that inherit identical D antigens. However, the association between LD identity and JOD is not absolute. This again suggests that the LD-linked genes are probably very important but not the sole determinants of the risk of developing JOD.

In a study by Morris *et al.* (1976), the previously demonstrated association between HLA-B8 and insulin-dependent diabetes was confirmed, but the association between HLA-BW15 or HLA-CW3 was not. The patients selected for this particular study were those who, for the most part, were islet-cell-antibody-positive (see Section 2.1.1.3b). Their findings support the earlier suggestion that different alleles determining susceptibility to diabetes may be associated with B8 and BW15 respectively. This study also showed an association between diabetes and HLA-A1 and HLA-B8. The increased frequency of HLA-A1 seen in these studies can be attributed to the known linkage disequilibrium between HLA-A1 and HLA-B8.

A possible unifying hypothesis is that in insulin-dependent diabetes, irrespective of age of onset, there are one or more immune response genes in linkage disequilibrium with HLA antigens that permit interaction of a virus with specific cell-membrane antigens, resulting in direct viral invasion and destruction of the beta cells. Alternatively, this interaction between the virus and the membrane receptor may result in antibody-mediated beta-cell destruction (Cudworth, 1976; Cudworth and Woodrow, 1976b; Nerup *et al.,* 1976).

In a Japanese population, an increased frequency of BW 22J was found in JOD, but not of B8 or BW15 as in Caucasian populations. *C* and *D* loci were not tested (Wakisaka *et al.,* 1976).

No abnormality in the frequency of HLA antigens has been found in the usual MOD. Nelson and Pyke (1976) HLA-typed 13 diabetics and 9 nondiabetic members of three maturity-onset-type diabetes of the young (MODY) families. They concluded that the gene in MODY is not linked to the *HLA-B* locus. On the other hand, Barbosa *et al.* (1976) reported data from study of two MODY families that seemed compatible with dominance of a gene in linkage with certain HLA haplotypes (A3-BW15).

2.1.1.2. Inheritance of (Genetic Susceptibility to) Virus-Induced Diabetes Mellitus

The possibility that individuals with genetic differences due to certain HLA types are more susceptible to or respond differently to environmental agents, such as viral infections, is an attractive hypothesis. Although indirect evidence has been cited to suggest that viral infection may play a role in the pathogenesis of JOD, as reviewed in last year's chapter, no direct evidence is available in man that a virus (one or more) is capable of attacking beta cells, associated with genetic susceptibility. Thus, studies in experimental models are particularly important to pursue this possibility. The "M" variant of encephalomyocarditis virus (EMC) infects pancreatic beta cells and causes the development of a diabetic syndrome in susceptible strains of mice. By examining the progeny of four F_1 crosses of susceptible and resistant strains of mice, Ross *et al.* (1976) concluded that the tendency to acquire diabetes after infection is inherited as a recessive trait. Analysis of the data from the F_2 generation indicated that more than one gene was involved in the development of EMC diabetes. The severity or frequency of abnormal glucose levels in EMC-infected animals appears to be markedly influenced by environmental factors.

Monolayer cultures of beta cells (85–95% beta cells) from susceptible mice supported replication of the "M" strain of EMC virus better than the beta cells from resistant strains of mice. Beta cells from susceptible mice that were infected *in vivo* with EMC virus showed higher viral titers, more severe degranulation, and lower concentrations of immunoreactive insulin than beta cells from resistant mice. Immunofluorescence and infectious center assays revealed that pancreas from susceptible mice contained at least 10 times more infected cells than pancreas from resistant mice (Yoon and Notkins, 1976). Monolayer beta cell cultures prepared from susceptible mice and infected *in vitro* also showed higher viral titers (50 times) and more severe cytopathological changes in beta-cell cultures from resistant mice. In contrast to beta-cell cultures, virus replicated equally well in primary embryo and kidney-cell cultures from susceptible and resistant strains of mice. It was concluded that the development of EMC-induced diabetes is related to genetically determined host differences in the capacity of the virus to infect beta cells. A variety of factors could influence viral titer in beta cells; e.g., genetically determined factors might control the number of viral receptors on the surface of beta cells, the ability of virus to replicate in beta cells, the rate of repair of damaged beta cells, or the responsiveness of beta cells to protection by interferon. Genetically determined factors may affect the susceptibility of one cell type to a particular virus infection without necessarily affecting the susceptibility of other cell types in the same host.

Further data showed that the differences between susceptible and nonsusceptible strains were due to differences in viral replication (Yoon *et al.,* 1976). Those with a higher viral replication were initially hyperinsulinemic and hypoglycemic after infection, due to acute beta-cell damage and a rapid release of insulin. At about 7 days after infection, these animals became hypoinsulinemic and hyperglycemic as a result of residual beta-cell damage and the decrease in the insulin content of the pancreas. Thus, EMC-induced hypoinsulinemia and hyperglycemia are secondary to genetically determined differences in the degree to which beta cells support viral replication.

2.1.1.3. Autoimmunity in Diabetes Mellitus

Evidence supporting an association between diabetes mellitus and autoimmunity was summarized briefly in last year's chapter. In 1976, further evidence was published that pancreatic-islet-cell antibodies (PICA or ICA) are commonly found in newly diagnosed JOD patients, that ICA may precede the onset of diabetes by several years, and that cell-mediated immunity may play a role in the pathogenesis of diabetes mellitus.

2.1.1.3a. Pancreatic-Islet-Cell Antibodies (PICA or ICA). Humoral antibodies in diabetes reacting specifically with pancreatic islet cells were first demonstrated only in diabetic patients with insulin-dependent diabetes plus coexisting autoimmunities (Bottazzo *et al.*, 1974; MacCuish *et al.*, 1974). Subsequently, further reports have appeared to show ICA in insulin-dependent diabetics without other coexistent autoimmune disease.

Irvine *et al.* (1976a) found that the prevalence of ICA was 0.5% in the general population but 70% in patients at the time of clinical diagnosis of JOD. ICA occurred irrespective of age at diagnosis in insulin-dependent patients. In insulin-independent diabetics requiring oral hypoglycemic agents, there was an 8% overall prevalence of ICA with a 20% prevalence at the time of progression. Those subjects who were ICA-positive had a strong tendency to develop insulin-dependent diabetes in subsequent years, suggesting different grades of disease severity and progression in autoimmune diabetes. The disease process that is associated with pancreatic autoimmunity and of which the terminal stage is JOD probably progresses at different rates in different people. Irvine *et al.* (1976a) reported the results of glucose tolerance tests (GTTs) in ICA-positive subjects not previously recognized as diabetic. ICA were detected in 31 patients with organ-specific autoimmune disorders, 4 first-degree relatives of ICA-positive diabetics, and 1 apparently normal subject. Of these 36 subjects, 14 were found to have abnormal GTTs and 22 had normal GTTs. An additional 2 patients had abnormal GTTs during pregnancy or thyrotoxicosis, while 2 subsequently developed insulin-dependent diabetes. The serum from 26 subjects had been stored for 1–11 years before the GTTs were performed. In addition to acting as markers for asymptomatic diabetes, the presence of ICA in serum may define a group of potential diabetics with normal GTTs. These findings occur mainly among subjects who have one or more organ-specific autoimmune diseases, but also occur among the first-degree relatives of ICA-positive patients (mainly insulin-dependent).

Another study (Lendrum *et al.*, 1976a) confirmed the strong association of ICA with insulin-dependent diabetes. The overall prevalence of ICA in 38% (319 of 829) of insulin-dependent diabetic patients compared with the lower prevalence of 5% (6 of 112 patients) in insulin-independent diabetics, and with 1.7% (3 of 177) in non-diabetic subjects. The prevalence of ICA declined as the duration of the disease increased. This decline was particularly rapid during the first 5 weeks of clinical disease, falling from 85 to 50%. Subsequently, the prevalence remained steady until the end of the first year. Over the next few years, the prevalence fell to between 10 and 20%, after which no further decline was observed. The decrease in antibody prevalence was independent of age of patients. There was no accompanying fall in the mean ICA titer of positive patients during this time, however, suggesting that in some patients, antibody disappeared completely, while in others it remained present at the same titer (in some patients for over 20 years; maximum 44 years). The initial high prevalence of ICA was undoubtedly due to selection of patients who had symptoms for only a short time; patients with symptomatic onset within 1 week of testing had probably undergone very recent islet-cell destruction. Others, in whom symptoms appeared more gradually, may have had more insidious damage going on for longer periods of time, and their antibodies may have already disappeared. In 1 of 10 nondiabetic subjects who were first-degree relatives of an insulin-dependent diabetic, overt diabetes developed 3½ years after detection of ICA. This suggests that the event that leads to diabetes occurs months or years before clinical features develop. There was no relationship between ICA and thyroid-microsomal- and gastric-parietal-cell antibodies. ICA thus seemed to have a different pattern of prevalence from other autoantibodies and may possibly be a simple by-product of islet-cell destruction rather than the cause of an autoimmune destructive process. The antibodies were directed against cytoplasmic components of islet cells, but not against insulin itself.

Another group (Christy *et al.*, 1976) found a 55% prevalence of ICA in JOD patients. No correlation was found between the occurrence of ICA and cell-mediated antipancreatic autoimmunity (APCI). Autoimmunity (ICA or APCI or both) was present in 73% of JODs and 89% of those who were HLA-B8-positive (Nerup *et al.*, 1976). Since ICA as well as APCI may decrease with increasing duration of the disease, an autoimmune phenomenon may be demonstratable with even higher prevalence at the time of diagnosis or during the months preceding clinical manifestation of the disease. Tingle *et al.* (1976) found the presence of ICA in a high proportion of recently diagnosed insulin-dependent JODs (77.8% positive within 0–1 years of insulin therapy, 25% within 1–5 years, 30% within 5–10 years, and 10% within 10–15 years). Another group found that ICA may be detected several years before the onset of diabetic symptoms and tend to persist for life (Bottazzo *et al.,* 1976). In a short communication, Bottazzo and Doniach (1976) suggest that where ICA positivity was temporary, it may be secondary to viral islet disease, while where it is permanent, it may be related to polyendocrine heredity and a genetic tendency to organ-specific autoimmunity not related to ordinary viruses.

Del Prete *et al.* (1976) confirm that ICA-positive patients with chemical diabetes may develop insulin dependency months after the first demonstration of ICA. They found ICA titers persistent in non-insulin-dependent MOD (8.3% of 373 patients) and in chemical diabetes (14.9% of 114 cases). These patients were said to have severely depressed insulin responses after oral or intravenous glucose. As will be discussed in Section 2.1.2, a low insulin response to glucose in a chemical or latent diabetic may be another prognostic indicator of the possible development of insulin-dependent diabetes in the future.

An intriguing finding, probably unrelated to the type of ICA just discussed, is the finding of separate autoantibodies to human pancreatic glucagon and somatostatin cells (Bottazzo and Lendrum, 1976). By double immunofluorescent technique, it was shown that 13 of 1279 serum samples contained antibodies reacting specifically with glucagon cells, while another 4 reacted with somatostatin cells. The antibodies were directed against intracellular components, not against the hormones themselves. Both types of antibodies occurred independently of ICA that have been described in diabetes mellitus. Baba *et al.* (1976) reported the presence of autoimmune glucagon antibodies in female diabetic patients who had been treated with tolbutamide but not with insulin. The significance of these findings is at present unknown.

2.1.1.3b. Relationship of HLA to ICA. There is still a difference of opinion whether there is an increased association between the increased prevalence of *HLA* antigens in JOD and that of ICA. The frequency of HLA-B8 was significantly increased in ICA-positive patients (61%) compared with ICA-negative patients (35%) and the control population (28%) (Morris *et al.,* 1976). This increased frequency of HLA-B8 was even more striking in diabetics in whom ICA persisted for more than 5 years (71%). The association with HLA-A1 and HLA-B8 appeared to be more strongly associated with the presence of ICA than with insulin dependence; the group of patients who were ICA-negative but insulin-dependent did not show a significant increase in the frequency of HLA-A1 and HLA-B8 (Morris *et al.,* 1976). Christy *et al.* (1976) also found ICA more frequently in HLA-B8 positive patients then in HLA-B8-negative patients. These findings appear to link the genetic marker for JOD and APCI.

On the other hand, Irvine *et al.* (1976a) found no correlation between the titer, change in titer, or duration of ICA and the presence of HLA-B8, -BW15, or -CW3. Likewise, in another study (Lendrum *et al.*, 1976b), no association between the presence of ICA and any particular *HLA* phenotype could be found.

2.1.1.3c. Cell-Mediated Immunity. Organ-specific cell-mediated autoimmunity has been detected in diabetes mellitus by two *in vitro* techniques (Irvine *et al.*, 1976b):

1. *Leukocyte migration-inhibition test:* Positive leukocyte migration-inhibition tests have been shown in JOD, using extracts of porcine, calf, and normal human pancreas (as well as insulinoma cells) as antigen. The same prevalence of positive migration-inhibition tests occurs irrespective of whether or not there are ICA in patients' serum and whether or not the patients have ever received insulin. The data presented indicate the presence in young diabetics of a state of cellular immunity to species-nonspecific antigens, pancreatic in origin but different from insulin.
2. *Lymphocyte transformation test:* Mitogen- or antigen-induced transformation of lymphocytes to blast cells is an alternative *in vitro* test of cellular immune function. Transformation studies using peripheral blood lymphocytes in control subjects and in diabetic patients showed that using either bovine insulin or porcine insulin as antigen, there was a significantly higher transformation index in newly diagnosed diabetics than in control subjects.

Using human insulinoma cells as model beta cells, Huang and McLaren (1976) developed an *in vitro* assay of lymphocyte-mediated cytotoxicity. Lymphocytes from 23 JOD patients demonstrated significant cytoadherence and cytotoxicity against human insulinoma cells *in vitro* as compared with lymphocytes from normal subjects. Of the 21 (*sic*) patients, 16 also had significant levels of circulating antibody against insulinoma cells. Serum antibodies failed to show any cytotoxicity with the cell suspension. Thus, cell-mediated immunity against cell-surface components of beta cells was postulated to play an important role in the pathogenesis of diabetes mellitus. This occurred before insulin therapy, which implies that sensitization to insulin is not a primary factor. The findings suggested to the authors that insulin-dependent diabetes may be a disease of autoaggression. They also postulated that infectious agents, particularly viruses, might trigger this process of autoimmune beta-cell destruction in a genetically predisposed individual.

The finding of a decreased percentage of peripheral thymus-dependent lymphocytes in JOD in comparison with MOD or normal subjects also suggested to Cattaneo *et al.* (1976) that an altered cell-mediated immunity existed in JOD. In another study, however, no significant differences in the precentages and the absolute numbers of total lymphocytes, thymus-dependent lymphocytes (T cells), or thymus-independent B lymphocytes (B cells) were found between children with JOD and the control children (Hann *et al.,* 1976). The T cells are primarily responsible for cell-mediated immunity and comprise a majority of the circulating lymphocytes. The B cells are thymus-independent and mainly responsible for humoral immunity. No significant quantitative differences in some populations of peripheral lymphocytes were found.

A new model of diabetes mellitus with a suggested pathogenesis of chemically initiated cell-mediated immune reaction was described by Like and Rossini (1976). Multiple small injections of streptozotocin in mice produced pancreatic insulitis characterized by mononuclear inflammatory cells (lymphocytes and macrophages) in and around the pancreatic islets. This was in contrast to the virtually inflammatory-free islet lesions observed after a single large injection. The time required for the first appearance of inflammatory cells was 5–6 days after the last injection, which is compatible with a cell-mediated immune reaction conceivably directed against beta cells modified by administration of streptozotocin. The reduction in beta-cell numbers and elevation of plasma glucose became progressively more pronounced during the 10–25 days after the last injection, long after streptozotocin is cleared from the bloodstream. The authors speculate that the mononuclear inflammatory cells are responsible for the progressive beta-cell destruction and the resulting increasingly severe hyperglycemia. Ultrastructural evidence of abundant type C virus within beta cells of treated mice suggested that streptozotocin may activate murine leukemia virus *in vivo* in susceptible hosts.*

2.1.1.4. Environmental Factors—Viruses and Other Infectious or Chemical Agents

The likely importance of environmental factors superimposed on genetic factors in the pathogenesis of diabetes mellitus was reviewed last year and again above. Evidence that viruses may play a pathogenetic role in some cases of JOD is still circumstantial (Craighead, 1976). Thus, findings of virus-induced diabetes in experimental animals serve as most useful models. Viral induction of diabetes employing EMC in mice was

*In contrast to the evidence of increased organ-specific cell-mediated autoimmunity presented in this section, the insulin-deficient diabetic state is associated with a general suppression of cell-mediated immune responses *in vivo* (Mahmoud *et al.,* 1976; Pallavicini and Nichols, 1976), a defect that is reversible with insulin treatment (Mahmoud *et al.,* 1976). It has also been suggested that there may be humoral immunodeficiency to bacterial antigens in patients with JOD (Ludwig *et al.,* 1976b).

reviewed in Section 2.1.1.2. In hamsters, a virus-induced pancreatic disease was induced by infection with Venezualan encephalitis virus (Rayfield *et al.,* 1976). Glucose intolerance occurred in hamsters in each of the infected groups associated with severely decreased insulin responses. Since pancreatic insulin content was within normal limits, a defect in insulin release was suggested. Spontaneous diabetes mellitus was also documented in a colony of guinea pigs (Lang and Munger, 1976). The contagious nature of the disease was verified, but the nature of the infectious agent is not known. The presence of significant islet pathology was reported. A new model of diabetes in which a chemical (repeated small doses of streptozotocin) was thought to have initiated a cell-mediated immune reaction by activating a murine virus was reviewed in Section 2.1.1.3c. These various findings lend additional support to the concept that infectious or other environmental agents could be operative in the etiology and pathogenesis of human diabetes mellitus.

2.1.2. Insulin Secretion

Although JOD is characterized by an absent insulin secretory response to glucose, insulin responses in the early stages of MOD are quite variable. Diminished initial rapid release of insulin has been reported, followed either by a subnormal later response or by a normal or even higher than normal insulin response. On the other hand, others have reported a normal or higher than normal initial response followed by a later supernormal insulin response. The finding of normal or even high insulin levels in mild diabetes has given rise to the conept of insulin resistance as the initial lesion in early MOD (see Section 2.1.3.1). That both types of insulin secretory responses are encountered indicates the existence of a heterogeneity of insulin responses to glucose in nonobese patients with latent diabetes and that the pathogenesis of glucose intolerance is heterogeneous.

2.1.2.1. Prognostic Significance of Heterogeneity of Insulin Responses to Glucose in Mild Diabetes

During a study of the natural history of latent or chemical diabetes in young people (for up to 22 years), it was found that at recognition of carbohydrate intolerance, patients with JOD and MODY may have identical abnormal GTTs. However, patients who were in the early stages of JOD usually progressed to insulin-requiring diabetes within 2 years of diagnosis, although longer intervals have been recorded (Fajans *et al.,* 1976). Among phenotypically latent diabetic patients, approximately 20% progressed to overt insulin-requiring diabetes. When the initial insulin responses to glucose determined at recognition of carbohydrate intolerance were examined, it was found that progression to diabetes that required insulin injections (some to ketosis-prone type) occurred only in those patients who initially had very low insulin responses to glucose or had insulin responses that were delayed and lower than the mean response of the control subjects. A low insulin response appears to be a more reliable prognostic indicator of decompensation to requirement of insulin at a later date than the degree of abnormality of carbohydrate intolerance. In preliminary studies, some of these patients had circulating ICA at recognition of mild carbohydrate intolerance. On the other hand, the *majority* of patients with low insulin responses to glucose have not progressed to insulin-requiring diabetes on long follow-up, and these patients were negative for ICA. They can be classified as MOD or MODY. In contrast, among a smaller group of patients with glucose intolerance who had supernormal insulin responses, not a single patient has progressed to insulin-requiring diabetes on long follow-up. This suggests that in these patients, hyperinsulinemia is secondary or compensatory to factors that cause glucose intolerance and that such a high insulin response to glucose appears to be a reliable prognostic indicator that the patient will not decompensate to diabetes requiring insulin at a later date. The heterogeneity of insulin responses in MOD and MODY patients demonstrates that plasma insulin levels during the GTT are not of diagnostic value although they may be of prognostic significance. The studies in the control subjects (Fajans *et al.,* 1976) demonstrate the great variability of insulin responses in the group of healthy subjects without a family history of diabetes mellitus (mean age 21.9 years; range 18–25 years). A similar wide range of insulin responses was seen in a group of healthy children ranging in age from 3 months to 15 years (Lestradet *et al.,* 1976), although insulin responses in children are lower than in adults, as previously reported.

2.1.2.2. Mechanism of Insulin Secretion Relevant to Clinical Diabetes Mellitus

It has been suggested that a defective acute insulin response in mild diabetes is due to a decreased sensitivity of the glucose receptors of the pancreatic beta cell to a rising plasma glucose level. Such a defect has been postulated to be genetically inherited. However, such findings are also compatible with the failure of adequate hormone output from stored insulin available for rapid release. The reproduction of similar insulin responses in mild alloxan-diabetic dogs has been interpreted to suggest that an early defect in insulin secretion is not necessarily on a genetic basis (Pupo *et al.,* 1976).

2.1.2.2a. Insulin Secretion in Experimental Alloxan Diabetes. The acute and late phases of insulin secretion were studied in mongrel dogs before and 7–10 days after the induction of mild alloxan diabetes (Pupo *et al.*, 1976). Mean fasting plasma glucose was 90 mg/dl before and 101 mg/dl after induction of alloxan diabetes. These differences were not significant. Fasting insulin levels were unchanged from pretreatment values. The alloxan-diabetic dogs had significantly decreased early-phase insulin responses to glucose pulses and slower plasma glucose disappearance rates. The authors concluded that the reduced early-phase insulin secretion is not dependent on genetic determinants even though it is similar to that reported in genetic human MOD. It is possible, however, that alloxan damages recognition sites on the beta-cell surface and thus simulates a genetic lesion in this area. In response to 4-hr glucose infusions, the alloxan-diabetic dogs had higher plasma glucose levels than normal dogs. Insulin levels were identical during the first 30 min of the infusion, but were then higher in the alloxan-diabetic dogs. The high glucose levels despite increased late-phase insulin secretion found in these dogs have also been observed in human genetic diabetes. The data in dogs do not provide a satisfactory explanation for the abnormally high insulin levels observed during the long-term glucose infusions, but the glucose intolerance is apparently associated with a diminished initial phase of insulin release.

2.1.2.2b. Basal Levels of Plasma Glucose and Acute Increases in Insulin Release to Glucose. Among a group of subjects with a wide range of fasting plasma glucose levels, the relationship was explored between fasting plasma glucose levels, glucose disappearance rates, and the acute insulin secretory response to a 20-g intravenous glucose stimulus (Brunzell *et al.*, 1976). The acute insulin response was present in subjects with fasting plasma glucose levels below 115 mg/dl, but was absent above this level. The glucose disappearance rate was related to the acute insulin response in subjects with fasting glucose below 115 mg/dl. All subjects with fasting glucose levels above 115 mg/dl had glucose disappearance rates below 1.06%/min. The authors state that these studies support epidemiological data indicating that a plasma glucose of 115 mg/dl is the upper limit of normal for fasting plasma glucose levels and that 1%/min is the lower limit of normal for the glucose disappearance rate. The studies give evidence for an important role for the acute insulin secretory response in the determination of glucose disappearance rates during intravenous GTTs (Brunzell *et al.*, 1976). Since the acute insulin secretory response to glucose is not only diminished but also disappears at a fasting plasma glucose level of 115 mg/dl, the basis of this definition of "upper limit of normal" coincides with a total absence of this essential physiological function. Although such patients have a marked attenuation of the early beta-cell response to intravenous glucose, they have a normal acute insulin response to arginine (Palmer *et al.,* 1976). This supports the previously reached conclusion that the mechanism by which arginine induces insulin release is different from that by which glucose induces this response (Fajans *et al.,* 1972).

2.1.2.2c. Adrenergic Activity. In nonketotic hyperglycemic diabetic patients, α-adrenergic blockade increased basal insulin levels to a greater extent than in normal subjects and also partially restored the acute insulin response to intravenous glucose stimulation in diabetics (Robertson *et al.,* 1976). The data also demonstrated that circulating catecholamine levels both in the basal state and immediately after glucose stimulation were greater in diabetics than in normal subjects, providing a likely hormonal mediator for the observed increases in endogenous α-adrenergic activity in these nonketotic diabetic patients. This is the first demonstration that circulating catecholamine levels in the basal state are elevated in nonketotic diabetics.

2.1.2.2d. Pharmacological Inhibition of Insulin Release and Stimulated Insulin Release. With severe reduction in beta-cell function or numbers, whether genetically determined or the result of a virus infection or autoimmunity, the resulting chronic overstimulation of the residual islet tissue may lead to impairment of the early insulin response either by interfering with normal beta-cell-membrane organization, islet energetics, or biosynthetic processes or by leading to depletion of preformed insulin stores. Interesting observations have been reported suggesting that reduction of elevated blood glucose or inhibition of basal insulin release may improve stimulated insulin secretion in diabetes.

Turner *et al.* (1976) gave infusions of insulin to patients with MOD and mild fasting hyperglycemia. This induced normal overnight fasting plasma glucose levels and lower-than-normal endogenous fasting plasma insulin levels. In response to intravenous glucose, these patients had a larger insulin reponse to glucose, including the first-phase insulin response, than before the insulin infusion. Thus, decreasing even slightly elevated plasma glucose levels improved the efficiency of insulin secretion in response to administered glucose. Applying these findings to therapy, a constant basal insulin supplement in patients with mild diabetes will reduce the basal plasma glucose concentration to normal and may allow a better stimulated beta-cell response. After acutely administered intravenous insulin, these authors' patients had normal decreases in plasma glucose following elevated or normal fasting plasma glucose levels. This finding does not support the suggestion of others (see Section 2.1.3.1) that insulin resistance is a universal feature of mild diabetes.

Greenwood *et al.* (1976) used another approach to improve the insulin response to secretory stimuli. They administered diazoxide to 4 normal subjects and 10 diabetic subjects for 5–7 days. Diazoxide selectively inhibits insulin release while allowing synthesis to continue in the fasting state, and thereby replenishes stored insulin. There was a reduction of basal insulin levels by diazoxide in the diabetic patients but not in the normal control subjects, which was interpreted as providing further evidence for chronic overstimulation of the beta cells in diabetes. In every case, there was substantial increase in the insulin response to combined stimulation of the pancreatic beta cells with 1 mg glucagon and 2 g tolbutamide given intravenously. It is likely that the observed improvement reflected increased insulin stores that resulted from diazoxide inhibition of insulin release. Thus, the poor insulin response to diabetes may be due at least in part to chronic overstimulation of the beta cells. The authors suggest the possibility of a treatment suppressing basal insulin release pharmacologically and administration of a potent sulfonylurea or other drug with meals to produce rapid insulin release. It should be noted that diazoxide exacerbated fasting hyperglycemia in the diabetic patients, and that this hyperglycemia may have potentiated glucagon- and tolbutamide-induced insulin release.

2.1.2.2e. Homeostasis of Basal Insulin Secretion in MOD. Although diabetic patients have an impaired insulin secretory response to a rise in plasma glucose, they have fasting basal plasma insulin concentrations similar to those of healthy subjects. Turner and Holman (1976) provided a hypothesis for an explanation of the normal basal plasma insulin concentration found in such diabetic patients despite impaired beta-cell function. The liver and beta cells are the major determinants in an integral feedback loop regulating both the plasma glucose and insulin concentrations. In diabetes, the insulin response to glucose is impaired, and the authors postulate that in the basal state, hepatic glucose efflux increases until the plasma glucose concentration is high enough to stimulate secretion of insulin so that basal portal vein insulin in concentration becomes normal. Insulin control of glucose efflux from the liver thus acts as an insulin sensor, and the basal plasm glucose would have the major role in regulating basal insulin secretion. Glucose regulation (hepatic glucose output) thus becomes of secondary importance to the maintenance of basal insulin secretion, which is teleologically needed for the anabolic requirements of cell growth (Turner and Holman, 1976). This maintenance of basal insulin secretion may account for the discrepancy between the marked hyperglycemia and the lack of ketosis and protein catabolism of MOD.

2.1.2.2f. Endogenous Gastric Inhibitory Polypeptide. In normal subjects, insulin secretion is greater in response to ingested glucose or intraduodenal perfusion of amino acids than after intravenously administered glucose or amino acids. The enhanced release of insulin evoked by the ingestion of these nutrients is generally attributed to one or more intestinal factors or hormones. It has been suggested that gastric inhibitory polypeptide (GIP) is the intestinal hormone that contributes primarily to insulin release after ingestion of food. GIP has been shown to have a potent insulinotropic effect both *in vivo* and *in vitro*. Increased GIP responses to a mixed meal have been observed in patients with MOD. They were also seen in patients with chronic pancreatitis, and were most marked in a group of patients with moderately impaired insulin release (Ebert *et al.*, 1976). In obese MODs with fasting hyperglycemia and a definite delay in glucose-stimulated insulin release, both fasting and glucose-stimulated GIP concentrations were higher than those found in normal subjects (Crockett *et al.*, 1976a). The findings of both groups of investigators suggest that insulin exerts a feedback control on the secretion of GIP and that the higher GIP levels in the two groups of patients may be due to the lack of feedback inhibition by insulin. In another study, Crockett *et al.* (1976b) made observations that were compatible with the interpretation that insulin exerts a feedback inhibition on GIP release in normal subjects. High GIP levels in diabetes may explain the exaggerated rise in plasma insulin in mild MODs after a second oral glucose load (Vinik *et al.*, 1976), confirming the earlier suggestion of Vinik and coworkers that there is overactivity of the enteroinsular axis in mild MOD.

2.1.2.3. Measurement of Beta-Cell Secretory Products—Connecting Peptide

The transformation of proinsulin to insulin and connecting peptide (C-peptide) begins in the Golgi apparatus and continues in the secretion granules of the pancreatic beta cells. An excellent brief review of circulating serum C-peptide (Horwitz *et al.*, 1976) reviews both the clinical indications for measuring circulating C-peptide and the interpretation of its serum concentrations. Also as reviewed last year, the availability of a radioimmunoassay for measuring serum C-peptide has greatly facilitated investigations concerning the differential diagnosis of insulinoma from factitious hypoglycemia and has been most useful in investigations concerning the natural history of beta-cell function in insulin-requiring diabetes, particularly in patients in whom the presence of circulating insulin antibodies interferes with insulin measurements. High insulin levels associated with low C-peptide levels suggests factitious or exogenous hyperinsulinism. Endogenous hyperinsulinism, on the other hand, is characterized by elevations of both insulin and C-peptide. In patients with insulinomas, the suppressibility of beta-cell secretion during insulin-induced hypoglycemia can be monitored by observation of serum C-peptide concentration. When compared with normal subjects, most patients with islet-cell tumors showed diminished or absent C-peptide suppression (Horwitz *et al.,* 1976).

As reviewed by Horwitz *et al.,* (1976), diabetic patients with stable or easily managed diabetes usually have retained beta-cell function as indicated by appreciable serum C-peptide levels. Other papers have appeared that confirm that measurement of C-peptide immunoreactivity (CPR) in blood and urine may be a useful measure of endocrine pancreatic function. T. Kuzuya *et al.* (1976) evaluated the use of this radioimmunoassay method employing synthetic human C-peptide and with the use of a Japanese C-peptide radioimmunoassay kit. The absence of any CPR in serum and urine of totally depancreatized patients suggested that this assay system really deals with endocrine pancreatic function. The authors confirmed that CPR responses to glucose were subnormal in diabetics, very low in JODs, and often poor in patients with insulin treatment. Fasting CPR levels were elevated in patients on corticosteroid treatment and with uremia. Urinary CPR was also very low in JOD patients.

Another study confirms that mild diabetics differ from juvenile diabetics in having significant residual pancreatic beta-cell function as measured by CPR (Lewis *et al.,* 1976). It has been assumed by some that insulin-requiring JODs have no residual insulin production shortly after the beginning of treatment. Ludvigsson and Heding (1976) report, however, that 35% of 96 patients with early-onset JOD of over 2 years' duration, i.e., beyond termination of any remission periods, showed measurable amounts of C-peptide in their serum, suggesting that there was some residual beta-cell function. As expected, patients with a remission had higher levels of C-peptide than those without. The longer the duration of diabetes, the lower were C-peptide levels.

Despite the higher molar concentration of CPR than insulin, the similarity of blood insulin and CPR response patterns in normal and diabetic subjects seems to indicate that assay of CPR in blood can be substituted for or used in addition to insulin assay. In the presence of insulin antibodies, some precipitation must be instituted to eliminate contributions from the cross-reacting endogenous antibody-bound proinsulin (Kuzuya, H., *et al.,* 1977).

2.1.3. Insulin Resistance

2.1.3.1. Evidence for Insulin Resistance

Some patients with chemical diabetes have greater absolute levels of circulating insulin during the GTT (the percentage depending on the series reported) than do healthy control subjects. This indicates that an insulin-resistant state must exist in these patients. Reaven and co-workers have published further papers in support of their thesis that nonketotic diabetes mellitus is associated with insulin resistance. Reaven *et al.* (1976) estimated both the insulin response to oral glucose and the glucose-lowering effect of exogenous insulin in 95 patients who were classified in five groups on the basis of their oral glucose tolerance: (1) those with normal GTTs; (2) those with borderline tolerance; (3) those with chemical diabetes (fasting plasma glucose <110 mg/dl, 1-hr >185 mg/dl, 2-hr >140 mg/dl; (4) those with fasting hyperglycemia (fasting plasma glucose 110–150 mg/dl; and (5) those with fasting hyperglycemia greater than 150 mg/dl. All four experimental groups, whose mean ages ranged from 47 to 53 years of age, had significantly higher plasma glucose levels than the control group. The group with borderline diabetes (group 2) had plasma insulin responses during the GTT similar to those of the controls. The patients with chemical diabetes (group 3) had insulin levels that were never lower than normal and were significantly elevated at ½, 1, and 2 hr after oral glucose. The mean insulin response of the group with fasting hyperglycemia (110–150 mg/dl) (group 4) was decreased at ½ hr and greater than normal at 2 hr. The patients with fasting hyperglycemia greater than 150 mg/dl (group 5) had significantly lower insulin levels at every time point. The authors concluded that the patients with borderline glucose intolerance and those with chemical diabetes must have insulin resistance and that abnormal carbohydrate tolerance in these subjects cannot be attributed to a deficiency of insulin. Since patients with fasting hyperglycemia do have an attenuated insulin response, insulin insufficiency must play a role in their carbohydrate intolerance. Subjects then received a constant infusion of insulin in combination with epinephrine, propranolol, and glucose. As reviewed last year, this study protocol is based on the assumption that endogenous insulin secretion is suppressed by epinephrine and propranolol (by α-adrenergic stimulation) and that hepatic glucose output is suppressed by the infusion of glucose and insulin. The rationale of this method is to measure the ability of similar plasma levels of insulin "steady-state plasma insulin" (SSPI)—to induce glucose uptake. All four patient groups with abnormal carbohydrate metabolism were more resistant than normal subjects to the action of insulin and had progressively higher steady-state plasma glucose (SSPG) levels. When a comparison was made of the calculated efficiency of "glucose uptake" (E_g) in the five patient groups, there was an increase in E_g only in the normal group and equal changes in the four abnormal groups, suggesting similar degrees of peripheral insulin resistance by this technique despite greatly different impairment of carbohydrate tolerance. Although the authors give alternative explanations, one of their main conclusions is that in nonketotic diabetes mellitus, insulin resistance is the primary lesion, that insulin deficiency results in some patients only as a secondary phenomenon to pancreatic exhaustion, and that patients with diabetes comprise a continuous spectrum of degrees of insulin resistance. That insulin infusion did not cause differing changes in glucose uptake in the groups of patients studied does not appear to support a difference in the degree of insulin resistance (see below). There can be no doubt that in these patients with borderline diabetes and chemical diabetes, insulin resistance must be responsible for carbohydrate intolerance. However, the authors' generalization or hypothesis that nonketotic diabetes mellitus is primarily a disease of insulin resistance is difficult to reconcile with several observations. First, several groups have reported patients with chemical diabetes and low insulin levels (see Section 2.1.2.1). Reaven (1976) confirmed this finding. Examination of the standard deviations calculated from plasma insulin levels during GTTs published in this group's previous papers also substantiates this. The authors do suggest that insulin deficiency may be the primary lesion in patients with severe fasting hyperglycemia and that insulin resistance can develop in these patients as a secondary phenonemon. Also, the authors' conclusions are based on cross-sectional studies, not on prospective studies. They concur that nonketotic diabetes need not comprise a homogenous entity but may be made up of distinct disease processes with a heterogeneity of insulin responses. On the basis of the results described above, this reviewer would agree that insulin resistance may be the primary lesion in some patients with mild nonketotic diabetes, but would add that insulin deficiency is a primary lesion not only in patients with fasting hyperglycemia, but also in some patients with chemical diabetes.

Reaven's group reported in another paper (Kimmerling *et al.*, 1976) their attempt to locate the site of insulin resistance in patients with nonketotic diabetes mellitus. They conclude that significant differences exist in the sensitivity of various tissues to the action of insulin. Insulin resistance and the ability of insulin to inhibit hepatic glucose production and to increase efficiency of glucose uptake were determined in 8 patients with normal oral glucose tolerance, 8 patients with chemical diabetes, and 8 nonketotic patients with fasting hyperglycemia ($>$150 mg/dl). Insulin resistance was estimated again by measuring the SSPG response to a continuous infusion of insulin, glucose, epinephrine, and propranolol. The study showed that SSPG was 113 mg/dl in normal subjects, 205 mg/dl in chemical diabetics, and 346 mg/dl in patients with fasting hyperglycemia. The authors concluded that insulin resistance exists in nonketotic diabetes, and the greater the degree of glucose intolerance, the greater the insulin resistance. In normal subjects, there was an 80% decrease in hepatic glucose production (HGP); in chemical diabetes, a 55% decrease in HGP; while in patients with fasting hyperglycemia, basal HGP did not fall during the infusion. Thus, the conclusion was reached that insulin had no suppressive effect in these patients. However, they infused only the pharmacological mixture used in these experiments and did not administer insulin alone. In nonketotic diabetic patients, Turner *et al.* (1976) found no evidence of insulin resistance, and as reviewed by them, other investigators were also able to suppress HGP in similar nonketotic diabetic patients with fasting hyperglycemia by the administration of insulin or glucose. Other authors, however, have also found that the ability of insulin to suppress hepatic glucose production seems to decrease with the severity of diabetes. Kimmerling *et al.* (1976) found that in patients with both chemical diabetes and fasting hyperglycemia, the basic infusion mixture containing insulin did not increase the efficiency of glucose uptake. They conclude that resistance to insulin-mediated glucose uptake seems to be the most basic lesion in patients with nonketotic diabetes, while resistance to insulin-mediated hepatic glucose production seems to occur only as the severity of diabetes increases. The possibility that healthy and diabetic patients have different counterregulatory responses to the pharmacological mixture administered rather than different degrees of resistance to insulin in the basal state was commented on last year.

2.1.3.2. Mechanism of Insulin Resistance: Decreased Insulin Binding to Insulin Receptors

Accepting that insulin resistance must play an important role in some patients with nonketotic diabetes mellitus, it becomes important to examine the mechanism for insulin resistance. The primary event in hormone action resides at the initial interaction with receptors at the plasma membrane. A series of other metabolic steps are interposed between the combination between hormones and receptor and the expression of final hormone action. Any of these steps could be rate-limiting.

Identification of insulin receptors has provided a major new tool for study of insulin action and of basic causes of diabetes (Maugh, 1976a). Binding of insulin to many types of cells is much lower than normal in both diabetic and insulin-resistant obese individuals. Insulin binding can be returned toward normal by regulation of the diet and by certain drugs.

2.1.3.2a. Insulin Receptors in Diabetes. Olefsky and Reaven (1976a) demonstrated again that the amount of insulin bound to monocytes and mononuclear leukocytes from diabetic patients was significantly less than that bound to similar cells from normal subjects. In a review article on the insulin receptor, Olefsky (1976) reported that mononuclear cells isolated from diabetic subjects with fasting hyperglycemia bound approximately 50% less insulin than cells from normal subjects, and that this decrease could be entirely accounted for by a decrease in the number of insulin receptors. The decreased binding may be related to insulin resistance in patients with chemical diabetes, but as the diabetic syndrome becomes more severe, additional factors causing insulin resistance may appear.

Olefsky and Reaven (1976b) also showed that when nonketotic diabetics with fasting hyperglycemia were treated for 1–3 months with the sulfonylurea chlorpropamide, hyperglycemia decreased and insulin receptors increased. Furthermore, patients whose hyperglycemia did not change showed no change in insulin binding. So far, it has not been demonstrated whether the increase in insulin binding is specifically related to sulfonylurea therapy or whether any treatment that improves the diabetic state will be associated with an increase in insulin receptors. Conceivably, glucose *per se* or other fuels might change configurational or replicative characteristics of the insulin receptors.

2.1.3.2b. Unusual Insulin-Receptor Disorders in Man. Kahn *et al.* (1976) described 6 female patients with acanthosis nigricans, varying degrees of glucose intolerance (normal glucose tolerance to symptomatic fasting hyperglycemia), hyperinsulinemia (80–300 μU/ml), and marked but variable resistance to exogenous insulin. Insulin resistance in these patients was due to marked decrease in insulin binding to its membrane receptors as demonstrated on circulating monocytes. When these patients were fasted, there was a fall in plasma insulin, but no increase in insulin binding as is observed in obesity under similar circumstances. This suggests that the receptor defect was not secondary to hyperinsulinemia. The clinical features shared by these 6 patients, and by others previously reported, may be divided into two unique clinical syndromes: Type A is a syndrome in younger or adolescent females with signs of virilization, accelerated growth, hirsutism, polycystic ovaries, clitoral enlargement, and coarse features, in whom the receptor defect may be primary, due to a decreased number of insulin receptors. Type B syndrome affects older females with signs of an immunological disorder with increased γ-globulin, proteinuria, leukopenia, alopecia, arthralgia, enlarged salivary glands, and positive antinuclear and anti-DNA antibodies. In all these patients, there was a marked decrease in insulin binding to its receptors. In Type A patients, this reduction appeared to be due to a change in number of receptors; in Type B patients, to decreased affinity of the receptor for insulin. In this condition, insulin resistance is due to circulating antibodies to the insulin receptor, as described in last year's review. A male patient with Type B syndrome was described by Pulini *et al.* (1976).

The circulating antibody or inhibitor of insulin receptors found in Type B patients was characterized by Flier *et al.* (1976). The inhibitor is an immunoglobulin by multiple criteria. Although predominantly IgG, some activity is found in the IgM fraction. The inhibitor immunoglobulins are polyclonal. Evidence suggests that these antibodies are directed at determinants on or near the insulin receptor and are responsible for the observed clinical insulin resistance.

2.2. Relationship of Fuels to Hormonal Release and Fuel Economy

This subject, which is important to the understanding of diabetes mellitus, is reviewed in Chapter 4.

2.3. Glucagon Secretion—Somatostatin

Glucagon secretion in diabetes mellitus and the effect of somatostatin on hormonal release are discussed in Chapter 3.

2.4. Epidemiological Findings

Epidemiological methods, particularly when applied longitudinally to natural populations, may lead to better understanding of the natural history, etiology, and pathogenesis of diabetes and its complications. Bennett *et al.* (1976) summarized the last 10 years of studies in the Pima Indians, who have the highest recorded prevalence of diabetes in the world. With a 2-hr post-glucose plasma level (PGPGL) over 160 mg/dl after a 75-g carbohydrate load as the criterion, 50% of the population over 35 years of age had diabetes. The prevalence of diabetes rose sharply to the age range of 45–55, but in subsequent decades, any increases were inconsistent or small. There was a sex difference in that the highest prevalence rate in males was 47%, while in females it was 69%. In contradistinction to other populations who have shown a unimodal distribution of 2hr PGPGL, Pima Indians in all decades aged 25 years or over showed an overlapping bimodal distribution of blood glucose levels. The presence of two components in the distribution indicated to the authors that there is a biological heterogeneity of glucose tolerance with two subgroups in that population. Cutoff points between the two subgroups in 2-hr PGPGL ranged from 204 to 227 mg/dl in males and from 225 to 245 mg/dl in females. These cutoff levels are 60 mg/dl or more higher than those frequently considered criteria for the diagnosis of diabetes. The authors believe that these cutoff points differentiate between "nondiabetes" and "diabetes" because of the finding of bimodality. They support their argument by noting that the frequency of diabetic retinopathy was low among subjects within the first component of the glucose distribution curve and high, reaching a plateau between 18 and 23%, in the patients at the beginning of the second component of the glucose distribution. The authors suggest that subjects falling into the hyperglycemic component represent the true diabetic segment of the population. Although retinal lesions were found 9 times less frequently in subjects with 2-hr PGPGL less than 200 mg/dl in comparison with those with levels greater than 200 mg/dl, the prevalence and gradual increase in prevalence of retinopathy at the lower levels (90–200 mg/dl) indicate that no sharp distinction can be made between diabetes and nondiabetes at the intersection of the two modes at approximately 200 mg/dl. Also, the frequency of retinopathy was related to duration of known diabetes, some 50% of those with diabetes of 10 years' or more duration having retinopathy. Proteinuria was also found in a much higher proportion of subjects in the hyperglycemic than in the lower component, and the frequency of renal disease was also related to the duration of known carbohydrate intolerance. As in diabetic Caucasians, there was an increased prevalence of perinatal mortality, high infant death rate, and high frequency of congenital anomolies in the diabetic pregnant Pimas (2-hr PGPGL >160 mg/dl). Up to the age of 35 years, the proportion of diabetes among the more obese was 2–3 times greater than those who were nonobese. This was not true of those over 35 years of age. The different patterns of association with age suggested to the authors that the degree of obesity perhaps influences the time at which diabetes appears rather than whether or not diabetes eventually develops.

Most American Indian tribes, such as the Pima and Papago, have diabetes rates 10–15 times the presumed frequency among whites, and health records have indicated that Indian diabetics have significantly greater frequencies of a large variety of illnesses (which extend well beyond the usual recognized complications) (Sievers, 1976). Standards have been developed for diabetes detection and treatment so that diabetes diagnosis is limited to persons with high probabilities of having the disease or to high-risk groups. In nonpregnant individuals, the criterion selected for making a diagnosis of diabetes on a modified GTT is a 2-hr PGPGL of greater than 200 mg/dl. The rationale for selecting this level includes the bimodal distribution mentioned above and an abrupt increase of specific diabetic complications (retinopathy, nephropathy) on follow-up evaluation of Pimas whose 2-hr PGPGLs were greater than 200 mg/dl (Sievers, 1976). On the other hand, in pregnant women during the first or second trimester, a 2-hr PGPGL of greater than 140 mg/dl was considered diagnostic for diabetes and had prognostic implications for the complications of diabetic pregnancies. In other words, for the pregnant patient, the Indian Health Service physicians do not accept the dividing line of 200 mg/dl derived from the bimodal distribution and the increased prevalence of specific diabetic complications as being the best criteria for separating nondiabetes from diabetes. Since pregnancy has a tendency to elevate 2-hr PGPGL in nondiabetic and diabetic patients, it is likely that a level of 140 mg/dl would also separate normal from abnormal in the nonpregnant individual.

Jarrett and Keen (1976) believe that the risk of specific diabetic complications becomes important only in people whth capillary whole blood sugar concentrations exceeding 200 mg/dl 2-hr after a 50-g oral glucose load ("clearly diabetes"). In the Bedford Study, the prevalence of retinopathy had increased greatly among the diabetics and in several had become florid with visual impairment, while by contrast, the "borderline diabetics" (2-hr PGPGL of 120–199 mg/dl) had only minor background retinopathy. Five years after the initial blood sugar measurements, they found a 3.3% frequency of diabetic retinopathy in subjects with 2-hr capillary blood sugar concentrations about 120 mg/dl, 11.8% in those with blood sugars over 200 mg/dl, 22.7% in those with blood sugars over 240 mg/dl, 26.3% in those with blood sugars over 285 mg/dl, and 33.3% in those with blood sugars over 330 mg/dl. Thus, as in the studies in the Pima Indians, the frequency of diabetic retinopathy was small in those with blood sugars below 200 mg/dl. On the other hand, in contrast to the Pima Indians, there was a continuing increase in prevalence of diabetic retinopathy with increasing blood sugar levels. Although diabetic retinopathy does not seem to be appreciable in frequency of severity in the "borderline diabetics," a 3.3% prevalence is greater than in a general population and suggests that these patients or some of them are indeed diabetic patients. Jarrett and Keen also state that as demonstrated from several epidemiological studies, borderline diabetes may be significant. In several studies, the prevalence of coronary heart disease was related to glucose intolerance rather than clinical diabetes.*

A 10-year follow-up report of the Birmingham Diabetes Survey of 1961 has been concluded (Birmingham Diabetes Survey Working Party, 1976). This study was concerned with the progress of minor abnormalities shown by the 50-g oral GTT. Obvious or florid diabetes was defined by a fasting blood sugar glucose level exceeding 130 mg/dl whether symptoms were present or not. GTT or chemical diabetes was defined as a peak blood glucose level of 180 mg/dl and a 2-hr level of 135 mg/dl using capillary blood. Minor and miscellaneous abnormalities, which deviated from normal glucose tolerance, were also noted. Patients who were classi-

*This does not apply to Pima Indians, since the prevalence of coronary heart disease is not increased significantly even in overt diabetes (see Section 2.6.2.1.).

fied originally as having GTT diabetes or other minor abnormalities were not treated over the period of 10 years. Of those with GTT diabetes, 45% had developed florid diabetes by the end of 10 years, while the others were unchanged or in nondiabetic categories. All of those who developed florid diabetes during the 10-year period showed minor abnormalities in the initial test, suggesting that most adults who present with MOD have had the disease in a form detectable by GTT for several years. This is compatible with the comparatively high prevalence of visible diabetic retinopathy at the time diabetes is diagnosed in middle-aged or elderly patients.

A mass screening program for diabetes mellitus was conducted by the Diabetes Association of Greater Cleveland with a 75-g oral load of carbohydrate (Genuth *et al.,* 1976). A 2-hr capillary blood glucose level of greater than 139 mg/dl was defined as positive. Of approximately 300,000 people screened, 4.1% had a positive test by these criteria (omitting 1968, when a state hospital for the mentally ill was included in the screened population, and the overall positivity rate fell to 3.6%). Of those retested, 65% were again positive by the same criterion. Of all the positives, 60% had blood glucose values between 140 and 179 mg/dl. Reproducibility clearly increased if the positive screening blood glucose level was greater than 200 mg/dl. Even with an initial screening blood glucose greater than 300 mg/dl, a small percentage of subjects failed to retest positive, confirming the fluctuating nature of early carbohydrate intolerance in diabetes (Genuth *et al.,* 1976). This detection experience is unique in scope and instructive in its implications. It suggests that screening by the 2-hr criterion of 140 mg/dl does not lead to a ridiculously large percentage of the population being labeled diabetic. If the overall positive rate of 4.1% is corrected for those who failed to retest positive, only 2.6% of Cleveland's screenees had firmly abnormal tests. These figures are very close to even the most conservative perception of the expected prevalence of diabetes. Furthermore, a screening glucose determination is not a formal GTT and would not be expected to give as high a reproducibility. The authors advise that selection of a positive cutoff point may depend on prevailing circumstances. If no ready means of reliable confirmation is available, then a higher cutoff point is probably reasonable for screening. Many normal subjects thereby escape the anxiety of being falsely labeled a diabetic suspect, and little immediate harm is likely to result to undetected diabetics who would have screened between 140 and 180 mg/dl. On the other hand, when rapid and more definite retesting can be provided either by a screening agency or by official referral to a physician, the cutoff point of 140 mg/dl may be more reasonable. Evidence is presented that florid diabetes will develop in some subjects with only borderline glucose abnormalities and that these abnormalities may be associated with a greater prevalence of cardiovascular abnormalities. This provokes some sense of responsibility for at least bringing persons with borderline glucose levels to medical recognizance. The authors give further recommendations for follow-up.

In an epidemiological study, with a test population of 10,559 subjects between the ages of 30 and 64 years, Mayer *et al.* (1976) evaluated the effects of time of day and time since last meal on blood sugar response to a standard oral glucose challenge. A significantly greater proportion of "abnormal" blood sugar elevations occurred during screening in the afternoon than in the morning. The proportion of "abnormal" responses at either time of day is lowest when the oral glucose is given shortly after a meal and highest when the challenge occurs 5–10 hr following prior alimentation. Thus, glucose tolerance is not fully restored until more than 7 hr have lapsed after the last meal. By its very nature, mass screening is usually incompatible with standardization of time of day or time since last meal. The effects of each parameter were exerted independently. The authors give a physiological explanation for these findings.

The prevalence of increased blood glucose levels clearly increases with advancing age, leading to the suggestion that criteria for the diagnosis of diabetes should be age-adjusted. Various suggestions for the degree of adjustment for age have been made, but they have been largely arbitrary. Adequate data are still not available to evaluate adjustment criteria. It is not known whether increasing blood glucose levels with age are due to (1) physiological deterioration of glucose tolerance, (2) increasing emergence of latent diabetes with advancing age, or (3) a combination of both factors.

In a group of lean subjects with no family history of diabetes mellitus and with normal glucose values during an oral GTT, significantly greater glucose levels were found in older subjects than in younger subjects (Duckworth and Kitabchi, 1976). Thus, even in subjects selected to have normal glucose tolerance, the process of aging decreased the ability to handle the oral glucose load. When the glucose responses were examined, however, in subjects of successive decades starting at 15 years of age, there was no increment in the 30-, 60-, 90-, or 120-min levels of the GTT or in the integrated areas under the curves for glucose, below 45 years of age. These findings suggest that age adjustment is not necessary in individuals under 45 or 50 years of age. Another group (Feldman and Plonk, 1976) detected no significant deterioration in the intravenous glucose tolerance of healthy volunteers between the ages of 22 and 67.

Another picture emerges when general populations including diabetics are screened. When the percentage distribution of those screened positive in Cleveland (Genuth *et al.,* 1976) was examined by age groups, there was a steady increase in prevalence from below 20 years to the range of 45–49 years of age, but thereafter, further increases were small and not consistent. In the Pima Indian, there was a similar increase in prevalence of diabetes with increasing age (Bennett *et al.,* 1976).

2.5. Control of Diabetes

Considerable controversy has marked the question whether blood glucose control is related to the development of long-term diabetic complications. This dilemma cannot be resolved at present due to, first, the impossibility of achieving physiological control of blood glucose with current therapeutic measures (Fajans and Freinkel, 1976) and, second, the inability to assess accurately the degree of hyperglycemia on a long-term basis. The hypothesis relating long-term optimal control of blood glucose to the prevention of diabetic complications has never been adequately tested, although a strong circumstantial case based on various studies in patients and experimental animals can be made (Gabbay, 1976). Third, since asymptomatic hyperglycemia (including fasting hyperglycemia) may exist for years or decades prior to the time of diagnosis of diabetes (Fajans *et al.,* 1976), any statement relating thickness of capillary basement membrane or microangiopathy to the "onset of diabetes" is inaccurate and does not take into account the natural history of hyperglycemia and diabetes.

2.5.1. General Considerations

In reviewing some data that are pertinent to the relationship of "control" to diabetic microvascular complications, Cahill *et al.* (1976) conclude:

> These data therefore place the burden of proof upon those who maintain that diabetes control is without effect. The goals of appropriate therapy should thus include a serious effort to achieve levels of blood glucose as close to those in the nondiabetic state as feasible. Obviously, patient needs and resources must also be carefully assessed, and the goals individualized accordingly. This concept is particularly applicable to the diabetic patient at greatest risk of the microvascular complication—the young and the middle-aged. It is well appreciated, however, that in some patients with juvenile-onset disease, it is most difficult, even with multiple insulin injections, to achieve real control of their hyperglycemia. Also, in certain elderly patients, their shorter life expectancy may preclude the need for achieving lower glucose levels, provided they are asymptomatic. . . . It can be concluded that the current means of therapy are only partly effective at best, and, therefore, a high priority must be assigned to the development of more physiologic insulin delivery

> systems or to approaches to the correction of the deficient insulin-producing mechanism itself. Finally, good diabetic management necessitates education and training of both patients and health professionals in the techniques involved, and close coordination and cooperation in patient management. Most important is a commitment to the view that better "control," when achievable, is beneficial.

Further examples linking control with complications are given below.

By a continuous blood-sampling procedure, previous results obtained by intermittent 24-hr sampling substantiated that good control of diabetes can lower elevated growth hormone (hGH) levels (Vigneria *et al.*, 1976). The hGH values in poorly controlled diabetes were higher and more fluctuating than in control subjects of corresponding age. After good control was reached, a significant decrease in hGH levels was observed. Such levels were normalized in middle-aged diabetics, but not in juvenile-onset-type diabetics. The authors conclude that hGH abnormalities in diabetes are a consequence of the metabolic abnormality.

At present, it can be recommended to the physician that he try to achieve the best control of blood glucose level possible in any diabetic patient in the absence of severe hypoglycemic reactions or disruption of the patient's psychosocial adjustment.

2.5.2. Glycosylated Hemoglobin and Diabetic Control

Recent work suggests that by measurement of concentration of hemoglobin $A_{1C'}$ long-term blood glucose regulation can be assessed objectively in the diabetic patient. Hemoglobin A_{1C} is one of three negatively charged minor hemoglobin components (HbA_{1A+B+C}) that are eluted on cation-exchange resin chromatography before the main hemoglobin A peak. Hemoglobin A_{1C}', the most abundant minor hemoglobin component in human erythrocytes, is increased in diabetes and is formed by having a hexose group attached as a ketamine to the N-terminal valines of the normal β chains of hemoglobin A (Bunn *et al.*, 1976). Glucose-6-phosphate hemoglobin may be an intermediate in the conversion of hemoglobin A to hemoglobin A_{1C} (Haney and Bunn, 1976). Because glycosylation of hemoglobin A_{1C} is a slow posttranslational event (Bunn *et al.*, 1976; Gabbay *et al.*, 1976) and a nearly irreversible process occurring continuously during the 120-day survival of the red cell, it is likely to be a nonenzymatic reaction (Haney and Bunn, 1976; Bunn *et al.*, 1976). The presence of hemoglobin and glucose in high concentrations and the relative irreversibility of the linkage results in the continuous formation and accumulation of these glycosylated hemoglobins. The rate of formation of hemoglobin A_{1C} should be directly proportional to the time-average concentration of glucose within the erythrocyte (Bunn *et al.*, 1976).

Koenig *et al.* (1976a) demonstrated that when diabetic patients are hospitalized and the blood glucose is optimally and carefully regulated, the hemoglobin A_{1C} levels are reduced toward normal with a lag time of 5–6 weeks. In 5 patients, mean fasting blood glucose levels of 343 mg/dl and hemoglobin A_{1C} concentration of 9.8% before treatment became 84 mg/dl and 5.8% after optimal diabetic control. The periodic monitoring of hemoglobin A_{1C} levels may provide a useful way of documenting the degree of control of glucose metabolism in diabetic patients over previous weeks and months, and provides a means for assessing the relation of carbohydrate control to the development of sequellae. Improvement in diabetes control results in proportionate decrease in hemoglobin A_{1C} concentration.

In another study by Koenig *et al.* (1976b), a highly significant correlation between hemoglobin A_{1C} concentration and response to an oral GTT was found in diabetic patients, independent of fasting blood sugar levels. Although a significant correlation was found between hemoglobin A_{1C} and fasting blood sugar concentrations, this probably reflects the interdependence of fasting blood sugar and glucose tolerance. Hemoglobin A_{1C} levels probably reflect best the mean daily blood sugar concentration and the degree of carbohydrate imbalance. There was a lack of correlation of hemoglobin A_{1C} levels with muscle capillary basement membrane thickness.

Paulsen and Koury (1976) show elevated levels of hemoglobin A_{1C} in insulin-dependent and -independent diabetics and patients with cystic fibrosis, who have marked suppression of insulin secretion. A group of 13 children with moderate impairment in glucose tolerance (fasting plasma glucose 97 ± 14 mg/dl; maximum level, 206 ± 40 mg/dl; 2-hr level, 155 ± 20 mg/dl) had significantly elevated hemoglobin A_{1C} levels. Seven hyperglycemic children, ages 9–14, were given an oral sulfonylurea for a 2-year period. At the end of this time, the glucose tolerance and hemoglobin A_{1C} levels were normal. Therapy was discontinued over the next 2 years; glucose intolerance reappeared, and hemoglobin A_{1C} returned to previously elevated levels.

Hemoglobin A_{1C} has a decreased reactivity to 2,3-diphosphoglycerate, and therefore an increased affinity for oxygen. Since an increase in hemoglobin A_{1C} may result in decreased oxygenation of tissues, the effects of pregnancy on hemoglobin A_{1C} in nondiabetic, gestational diabetic, and diabetic women were ascertained (Schwartz *et al.*, 1976). Hemoglobin A_{1C} was found to be slightly elevated in pregnant normal (6.97%), pregnant nondiabetic obese (6.89%), and gestational diabetic subjects (8.77%) above the level in normal females (5.68%). A remarkable difference was observed between the nonpregnant diabetics (12.77%) and the pregnant diabetics (8.46%). This decrease in the level of hemoglobin A_{1C} in pregnant diabetics as compared with nonpregnant diabetics may reflect either a better state of diabetic control—although no quantitative data were obtained in this regard in the subjects—or compensatory mechanisms to protect the fetus by facilitating oxygen exchange from mother to fetus, or both.

Koenig *et al.* (1976c) found that hemoglobin A_{1C} was elevated approximately 2-fold in genetically diabetic mice or in alloxan- and streptozotocin-diabetic mice.

In addition to diabetes, cell age is a significant determinant of the amount of hemoglobin A_{1A+B} and HbA_{1C} in erythrocytes (Fitzgibbons *et al.,* 1976). Both normal and diabetic erythrocytes contain increased amounts of these minor hemoglobin components in old as compared with young cells. In diabetes, the increase is significantly greater than in normal and appears to be related to the degree of hyperglycemia.

2.6. Long-Term Complications

2.6.1. Diabetic Microangiopathy

At a conference on diabetic microangiopathy (McMillan and Ditzel, 1976), data and a series of hypotheses about the pathogenesis and treatment of diabetic microangiopathy were presented. Some of the data were reviewed in last year's chapter on diabetes mellitus, and others will be referred to below. Those interested in the subject will find the proceedings interesting and provocative. In addition, other pertinent articles will be reviewed.

2.6.1.1. Changes in Plasma Proteins

McMillan (1976) suggests that changes in plasma proteins in diabetics and their effects on blood flow play a role in accelerating the rate of progression of diabetic microangiopathy by raising plasma viscosity and by increasing aggregation of erythrocytes. In addition to an increase in α_2-globulin and fibrinogen and a decrease in serum albumin, the levels of the majority of serum proteins are altered in diabetes. Although these changes are not specific to diabetes, their interaction with other defects in the diabetic state may promote the development of diabetic microangiopathy.

Almér and Pandolfi (1976) also reported that increased levels of fibrinogen and α_2-macroglobulin, a protein that acts as an inhibitor of fibrinolysis, are found in diabetic patients with retinopathy. The spontaneous fibrinolytic activity of the blood is abnormally low more often in persons with diabetes mellitus than in nondiabetic controls. These findings imply a poor defense mechanism against fibrin deposition in the vessel walls in diabetes, which might contribute to the development of diabetic microangiopathy.

Glycoproteins in plasma were measured in 280 diabetic patients (Terrasse *et al.*, 1976). The authors confirmed that the α-macroglobulins were increased in patients with microangiopathy. In another study, Jonsson and Wales (1976) measured five glycoproteins in the blood of 145 diabetic patients, with and without clinical evidence of complications. Patients with diabetic complications had higher glycoprotein levels, particularly when the levels were expressed as a ratio to serum albumin levels. α_2-Macroglobulins and serum β-lipoprotein levels were not as elevated as the other glycoproteins, haptoglobulin, caeruloplasmin, and particularly fibrinogen levels. However, the results in the small number of patients with retinopathy alone do not suggest that these measurements would be of value in detecting this diabetic complication. Only prospective studies, still to be performed, would indicate whether rising levels of certain glycoproteins in the blood of diabetic patients may indicate the development of diabetic vascular complications and predate the clinical appearance of the complications.

2.6.1.2. Changes in Microvascular Permeability

The microvascular permeability to small and large molecules was studied during good and poor metabolic regulation in 10 short-term juvenile diabetics (Parving *et al.*, 1976). The following variables were measured: daily urinary albumin and β_2-microglobulin excretion rates, whole-body transcapillary escape rate of albumin, glomerular filtration rate, capillary filtration coefficient, and capillary diffusion capacity. All these variables except capillary diffusion capacity were significantly increased during poor diabetic control, indicating a functional microangiopathy. Increased transcapillary escape rate of albumin during poor metabolic regulation demonstrates that increased extravasation of albumin occurs in the microvasculature of the extrarenal organs. The increased capillary filtration coefficient in the subcutaneous tissues of the forearm during poor metabolic control emphasizes the leakiness of the microvasculature. The author suggests that increased microvascular protein passage with subsequent deposition into the vascular wall at the onset of diabetes, and before thickening of the basement membrane can be demonstrated, may be an initial and important event in the morphogenesis of diabetic microangiopathy. Short periods of poor metabolic control could initiate these abnormalities. These findings support the case for the most effective possible control of diabetes. Parving (1976) also suggests that effective treatment of hypertension may arrest development of the microvascular lesions.

2.6.1.3. Biochemical Studies

In a review article, Spiro (1976) evaluates the biochemical events that could be responsible for the basement membrane lesions of diabetes. He reviews some evidence that hyperglycemia or elevation in plasma hGH levels alone or in combination may play an important role in the development of microvascular disease.

In chronic streptozotocin-induced diabetes in rats, Beisswenger (1976) was not able to find changes in the biosynthesis, chemical composition, or morphology of the glomerular basement membrane in comparison with age-matched control animals.

Westberg (1976) describes his findings of biochemical alterations of the human glomerular basement membrane in diabetes, which differ from those described by Spiro. Immunofluorescent studies indicate the presence of serum proteins in the diabetic glomerular basement membrane, probably as a result of increased membrane permeability.

The activities of the four enzymes catalyzing intracellular posttranslational modifications of collagen polypeptide chains were assayed in the kidneys of rats with streptozotocin diabetes (Risteli *et al.,* 1976). If changes were expressed as total enzyme activities per two kidneys, significant increases were found in all four enzyme activities at 12 weeks of diabetes. These data would be consistent with an increased collagen synthesis in diabetic kidneys. They do not support the hypothesis that there might be specific changes in some of these enzyme activities or in the level of certain modifications of the collagen polypeptide chains in this disease.

2.6.1.4. Muscle Capillary Basement Membrane Thickening

2.6.1.4a. Technique of Measurement. Controversy continues about different methods of fixation and of measuring and estimating capillary basement membrane width. Williamson *et al.* (1976) reviewed the previous and current investigations as well as those of other investigators and came to the conclusion, in contrast to that of Siperstein *et al.* (1973), that various methods gave comparable results. Yet they state that values of basement membrane width derived by Siperstein from control subjects are anomalously low and may explain the high prevalence of basement membrane thickening reported by the latter in diabetic and prediabetic subjects.

2.6.1.4b. Studies in Diabetic Patients. In a pair of 19-year-old monozygotic twin girls, one developed insulin-dependent, ketosis-prone diabetes at the age of 3 and has required insulin for the past 16 years (Karam *et al.,* 1976). Her identical twin has maintained normal oral and intravenous glucose tolerance with normal insulin release and glucagon suppression. An unequivocal hypertrophy of the muscle capillary basement membrane (1800 ± 148 Å) was found in the diabetic, while membrane thickness in the nondiabetic sister was normal (1149 ± 62 Å). These findings suggest that capillary basement membrane thickness is not an independent marker for genetic diabetes mellitus and is predominantly genetically determined, but that it is consequent to long-standing hyperglycemia or other metabolic effects secondary to insulin insufficiency. Follow-up of the present subjects and data from other discordant identical twins are necessary to reach definite conclusions.

Findings of capillary basement membrane widths in diabetic children by one group were reviewed in last year's chapter on diabetes mellitus. Sheikholislam *et al.* (1976a,b) report cross-sectional and longitudinal studies of carbohydrate metabolism and capillary basement membrane widths in children. In the cross-sectional studies, there were 19 diabetic children, 7 with "suspect" diabetes (abnormal glucose tolerance without fasting hyperglycemia) and 13 control subjects. Average basement membrane thickness (ABMT) and minimum basement membrane thickness (MBMT) correlated well, but did not correlate with age or, in the diabetics, with duration of clinical disease. Diabetics had the greatest and the control subjects the least mean ABMT and MBMT, but the differences were not statistically significant. High values were much more common among the suspected diabetics and the diabetics. Longitudinal, biochemical, and histological studies were carried out in 11 children receiving oral hyperglycemic agents. Changes in capillary basement membrane thickness were found to be statistically significant in a number of individual patients. Decreasing BMTs are associated with increasing glucose disappearance rate (K), and vice versa. A similar trend was apparent among other patients. When the data were pooled, K and ABMT and MBMT were found to change in opposite directions significantly. Although BMT and K may be influenced by many variables, the findings suggest that glucose tolerance and BMT have a close interdependence.

2.6.1.4c. Studies in Animal Models. Significant muscle capillary basement membrane thickening has been found in another model of spontaneously diabetic animals, in *Mystromys albicaudatus* (Yesus *et al.,* 1976). MBMT was 482.6 ± 48.7 Å in nondiabetic animals as against 779 ± 319.9 Å in the diabetic ones. Although there was overlap in MBMT between nondiabetic and diabetic animals, 75% of the diabetic animals showed significant basement membrane thickening. There was also greater segmental variation in basement membrane thickness among diabetic than among nondiabetic animals, as was found by Williamson *et al.* (1976) in man. Likewise, there was a high positive correlation between MBMT and duration of diabetes. In Caucasians and in Pima Indians, a significant correlation between duration of diabetes and BMT was found by both ABMT and MBMT techniques (Aronoff *et al.*, 1976). The same correlation was found in latent diabetic patients (Fajans *et al.*, 1976). These preliminary observations show that diabetes-related basement membrane thickening similar to that seen in human diabetes was present in this animal model.

2.6.1.5. Diabetic Retinopathy

2.6.1.5a. Pathogenetic Factors. The sorbitol, fructose, and glucose contents of the retina, blood, and liver from normal and streptozotocin-diabetic rats fed either starch- or sucrose-rich diets for 15 days were determined (Heath and Hamlett, 1976). Sorbitol and fructose levels in the retina were much higher than in either the liver or blood and were significantly increased in the diabetic rat on either diet. The sorbitol concentration of either the liver or the blood did not increase in diabetic animals on either diet. The possibility that the sorbitol pathway can play an important metabolic role in the diabetic retina was considered. The levels of sorbitol found in the retina in this investigation are considerably higher than those previously reported, and are of an order similar to those occurring in neural tissue from diabetic animals.

Normal and streptozotocin-diabetic rats were fed diets high in cornstarch or sucrose for 6–11 months (Papachristodoulous *et al.*, 1976). Retinal lesions similar to those seen in human diabetic retinopathy did not occur in normal rats fed starch-rich diets, but developed to a similar extent in sucrose-fed normal rats and starch-fed diabetic rats. The changes were most severe in sucrose-fed diabetic rats after 6 months. Superimposition of sucrose feeding on streptozotocin-induced diabetes led to an acceleration in the appearance of retinal alterations. The retinopathy of all three groups progressed to a similar degree by the ninth month. These studies suggest that environmental factors may contribute to the development of retinopathy. That human diabetic retinopathy may be due to both genetic and environmental factors was discussed last year.

2.6.1.5b. Prevalence. The occurrence of retinopathy and its relationship to diabetes in 1640 Pima Indians, ages 15 and over, was reported by Dorf *et al.* (1976). Of those with 2-hr PGPGLs of 200 mg/dl, or higher, 18% had some evidence of retinopathy. Of those with retinopathy and diabetes, 7% were found to have proliferative or neovascular changes. The prevalence of each element of retinopathy was related to the duration of diabetes. The frequency of retinopathy increased from 3% among newly diagnosed diabetics to 11% of those who had diabetes for less than 5 years and to 47% among those with diabetes of 10 or more years' duration. No relationship was found between the frequency of retinopathy and sex, the age at diagnosis, or age at time of examination when duration of diabetes was taken into account. No proliferative or neovascular changes were found in diabetics with duration of less than 10 years. The authors state that estimation of duration of diabetes was more accurate in younger than in older people. The relationship of prevalence of retinopathy to blood glucose levels was discussed in Section 2.4.

A rapid onset of proliferative retinopathy in young patients with MOD was described by Steel *et al.* (1976). Five patients who were diagnosed as diabetic between the ages of 34 and 39 years developed an accelerated type of proliferative retinopathy within 1 or 2 to 7–10 years of diagnosis. They were insulin-independent and controlled on diet or diet and oral agents. One became blind, and the others had severe visual impairment; two had severe renal involvement; three of four patients described in greater detail had a family history of diabetes of apparently insulin-independent type. In one patient, there was a three-generation history of MOD. Two patients had first-degree relatives with uncomplicated MOD, with one mother and grandmother being involved in one and a grandmother having had that diagnosis in the other. This report indicates that proliferative retinopathy may occur in MODY. Four of these patients suffered from recurrent foot ulcers. Although they were described as being "well controlled," they had midmorning blood sugar levels greater than 180 mg/dl. Since the duration of carbohydrate intolerance may have preceded the diagnosis by years or decades, the "rapid" onset of proliferative retinopathy applies only to the time of diagnosis, not necessarily to duration of diabetes. Although most families of MODY have been described as being relatively free of complications, this conclusion may not apply to all. The reviewer has seen one family with three generations of MODY in which the grandfather had been blind due to retinopathy and had had an amputation.

2.6.1.5c. Treatment—Ophthalmological and Medical. Two excellent reviews (Morse and Duncan, 1976; Maugh, 1976b) describe the ophthalmological management of diabetic retinopathy and review briefly but succinctly clinical findings, natural history, studies of experimental retinopathy, methods of examination and evaluation, and methods of treatment with photocoagulation and vitrectomy. A diabetic retinopathy study (Diabetic Retinopathy Study Research Group, 1976) was begun in 1971 and is a controlled clinical trial involving more than 1700 patients enrolled in 15 medical centers. It is designed to evaluate whether or not photocoagulation therapy is a useful means of preserving vision in patients with diabetic retinopathy. Only diabetic patients with visual acuity of 20/100 or better in each eye but with evidence of proliferative retinopathy in at least one eye or evidence of severe nonproliferative diabetic retinopathy in both eyes were eligible for enrollment. One eye from each patient was randomly chosen for treatment. The patients enrolled were randomly assigned to treatment with either argon laser or xenon arc. Based on an analysis of 2-year follow-up data, the occurrence of visual acuity of less than 5/200 for two consecutive completed 4-month visits was reduced from 16.3% in all untreated eyes to 6.4% in treated eyes after 2 years of follow-up observation. These data have necessitated some changes in the research protocol of this therapeutic trial. They led to consideration of treatment of the eye originally assigned to no treatment when certain conditions were present. Minor losses of acuity were more frequent in treated than in untreated eyes, though after 2 years the difference was very small. This study shows that the risk of blindness can be reduced by 61% by the introduction of photocoagulation in certain selected eyes afflicted with diabetic retinopathy. Photocoagulation is of significant benefit to the patients with little risk of complications or side effects other than a mild reduction in the visual field following the procedure.

Although photocoagulation has replaced pituitary ablation for the treatment of diabetic retinopathy of most types, it appears that in a rare type of "florid" form of diabetic retinopathy, pituitary ablation remains the treatment of choice (Kohner *et al.,* 1976). The 1- and 2-year visual acuities were significantly better in the pituitary-ablated eyes than in the untreated or photocoagulated ones. It is suggested that for this rare form of retinopathy, pituitary ablation remains the treatment of choice if vision is to be maintained.

As reviewed last year and again by Job *et al.* (1976), there are a few experimental and clinical studies that suggest that there is less progression in the clinical manifestations of microangiopathy in well-controlled than in poorly controlled experimental animals or patients. There is, however, no unanimity of opinion that improvement in control of hyperglycemia may have a beneficial effect on the development or progression of clinical manifestations of retinopathy. Job *et al.* (1976) reported a clinical trial that was undertaken to compare the effect of divided daily insulin administration vs. one daily insulin injection on the course of early diabetic retinopathy. The patients selected for study were insulin-dependent, were treated by one daily insulin injection, and had early-stage diabetic retinopathy without proliferative changes. The patients were not asked about their willingness to accept multiple daily insulin injections in the future, but were randomized in one of two insulin programs: single (S) or multiple (M) doses of daily insulin. Of the 52 insulin-dependent diabetics selected, 6 patients of the S- and 4 of the M-dose group were lost to follow-up.

Twenty-one patients in each group were followed for 1–4 years. Although there were some changes in treatment during follow-up in both groups, finally 16 of 21 subjects in the S group were treated during the entire trial with one injection and 17 of the 21 subjects in the M group were on two or three divided doses during the entire trial. Retinal changes were quantitatively estimated by counting the microaneurysms (MAs) observed on fluorescent angiograms at the posterior pole of the more diseased eye. During the follow-up period (mean duration of 3 years), the mean yearly progression in the number of MAs was significantly less in the M than in the S injection group—1.8 ± 0.7 vs. 7.2 ± 1.9—though final values were, respectively, 15.2 ± 4.9 and 33.0 ± 79 MAs. These differences were significant. Comparison of fasting blood sugar levels between the two groups at base line was 210 ± 12 and 200 ± 19 mg/dl for the two groups (P-NS). The mean survey plasma glucose values were 197 ± 9 and 171 ± 10 mg/dl ($P < 0.06$) for the S and M group, respectively, whereas the last-year values were 195 ± 11 and 154 ± 15 mg/dl ($P < 0.05$) for the two groups, respectively. Thus, in this clinical trial made under routine treatment conditions, the use of divided daily insulin injections was effective in achieving a slight improvement in diabetes control and in delaying retinal changes in insulin-dependent diabetics. This study cannot settle the question of the value of control on influencing diabetic retinopathy in view of the relatively small number of patients, the limited number of years of follow-up, and the change in treatment programs in several patients. It constitutes a good beginning, however, and should give encouragement to mounting larger well-controlled trials of the effect of improved control as achieved by two or more insulin injections. The ultimate judgment may not be possible until physiological control can be achieved (Fajans and Freinkel, 1976).

2.6.1.6. Diabetic Nephropathy

Mauer *et al.* (1976b) reviewed publications mentioned in last year's chapter and presented further studies by their Minnesota group performed in diabetic animals and in man to elucidate the pathogenesis of diabetic nephropathy.

2.6.1.6a. Nature of Lesions and Pathogenesis. There is controversy as to whether diabetic nephropathy, another manifestation of microangiopathy, is secondary to carbohydrate intolerance or is determined by a separate genetic factor. Further evidence supports the concept that the renal lesions develop in the abnormal metabolic environment of the diabetic patients and are not a separately inherited disorder, unrelated to abnormalities in carbohydrate metabolism. Miller and Michael (1976) documented the presence of intensive linear immunofluorescence staining for IgG and albumin of renal extracellular membranes, primarily the tubular basement membranes, but also glomerular basement membranes and Bowman's capsule of patients with severe diabetic nephropathy. There is no evidence that an immunological process is responsible for these findings. These immunofluorescent findings are *specific* for severe diabetic nephropathy and distinguish it clearly from other renal disease. The observations of increased immunofluorescence for IgG and albumin and nonvascular extracellular basement membrane would suggest that all renal extracellular membranes are uniquely abnormal in advanced diabetic nephropathy.

In another paper, Mauer *et al.* (1976a) report that the immunopathological findings described above in renal extracellular membranes in diabetes develop in normal kidneys transplanted into diabetic patients. Immunofluorescent studies were carried out on kidney tissue obtained from 12 diabetic and 17 nondiabetic patients from 2 to 12 years following renal transplantation. The frequency and intensity of IgG and albumin staining of these membranes were significantly greater in the diabetic than in the nondiabetic patients. Basement membrane staining did not occur in any of the seven kidneys studied at the time of the transplantation into diabetic recipients. The abnormalities leading to the deposition or trapping of proteins in the renal extracellular membranes occur early (2 or more years) after the placement of normal kidneys into the abnormal metabolic environment of the diabetic transplant recipient and occur early in the natural history of the disease.

Furthermore, the development of diabetic vascular lesions in normal kidneys transplanted into patients with diabetes mellitus was observed by Mauer *et al.* (1976c). The authors examined renal transplant tissue from diabetic and nondiabetic patients who had had renal grafts for at least 2 years. In 10 of 12 diabetic patients, arteriolar hyalinosis lesions developed from 2 to 5 years after transplantation. In 6, these lesions involved both afferent and efferent limbs of glomerular arterioles, a pathological finding virtually diagnostic of diabetes mellitus. Only 3 of 28 nondiabetic patients had hyaline vascular changes, which occurred only rarely, did not appear within the first 5 years after transplantation, and did not involve both afferent and efferent arterioles. One diabetic patient developed nodular glomerulosclerosis. The first clearly distinguishable vascular lesion of diabetes that occurs with frequency in normal kidneys transplanted into diabetic patients is arteriolar hyalinosis. These observations support the concept that basement membrane alterations in diabetes and hyalin vascular lesions develop as a consequence of placement of a normal kidney into an abnormal metabolic environment of the diabetic patient, rather than being due to a separate inherited disorder.

In addition to the finding of structural changes in the kidney early in the natural history of diabetes, Mogensen (1976) presented data and reviewed studies showing that a number of functional abnormalities are present in the kidney in early diabetes, especially in the uncontrolled state. There was an elevated basal albumin excretion, increased glomerular filtration rate, increase in filtration fraction, and increase in kidney size and calculated kidney weight. During improved control of the diabetes, there was normalization of these functions and decrease in renal size, supporting the desirability of maintaining the best possible control in diabetic patients. Mogensen's study also indicated that antihypertensive therapy may be beneficial for young proteinuric diabetics and may postpone the stage of renal insufficiency. A state of "functional" microangiopathy was discussed in Section 2.6.1.2 in reference to the data of Parving (1976) and Parving *et al.*, (1976).

Nodular intercapillary glomerulosclerosis was found at autopsy in a 47-year-old man who had been a diabetic secondary to chronic fibrocalcific pancreatitis for 20 years (Wellman and Volk, 1976). The family history for diabetes was negative. The patient also had diabetic retinopathy. Since this is only the fourth recorded case of histologically documented nodular glomerulosclerosis occurring in a patient with pancreatogenic diabetes, this finding, although suggestive, adds little to settling the controversy whether environmental or genetic causes are more important in the pathogenesis of this lesion.

2.6.1.6b. Clinical Course. Kussman *et al.* (1976) reported a retrospective record analysis of 112 JOD patients with nephropathy to describe their clinical course. Since diabetic patients with chronic renal failure have been accepted with increasing frequency as candidates for treatment by chronic hemodialysis or renal transplantation, precise knowledge of the natural course of diabetic nephropathy is needed as a basis for judgment as to proper time and mode of therapeutic intervention. The mean duration of diabetes at the onset of proteinuria was 17.3 ± 6 years. Apparent renal failure appeared 2 years after the onset of proteinuria, and severe or late renal failure (mean serum creatinine 8.5 ± 3.9 mg/dl), 4 years after the onset of proteinuria. Mean duration of life after the onset of proteinuria was 4.8 years, the longest survival being 13.3 years. Mean survival after the onset of early renal failure was 2.7 years, the longest survival being 5.7 years. The time between the onset of late renal failure to death was only 7 months, and no patient survived for more than 12 months. All patients experienced progressive deterioration of renal function and the other complications of diabetes, the rate of progression being accelerated toward the end of the course.

2.6.1.6c. Treatment. The rationale for best possible control in the hope of preventing or delaying renal lesions is based on the findings reviewed in Sections 2.6.1.2 and 2.6.1.6a. Since diabetic nephropathy is steadily progressive to death, and renal transplantation is a feasible form of treatment, patients should be considered for transplantation before the serum creatinine reaches 8.5 mg/dl. Kussman *et al.* (1976) state that at the Joslin Clinic, evaluation of renal transplantation is begun when serum creatinine levels reach 5.0 mg/dl, which, in most patients, occurs prior to the need for hemodialysis.

Shideman *et al.* (1976) described the complications of hemodialysis in 67 insulin-dependent diabetic patients accepted for renal transplantation. These were compared with the complications in 67 nondiabetic hemodialysis patients. Of the 67 diabetic patients, 11 died before receiving renal transplants—4 of myocardial infarction, 3 of dialysis-related causes, and 4 of infection. Of the 67 nondiabetic patients, 1 died of infection before transplantation. The diabetic patients experienced more complications on dialysis; they were more hypertensive, required more ultrafiltration during dialysis, and had a higher incidence of hypertensive episodes during dialysis, as well as a high incidence of predialysis hyperglycemia. These findings suggested to the authors that diabetic patients with renal failure should be dialyzed more frequently and should receive transplants at creatinine levels of 6–8 mg/100 ml to avoid the complications associated with hemodialysis.

2.6.1.6d. Plasma Renin Activity in Diabetes. In a review article, Christlieb (1976) presents data and speculates about alteration in the renin–angiotension–aldosterone system in diabetes mellitus. This system appears to function normally in uncomplicated diabetes, but is altered when there are microvascular and electrolyte complications.

Christlieb *et al.* (1976b) reported their experience with the determination of plasma renin activity (PRA) in patients with diabetes. The results suggest that the mean PRA is normal in normotensive diabetics and that upright PRA in diabetics with hypertension but no nephropathy is similar to that in essential hypertension. On the other hand, patients with diabetes, hypertension, and nephropathy have "low renin hypertension," possibly explaining the virtual absence of malignant hypertension in this group. The authors state that although the major mechanism for this low PRA may be volume expansion, indicating the need for potent diuretics, other mechanisms include hyalinization of the afferent arterioles, decreased catecholamine stimulation of renin release, and inadequate conversion of prorenin to renin.

DeLeiva *et al.* (1976) reported two female patients with diabetes mellitus and selective hypoaldosteronism. They demonstrated a block in conversion from prorenin—a relatively inactive precursor of renin with a higher molecular weight—to renin, as well as blockade of aldosterone synthesis with defective conversion of an aldosterone precursor to aldosterone. The authors suggest that in these two diabetic patients, and in others reported, hypoaldosteronism resulted from the combined actions of two distinct defects. Diabetic renal disease was offered as a possible cause for the defect in renin production. The authors reviewed the literature and state that 19 of 67 (28%) patients with selective hypoaldosteronism also had diabetes mellitus. In most of these cases, there was some degree of renal disease and decreased PRA. Possible causes of abnormalities in the renin–angiotensin–aldosterone system in diabetic patients include renal disease, enzymatic defects in aldosterone biosythesis, decreased circulating levels of catecholamines, autonomic neuropathy, and defective conversion from prorenin to renin.

Decreased PRA and hypoaldosteronism have been found in diabetic patients with neuropathy, orthostatic hypotension, and renal disease. Diabetic patients with hyperkalemia out of proportion to the degree of renal dysfunction should be evaluated for hypoaldosteronism.

Christlieb *et al.* (1976a) reported that diabetics with retinopathy have increased vascular reactivity to both angiotensin II and norepinephrine when compared with diabetics with no evidence of diabetic complications. Neither diabetic group, however, was significantly different from normal subjects. The various possibilities responsible for the differences between the two diabetic groups are discussed, but any possible relationship between the observed alterations and vascular reactivity and the vascular complications of diabetes remain to be determined.

In diabetic ketoacidosis, PRA and aldosterone are stimulated secondary to the associated dehydration with hypovolemia.

2.6.2. Diabetic Macroangiopathy

2.6.2.1. Prevalence

The frequency of electrocardiographic evidence of coronary heart disease and the rate of autopsy-proved myocardial infarction were determined in the Pima Indians, a tribe with a high prevalence of diabetes mellitus (see Section 2.4). The frequency of coronary heart disease was about one-half that found in Tecumseh, Michigan (Ingelfinger *et al.*, 1976). Subjects with diabetes had a higher rate of coronary heart disease than nondiabetics, both electrocardiographically and at postmortem examination, although the differences were not statistically significant. Serum cholesterol levels in the Pima aged 40 years or older were low, averaging 189 and 188 mg/dl, respectively, in the male and female nondiabetics, and 197 and 198 mg/dl, respectively, in the male and female diabetics. Despite the high prevalence of diabetes mellitus, the Pima Indians have a lower frequency of coronary heart disease than the predominantly Caucasian populations of the United States. This implies that coronary heart disease may not be an inevitable complication of diabetes mellitus.

In a more detailed investigation of cholesterol levels in Pima Indians, Savage *et al.* (1976) found that cholesterol levels at birth were similar in Pimas and Caucasians, but levels in Pimas from 5 to 16 years of age were 10–30 mg lower than among most white populations. Cholesterol levels in adult Pimas were 50–60 mg/dl lower than in American whites and showed little increase after age 25. Evidence of a causal relationship between the relatively lower levels of serum cholesterol and lower rates of coronary heart disease remains to be established.

A brief clinical note emphasizes the value of perfusion scanning in combination with arteriography in the diagnostic workup of the diabetic patient who, because of peripheral vascular complications, is a candidate for surgery (Rhodes *et al.*, 1976). Abnormal arteriograms with normal scans indicate large-vessel disease without significant small-vessel involvement. On the other hand, normal arteriograms with abnormal scans indicate small-vessel disease without significant large-vessel involvement. The latter patients are not candidates for vascular reconstruction.

2.6.2.2. Pathogenetic Factors

The reason that accelerated macroangiopathy or atherosclerosis occurs in diabetic patients at an earlier age, is more frequent, and progresses more rapidly than in nondiabetic patients is not clear. Recent studies have shown that the smooth muscle cell is primarily involved in the development of the atherosclerotic lesions. To explore aspects of diabetic macroangiopathy in an *in vitro* model, the growth rate and the morphology of aortic smooth muscle cells from normal and diabetic rabbits, in primary explants incubated in normal, diabetic, and hyperlipemic sera, as well as in normal serum with added glucose, were investigated. Smooth muscle cell cultures were grown from thoracic aortas of normal and diabetic rabbits. Media containing diabetic serum stimulated the growth of both cultures significantly. Control media containing normal serum with added glucose had no such effect. The growth-promoting effects of diabetic serum and of hyperlipemic serum from nondiabetic rabbits were of the same magnitude, although the latter resulted in smaller cells. These results indicate that diabetic serum contains a factor or factors that stimulate the arterial medial cell to excessive growth. The factor is not glucose, insulin, or lipid (Ledet *et al.*, 1976). In further experiments, Ledet (1976) demonstrated that supplementation of normal serum with hGH (final concentration 1.5 ng/ml medium, i.e., a concentration that occurs in diabetic plasma) resulted in a significant enhancement of growth of rabbit aortic medial cell cultures. The results imply that the growth-stimulating factor(s) in diabetic serum is not insulin, but may be hGH.

2.6.3. Diabetic Neuropathy

2.6.3.1. Clinical Aspects

The remarkable frequency, the clinical impact, and the clinical aspects of diabetic neuropathies were comprehensively reviewed by Ellenberg (1976). A classification is given and the clinical aspects are reviewed in detail.

Urodynamic and electrophysiological techniques were applied to assess the frequency and extent of autonomic and peripheral neuropathy in 60 subjects with diabetes mellitus (Buck *et al.*, 1976). Of the subjects, 38 were diabetic patients with suggestive symptoms and the others were representative newly diagnosed or treated diabetics. Objective evidence of neuropathic bladder dysfunction was detected in 72%. Eletrophysiological studies found a sensory defect in the lower limbs in all tested patients (100%) and an associated motor conduction abnormality, more frequent and marked in the lower than in the upper extremities, in 41 patients (69%). These functional abnormalities appear to be related to the severity of diabetes but less to its duration. The high incidence of bladder dysfunction and peripheral neuropathy in this series indicates the frequency of subclinical diabetic neuropathy.

An electrophysiological study of bladder and urethral innervation showed slowing of conduction velocities indicative of neuropathy when conventional diagnostic modalities such as gas cystometry did not show any abnormality in asymptomatic patients (Andersen and Bradley, 1976). Spinal involvement may be a neglected disturbance of bladder innervation in patients with diabetes.

Diabetic autonomic neuropathy may affect the cardiovascular system, the main clinical manifestation being postural hypotension. The effect of administration of insulin on postural hypotension in 8 diabetics with autonomic neuropathy was investigated by Page and Watkins (1976). Systolic and diastolic pressures fell considerably after insulin in all patients, and this fall was aggravated by tilting to the vertical position. The hypotensive effect of insulin occurred whether it was administered intravenously, intramuscularly, or subcutaneously. It coincided with a fall in blood glucose levels but occured before hypoglycemic levels were reached, and might have been present when the blood glucose level was elevated. Some patients were unable to differentiate between symptoms of hypoglycemia and hypotension. Postural hypotension may account for some episodes of sudden loss of consciousness without warning, usually attributed to hypoglycemia. The effect of insulin was not due to hypoglycemia, and its exact mode of action is unknown.

Autonomic neuropathy is associated with a high mortality rate in diabetic patients. A group of 38 diabetics with symptoms and clinical features suggestive of autonomic neuropathy were followed prospectively for 33 months (Ewing *et al.*, 1976). More than 25% were dead within 2½ years. Of the 20 with abnormal Valsalva or hand grip tests initially, 10 (50%) were dead within this time. The causes of death were renal failure (6 patients), cerebral vascular accident (2 patients), hypoglycemic coma (1 patient), and sudden death (1 patient). In patients with diabetes with the clinical features of autonomic neuropathy, simple autonomic function tests give a good guide to prognosis. Patients who survived had considerable morbidity and worsening of autonomic symptoms.

Peripheral and autonomic nerve function was assessed in 7 diabetic patients during and for 3 months after diabetic ketoacidosis (Campbell *et al.*, 1976). There was marked improvement in motor nerve conduction velocity and terminal latency of both ulnar and common perineal nerves in all patients. Five had one or more abnormal autonomic function tests, but there was no consistent change during the same period. The authors postulate that peripheral nerves may be more susceptible to acute metabolic damage than autonomic nerve fibers.

Autonomic neuropathy may effect the regulation of the heart rate. Lloyd-Mostyn and Watkins (1976) reported a patient with severe autonomic neuropathy whose heart behaved as if totally denervated. There were no changes in heart rate that could be attributed to attempts to stimulate, inhibit, or pharmacologically block autonomic nerves to the heart. The behavior of the patient's heart was similar to that of the transplanted heart. Although total cardiac denervation must be a rare diabetic complication, the same investigators previously described 13 diabetic patients with autonomic neuropathy in whom heart-rate responses to autonomic stimulation and inhibition were impaired to a varying degree (Lloyd-Mostyn and Watkins, 1975). Fekete *et al.* (1976) compared the frequency of sinus arrhythmia in 26 diabetic patients with that in 26 nondiabetic controls. Forced inspiration–expiration failed to provoke sinus arrhythmia in 11 of the diabetic patients, but in only 1 nondiabetic control. Mean duration of diabetes was 4 years in patients who manifested sinus arrhythmia, as contrasted to the mean of 8 years in those who did not. A correlation of duration of diabetes with the absence of sinus arrhythmia was also demonstrated by Neubauer and Gundersen (1976). The majority of long-term diabetics showed no respiratory arrhythmia.

2.6.3.2. Pathogenetic Factors

Winegrad and Green (1976) reviewed the importance of insulin deficiency, hyperglycemia, and alteration in myoinositol metabolism in the pathogenesis of diabetic polyneuropathy. The original studies that formed the basis of this review article were discussed in last year's chapter.

Timperely *et al.* (1976) believe that fibrin deposition within small vessels, within vasa nervora, could play a part in damaging the diabetic nerve. They performed serial nerve biopsies in 24 diabetic patients with clinical and electrophysiological evidence of diabetic neuropathy. Vessels plugged with fibrin were seen within the nerve in 9 patients.

2.6.4. Disturbance of Growth and Accelerated Aging in Diabetes Mellitus

Poor growth occurs in severe diabetes mellitus despite elevation of plasma hGH. The mechanism for poor growth in insulin deficiency was investigated in acute streptozotocin-induced diabetes in rats (Phillips, L. S., and Young, 1976). In these animals, there was a significant decrease in both serum somatomedin and cartilage growth activity; these changes were not ameliorated by administration of growth hormone. Insulin therapy could both prevent and reverse the fall in somatomedin and cartilage growth activity. The authors concluded that growth failure in insulin deficiency, as in malnutrition, may be due to the decreased somatomedin activity.

Evidence for accelerated aging in diabetes mellitus was reviewed last year. Aging changes in the intervertebral disks were similar in diabetic Chinese hamsters and nondiabetic animals (Silberberg and Gerritsen, 1976). In diabetic hamsters, however, the incidence of spondylosis was significantly increased and appearance of lesions was accelerated. The bone changes could be due to defective synthesis of mucopolysaccharides or could be interpreted as a manifestation of accelerated aging.

Skeletal mass in the forearm was assessed in 35 patients with insulin-dependent JOD and in 101 stable patients with MOD on diet alone, insulin, or oral hypoglycemic agents (Levin *et al.,* 1976). Bone mass was determined by a direct photon-absorption method. There was a significant loss of bone mass in both JOD and MOD as compared with controls matched for age and sex. The decrease was present in patients with diabetes of less than 5 years' known duration. There was no correlation between bone loss and duration of diabetes. The authors suggest that osteopenia in diabetes may be due to a decrease in bone formation rather than to increased bone loss, and may be a manifestation of early senescence of all cells as a basic defect of diabetes. Insulin-treated patients had a lesser decrease in bone mass than those treated by diet, while patients treated with sulfonylurea had the greatest loss in bone mass. Since activation of adenylate cyclase and the AMP system has been shown to increase bone resorption and insulin has an inhibitory effect on this system, while sulfonylurea agents may produce an increase in AMP, the authors postulate that the opposite effects of insulin and sulfonylurea on AMP may explain the greatest difference in bone mass between the group taking insulin and that taking oral agents. These factors would operate independent of the inherent defect in diabetic bone.

In another study, Ringe *et al.* (1976) also found an abnormally reduced mineral content in 21 of 57 insulin-requiring diabetic patients by direct photon absorption. These authors interpreted the findings as being a late complication of diabetes.

2.6.5. Prevention and Treatment—Islet and Pancreas Transplantation

Several observations in experimental animals (see last year's chapter), as well as in diabetic patients, support the hypothesis that angiopathic and neuropathic lesions associated with diabetes are secondary to abnormal metabolism. Precise regulation of insulin secretion and carbohydrate metabolism await the development of approaches or techniques that simulate physiological insulin delivery. Matas *et al.* (1976) reviewed the current status of islet and pancreas transplantation in diabetes. The literature on experimental transplantation of the whole pancreas, clinical transplantation of the whole pancreas, experimental transplantation of islet tissue, preparation of human islet tissue, clinical islet transplantation, and prospects of clinical transplantation is cited and discussed. In a separate communication, Sutherland *et al.* (1976) presented evidence that the infant human cadaver pancreas may be an ideal source of islet tissue for transplantation to selected diabetic patients.

2.7. Diabetes in Pregnancy

An editorial in *The Lancet* (1976) reviews the undesirable effects of hyperglycemia and hypoglycemia during pregnancy. The GTT will identify the small percentage of the pregnant population who develop mild diabetes. Among these women, the risk of perinatal loss is increased, especially if they are over 25 years old or obese. From an analysis of a large series of GTTs in the third trimester, Abell and Beischer (1976) found a normal range and took single plasma glucose levels above the

95th percentile or below the 5th percentile as indicating hyperglycemia or hypoglycemia—14.8% and 11.7%, respectively, of pregnant women falling in these two categories. While hyperglycemia was associated with increased placental growth and perinatal mortality, hypoglycemia led to placental and fetal growth retardation and incresed perinatal mortality. When urinary estriol excretion was persistently abnormal in the presence of hypoglycemia or hyperglycemia, the risk of perinatal loss was still greater. The oral GTT, analyzed as a total area under the GTT curve, is a good reflection of mean blood sugar levels. Abell and Beischer concluded that hyperglycemia of a lesser degree than that indicating diabetes mellitus is also associated with increased perinatal mortality. Whether a single blood sugar value during a GTT is enough to point to a fetus in danger of glucose starvation seems open to question, but a subnormal estriol level may be of additional prognostic value.

Perinatal data on 805 infants of diabetic mothers and 10,152 infants of nondiabetic mothers were examined for a relationship between maternal diabetes and respiratory-distress syndrome of the newborn (Robert *et al.*, 1976). The syndrome occurred in 23.4% of the diabetics vs. 1.3% of the nondiabetic group. When features associated with diabetes that are in themselves risk factors, such as gestational age and route of delivery, were considered, a respiratory-distress syndrome in infants of diabetics mothers was 5.6 times as likely to develop as in infants of nondiabetic mothers. This observation suggests that maternal diabetes *per se* predisposes an infant to the syndrome. The authors speculate on the mechanism by which maternal diabetes delays normal fetal lung maturation. The timing of normal lung maturation depends on elevation of fetal glucocorticoids late in gestation. It has been shown that insulin can block the enzyme-inductive action of cortisol in the liver in various animal models. It is postulated that fetal hypersecretion of insulin in the offspring of diabetic mothers could block the enzyme-inductive capability of cortisol in the fetal lung, and thus, an impairment in synthesis of the pulmonary surfactant could result in an infant with surfactant deficiency. Surfactant deficiency is essential to the development of the respiratory-distress syndrome.

2.8. Treatment of Diabetes Mellitus

2.8.1. Dietary Treatment

It is a dictum that diet is the first line of management in newly diagnoised nonketotic diabetic patients. Plasma glucose and plasma insulin during the oral GTT were determined in 118 newly diagnosed MOD patients before and after treatment with diet alone for periods of 2 and 6 months (Doar *et al.,* 1976). The patients were 33–73 (mean 56) years of age. Patients with ketonuria or random blood sugars greater than 350 mg/dl at the first visit were excluded. The patients were instructed in a diet designed to reduce the intake of sugar and to reduce body weight when obese. Mean fasting blood glucose was approximately 250 mg/dl initially and approximately 170 mg/dl after 2 months. There was a corresponding decrease in glucose intolerance. The mean OGTT-sugar area improved from 2247 ± 481 to 1677 ± 462 (S.D.) U ($P < 0.001$), and the mean insulin area rose from 185 ± 183 to 207 ± 161 U ($P < 0.005$). The mean fasting plasma insulin fell slightly (2.62 ± 7.24 μU/ml; $P < 0.001$). Of the 118 patients, 112 (95%) obtained some improvement in glucose tolerance. While only 14% of the group achieved normal glucose tolerance curves after 2 months of dietary treatment, the diabetic clinic random blood sugar levels were below 150 mg/dl in 59% of the patients. The mean degree of obesity of the group was 129 ± 21% initially, and the mean weight loss between the two tests was 5.1 ± 4.0 k ($P < 0.01$). Optimal multiple regression analysis showed that the OGTT-sugar area during the second test was predicted by a combination of the first OGTT-sugar area and the weight loss between the two tests. This prediction was not improved by the addition of further variables including age, obesity, and plasma insulin levels during the first test. The study confirms that diet alone should be the first type of management for patients with newly diagnosed MOD. Some obese patients obtained good diabetic control without weight reduction, presumably by reducing their carbohydrate intake while maintaining their previous total caloric intake.

In a study extending over 5 years, 35 of 70 excessively overweight patients with subclinical diabetes who had not significantly changed their weight demonstrated further deterioration in glucose tolerance, and manifest diabetes occurred in 10 (Berger *et al.,* 1976). In the remaining 35 patients, who had achieved 20% weight reduction, glucose tolerance had become normal. The two groups were similar in age, initial weight, and original degree of glucose intolerance. There was a significant correlation between the loss of weight and increased glucose tolerance. No such correlation occurred with subgroups of patients whose initial overweight was more than 100% and who had been more than 50 years of age at the start of the study.

Bistrian *et al.* (1976) reported on a protein-sparing modified fast (PSMF), which is a total fast modified by the intake of 1.2–1.4 g protein/kg ideal body weight, fluids *ad libitum,* and vitamin and mineral supplementation. When 7 obese MOD patients who were receiving 30–100 U insulin/day were put on this fast, insulin could be discontinued after 0–19 (mean 6.5) days. In the 3 patients who had extensive nitrogen balance studies, balance could be maintained chronically by 1.3 g protein/kg ideal body weight despite the gross caloric inadequacy of the diet. The PSMF was tolerated well in an outpatient setting after the initial insulin-withdrawal phase had occurred in the hospital. Significant improvement in blood pressure, lipid abnormality, parameters of carbohydrate metabolism, and cardiorespiratory symptoms was associated with weight loss or PSMF or both. For diabetics with some endogenous insulin reserve, the PSMF offered significant advantages for weight reduction, including preservation of lean body mass (as reflected in nitrogen balance) and withdrawal of exogenous insulin. Of the 7 patients, 5 achieved weight loss of greater than 40 pounds, primarily as outpatients. At intervals of 5–12 months, substantial weight loss was maintained.

The effects on postprandial plasma glucose and insulin responses of different kinds of dietary carbohydrates when given alone and in combination with other nutrients in a test meal were compared by Crapo *et al.* (1976). Glucose, sucrose, and various starches were compared, all calculated to contain the equivalent of 50 g glucose. Glucose and sucrose elicited similar plasma glucose response curves, but sucrose elicited a greater plasma insulin response. Raw starch ingestion resulted in a 44% lower glucose and a 35–65% lower insulin response than did either glucose or sucrose ingestion. When carbohydrate was given as a mixed meal, the plasma glucose response was 40–60% lower than when the same carbohydrate was given alone, while the insulin responses were generally comparable. Complex carbohydrates (starches) resulted in lower glucose and insulin responses than equivalent amounts of glucose as mono- and disaccharides. An unexpected finding was that when different cooked starches were compared, the plasma glucose and insulin responses to rice were significantly lower (50%) than the responses to potato starch. Apparently not all starches are treated identically by gastrointestinal digestive and absorptive processes.

The effect of raising the fiber or unabsorbable carbohydrate content of the diabetic diet was explored by Jenkins *et al.* (1976). Guar and pectin, gel-forming carbohydrates of vegetable origin, were incorporated in a controlled meal containing 106 g carbohydrate. In the test meal, each portion of bread also contained 16 g guar powder (a storage polysaccharide of an Indian legume), and 10 g pectin (a constituent of cell walls of citrus fruit and apple) was added to marmalade. Neither of these substances is hydrolyzed by the digestive juices of man. Addition of these unabsorbable carbohydrates into the test meal significantly decreased postprandial hyperglycemia in 8 non-insulin-requiring diabetics and in 3 insulin-dependent diabetic patients. There was a 40–60% decrease in the rise in blood sugar over a 50- to 90-min period. Insulin responses to the carbohydrate meals were also reduced in the non-insulin-requiring diabetics after taking fiber-enriched test meals. The addition of unavailable carbohydrate to carbohydrate meals may prove useful in the dietary control of diabetes, by decreasing postprandial hyperglycemia and reducing insulin requirements in insulin-dependent diabetics.

2.8.2. Insulin Treatment

2.8.2.1. Ketoacidosis

A comparison of low-dose insulin treatment for diabetic ketoacidosis—either by intramuscular injection or by continuous intravenous infusion—with insulin treatment of large intravenous boluses was reviewed in last year's chapter. This reviewer concluded (Fajans, 1976, pp. 57–58):

> In a majority of patients with moderately severe diabetic ketoacidosis, the mode of administration of insulin appears to be of limited significance, and small doses, although effective in most cases, are not clearly superior to conventional treatment with larger doses. The possibility of larger insulin requirements in a few severely ketoacidotic, comatose patients should be recognized and anticipated. Individualization of insulin administration superimposed on any of a number of conventional regimens appears most important in the successful management of any given patient with severe ketoacidosis.

Kitabchi *et al.* (1976) state that a well-controlled randomized prospective study comparing the efficacy of conventional high-dose vs. low-dose intramuscular insulin therapy was not available in the literature, and that their study provides for the first time a randomized prospective study to settle the question objectively. The effect of low-dose intramuscular insulin therapy was compared with that of "high-dose" insulin therapy by intravenous and subcutaneous routes in 48 patients with diabetic ketoacidosis. The authors claim that they found comparable results in both groups, but that hypoglycemia was a significant complication in the high-dose group, occurring in 25%, and that slight hypokalemia was seen more frequently in the high-dose group (29%) than in the low dose group (4%). Neither of these complications of therapy resulted in fatality or in any apparent increase in morbidity. None of these patients was in shock or was hypotensive, and all were able to sign "informed consent" before being admitted to the Clinical Research Center. Thus, this comparison does not include patients with severe diabetic ketoacidosis and coma, and does not address itself to the efficacy of the two regimens in such patients. Furthermore, the "high-dose" insulin schedule contained relatively small amounts of intravenous insulin (25 U for initial plasma glucose of 600–1,000 mg/dl) and consisted primarily of subcutaneous insulin. Although the rate of glucose fall in the two groups was not significantly different at any period examined, the fall in ketone bodies was significantly greater in the high-dose group at the 1st, 3rd, and 5th hr of therapy, but not at the 7th hr. The mean pH on admission was 7.15 ± 0.02 and 7.13 ± 0.02 in the two groups. The potassium replacement therapy consisted of only 15–20 mEq potassium chloride/liter intravenous fluid.

As Madison (1976) pointed out in an editorial, the major fatality in diabetic ketoacidosis is related to the presence of deep coma or severe complicating disease, and a large prospective randomized study comparing conventional high-dose intravenous insulin regimens with the low-dose continuous-infusion technique or intramuscular technique must also be conducted in severely ill patients before the relative efficacy of the various programs can be settled. Patients with mild or moderately severe diabetic ketoacidosis will recover whatever insulin and fluid program is administered.

Holt and Cudworth (1976) described a patient in severe ketoacidotic hyperglycemic coma who received an initial bolus of 100 U i.v. followed by continuous infusion of insulin at the rate of 6 U/hr. Despite continuous insulin infusion for 2½ hr, plus a further bolus of 100 U bovine insulin i.v. at 2 hr and steady fluid replacement, the patient's general condition remained poor and plasma glucose remained unchanged. The insulin was then changed to soluble porcine monocomponent insulin at a constant infusion rate of 12 U/hr coupled with an initial bolus injection of 100 U i.v. Within an hour, the plasma glucose fell steadily. The authors claim that this case is evidence that insulin resistance may occur during continuous infusion of insulin, and they state that the prompt fall in plasma glucose when insulin was changed to porcine soluble monocomponent insulin suggests the real possibility of insulin resistance to the bovine insulin antibodies. The authors believe that the insulin of choice in the management of diabetic coma should be monocomponent porcine insulin when a low-dose infusion is used. Unfortunately, it is impossible to gauge whether there might have been a fall in plasma glucose at 3½ hr with continuation of the initial insulin program.

In a study to compare the effectiveness of various routes of insulin administration, Guerra and Kitabchi (1976) found that in normal lean subjects, insulin injected by the intramuscular route provides a fast absorption of insulin and can account for a greater drop in plasma glucose than does injection by the subcutaneous route. As expected, intravenous insulin produced the highest pharmacological levels of insulin in 2 min. When rapid insulinization is desirable in the treatment of diabetic ketoacidosis, the advantage of an initial intravenous bolus of insulin is obvious as compared with even intramuscular insulin, with which peak plasma insulin levels may not be reached for a mean of 50 min after administration.

A pharmacokinetic model of the insulin–glucose system was used to examine the effectiveness of insulin administered by a variety of routes and regimens for the treatment of diabetic ketoacidosis (Hayton and Grisafe, 1976). The results of this analysis show that an initial intravenous bolus of insulin followed immediately by an intravenous infusion or an intermittent bolus may provide the optimum therapeutic response to insulin for patients with diabetic ketoacidosis. The initial decline of the plasma glucose level was relatively slow with both the intramuscular and constant-rate infusion regimens (without initial bolus). An additional problem with the intramuscular route was the accumulation of insulin at sites of administration, making judgment of the appropriate time to discontinue insulin difficult. Both regimens, the hourly intravenous bolus and the constant-rate infusion with loading dose, caused a prompt decline in the plasma glucose level. The potential for causing hypoglycemia was low provided insulin was discontinued when plasma glucose reached 180 mg/dl. It should be noted that the insulin–glucose model used was determined in normal subjects, not in patients with diabetic ketoacidosis.

Insulin is adsorbed to the solid surfaces of commonly used infusion sets (Peterson *et al.,* 1976). Because of the interest in the use of insulin infusions for ketoacidosis, the need for protein other than insulin in the infusion solution to prevent loss of insulin by adsorption was evaluated. It was concluded that if an insulin concentration of at least 25 U/500 ml is used and if 50 cc is washed through the infusion apparatus before treatment of a hyperglycemic patient is instituted, the sites of nonspecific binding of insulin are saturated and further loss of insulin through adsorption is minimal. Under these conditions, the authors conclude that no extra protein additives are necessary.

Cerebral edema has been an unpredictable and generally fatal complication of diabetic ketoacidosis, particularly in children. Duck *et al.* (1976) reported four cases of cerebral edema associated with therapy for diabetic ketoacidosis and reviewed the common characteristics of other reported cases. They conclude that (1) patients admitted with diabetic ketoacidosis who have or who develop hypernatremia may be at an increased risk of developing cerebral edema; (2) cerebral edema associated with therapy of diabetic ketoacidosis has not been reported with rates of fluid administration less than 4 liters/m^2 per 24 hr; and (3) if recognized early, cerebral edema associated with therapy for ketoacidosis may be reversible.

Lim and Walsh (1976), reported two patients who were diagnosed as having diabetic ketoacidosis on admission and who were actually found to have a metabolic alkalosis. Both patients had been vomiting and one had diarrhea in addition. One had been taking alkali. Both patients were dehydrated and had ketonuria. Both were tachypneic. These patients demonstrated the importance of a hydrogen-ion measurement in the initial investigation of patients thought to be in diabetic ketoacidosis. The use of alkali in replacement therapy of these patients would have been inappropriate.

2.8.2.2. Chronic Therapy

In the United States, the insulins available at present are of the single-peak variety, which are purer insulin preparations than the older commercially available ones. More highly purified preparations such as monocomponent porcine insulin is available only on special request in the United States. Danish manufacturers have made available monocomponent preparations for routine therapy in Europe, as well as "fractionated" insulin in soluble and isophane (NPH) preparations. An editorial in *The Lancet* (1976) reviews the relative advantages and disadvantages of high-purity insulins. With their use, plasma insulin-binding capacity by insulin antibodies is usually but not uniformly reduced, resulting in lower daily insulin dosages. Allergic reactions are fewer, lipoatrophy does not occur, and the remission phase of the initial insulin treatment may be longer. These advantages are offset by production losses of considerable insulin with possible future worldwide shortages of insulin preparations, the higher price of pure products, and the possible hazard of changing to a new insulin at the same dose. This hazard has not been a problem. No convincing change in the quality of diabetic control has been reported when patients have switched to new insulins. There is no evidence that high-purity monospecies insulins will result in a reduction in incidence of diabetic complications. An anaphylactoid reaction to a monocomponent pork insulin was reported in a patient in whom desensitization was attempted with monocomponent regular pork insulin (Goldman *et al.*, 1976). The patient had exhibited local skin erythemia with the monocomponent pork insulin.

Insulin-induced lipoatrophy, a sharply defined disappearance of subcutaneous fat without exudative reactions and appreciable fibrosis, occurs commonly, particularly in girls under 20 years of age. Hulst (1976) reports the successful treatment of 20 children with insulin-induced lipoatrophy by injecting the insulin into the lipoatrophic area. In 10 children, insulin therapy with monocomponent insulin resulted in a disappearance of the lipoatrophy after 2 months of treatment. In 10 other children in whom the previously used insulin was injected into the lipoatrophic area, essentially the same type of recovery resulted. Lipoatrophy could still be observed after 2 months of treatment, however, and complete disappearance was found only after 6 months. These data suggest that the primary factor in treating insulin-induced lipoatrophy is the careful injection of insulin into the atrophic area. Since no lipoatrophy has yet been reported in patients treated with monocomponent insulin, it may be advisable to start insulin treatment in young diabetics with monocomponent insulins in countries in which it is available. Less purified insulins, however are also suitable for treating this complication of insulin therapy when the insulin is injected carefully into the lipoatrophic area.

Under normal physiological circumstances, insulin is secreted into the portal circulation. For the treatment of diabetes, insulin is administered via the peripheral circulation. Insulin administered by artificial endocrine pancreas restored glucose homeostasis in anesthetized pancreatectomized dogs and in labile human diabetics given regular meals. Insulin has been infused under computer control into a peripheral vein. Botz *et al.* (1976) assessed whether intraportal rather than a peripheral route of administration would more closely approximate the physiological situation. In anesthetized normal and pancreatectomized dogs, the results show no significant difference between intraportal and peripheral intravenous insulin infusion in terms of glycemic response, peripheral plasma insulin levels, insulin infusion patterns, and total insulin requirements during the steady state or during the changing glucose concentrations that result from the glucose loading test. It is apparent that the peripheral route, which is more readily accessible than the portal route, may be an appropriate infusion site for an implantable or portable prosthesis for controlling blood glucose concentrations.

Near-normal blood glucose fluctuations can be achieved in brittle diabetics by preplanned insulin infusion without blood glucose monitoring. An important prerequisite for successful insulin infusion treatment was a fairly good estimate of the daily insulin requirement (Deckert and Lørup, 1976). Insulin was infused intravenously over 24-hr periods but at varying rates that could imitate physiological plasma insulin variations in nondiabetics.

2.8.3. Oral Hypoglycemic Therapy

2.8.3.1. Sulfonylureas

There was published by the University Group Diabetes Program (1976) a supplementary report dealing with the development of nonfatal events in patients assigned to placebo (PL), tolbutamide (Tolb), insulin-standard (ISTD), or insulin-variable (IVAR) groups based on observations reported at all quarterly examinations completed up to and including the time when Tolb therapy was discontinued. Review of all findings for fatal and nonfatal events provides no evidence of benefit associated with the long-term use of Tolb. There were few differences among the groups in the occurrence of nonfatal events or conditions. The occurrence of myocardial infarctions as well as other vascular changes was about the same in all treatment groups, even though the Tolb and IVAR groups had lower blood glucose levels. The investigators state that attempts to normalize blood glucose levels in the MOD patient will not alter the incidence of vascular complications. They recognize that few patients were found to have renal or occular disorders over the period covered by this report. They do not state that good control, by their own criteria, was obtained in only 49% of the patients treated with IVAR. The excess mortality in the Tolb group over that of patients treated with diet plus insulin appears to be the result of increased mortality among Tolb patients who had sustained a myocardial infarction. The mortality for patients who had at least one myocardial infarction during the course of follow-up was 50% for patients in the Tolb group and 18% for patients in the PL group ($P < 0.01$) The mortality for such patients in the insulin-treated groups was 35% for ISTD and 40% for IVAR (NS). The investigators state that these observations are consistent with previously published observations that sulfonylurea drugs may produce an enhanced inotropic effect on heart muscle and increased automaticity of the Purkinje fibers, since these factors may increase the extent of ischemic myocardial damage and lead to arrhythmias.

In another study of the cardiac pharmacology of tolbutamide, Curtis *et al.* (1975) concluded that there is a small species-specific inotropic effect in the rabbit but not in the cat or dog, and, in addition, that this inotropic effect is small compared with the maximum response, which is observed only *in vitro.* Tolbutamide had no effect on cardiac pacemaker activity. The investigators concluded that their data failed to support previous conclusions suggesting deleterious cardiac effects of tolbutamide.

2.8.3.2. Phenformin

Phenformin-associated or -induced lactic acidosis continues to be reported (Fulop and Hoberman, 1976; Fulop *et al.,* 1976; Conlay and Loewenstein, 1976; Blumenthal and Streeten, 1976). Fulop and Hoberman (1976) reported on 18 consecutive phenformin-treated diabetic patients admitted to their medical service acutely ill with metabolic acidosis. Lactic acidosis was documented in all. All had coexisting elevation of plasma 3-hydroxybutyrate. The authors suggest that treatment of these patients should include insulin and glucose, since most do not have marked hyperglycemia and some of these patients have hypoglycemia. The patients ranged in age from 45 to 88 years, with a mean of 72 years. Nine patients died; survival correlated closely with the absence of shock on arrival. In 10 patients, there was no discernible cause for the acute illness apart from the teatment with phenformin. Conditions that lead to vascular insufficiency may cause an accumulation of phenformin and aggravate or cause severe lactic acidosis. In the absence of such predisposing factors, a mild intercurrent illness can cause dehydration leading to a decrease in glomerular filtration and retention of phenformin, which can cause lactic acidosis. The authors conclude that since this disorder can occur in the absence of other acute life-threatening illness and because patients treated with phenformin are often elderly with other disorders that may limit their ability to compensate for physiological disturbances, the use of phenformin in the treatment of diabetes mellitus should be avoided. In another report, Fulop *et al.* (1976) documented coexisting lactic acidosis in 7 of 39 patients with ketoacidosis.

Conlay and Loewenstein (1976) reported that 5 patients, aged 49–86 years, with severe lactic acidosis admitted to a university teaching hospital during a 17-month period were taking phenformin hydrochloride. Prerenal azotemia was present at the time of admission in all, since renal function was normal at the time of discharge in those patients who survived the lactic acidosis. The authors also concluded that phenformin should be restricted severely or removed from use. Lactic acidosis may occur in young patients as well. Blumenthal and Streeten (1976) reported a 30-year-old man, treated with 250 mg phenformin, who developed lactic acidosis. The patient was severely dehydrated, impairing renal excretion of phenformin, which in turn led to higher plasma and tissue concentration of the drug. The patient also received tetracycline, also potentially nephrotoxic. Other cases of lactic acidosis in phenformin- and tetracycline-treated patients have been reported, and an interaction between the two drugs in predisposing to lactic acidosis was suggested by P. J. Phillips and Pain (1977).

In reviewing the University Group Diabetes Program (1975) report on increased mortality observed in the phenformin treatment group, Williams and Palmer (1975) suggested that the excess mortality, elevated blood pressure, and occurrence of lactic acidosis observed in the phenformin-treated patients make it extremely difficult to justify further treatment of diabetes with this drug. Indeed, the manufacturer of phenformin, Geigy Pharmaceuticals, has issued an important new warning on the use of phenformin in the treatment of diabetes. Since there have been numerous reports of lactic acidosis associated with phenformin therapy and since lactic acidosis is an often fatal metabolic acidosis, the manufacturers stress the increased risk of lactic acidosis in recommending a severely restricted use of the drug. These warnings, which are reproduced in the drug package insert, should be read by all physicians when considering the use or continued use of phenformin in any patient. For practical purposes, phenformin should not be employed in the management of patients with diabetes mellitus.

References

Abell, D. A., and Beischer, N. A., 1976, Effects of hypoglycaemia and hyperglycaemia on pregnancy outcome, *Aust. N. Z. J. Obstet. Gynaecol.* **16**:75.

Almér, L.-O., and Pandolfi, M., 1976, Fibrinolysis and diabetic retinopathy, *Diabetes* **25** (Suppl. 2): 807.

Andersen, J. T., and Bradley, W. E., 1976, Early detection of diabetic visceral neuropathy: An electrophysiologic study of bladder and urethral innervation, *Diabetes* **25**:1100.

Aronoff, S. L., Bennett, P. H., Williamson, J. R., Siperstein, M. D., Plumer, M. E., and Miller, M., 1976, Muscle capillary basement membrane (MCBM) measurements in prediabetic, diabetic, and normal Pima Indians and normal Caucasians, *Clin. Res.* **24**:455A.

Baba, S., Morita, S., Mizuno, N., and Okada, K., 1976, Autoimmunity to glucagon in a diabetic not on insulin, *Lancet* **2**:585.

Barbosa, J., Noreen, H., Doe, R. P., and Yunis, E. J., 1976, The genetic heterogeneity of diabetes: Histocompatibility antigens *(HLA)* in families with maturity-onset type diabetes of the young (MODY) and juvenile, insulin dependent diabetes (JID), *Diabetes* **25**:336.

Beisswenger, P. J., 1976, Glomerular basement membrane: Biosynthesis and chemical composition in the streptozotocin diabetic rat, *J. Clin. Invest.* **58**:44.

Bennett, P. H., Rushforth, N. B., Miller, M., and LeCompte, P. M., 1976, Epidemiologic studies of diabetes in the Pima Indians, *Rec. Prog. Horm. Res.* **32**:333.

Berger, M., Baumhoff, E., and Gries, F. A., 1976, Gewichtsreducktion und Glucose-intoleranz bei Adipositas, *Deutsch. Med. Wochenschr.* **101**:307.

Birmingham Diabetes Survey Working Party (Report by the), 1976, Ten-year follow-up report on Birmingham Diabetes Survey of 1961, *Br. Med. J.* **2**:35.

Bistrian, B. R., Blackburn, G. L., Flatt, J. P., Sizer, J., Scrimshaw, N. S., and Sherman, M., 1976, Nitrogen metabolism and insulin requirements in obese diabetic adults on a protein-sparing modified fast, *Diabetes* **25**:494.

Blumenthal, S. A., and Streeten, D. H. P., 1976, Phenformin-related lactic acidosis in a thirty-year-old man, *Ann. Intern. Med.* **84**:55.

Bottazzo, G. F., and Doniach, D., 1976, Pancreatic autoimmunity and *HLA* antigens, *Lancet* **2**:800.

Bottazzo, G. F., and Lendrum, R., 1976, Separate autoantibodies to human pancreatic glucagon and somatostatin cells, *Lancet* **2**:873.

Bottazzo, G. F., Florin-Christensen, A., and Doniach, D., 1974, Islet-cell antibodies in diabetes mellitus with autoimmune polyendocrine deficiencies, *Lancet* **2**:1279.

Bottazzo, G. F., Doniach, D., and Pouplard, A., 1976, Humoral autoimmunity in diabetes mellitus, *Acta Endocrinol. (Copenhagen),* Suppl. 205, pp. 55–61.

Botz, C. K., Leibel, B. S., Zingg, W., Gander, R. E., and Albisser, A. M., 1976, Comparison of peripheral and portal routes of insulin infusion by a computer-controlled insulin infusion system (artificial endocrine pancreas), *Diabetes* **25**:691.

Brunzell, J. D., Robertson, R. P., Lerner, R. L., Hazzard, W. R., Ensinck, J. W., Bierman, E. L., and Porte, D., Jr., 1976, Relationships between fasting plasma glucose levels and insulin secretion during intravenous glucose tolerance tests, *J. Clin. Endocrinol. Metal.* **42**:222.

Buck, A. C., Reed, I., Siddiq, Y. K., Chisholm, G. D., and Fraser, T. R., 1976, Bladder dysfunction and neuropathy in diabetes, *Diabetologia* **12**:251.

Bunn, H. F., Haney, D. N., Kamin, S., Gabbay, K. H., and Gallop, P. M., 1976, The biosynthesis of human hemoglobin $A_{1C'}$, *J. Clin. Invest.* **57**:1652.

Burch, P. R. J., 1976, Diabetes mellitus: Concordance in monozygotic twins, *Lancet* **2**:632.

Cahill, G. F., Etzwiler, D. D., and Freinkel, N., 1976, "Control" and diabetes (editorial), *N. Engl. J. Med.* **294**:1004.

Campbell, I. W., Ewing, D. J., Harrower, A. B. D., Neilson, J. M. M., Faser, D. M., Baldwa, V. S., Murray, A., and Clarke, B. F., 1976, Peripheral and autonomic nerve function in diabetic ketoacidosis, *Lancet* **2**:167.

Cattaneo, R., Saibene, V., and Pozza, G., 1976, Peripheral T-lymphocytes in juvenile-onset diabetes (JOD) and in maturity-onset diabetes (MOD), *Diabetes* **25**:223.

Christlieb, A. R., 1976, Renin–angiotensin–aldosterone system in diabetes mellitus, *Diabetes* **25** (Suppl. 2): 820.

Christlieb, A. R., Janka, H. U., Kraus, B., Gleason, R. E., Icasas-Cabral, E. A., Aiello, L. M., Cabral, B. V., and Solano, A., 1976a, Vascular reactivity to angiotensin II and to norepinephrine in diabetic subjects, *Diabetes* **25**:268.

Christlieb, A. R., Kaldany, A., and D'Elia, J. A., 1976b, Plasma renin activity and hypertension in diabetes mellitus, *Diabetes* **25**:969.

Christy, M., Nerup, J., Bottazzo, G. F., Doniach, D., Platz, P., Svejgaard, A., Ryder, L. P., and Thomsen, M., 1976, Association between HLA-B8 and autoimmunity in juvenile diabetes mellitus, *Lancet* **2**:142.

Conlay, L. A., and Loewenstein, J. E., 1976, Phenformin and lactic acidosis, *J. Am. Med. Assoc.* **235**:1575.

Craighead, J. E., 1976, Virus induced insulitis in experimental animal models, *Acta Endocrinol.* **83** *(Suppl. 205)*:123.

Crapo, P. A., Reaven, G., and Olefsky, J., 1976, Plasma glucose and insulin responses to orally administered simple and complex carbohydrates, *Diabetes* **25**:741.

Creutzfeldt, W., Köbberling, J. and Neel, J. V. (eds.), 1976, *The Genetics of Diabetes Mellitus*, p. 248, Springer-Verlag, Heidelberg, Berlin, and New York.

Crockett, S. E., Mazzaferri, E. L., and Cataland, S., 1976a, Gastric inhibitory polypeptide (GIP) in maturity-onset diabetes mellitus, *Diabetes* **25**:931.

Crockett, S. E., Cataland, S., Falko, J. M., and Mazzaferri, E. L., 1976b, The insulinotropic effect of endogenous gastric inhibitory polypeptide in normal subjects, *J. Clin. Endocrinol. Metab.* **42**:1098.

Cudworth, A. G., 1976, The aetiology of diabetes mellitus, *Br. J. Hosp. Med.* **16**:207.

Cudworth, A. G., and Woodrow, J. C., 1976a, Genetic susceptibility in diabetic identical twins, *Lancet* **2**:518.

Cudworth, A. G., and Woodrow, J. C., 1976b, Genetic susceptibility in diabetes mellitus: Analysis of the *HLA* association, *Br. Med. J.* **2**:846.

Curtis, G. P., Setchfield, J., and Lucchesi, B. R., 1975, The cardiac pharmacology of tolbutamide, *J. Pharmacol. Exp. Ther.* **194**:264.

Deckert, T., and Lørup, B., Regulation of brittle diabetics by a preplanned insulin infusion programme, *Diabetologia* **12**:573.

DeLeiva, A., Christlieb, A. R., Melby, J. C., Graham, C. A., Day, R. P., Luetscher, J. A., and Zager, P. G., 1976, Big renin and biosynthetic defect of aldosterone in diabetes mellitus, *N. Engl. J. Med.* **295**:639.

Del Prete, G. F., Betterle, C., Bersani, G., Romano, M., and Tiengo, A., 1976, Pancreatic islet-cell autoimmunity, *Lancet* **2**:1090.

Diabetic Retinopathy Study Research Group, 1976, Preliminary report on effects of photocoagulation therapy, *Am. J. Ophthalmol.* **81**:383.

Doar, J. W. H., Thompson, M. E., Wilde, C. E., and Sewell, P. F. J., 1975, Influence of treatment with diet alone on oral glucose-tolerance test and plasma sugar and insulin levels in patients with maturity-onset diabetes mellitus, *Lancet* **1**:1263.

Dorf, A., Ballintine, E. J., Bennett, P. H., and Miller, M., 1976, Retinopathy in Pima Indians, *Diabetes* **25**:554.

Duck, S. C., Weldon, V. V., Pagliara, A. S., and Haymond, M. W., 1976, Cerebral edema complicating therapy for diabetic ketoacidosis, *Diabetes* **25**:111.

Duckworth, W. C., and Kitabchi, A. E., 1976, The effect of age on plasma proinsulin-like material after oral glucose, *J. Lab. Clin. Med.* **88**:359.

Ebert, R., Creutzfeldt, W., Brown, J. C., Frerich, S. H., and Arnaud, R., 1976, Response of gastric inhibitory polypeptide (GIP) to test meal in chronic pancreatitis—relationship to endocrine and exocrine insufficiency, *Diabetologia* **12**:609.

Ellenberg, M., 1976, Diabetic neuropathy: Clinical aspects, *Metabolism* **25**:1627.

Ewing, D. J., Campbell, I. W., and Clarke, B. F., 1976, Mortality in diabetic autonomic neuropathy, *Lancet* **1**:601.

Fajans, S. S., 1976, Diabetes mellitus, in: *The Year in Metabolism 1975–1976* (N. Freinkel, ed.), Chapt. 2, pp. 45–71, Plenum Publishing Corp., New York.

Fajans, S. S., and Freinkel, N., 1976, The problem of diabetes mellitus, in: *Diabetes Mellitus,* Fogarty International Center Series on Preventative Medicine, Vol. 4, Chapt. 1, p. 1, DHEW, Publ. No. 76-854, National Institutes of Health, Bethesda, Maryland.

Fajans, S. S., Floyd, J. C., Jr., Knopf, R. F., Pek, S., Weissman, P. N., and Conn, J. W., 1972, Amino acids and insulin release *in vivo, Isr. J. Med. Sci.* **8**:223.

Fajans, S. S., Floyd, J. C., Jr., Tattersall, R. B., Williamson, J. R., Pek, S., and Taylor, C. I., 1976, The various faces of diabetes in the young, *Arch. Intern. Med.* **136**:194.

Fekete, T., Rub, D., and Bogdan, E., 1976, Absence of respiratory arrhythmia: A possible symptom of cardiac autonomic neuropathy in diabetes mellitus, *Diabetologia* **12**:390.

Feldman, J. M., and Plonk, J. W., 1976, Effect of age on intravenous glucose tolerance and insulin secretion, *J. Am. Geriatr. Soc.* **24**:1.

Fitzgibbons, J. F., Koler, R. D., and Jones, R. T., 1976, Red cell age-related changes of hemoglobins A_{Iab} and A_{Ic} in normal and diabetic subjects, *J. Clin. Invest.* **58**:820.

Flier, J. S., Kahn, R., Jarrett, D. B., and Roth, J., 1976, Characterization of antibodies to the insulin receptor, *J. Clin. Invest.* **58**:1442.

Fulop, M., and Hoberman, H. D., 1976, Phenformin-associated metabolic acidosis, *Diabetes* **25**:292.

Fulop, M., Hoberman, H. D., Rascoff, J. H., Bonheim, N. A., Dreyer, N. P., and Tannenbaum, H., 1976, Lactic acidosis in diabetic patients, *Arch. Intern. Med.* **136**:987.

Gabbay, K. H., 1976, Glycosylated hemoglobin and diabetic control, *N. Engl. J. Med.* **295**:443.

Gabbay, K. H., Haney, D. N., Hasty, K., Gallop, P. M., and Bunn, H. F., 1976, Glycosylation of hemoglobin *in vivo:* A monitor of diabetic control?, *Diabetes* **25**:335.

Genuth, S. M., Houser, H. B., Carter, J. R., Jr., Merkatz, I., Price, J. W., Schumacker, O. P., and Wieland, R. G., 1976, Community screening for diabetes by blood glucose measurement, *Diabetes* **25**:1110.

Goldman, R. A., Lewis, A. E., and Rose, L. I., 1976, Anaphylactoid reaction to single-component pork insulin, *J. Am. Med. Assoc.* **236**:1148.

Greenwood, R. H., Mahler, R. F., and Hales, C. N., 1976, Improvement in insulin secretion in diabetes after diazoxide, *Lancet* **1**:444.

Guerra, S. O., and Kitabchi, A. E., 1976, Comparison of the effectiveness of various routes of insulin injection: Insulin levels of glucose response in normal subjects, *J. Clin. Endocrinol. Metal.* **42**:869.

Haney, D. N., and Bunn, H. F., 1976, Glycosylation of hemoglobin *in vitro:* Affinity labeling of hemoglobin by glucose-6-phosphate, *Proc. Natl. Acad. Sci. U.S.A.* **73**:3534.

Hann, S., Kaye, R., and Falkner, B., 1976, Subpopulations of peripheral lymphocytes in juvenile diabetes, *Diabetes* **25**:101.

Hayton, W. L., and Grisafe, J. A., 1976, Pharmacokinetic evaluation of dosing regimens for insulin in diabetic ketoacidosis, *Diabetes* **25**:771.

Heath, H., and Hamlett, Y. C., 1976, The sorbitol pathway: Effect of streptozotocin induced diabetes and the feeding of a sucrose-rich diet on glucose, sorbitol and fructose in the retina, blood and liver of rats, *Diabetologia* **12**:43.

Holt, S., and Cudworth, A. G., 1976, Insulin resistance during continuous infusion, *Lancet* **1**:44.

Horwitz, D. L., Kuzuya, H., and Rubenstein, A. H., 1976, Circulating serum C-peptide, *N. Engl. J. Med.* **295**:207.

Huang, S.-W., and McLaren, N., 1976, Insulin-dependent diabetes: A disease of autoaggression, *Science* **192**:64.

Hulst, S. G. T., 1976, Treatment of insulin-induced lipoatrophy, *Diabetes* **25**:1052.

Ingelfinger, J. A., Bennett, P. H., Liebow, I. M., and Miller, M., 1976, Coronary heart disease in the Pima Indians: Electrocardiographic findings and postmortem evidence of myocardial infarction in a population with a high prevalence of diabetes mellitus, *Diabetes* **25**:561.

Irvine, W. J., Gray, R. S., and McCallum, C. J., 1976a, Pancreatic islet-cell antibody as a marker for asymptomatic and latent diabetes and prediabetes, *Lancet* **2**:1097.

Irvine, W. J., MacCuish, A. C., Campbell, J., and Duncan, L. J. P., 1976b, Organ specific cell-mediated autoimmunity in diabetes mellitus, *Acta. Endocrinol. (Copenhagen)*, Suppl. 205, p. 65.

Jarrett, R. J., and Keen, H., 1976, Hyperglycemia and diabetes mellitus, *Lancet* **2**:1009.

Jenkins, D. J. A., Leeds, A. R. Wolever, T. M. S., Goff, D. V., Alberti, K. G. M. M., Gasull, M. A., and Hockaday, T. D. R., 1976, Unabsorbable carbohydrates and diabetes: Decreased postprandial hyperglycemia, *Lancet* **2**:172.

Job, D., Eschwege, E., Guyot-Argenton, C., Aubry, J.-P., and Tchobroutsky, G., 1976, Effect of multiple daily insulin injections on the course of diabetic retinopathy, *Diabetes* **25**:463.

Jonsson, A., and Wales, J. K., 1976, Blood glycoprotein levels in diabetes mellitus, *Diabetologia* **12**:245.

Kahn, C. R., Flier, J. S., Bar, R. S., Archer, J. A., Gorden, P., Martin, M. M., and Roth, J., 1976, The syndromes of insulin resistance and acanthosis nigricans: Insulin-receptor disorders in man, *N. Engl. J. Med.* **294**:739.

Karam, J. H., Rosenthal, M., O'Donnell, J. D., Tsalikian, E., Lorenzi, M. Gerich, J. E., Siperstein, M. D., and Forsham, P. H., 1976, Discordance of diabetic microangiopathy in identical twins, *Diabetes* **25**:24.

Kimmerling, G., Javorski, W. C., Olefsky, J. M., and Reaven, G. M., 1976, Locating the site(s) of insulin resistance in patients with nonketotic diabetes mellitus, *Diabetes* **25**:673.

Kitabchi, A. E., Ayyagari, V., Guerra, S. M. O., and Medical House Staff, Memphis, Tennessee, 1976, The efficacy of low-dose versus conventional therapy of insulin for treatment of diabetic ketoacidosis, *Ann. Intern. Med.* **84**:633.

Koenig, R. J., Peterson, C. M., Jones, R. L., Saudek, C., Lehrman, M., and Cerami, A., 1976a, Correlation of glucose regulation and hemoglobin A_{IC} in diabetes mellitus, *N. Engl. J. Med.* **295**:417.

Koenig, R. J., Peterson, C. M., Kilo, C., Cerami, A., and Williamson, J. R., 1976b, Hemoglobin A_{IC} as an indicator of the degree of glucose intolerance in diabetes, *Diabetes* **25**:230.

Koenig, R. J., Araujo, D. C., and Cerami, A., 1976c, Increased hemoglobin A_{IC} in diabetic mice, *Diabetes* **25**:1.

Kohner, E. M., Hamilton, A. M., Joplin, G. F., and Fraser, T. R., 1976, Florid diabetic retinopathy and its response to treatment by photocoagulation or pituitary ablation, *Diabetes* **25**:104.

Kussman, M. J., Goldstein, H., and Gleason, R. E., 1976, The clinical course of diabetic nephropathy, *J. Am. Med. Assoc* **236**:1861.

Kuzuya, H., Blix, P. M., Horwitz, D. L., Steiner, D. F., and Ruberstein, A. H., 1977, Determination of free and total insulin and C-peptide in insulin-treated diabetics, *Diabetes* **26**:22.

Kuzuya, T., Matsuda, A., Saito, T. and Yoshida, S., 1976, Human C-peptide immunoreactivity (CPR) in blood and urine-evaluation of a radioimmunoassay method and its clinical applications, *Diabetologia* **12**:511.

Lancet, 1976, Hyperglycemia and hypoglycemia during pregnancy (editorial), **2**:889.

Lang, C. M., and Munger, B. L., 1976, Diabetes mellitus in the guinea pig, *Diabetes* **25**:434.

Ledet, T., 1976, Growth hormone stimulating the growth of arterial medial cells *in vitro:* Absence of effect of insulin, *Diabetes* **25**:1011.

Ledet, T., Fisher-Dzoga, K., and Wissler, R. W., 1976, Growth of rabbit aortic smooth-muscle cells cultured in media containing diabetic and hyperlipemic serum, *Diabetes* **25**:207.

Lendrum, R., Walker, G., Cudworth, A. G., Theophanides, C., Pyke, D. A., Bloom, A., and Gamble, D. R., 1976a, Islet-cell antibodies in diabetes mellitus, *Lancet* **2**:1273.

Lendrum, R., Walker, G., Cudworth, A. G., Woodrow, J. C., and Gamble, D. R., 1976b, *HLA*-linked genes and islet-cell antibodies in diabetes mellitus, *Br. Med. J.* **1**:1565.

Lestradet, H., Deschamps, I., and Giron, B., 1976, Insulin and free fatty acid levels during oral glucose tolerance test and their relation to age in 70 healthy children, *Diabetes* **25**:505.

Levin, M. E., Boisseau, V. C., and Avioli, L. V., 1976, Effects of diabetes mellitus on bone mass in juvenile and adult-onset diabetes, *N. Engl. J. Med.* **294**:241.

Lewis, S. B., Wallin, J. D., Kuzuya, H., Murray, W. K., Coustan, D. R., Daane, T. A., and Rubenstein, A. H., 1976, Circadian variations of serum glucose, C-peptide immunoreactivity and free insulin in normal and insulin-treated diabetic pregnant subjects, *Diabetologia* **12**:343.

Like, A. A. and Rossini, A. A., 1976, Streptozotocin-induced pancreatic insulitis: New model of diabetes mellitus, *Science* **193**:415.

Lim, K. C., and Walsh, C. H., 1976, Diabetic ketoalkalosis: Readily mid-diagnosed entity, *Br. Med. J.* **2**:19.

Llovd-Mostyn, R. H., and Watkins, P. J., 1975, Defective innervation of heart in diabetic autonomic neuropathy, *Br. Med. J.* **3**:15.

Lloyd-Mostyn, R. H., and Watkins, P. J., 1976, Total cardiac denervation in diabetic autonomic neuropathy, *Diabetes* **25**:748.

Ludvigsson, J., and Heding, L. G., 1976, C-Peptide in children with juvenile diabetes: A preliminary report, *Diabetologia* **12**:627.

Ludwig, H., Eibl, M., Schernthaner, G., Erd, W., and Mayr, W. R., 1976a, Humoral immunodeficiency to bacterial antigens in patients with juvenile onset diabetes mellitus, *Diabetologia* **12**:259.

Ludwig, H., Schernthaner, G., and Mayr, W. R., 1976b, Is HLA-B7 a marker association with a protective gene in juvenile-onset diabetes mellitus?, *N. Engl. J. Med.* **294**:1066.

MacCuish, A. C., Irvine, W. J., Barnes, E. W., and Duncan, L. H., 1974, Antibodies to pancreatic islet cells in insulin-dependent diabetics with coexistent autoimmune disease, *Lancet* **2**:1529.

Madison, L. L., 1976, Low-dose insulin: A plea for caution (editorial), *N. Engl. J. Med.* **294**:393.

Mahmoud, A. A. F., Rodman, H. M., Mandel, M. A., and Warren, K. S., 1976, Induced and spontaneous diabetes mellitus and suppression of cell-mediated immunologic responses: Granuloma formation, delayed dermal reacitivty, and allograft rejection, *J. Clin. Invest.* **57**:362.

Matas, A. J., Sutherland, D. E. R., and Najarian, A. S., 1976, Current status of islet and pancreas transplantation in diabetes, *Diabetes* **25**:785.

Mauer, S. M., Miller, K., Goetz, F. C., Barbosa, J., Simmons, R. L., Najarian, J. S., and Michael, A. F., 1976a, Immunopathology of renal extracellular membranes in kidneys transplanted into patients with diabetes mellitus, *Diabetes* **25**:709.

Mauer, S. M., Steffes, M. W., Michael, A. F., and Brown, D. M., 1976b, Studies of diabetic nephropathy in animals and man, *Diabetes* **25** (Suppl. 2):850.

Mauer, S. M., Barbosa, J., Vernier, R. L., Kjellstrand, C. M., Buselmeier, T. J., Simmons, R. L., Najarian, J. S., and Goetz, F. C., 1976c, Development of diabetic vascular lesions in normal kidneys transplanted into patients with diabetes mellitus, *N. Engl. J. Med.* **295**:916.

Maugh, T. H., II, 1976a, Hormone receptors: New clues to the cause of diabetes, *Science* **193**:220.

Maugh, T. H., II, 1976b, Diabetic retinopathy: New ways to prevent blindness, *Science* **192**:539.

Mayer, K. H., Stamler, J., Dyer, A., Freinkel, N., Stamler, R., Berkson, D. M., and Farber, B., 1976, Epidemiologic findings on the relationship of time of day and time since last meal to glucose tolerance, *Diabetes* **25**:936.

McMillan, D. E., 1976, Plasma protein changes, blood viscosity, and diabetic microangiopathy, *Diabetes* **25**:858.

McMillan, and Ditzel, J. (eds.), 1976, Proceedings of the conference on diabetic microangiopathy, *Diabetes* **25** (Suppl. 2): 805.

Miller, K., and Michael, A. F., 1976, Immunopathology of renal extracellular membranes in diabetes mellitus—specifically of tubular basement-membrane immunofluorescence, *Diabetes* **25**:701.

Mogensen, C. E., 1976, Renal function changes in diabetes, *Diabetes* **25**:872.

Morris, P. J., Irvine, W. J., Gray, R. S., Duncan, L. J. P., Vaughan, H., McCallum, F. J., Campbell, C. J., and Farguhar, J. W., 1976, *HLA* and pancreatic islet cell antibodies in diabetes, *Lancet* **2**:652.

Morse, P. H., and Duncan, T. G., 1976, Ophthalmologic management of diabetic retinopathy, *N. Engl. J. Med.* **295**:87.

Nelson, P. G., and Pyke, D. A., 1976, Genetic diabetes not linked to the *HLA* locus, *Br. Med. J.* **1**:196.

Nerup, J., Ortved-Anderson, O., Christy, M., Platz, P., Ryder, L., Thomsen, M., and Svejgarrd, A., 1976, *HLA,* autoimmunity, virus and the pathogenesis of juvenile diabetes mellitus, *Acta Endocrinol (Copenhagen),* Suppl. 205, p. 167.

Neubauer, B., and Gundersen, H. G., 1976, Early and progressive loss of autonomic control of the heart in diabetics measured on a standard, resting ECG, *Diabetologia* **12**:412.

Olefsky, J. M., 1976, The insulin receptor: Its role in insulin resistance of obesity and diabetes, *Diabetes* **25**:1154.

Olefsky, J. M., and Reaven, G., 1976a, Insulin binding to monocytes and total mononuclear leukocytes from normal and diabetic patients, *J. Clin. Endocrinol. Metab.* **43**:226.

Olefsky, J. M., and Reaven, G. M., 1976b, Effects of sulfonylurea therapy on insulin binding to mononuclear leukocytes of diabetic patients, *Am. J. Med.* **60**:89.

Page, M. McB., and Watkins, P. J., 1976, Provocation of postural hypotension by insulin in diabetic autonomic neuropathy, *Diabetes* **25**:90.

Pallavicini, M. G., and Nichols, W. K., 1976, Inhibition of lymphocyte blastogenesis by factor(s) in alloxan-diabetic rat plasma, *Diabetes* **25**:614.

Palmer, J. P., Benson, J. W., Walter, R. M., and Ensinck, J. W., 1976, Arginine-stimulated acute phase of insulin and glucagon secretion in diabetic subjects, *J. Clin. Invest.* **58**:565.

Papachristodoulous, D., Heath, H., and Kang, S. S., 1976, The development of retinopathy in sucrose-fed and streptozotocin-diabetic rats, *Diabetologia* **12**:367.

Parving, H.-H., 1976, Increased microvascular permeability to plasma proteins in short- and long-term juvenile diabetes, *Diabetes* **25**:884.

Parving, H.-H., Noer, I., Deckert, T., Evrin, P.-E., Nielsen, S. L., Lyngsøe, J., Mogensen, C. E., Rørth, M., Svendsen, P. A., Trap-Jensen, J., and Lassen, N. A., 1976, The effect of metabolic regulation on microvascular permeability to small and large molecules in short-term juvenile diabetics, *Diabetologia* **12**:161.

Paulsen, E. P., and Koury, M., 1976, Hemoglobin A_{IC} levels in insulin-dependent and -independent diabetes mellitus, *Diabetes* **25**:890.

Peterson, L., Caldwell, J., and Hoffman, J., 1976, Insulin absorbance to polyvinylchloride surfaces with implications for constant-infusion therapy, *Diabetes* **25**:72.

Phillips, L. S., and Young, H. S., 1976, Nutrition and somatomedin. II. Serum somatomedin activity and cartilage growth activity in streptozotocin-diabetic rats, *Diabetes* **25**:516.

Phillips, P. J., and Pain, R. B., 1977, Phenformin, tetracycline and lactic acidosis, *Ann. Intern. Med.* **86**:111.

Pulini, M., Raff, S., Chase, R., and Gordon, E. E., 1976, Insulin resistance and acanthosis nigricans: Report of a case with antibodies to insulin receptors, *Ann. Intern. Med.* **85**:749.

Pupo, A. A., Ursich, M. J. M., Iamaguchi, E., and Vasconcellos, F. G., 1976, Acute- and late-phase insulin secretion and glucose tolerance in mild alloxan diabetes in dogs, *Diabetes* **25**:161.

Pyke, D. A., Theophanides, C. G., and Tattersall, R. B., 1976a, Genetic origin of diabetes: Re-evaluation of twin data, *Lancet* **2**:464.

Pyke, D. A., Theophanides, C. G., and Tattersall, R. B., 1976b, Genetic origin of diabetes, *Lancet* **2**:1201.

Rayfield, E. J., Gorelkin, L., Curnow, R. T., and Jahrling, P. B., 1976, Virus-induced pancreatic disease by Venezuelan encephalitis virus: Alterations in glucose tolerance and insulin release, *Diabetes* **25**:623.

Reaven, G. M., 1976, Relationship between heterogeneity of insulin responses and insulin resistance in normal subjects and patients with chemical diabetes, *Diabetes* **25**:383.

Reaven, G. M., Bernstein, R., David, B., and Olefsky, J. M., 1976, Nonketotic diabetes mellitus: Insulin deficiency or insulin resistance?, *Am. J. Med.* **60**:80.

Rhodes, B. A., Bader, P., Stolz, K., White, R. I., and Siegel, M. E., 1976, Assessment of peripheral vascular disease in patients with diabetes: Two case studies, *Diabetes* **25**:307.

Rimoin, D. L., and Rotter, J. I., 1976, Inheritance of diabetes mellitus, *N. Engl. J. Med.* **295**:1321.

Ringe, J.-D., Kuhlencordt, F., and Kühnau, J., 1976, Mineralgehalt des Skeletts bei Langzeitdiabetikern, *Deutsch. Med. Wochenschr.* **101**:280.

Risteli, J., Koivisto, V. A., Åkerblom, H. K., and Kivirikko, K. I., 1976, Intracellular enzymes of collagen biosynthesis in rat kidney in streptozotocin diabetes, *Diabetes* **25**:1066.

Robert, M. F., Neff, R. K., Hubbell, J. P., Taeusch, H. W., and Avery, M. E., 1976, Association between maternal diabetes and the respiratory distress syndrome in the newborn, *N. Engl. J. Med.* **294**:357.

Robertson, R. P., Halter, J. B., and Porte, D., Jr., 1976, A role for alpha-adrenergic receptors in abnormal insulin secretion in diabetes mellitus, *J. Clin. Invest.* **57**:791.

Rosenthal, M. B., Goldfine, I. D., and Siperstein, M. D., 1976a, Genetic origin of diabetes: Re-evaluation of twin data, *Lancet* **2**:250.

Rosenthal, M. B., Goldfine, I. D., and Siperstein, M. D., 1976b, Genetic origin of diabetes, *Lancet* **2**:908.

Rosenthal, M. B., Goldfine, I. D., and Siperstein, M. D., 1976c, Inheritance of diabetes mellitus, *N. Engl. J. Med.* **295**:1321.

Ross, M. E., Onodera, T., Brown, K. S., and Notkins, A. L., 1976, Virus-induced diabetes mellitus. IV. Gentic and environmental factors influencing the development of diabetes after infection with the M variant of encephalomyocarditis virus, *Diabetes* **25**:190.

Rubinstein, P., Suciu-Foca, N., Nicholson, J. R., Fotina, M., Molinaro, A., Harisiadis, L., Hardy, M. A., Reemstsma,K., and Allen, F. H., Jr., 1976, The *HLA* system in the families of patients with juvenile diabetes mellitus, *J. Exp. Med.* **143**:1277.

Savage, P. J., Hamman, R. F., Bartha, G., Dipper, S. E., Miller, M., and Bennett, P. H., 1976, Serum cholesterol levels in American (Pima) Indian children and adolescents, *Pediatrics* **58**:274.

Schwartz, H. C., King, K. C., Schwartz, A. L., Edmunds, D., and Schwartz, R., 1976, Effects of pregnancy on hemoglobin A_{IC} in normal, gestational diabetic and diabetic women, *Diabetes* **25**:1118.

Seignalet, J., Mirouze, J., Jaffiol, C., Selan, J. L., and Lapinski, H., 1975, *HL-A* in Grave's disease and in diabetes mellitus, insulin-dependent, *Tissue Antigens* **6**:272.

Sheikholislam, B. M., Irias, J. J., Lin, H. J., Lowrey, G. H., Stephenson, S. R., Peterson, G. E., Devereaux, D. F., and Volk, T. L., 1976a, Carbohydrate metabolism and capillary basement-membrane thickness in children. I. Cross-sectional studies, *Diabetes* **25**:650.

Sheikholislam, B. M., Irias, J. J., Lowrey, G. H., and Lin, H. J., 1976b, Carbohydrate metabolism and capillary basement-membrane thickness in children. II. Longitudinal studies, *Diabetes* **25**:661.

Shideman, J. R., Buselmeier, T. J., and Kjellstrand, C. M., 1976, Hemodialysis in diabetics: Complication in insulin-dependent patients accepted for renal transplantation, *Arch. Intern. Med.* **136**:1126.

Sievers, M. L., 1976, Diabetes mellitus in American Indians—standards for diagnosis and management, *Diabetes* **25**:528.

Silberberg, R., and Gerritsen, G., 1976, Aging changes in intervertebral discs and spondylosis in Chinese hamsters, *Diabetes* **25**:477.

Siperstein, M. D., Raskin, P., and Burns, H., 1973, Electron microscopic quantification of diabetic microangiopathy, *Diabetes* **22**:514.

Spiro, R. G., 1976, Search for a biochemical basis of diabetic microangiopathy, Claude Bernard lecture, *Diabetologia* **12**:1.

Steel, J. M., Shenfield, G. M., and Duncan, L. J. P., 1976, Rapid onset of proliferative retinopathy in young insulin-independent diabetics, *Br. Med. J.* **2**:852.

Sutherland, D. E. R., Matas, A. J., Steffes, M. W., and Najarian, J. S., 1976, Infant human pancreas: A potential source of islet tissue for transplantation, *Diabetes* **25**:1123.

Svejgaard, A., 1976, *HLA* facts and immune function, *Acta Endocrinol. (Copenhagen)*, Suppl. 205, p. 77.

Terrasse, J., Moinade, S., Gentou, C., and Marre, L., 1976, Les glycoproteins et les complications vasculaires du diabete, *Sem. Hop. Paris* **52**:739.

Timperely, W. R., Ward, J. D., Preston, F. E., Duckworth, T., and O'Malley, B. C., 1976, Clinical and histological studies in diabetic neuropathy: A reassessment of vascular factors in relation to intra-vascular coagulation, *Diabetologia* **12**:237.

Tingle, A. J., Guasparini, R., Tze, W. J., and Colle, E., 1976, Islet cell antibodies in juvenile onset diabetes mellitus, *Clin. REs.* **24**:188A.

Turner, R. C., and Holman, R. R., 1976, Insulin rather than glucose homeostasis in the pathophysiology of diabetes, *Lancet* **1**:1272.

Turner, R. C., McCarthy, S. T., Holman, R. R., and Harris, E., 1976, Beta-cell function inproved by supplementing basal insulin secretion in mild diabetes, *Br. Med. J.* **1**:1252.

University Group Diabetes Program, 1975, A study of the effects of hypoglycemic agents on vascular complications in patients with adult-onset diabetes. V. Evaluation of phenformin therapy, *Diabetes* **24** *(Suppl. 1)*:65.

University Group Diabetes Program, 1976, A study of the effects of hypoglycemic agents on vascular complications in patients with adult-onset diabetes. VI. Supplementary report on nonfatal events in patients treated with tolbutamide, *Diabetes* **25**:1129.

Van De Putte, I., Vermylen, C., Decraene, P., Vlietinck, R., and Van Den Berghe, H., 1976, Segregation of HLA B7 in juvenile-onset diabetes mellitus, *Lancet* **2**:251.

Vigneri, R., Squatrito, S., Pezzino, V., Filetti, S., Branca, S., and Polosa, P., 1976, Growth hormone levels in diabetes: Correlation with the clinical control of the disease, *Diabetes* **25**:167.

Vinik, A. I., Kalk, W. J., Botha, J. L., Jackson, W. P. U., and Blake, R. C. H., 1976, The inexhaustible beta cell, *Diabetes* **25**:11.

Wakisaka, A., Aizawa, M., Matsuura, N., Nakagawa, S., Nakayama, E., Itakura, K., Okuno, A., and Wagatsuma, Y., 1976, *HLA* and juvenile diabetes mellitus in the Japanese, *Lancet 2*:970.

Wellman, K. F., and Volk, B. W., 1976, Nodular intercapillary glomerulosclerosis in diabetes secondary to chronic calcific pancreatitis, *Diabetes* **25**:713.

Westberg, N. G., 1976, Biochemical alterations of the human glomerular basement membrane in diabetes, *Diabetes* **25**:920.

Williams, R. H., and Palmer, J. P., 1975, Farewell to phenformin for treating diabetes mellitus, *Ann. Intern. Med.* **83**:567.

Williamson, J. R., Rowold, E., Hoffman, P., and Kilo, C., 1976, Influence of fixation and morphometric techniques on capillary basement membrane thickening prevalence data in diabetes, *Diabetes* **25**:604.

Winegrad, A. E., and Greene, D. A., 1976, Diabetic polyneuropathy: The importance of insulin deficiency, hyperglycemia and alterations in myoinositol metabolism in its pathogenesis, *N. Engl. J. Med.* **295**:1416.

Yesus, Y. W., Esterly, J. A., Stuhlman, R. A., and Townsend, J. F., 1976, Significant muscle capillary basement membrane thickening in spontaneously diabetic *Mystromys albicaudatus, Diabetes* **25**:444.

Yoon, J. W., and Notkins, A. L., 1976, Virus-induced diabetes mellitus. VI. Genetically determined host differences in the replication of encephalomyocarditis virus in pancreatic beta cells, *J. Exp. Med.* **143**:1170.

Yoon, J. W., Lesniak, M. A., Fussganger, R., and Notkins, A. L., 1976, Genetic differences in susceptibility of pancreatic B-cells to virus-induced diabetes mellitus, *Nature (London)* **264**:178.

Zonana, J., and Rimoin, D. L., 1976, Current concepts in genetics: Inheritance of diabetes mellitus, *N. Engl. J. Med.* **295**:603.

3

Glucagon and Somatostatin

Roger H. Unger

3.1. Immunoreactive Glucagons in Tissues and Plasma

3.1.1. Primary Structure of Glucagon

The primary structure of true glucagon, the biologically active 3485-molecular-weight polypeptide, is identical in all mammalian species thus far studied, with the exception of the guinea pig. Porcine (Bromer *et al.*, 1957), bovine (Bromer *et al.*, 1971), and human (Thomsen *et al.*, 1972) glucagons have identical sequences, and it is likely that rabbit (Sundby and Markussen, 1972), camel, and rat (Sundby and Markussen, 1971) glucagons are also identical. The guinea pig glucagon, however, has a molecular weight of 4000–5000 and appears to differ from porcine glucagon (Sundby, 1976).

All three avian glucagons thus far studied—duck (Sundby *et al.*, 1972), turkey (Markussen *et al.*, 1972), and chicken (Pollock and Kimmel, 1975)—differ slightly from mammalian glucagons in their primary structure. The substitution of a serine residue for asparagine at position 28

ROGER H. UNGER • Veterans Administration Hospital, Dallas, Texas; The University of Texas Southwestern Medical School, Department of Internal Medicine, Dallas, Texas 75216.

appears to alter the immunologic properties of avian glucagon; it reacts weakly with so-called "specific" C-terminal-reacting antisera for glucagon, while "cross-reacting" with N-terminal-reacting antiglucagon sera (Sundby, 1976). Fish glucagons resemble avian glucagons in this respect (Sundby, 1976).

3.1.2. 'Glucagonlike Immunoreactivity'

The relationship of "glucagonlike immunoreactivity" (GLI) to true glucagon has long been a matter of uncertainty. GLI refers to a group of polypeptides, some of which possess certain of the biological properties of glucagon; most GLIs are more basic than glucagon (Sasaki *et al.*, 1975b), and all react poorly with so-called "specific" antisera that recognize the *C*-terminal segment of the glucagon molecule (Assan and Slusher, 1972; Heding *et al.*, 1976). GLI is most abundant in the postduodenal small bowel (Unger *et al.*, 1968; Valverde *et al.*, 1975), and has been localized by immunocytochemical techniques (Polak *et al.*, 1971) to so-called "A-like" cells (Orci *et al.*, 1968) or EG cells in the gut. Sundby *et al.* (1976) characterized a member of the GLI family with a molecular weight of 11,625, and its N- and C-terminal amino acid composition differ from true glucagon. But a surprising new development is the recent identification of GLI in glucagon-containing cells of the pancreas (Moody *et al.*, 1976) and of the canine gastric fundus (Ito and Kobayashi, 1976). If GLI moieties coexist in the same pancreatic and gastric A-cells as glucagon, they could be precursors of glucagon or constitute a separate secretion product. A glucagon-sized GLI with an isoelectric point greater than 9.0 is present in pancreatic extracts and in relatively pure commercial preparations of glucagon (Srikant and Unger, 1976; Srikant *et al.*, 1977). Moody *et al.* (1976) suggested that the GLI moieties of a given animal species contain the full sequence of its glucagon, and that biosynthesis of glucagon proceeds via a molecule having extensive chemical similarities to gut GLI. In any case, the possibility that GLI is an unrecognized component of relatively pure "glucagon" preparations and accounts for some of the biological actions hitherto ascribed to glucagon must be considered.

3.1.3. Glucagon Biosynthesis

Our understanding of the biosynthetic pathway of glucagon remains rudimentary. Noe (1976) proposed that the biosynthetic precursor for glucagon, at least in the anglerfish, is a polypeptide of approximately 12,000 molecular weight, although a larger precursor is possible (see Section 3.1.4). In any case, the 12,000-molecular-weight polypeptide is rapidly cleaved to a 9000-dalton moiety, probably the same polypeptide previously referred to as *proglucagon* by Noe and Bauer (1971) and Noe *et al.* (1975), and as *large glucagon reactivity* by Rigopoulou *et al.* (1970). The 9000-molecular-weight intermediate is probably then cleaved to a polypeptide of about 4900, which is then in turn converted to a 3500-molecular-weight glucagon. The 4900-molecular-weight polypeptide may be similar to the fragment of proglucagon isolated from crystalline and mammalian glucagon and characterized by Tager and Steiner (1973). Preliminary experiments by Noe (1976) indicate that the microsomal fraction of the A-cell is the site of synthesis for the 12,000-molecular-weight component, and that portions of the 12,000- and 9000-molecular-weight components are transported to the secretory granule fractions prior to cleavage to smaller products.

O'Connor and Lazarus (1976) suggest a somewhat different relationship between the large and small IRG moieties, having failed to establish a precursor–product relationship. They found that both little and big immunoreactive glucagons were actively secreted, and that the synthesis of both was inhibited by high concentrations of glucose. Big glucagon was estimated to have a molecular weight of 20,000. It seems likely that much of the present confusion in this area is the consequence of the use of different species, different conditions, and antisera that recognize different portions of the glucagon and GLI molecules.

3.1.4. Tissue Immunoreactive Glucagon

Glucagon-containing tissues such as the pancreas (Srikant *et al.,* 1977) and the fundus of the canine stomach (Srikant *et al.,* 1977) contain four major immunoreactive components (Table I): (1) true biologically active glucagon; (2) an immunoreactive glucagon (IRG) of about 2000 daltons; (3) an IRG of about 9000 daltons (Rigopoulou *et al.,* 1970) that does not bind to hepatic glucagon receptors or activate hepatic adenylate cyclase and that corresponds to the 9000-molecular-weight "proglucagon" of Noe and Bauer (1970); (4) an IRG of about 65,000 present in extracts of canine fundus that binds to hepatic glucagon receptors, activates adenylate cyclase, and has approximately the same glycogenolytic activity as glucagon (Srikant *et al.,* 1977), but that could not be detected in extracts of whole pancreas. Using different extraction methods, Tager and Markese (1976) recovered from isolated rat islets large IRG components, including one of 50,000 daltons. Their results suggest that high-molecular-weight IRGs are being overlooked because of inadequate extraction methods.

3.1.5. Plasma Immunoreactive Glucagon

Valverde *et al.* (1970, 1974, 1975) identified four IRG fractions in plasma. Three correspond to IRG components present in glucagon-secreting tissues: $IRG^{\sim 2000}$, an $IRG^{\sim 3500}$ presumed to be true glucagon,

Table I. IRG Moieties of Canine Tissues

Molecular size	Biological activity (100% glucagon)			Isoelectric point
	Glycogenolytic	Adenylate-cyclase activating	^{125}I Glucagon-displacing	
Pancreas				
IRG^{2000}				
IRG^{3500} (true glucagon)	100	100	100	6.25
IRG^{9000}	0	0	~10	4.65
$IRG^{65,000}$ [a]				
Fundus				
IRG^{2000}				
IRG^{3500}	120	180	107	6.15
IRG^{9000}	0	0	~10	4.50
$IRG^{65,000}$	110	83	98	6.40

[a] Too little to measure; an $IRG^{50,000}$ was identified by Tager and Markese (1976).

and an $IRG^{\sim 9000}$ thought to correspond to "proglucagon." The fourth is "big plasma glucagon" (BPG), a globulin-sized immunoreactive substance referred to variously as *interfering factor* (Weir *et al.*, 1973) and *macro-IRG* (Valverde *et al.*, 1975). Ensinck and Palmer (1976) reported the inheritance of this BPG species in three generations of a family in a pattern consistent with an autosomal dominant trait, causing "hyperglucagonemia," which on dilution gave radioimmunoassay readings as high as 9000 pg/ml. In involved family members, however, abnormally high levels of $IRG^{\sim 9000}$ and $IRG^{\sim 20,000}$ were observed without increased levels of BPG. None of the members of this prepositus had diabetes mellitus or any disorder that might be related to this abnormality. This family is reminiscent of the pedigree reported by Gabbay *et al.* (1976) in which hyperproinsulinemia was reported without a manifest metabolic abnormality.

The 9000-molecular-weight IRG was reported by several workers to be increased in patients with glucagonoma (Valverde *et al.*, 1976; Jaspan *et al.*, 1976; Danforth *et al.*, 1976) and in renal insufficiency (Kuku *et al.*, 1976). In addition, chronic hypersecretion of glucagon may be accompanied by increased levels of $IRG^{\sim 9000}$ (Valverde *et al.*, 1975).

3.2. Structure–Function Relationships of Glucagon

3.2.1. Biological

Some or all of the three C-terminally located residues to glucagon may be necessary for glucagon to assume a helical conformation and to be biologically active (Bromer, 1976). Hruby *et al.* (1976) reported that the C-terminal portion of glucagon is concerned primarily with binding to the receptor, while the N-terminal and perhaps the central portion of the molecule are important both for binding to the receptor and for activation of adenylate cyclase. Epand *et al.* (1976) suggested that the binding phenomenon is determined by interaction of the membrane receptor with most, if not all, of the glucagon molecule, rather than with any specific region.

Blundell *et al.* (1976) reported that the structure of glucagon crystals is largely helical, with molecules associated in a complex arrangement of trimers. They now believe the evidence favors the existence of such helical trimers in the α-granules of the A_2 cells and the formation of a helical conformer at the glucagon receptor. They point out that the molecule is α-helical between residues 6 and 27, two hydrophobic patches interacting to form trimers in the crystals and, in addition, providing for interaction between glucagon and its receptors. Blundell speculates that the glucagon–receptor complex arises from hydrophobic side chains brought together in the helical conformer by means of the receptor through the two hydrophobic patches with the intermediate residues initially flexible. The demonstration that iodinated glucagon at pH 7 binds to the glucagon receptor and activates adenylate cyclase with an affinity about threefold higher than native glucagon may reflect increased hydrophobic interaction of the hormone with the receptor and point to critical involvement of the tyrosine residues in the function of the hormone (Lin *et al.*, 1976). The consensus is that the C-terminal portion of glucagon is concerned primarily with binding to the receptor, while the amino terminal and perhaps the central portion of the molecule are important to both binding to the receptor and activation of adenylate cyclase. The recent evidence that insulin–receptor complex of rat liver cells is present not only on the cell surface but also within the cell itself, even on nuclei, does not appear to apply to glucagon (Goldfine and Smith, 1976).

3.2.2. Immunologic

Heding *et al.* (1976) extended previous evidence of Assan and Slusher (1972) and Faloona (1972) that glucagon fragments 1–21, 1–23, and 1–27 react with "nonspecific" antiserum more avidly than with so-called "pancreatic-specific" antiserum. Studies reviewed by Heding *et al.* (1976) suggest that the antigenic site of glucagon for "specific" antisera is located within the 24–29 section of the molecule, while that of the cross-reacting sera occupies the 2–23 segment. It is also clear that biologically inactive glucagon may retain its immunoreactivity despite the loss of receptor binding activity, an issue of great importance in interpreting certain clinical studies on glucagon's role in diabetes (Sherwin *et al.*, 1976; Unger *et al.*, 1976).

3.3. Molecular Basis for Glucagon Actions

Hammes and Rodbell (1976) suggest that the adenylate cyclase system can exist in two states, an A and a B state (Fig. 1). Activating ligands bind preferentially to the B state, and only the B state is active. Rodbell and Londos (1976) propose that the adenylate cyclase system in rat liver membranes contains four effector sites, three of which (glucagon, GTP, and divalent cations) enhance activity, while occupation of the adenosine site results in inhibition of enzyme activity. All the sites are allosterically linked to give a finely controlled regulatory system; control is exerted by a shift in equilibrium between inactive (A) and active (B) states of the enzyme, and preferential binding of the effectors to the B state, as shown in Fig. 1. As for the specific role of the hormone, they propose that it serves a permissive role when combined with GTP and metal ions. These and similar proposals may have profound implications for the control of glucagon action.

3.4. Glucagon Metabolism, Clearance, and Degradation

Valverde *et al.* (1975) estimate the half-time of disappearance of endogenous true glucagon to be approximately 3 min, whereas that of $IRG^{\sim 9000}$ is approximately 16 min. The fact that studies of IRG gradients across the liver have ignored the individual IRG fractions and have measured only total plasma IRG may account for the wide differences in the reported IRG gradient across the human liver. Felig *et al.* (1974) reported a portal–peripheral venous gradient of only 1.3 in the basal state, when true glucagon makes up only a small percentage of total IRG. In contrast, during arginine infusion, which stimulates true glucagon secretion, Blackard *et al.* (1974) noted portal vein IRG levels of more than 1000 pg/ml without a rise in peripheral vein plasma IRG. Also, Dencker *et al.* (1975) observed increases in portal vein IRG after an ordinary meal at a time when no measurable change in plasma IRG occurred. Srikant *et al.* (unpublished) noted a ratio as high as 2.5 for the IRG^{3500}, true glucagon, across the liver of diabetic dogs during alanine stimulation. In sheep, Brockman *et al.* (1975) estimate that the liver removes from 31 to 35% of the portal vein IRG secretory rate. It appears that transhepatic gradients of whole IRG do not reflect accurately the hepatic extraction of biologically active true glucagon, particularly under conditions in which true glucagon makes up only a small fraction of the total IRG.

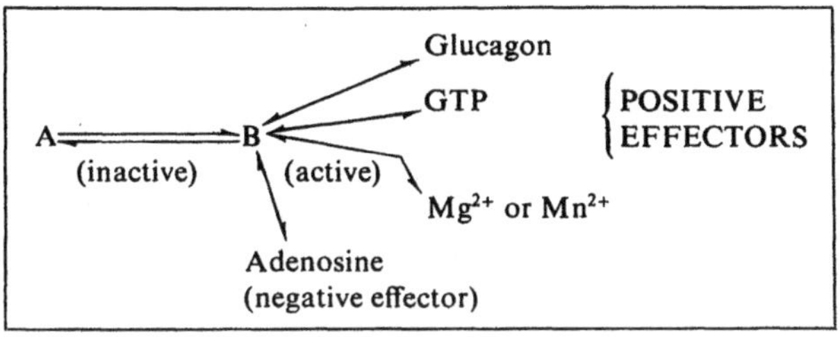

Fig. 1. Model of adenylate cyclase system of Rodbell and Londos. Control is exerted by the shift in equilibrium between inactive (A) and active (B) states of the enzyme and the preferential binding of the effectors to the B state. Reprinted from Rodbell and Londos (1976) with permission of *Metabolism*.

Removal of glucagon from the plasma may involve its degradation within the liver at a site considered separate from the glucagon receptor. Kakiuchi and Tomizawa (1964) reported a glucagon-degrading enzyme purified from hepatic glutathione insulin transhydrogenase. Duckworth and Kitabchi (1974) identified an "insulin–glucagon specific protease" in muscle, but as yet this has not been reported in liver. Some evidence that glucagon and insulin may interact in insulin-degrading systems was already advanced in early studies of insulin degradation by human placenta (Freinkel and Goodner, 1960). About 0.5 mg glucagon/day is excreted in the bile (Assan, 1972), but the kidneys appear to be the major site of glucagon removal (Lefebvre and Luyckx, 1975, 1976). The rise in plasma IRG that follows bilateral kidney exclusion is due, not to an increase in secretion, but rather to an abrupt cessation of glucagon uptake (Lefebvre and Luyckx, 1976). The hyperglucagonemia of renal insufficiency (Bilbrey *et al.*, 1974) is believed to result in large part from the decreased removal of glucagon; most of this increase in IRG is the result of a disproportionate increase in $IRG^{\sim 9000}$ (Kuku *et al.*, 1976).

Fisher *et al.* (1976) reported that starvation changes the kinetics of glucagon in man and lowers the metabolic clearance rate, perhaps accounting for the increased IRG concentrations.

3.5. Physiologic Actions of Glucagon

3.5.1. Hepatic Glycogenolysis

The glycogenolytic actions of glucagon are demonstrated with ease in all *in vivo* and *in vitro* models employed. There seems to be little quarrel with the classic concept of phosphorylase activation mediated by glucagon-enhanced cyclic AMP (cAMP) production and the cAMP-dependent protein kinase (for a review, see Cherrington and Exton, 1976). While glucagon-induced glycogenolysis appears to be mediated by cAMP and cAMP-dependent protein kinase, epinephrine stimulates glycogen breakdown via alpha receptors, which cause rapid activation of phosphorylase and inactivation of glycogen synthase without accumulation of cAMP or activation of cAMP-dependent protein kinase (Hutson *et al.,* 1976; Cherrington and Exton, 1976).

3.5.2. Gluconeogenesis

3.5.2.1. Molecular

The site of action of glucagon in the gluconeogenic pathway remains unknown (for a review, see Pilkis *et al.,* 1976). Earlier studies by Exton and Park (1969) had pointed to a site of action somewhere between pyruvate and phosphoenolpyruvate; more recently, however, attention has been directed toward the enzyme pyruvate kinase, which, if inhibited by glucagon, would reduce the amount of phosphoenolpyruvate converted to pyruvate and thus favor glucose formation. Blair *et al.* (1976) also found similar inhibition of this enzyme, and reported reversible interconversion of two kinetically distinct forms of hepatic pyruvate kinase regulated by glucagon and insulin in the perfused rat liver. Glucagon and cAMP inhibit pyruvate kinase via phosphorylation of pyruvate kinase by cAMP-dependent protein kinase (Feliu *et al.,* 1976), while insulin counteracts the glucagon-induced inhibition of pyruvate kinase. Glucose can inhibit gluconeogenesis without changing protein kinase activity. Veneziale *et al.* (1976) also demonstrated inhibition by glucagon of both pyruvate·kinase and phosphofructokinase.

3.5.2.2. Physiologic

Evidence of glucagon's physiologic importance as a regulator of gluconeogenesis continues to accumulate. Direct stimulation by glucagon of net hepatic uptake of alanine, glycine, glutamine, arginine, asparagine, threonine, syrine, and lactate has been demonstrated (Brockman *et al.,* 1975), but in addition, increased intrahepatic shunting of alanine into gluconeogenic pathways appears to be an important effect of glucagon (Chiasson *et al.,* 1975). The importance of glucagon in neonatal gluconeogenesis has been stressed (Girard *et al.,* 1976), and the rapid rise in plasma IRG within 2 hr of life in newborn lambs and humans suggests that the neonatal surge in IRG associated with a coexisting low insulin level may be an important event in the adjustment of glucose homeostasis in perinatal life (Sperling *et al.,* 1976). Glucagon appears to influence protein and amino acid metabolism within the liver, enhancing ureogenesis and depressing albumin synthesis (Dich and Glund, 1976; Miller, 1976), effects that are inhibited by insulin.

3.5.3. Ketogenesis

Glucagon appears to be essential for hepatic ketogenesis. The studies of McGarry *et al.* (1976) suggested that maximal activation of hepatic fatty acid oxidation requires both an increase in hepatic carnitine and depletion of hepatic glycogen content. These workers believe that glucagon is of critical importance in "switching" the liver to a high ketogenic capacity, which in the presence of an abundant supply of substrate, free fatty acids, will result in ketogenesis. While the mechanism by which ketogenesis is induced by glucagon remains obscure, an essential role of glucagon in ketoacidosis in man appears likely (Gerich *et al.,* 1975b).

3.6. Physiologic Roles of Glucagon in Fuel Homeostasis

3.6.1. Maintenance of Basal Hepatic Glucose Production

The elegant studies of Liljenquist *et al.* (1976) at Vanderbilt delineated quantitatively the contribution of glucagon and insulin to the regulation of hepatic fuel production. Using somatostatin as a tool for the suppression of both insulin and glucagon, they observed during a deficiency of both hormones a 40% decline in hepatic glucose production; this is not further decreased when insulin is replaced. When insulin deficiency without concomitant glucagon deficiency is produced by infusing somatostatin plus replacement doses of glucagon, hepatic glucose production increases 80% and hyperglycemia appears. They conclude that the basal glucagon concentration plays a role in maintaining basal hepatic glucose production *in vivo* through interaction between the stimulatory effect of glucagon and the inhibitory effect of insulin. Like others (Cherrington and Vranic, 1974; Felig *et al.,* 1976), however, this group finds that the action of a constant infusion of glucagon on hepatic overproduction of glucose is evanescent.

3.6.2. Increase in Hepatic Glucose Production during Protein Meals

A second important physiologic role of glucagon is in preventing protein-induced hypoglycemia by augmenting the production of glucose during the ingestion of a protein meal. Protein elicits an increase in insulin secretion necessary for an anabolic disposition of the ingested amino acids. Insulin increases glucose utilization, however, and would result in hypoglycemia were it not for appropriate secretion of glucagon (Unger *et al.*, 1969; Wahren *et al.*, 1976; Metzger *et al.*, 1977).

3.6.3. Increase in Hepatic Glucose Production during Exercise

Exercise-induced hyperglucagonemia (Bottger *et al.*, 1972; Luyckx and Lefebvre, 1972; Harvey *et al.*, 1974) may, together with adrenergic influences, maintain glucose production during exercise. When exercising rats are treated with antiglucagon serum, hepatic glycogen depletion is reduced to 50% of control rats treated with nonimmune serum, thus underscoring the importance of glucagon in glucose delivery during exercise (Galbo and Holst, 1976).

3.6.4. Effects of Glucagon on Lipids and Ketones

Gerich *et al.* (1976c) studied the effects of glucagon on human lipid and amino acid metabolism by infusing glucagon in juvenile-type diabetics during a constant insulin infusion, thereby raising IRG levels to about 200 pg/ml. Mild hyperglycemia appeared, and when insulin was withdrawn, it became more severe. Glucagon had no effect on β-hydroxybutyrate, free fatty acids, or glycerol levels in the presence of insulin, but caused an increase in all the foregoing measurements when insulin was withdrawn.

3.7. Concept of the Bihormonal Unit

The concept of the islet as a bihormonal regulator of nutrient homeostasis involving coordinated secretion of biologically antagonistic hormones, insulin and glucagon (Unger, 1971b, 1976), has its roots in the classic studies of Park and Exton (1972) and Mackrell and Sokal (1969) and is supported by a host of biochemical, physiologic, morphologic, and pathophysiologic observations. It is proposed that within a given metabolic setting, the molar ratio of insulin to glucagon, rather than the concentration of one hormone alone, determines the rate and directions of metabolic processes in target tissues on which both hormones act such as the liver—at least within a broad physiologic and pathophysiologic range of concentrations.

The islets of Langerhans, through these two hormones, and perhaps other hormones, play the principal role in regulation of nutrient flux rates. Of the key fuels, however, only one, glucose, the critical fuel of the CNS, is maintained within the remarkably narrow limits of concentration that clinicians regard as normal, and this requires an exquisitely sensitive glucose sensor to govern the hormonal responses appropriately. The priority and precision of glucose homeostasis over that of other fuels is attributed to the glucose dependence of the CNS. This requires that major reductions in extracellular glucose concentration be avoided even though glucose flux rates are changed; i.e., glucose entry into and exit from the extracellular space must always be close to equal. When glucose enters at mealtime, insulin augments the rate of glucose efflux from the extracellular space into insulin-responsive tissues, principally liver, fat, and muscle, thus preventing hyperglycemia; but when glucose influx is low, as in fasting, and when glucose efflux is high, as during protein ingestion or exercise, enhanced glucagon secretion augments hepatic glucose production, thereby preventing hypoglycemia. If deprivation of exogenous carbohydrate is prolonged and hepatic glycogen stores are depleted, the continued influence of high glucagon levels relative to insulin levels will increasingly augment gluconeogenesis to meet the need for glucose. But, ultimately, this glucagon/insulin mixture will promote ketone production as an alternative fuel for the CNS and other tissues, thereby sparing protein and prolonging survival (Cahill, 1971).

The validity of the basic concept of the insulin/glucagon ratio is supported by short-term studies demonstrating relationships to gluconeogenesis (Parrilla *et al.*, 1975) and hepatic cAMP concentrations (Seitz *et al.*, 1976). In general, however, it should be regarded as a semiquantitative guide, reflecting the dominance of one hormone over the other; ratios of 1.0 or less are well correlated with "glucagon-dominated" catabolic states and ratios of more than 5.0 constitute "insulin-dominated" anabolic states (Unger, 1971b). A ratio of less than 1.0 is normal during starvation, strenuous exercise, or stress, but failure of the ratio to rise during feeding is distinctly abnormal and would be regarded as likely evidence of a catabolic disorder.

3.8. Control of Glucagon Secretion

3.8.1. Glucose

The physiologic importance of glucose as a fuel is reflected by the fact that the arterial glucose level appears to dominate the secretory responses of the islet cells in an obligatory fashion. By this is meant that hyperglycemia is the most potent physiologic suppressor of glucagon among the nutrients, and that in normal subjects, the glucagon response to various stimuli, such as protein and exercise, is abolished by hyperglycemia. The priority of glycemia also obtains for insulin secretion; stimulation of insulin secretion by nonglucose secretagogues is greatly obtunded by glucose lack and enhanced by glucose secretion.

The mechanism by which glucose blocks the secretion of glucagon is unknown. The concept of an A-cell glucoreceptor is supported to a degree by the fact that the α-anomer of glucose is more potent than the β-anomer in suppressing glucagon secretion, just as it is in stimulating insulin secretion (Matschinsky *et al.,* 1975). This would be compatible with a stereospecific site, perhaps on the A-cell membrane, that evokes the negative A-cell response. The original notion that intracellular ATP accumulation "turns off" the secretion of glucagon and that it is stimulated by an energy deficit within the A-cell is challenged by Matschinsky *et al.* (1976), who find that the "glucose blindness" of diabetic A-cells cannot be explained on the basis of differences in their glucose or ATP content. Because insulin failed to increase the glucose space or the ATP content of diabetic islets, which consist largely of A-cells, these workers consider that lack of intracellular glucose entry is not the cause of the defect of the A-cell in diabetes; indeed, they were able to suppress the A-cells in diabetes with as little as 2.5 mM glucose. Their studies are in apparent conflict with *in vivo* studies (Braaten *et al.,* 1974), and with the *in vitro* work of Weir *et al.* (1976), who find the same paradoxical increase in glucagon release during perfusion of rat pancreases with a glucose concentration of 300 mg/dl that is observed in human diabetics (Buchanan and McCarroll, 1972). Insulin in very large concentrations intended to simulate within-islet insulin concentrations (20,000 mU/ml) suppressed glucagon secretion. The results were compatible with the hypothesis that local within-islet insulin secretion can exert a significant suppressive effect on the A-cell and that inhibition of glucagon secretion by glucose is at least partially mediated by this mechanism; if so, the abnormal glucagon secretion of diabetes may then be secondary to abnormal insulin secretion. The fact that glucagon secretion by extrapancreatic A-cells in the gastric fundus is suppressed by insulin (Blazquez *et al.,* 1976), but not by hyperglycemia, tends to support their view. Also, insulin reportedly decreased glucagon release by a glucagonoma, whereas glucose alone did not (Tiengo *et al.,* 1976). The glucose-sensing machinery of the A-cell may require the presence of insulin, and insulin might even be the mediator of the response of glucagon to glucose. Indeed, in both normal and diabetic subjects, small increases in insulin lower plasma IRG levels without any increase in plasma glucose concentration (Raskin *et al.,* 1975). It would seem that insulin plays a major role in the A-cell response to hyperglycemia.

The islets of rats fed a high-protein diet for 5 days exhibit a loss of the suppressive effect of high glucose concentrations on glucagon secretion, alterations in A-cell function similar to those found in human and experimental diabetes (Eisenstein and Strack, 1976). This would suggest that during deprivation of exogenous carbohydrate, islet-cell behavior is altered so as to maintain a high rate of endogenous fuel production through a fixed low insulin/glucagon ratio. In man, Permutt *et al.* (1976) observed impaired glucagon suppression in response to glucose ingestion following a period of carbohydrate restriction.

The role of calcium in glucose-induced suppression of glucagon secretion (Leclercq-Meyer *et al.*, 1975) is a matter of continuing investigation, and Lundquist *et al.* (1976b) reported that glucagon suppression by glucose requires calcium.

Since pancreatic somatostatin release is stimulated by glucose concentrations of 150 mg/dl or more (Schauder *et al.*, 1976; Ipp *et al.*, 1977), the same levels that suppress glucagon, this polypeptide might also be involved in A-cell suppression.

3.8.2. Amino Acids

Infused amino acids, particularly arginine, alanine, and several others, are powerful stimuli of pancreatic glucagon secretion (Rocha *et al.*, 1972), as are ingested protein hydrolysates or protein. The function of aminogenic release of glucagon is to prevent hypoglycemia secondary to aminogenic insulin secretion (Unger *et al.*, 1969; Wahren *et al.*, 1976). This action is believed to be vital in preventing an insulin-mediated decrease in hepatic glucose production and hypoglycemia.

3.8.3. Free Fatty Acids

An increase in free fatty acids suppresses plasma IRG levels (Madison *et al.*, 1968). Lefebvre and Luyckx (1972) showed that plasma IRG levels rise when plasma free fatty acids are reduced by nicotinic acid and fall when they are raised by an intravenous infusion of heparin and triglyceride. In juvenile diabetics in whom the normal suppression of glucagon secretion by glucose is lost, an increase in free fatty acid concentration results in normal suppression of glucagon, evidence that the defect in the diabetic A-cell is selective for glucose and does not involve loss of suppression by free fatty acids (Gerich *et al.*, 1976b).

3.8.4. Calcium

Lundquist *et al.* (1976a) demonstrated that staircase increments of calcium from 0.5 to 15 mEq/liter caused large spikes in glucagon release from the isolated perfused rat pancreas, particularly at low and high concentrations. This response was suppressed by destruction of peripheral adrenergic neurons, suggesting that glucagon secretion is modulated by a stimulant effect of the pancreatic adrenergic nerves, perhaps via norepinephrine, and that calcium in part positively effects the release of glucagon by permitting the neural stimulation. Studies by Ashby and Speake (1975) using calcium ionophores suggest that calcium is involved in the secretion of glucagon. Wollheim *et al.* (1976b) also concluded that calcium plays an essential role in stimulus-secretion coupling of the pancreatic A-cells (see also Section 3.8.1).

3.8.5. Cyclic 3′,5′-Adenosine Monophosphate

Conflicting data concerning the role of cAMP in glucagon secretion may, in part, have been clarified by the studies of Wollheim *et al.* (1976a), demonstrating that the effect of cAMP on glucagon release can be either stimulatory or inhibitory depending on the calcium concentration of the medium and the duration of the exposure to the raised cAMP levels.

3.8.6. Adrenergic Stimulation—Stress and Exercise

The sympathetic nervous system is considered to stimulate glucagon by a β-adrenergic mechanism that can be blocked by propranolol (Marliss *et al.*, 1973). The increase in glucagon secretion that occurs in exercise and stress may be mediated by this system. Stress- and exercise-induced hyperglycemia may in large part be the consequence of the rise in glucagon. Gerich *et al.* (1976a) provided evidence that epinephrine-induced hyperglucagonemia participates in the hyperglycemic, although not in the lipolytic, response to epinephrine. In exercising man, catecholamines and glucagon levels rise progressively and insulin declines; β-adrenergic blockade does not diminish the glucagon response, nor is it increased by α-receptor stimulation, suggesting that decreased glucose availability in prolonged exercise is the basis for the response (Galbo *et al.*, 1976).

Release of norepinephrine from the sympathetic nerve endings in the pancreas can be induced by scorpion toxin, which stimulates glucagon secretion (Johnson and Ensinck, 1976), an effect that is blocked by propranolol, pentolamine, and phenoxybenzine, but not atropine; somatostatin does not alter the release of norepinephrine by the scorpion toxin, but does block the glucagon response. The importance of sympathetic nervous control over the moment-to-moment secretory activity of A- and B-cells was emphasized by the studies of Girardier *et al.* (1976).

3.8.7. Hormones

3.8.7.1. Gastrointestinal Hormones

Gastrin (Unger *et al.*, 1967), pancreozymin-cholecystokinin (Unger *et al.*, 1967; Frame *et al.*, 1975), GIP (Rabinovitch and Dupre, 1974), and

VIP (Schebalin *et al.,* 1977) have been identified as glucagon secretagogues. An unexplained tenfold increase in basal and stimulated plasma IRG levels without any change in basal or stimulated insulin levels has been reported following portacaval shunt surgery in a normal child treated for homozygous familial hypercholesterolemia (Bilheimer *et al.,* 1975). Perhaps it is the consequence of failure of the liver to remove a potent secretagogue of pancreatic IRG release. The hyperglucagonemia of cirrhosis (Marco *et al.,* 1973; Wise *et al.,* 1973; Soeters and Fischer, 1976) could have a similar etiology.

3.8.7.2. Growth Hormone

A direct stimulatory effect of bovine growth hormone on the release of glucagon and insulin from perfused rat pancreas has been observed at physiologic as well as at pharmacologic concentrations by Tai and Pek (1976). It is well known that glucagon and insulin levels are increased in acromegaly.

3.8.7.3. Neurotensin and Substance P

Neurotensin and substance P have a hyperglycemic, hyperglucagonemic effect *in vivo,* and less consistently, they suppress insulin levels (Brown and Vale, 1976; Nagai and Frohman, 1976; Ishida *et al.,* 1976; Brown *et al.,* 1976a,b). In the isolated perfused canine pancreas generally similar findings are reported (Patton *et al.,* 1976a).

3.8.7.4. Glucocorticoids

The chronic administration of glucocorticoids increases aminogenic glucagon secretion (Wise *et al.,* 1973; Marco *et al.,* 1973) in addition to increasing sensitivity of the liver to glucagon's effects. Marco *et al.* (1976) observed that in isolated islets obtained from prednisolone-pretreated mice, the secretory activity of the A-cell in response to arginine was increased, but that direct addition of glucocorticoids to the islets of untreated mice had no such effect.

3.8.7.5. Prostaglandins

In the isolated perfused rat pancreas, PGE_2 elicited dose-related increases in glucagon and insulin secretion (Pek *et al.,* 1975). The increase in glucagon occurred within 24 sec, while the rise in insulin required 48 sec, and a biphasic pattern of release was observed for both islet hormones. Prostaglandins may play a physiologic role in mediating or modifying the islet hormone response to other secretagogues.

3.9. Extrapancreatic Glucagon

The pancreas is not the sole source of immunologically and biologically active glucagon. Sutherland and DeDuve (1948) first reported the hyperglycemic effect of extracts of canine gastric fundus and duodenum. Subsequently, Ferner (1953) proposed the existence of extrapancreatic A-cells. Vranic *et al.* (1974), Matsuyama and Foa (1975), and Mashiter *et al.* (1975) observed residual glucagonemia in insulin-deprived dogs following total pancreatectomy, following which it was reported that IRG with the immunologic, physicochemical, and biologic properties of pancreatic glucagon are present in extracts of gastrointestinal tissues (Dobbs *et al.*, 1975; Sasaki *et al.*, 1975a; Vranic *et al.*, 1976; Srikant *et al.*, 1977) (see Section 3.1.4). A-cells have been found in abundance in the fundus and corpus of the stomach of animals (Larsson *et al.*, 1975; Baetens *et al.*, 1976b), but in man, their presence has been difficult to identify. Only one of eight human stomachs obtained at autopsy contained immunohistochemically identifiable glucagon-containing cells (Muñoz-Barragan *et al.*, 1977), and recent attempts by Orci *et al.* (personal communication) and Shannon *et al.* (private communication) to establish the existence of glucagon-containing cells in fundi obtained from surgical resection of the gastric fundus have been thus far negative. Sasagawa *et al.* (1973) and Baetens *et al.* (personal communication) both observed electron-microscopically identifiable cells containing alpha granules in the duodenum of human subjects, and Orci observed the presence of such cells in the stomach of human abortuses (personal communication). Lawrence *et al.* (1976) reported morphological and biochemical evidence of an IRG fraction that reacts proportionately with C-terminal-reacting antiglucagon serum, but that has a molecular size considerably greater than glucagon. This material had hyperglycemic activity and was released from incubated slices of submaxillary glands subjected to low glucose concentration or stimulated with arginine (Lawrence *et al.*, 1976). Conceivably, this explains the observation of Penhos *et al.* (1975) of a rise in circulating IRG levels following total eviscerectomy in rats.

The foregoing observations fail to reveal the source of the circulating IRG present after total resection of the pancreas in humans. The question is of more than theoretical interest in view of the demonstration that in the insulin-deprived state in both totally depancreatized dogs (Blazquez *et al.*, 1976) and alloxan-diabetic dogs (Blazquez *et al.*, 1977), the stomach is a major contributor to the circulating IRG and that its suppression is accompanied by a reduced hyperglycemia (Sakurai *et al.*, 1975b).

In man, Barnes and Bloom (1976) reported zero levels of circulating glucagon in the plasma of totally depancreatized subjects, but they employed an unusual radioimmunoassay designed to measure only IRG moieties with the highest affinity for the antibody employed; it is possible, therefore, that circulating IRG and GLI moieties with glucagonlike biological activity were present but not measured. Moreover, their patients had received insulin 24 hr earlier, and it is likely that in man, as in the dog, extrapancreatic glucagon secretion is readily suppressed by insulin. Using conventional radioimmunoassays for IRG, all other workers have observed circulating IRG in the plasma of totally depancreatized patients. Miyata *et al.* (1976) made serial measurements of "true glucagon" and GLI during and after total resection of the pancreas in a 62-year-old man with calcific pancreatitis. Within 30 min after resection of the pancreas, IRG disappeared from the blood. Despite evidence that no pancreatic tissue was present in the abdomen, IRG became detectable 18 hr after pancreatectomy, but arginine did not stimulate a further rise in plasma IRG levels. GLI decreased initially, then rose abruptly on the second postoperative day and remained elevated thereafter. Palmer *et al.* (1976) studied three pancreatectomized humans 24 hr after their previous dose of insulin. "Glucagon" was present in all three. In one patient, glucagon rose from 35 to 91 pg/ml during arginine infusion and glucose rose 50 mg/dl during this 90-min study. In a second patient, arginine induced a 45 pg/ml rise in glucagon, but only a slight rise in glucose. In the third patient, arginine elicited no rise in glucagon. High levels of GLI were also present in these patients (Werner and Palmer, 1977).

On the basis of the evidence available at present, it would appear reasonable to conclude that in most totally depancreatized patients, circulating IRG and GLI are both present to a varying degree. IRG levels will be low if the patient has recently received insulin. In some, but not all, patients, arginine stimulates a rise in extrapancreatic IRG concentrations, and this may be associated with a rise in plasma glucose concentration. The tissue of origin of circulating IRG in depancreatized humans remains unclear. Just how much of the plasma "IRG" is GLI is also uncertain; 2% of GLI can react in so-called "highly specific" radioimmunoassays employing *C*-terminal-reacting antisera such as 30K. Plasma GLI levels 2–4 times normal could therefore account for much, most, or all of the measured IRG. GLI levels as high as 4 ng/ml have been observed in totally depancreatized patients and would give an "IRG" reading of 100 pg/ml in the 30K assay. GLI is said to have approximately half the biological activity of true glucagon when perfused in the isolated rat liver (Sasaki *et al.*, 1975b).

3.10. Somatostatin

The 14-amino-acid polypeptide somatostatin discovered in 1973 by Brazeau *et al.* (1973) is widely distributed throughout the CNS, gastrointestinal tissues, and pancreas (Vale *et al.*, 1976). Its ability to inhibit both insulin and glucagon secretion (Koerker *et al.*, 1974; Mortimer *et al.*, 1974) has made it an invaluable tool for the study of isolated insulin and glucagon deficiency, and has generated much of the new information concerning the physiologic roles of these hormones reviewed in the preceding sections of this chapter.

3.10.1. Pancreatic Somatostatin

3.10.1.1. Paracrine Actions of Somatostatin

The subsequent discovery of somatostatin (Arimura *et al.*, 1975) and somatostatin-containing cells in the islets of Langerhans (Luft *et al.*, 1974; Dubois, 1975) has opened a new phase in our understanding of islet physiology. Their subsequent identification as D-cells (Orci *et al.*, 1975a; Polak *et al.*, 1975) has led to the hypothesis (Orci and Unger, 1975; Unger and Orci, 1977) that the location of somatostatin-containing D-cells between A- and B-cells may signify that they inhibit by direct local action the secretion of glucagon and insulin. Additionally, insulin is known to suppress glucagon (Samols *et al.*, 1972; Raskin *et al.*, 1975), and glucagon stimulates both insulin (Samols *et al.*, 1965) and somatostatin (Patton *et al.*, 1976b, 1977). A within-islet "paracrine" system as depicted in Fig. 2 could therefore exist. Barden *et al.* (1977) reported that exposure of cultured islets to antisomatostatin serum is associated with an increase in secretion of glucagon, but not insulin, a finding compatible with a restraining role of the polypeptide on glucagon secretion. The restraining role of insulin on glucagon secretion is firmly established, and in rats, antiinsulin serum elicits a rise in glucagon (Müller *et al.*, 1971). Perhaps only the A-cells and the outer layer of the central mass of insulin-producing cells, the probable pacemaker area of the islet of Langerhans (Meissner, 1976) where autonomic nerves and afferent blood vessels enter, are influenced by local release of somatostatin. In any case, the D-cell could be part of an intraislet "paracrine" system in which the secretory products of A-, B-, and D-cells influence the release of secretory products of one or more of the neighboring cells and thus regulate the composition of the secretory mixture of hormones released by the pancreas.

3.10.1.2. Endocrine Actions of Somatostatin

Evidence that pancreatic somatostatin may have an endocrine role has recently been presented. The perfusion of the isolated dog pancreas with high concentrations of arginine (Patton *et al.*, 1976c, 1977) is accompanied by an increased immunoreactive somatostatin concentration in the

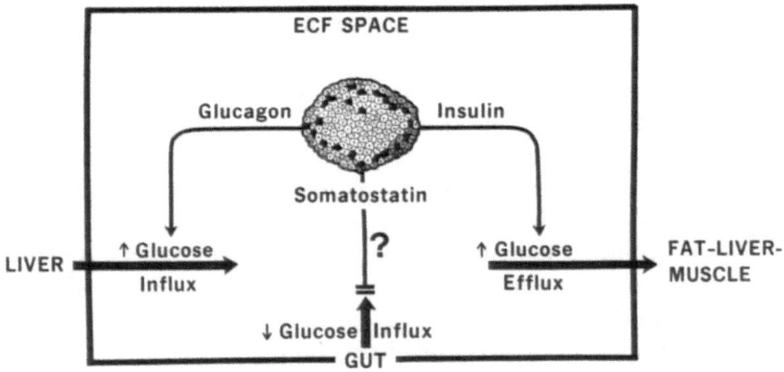

Fig. 2. Scheme in which the islets maintain regulatory influence over routes of nutrient influx and efflux. According to this scheme, somatostatin slows the rate at which glucose and other ingested nutrients enter the circulation, glucagon promotes production of glucose or ketones from the liver, and insulin promotes uptake of ingested nutrients and in the postabsorptive state restrains release of endogenous nutrients from the liver, fat, and muscle.

pancreatic effluent. Several groups have shown that glucose (Schauder *et al.*, 1976; Ipp *et al.*, 1977; Weir *et al.*, 1977), leucine (Ipp *et al.*, 1977), amino acid mixtures (Ipp *et al.*, 1977), and pancreozymin-cholecystokinin (Ipp *et al.*, 1977), all of which stimulate insulin, also stimulate somatostatin, while epinephrine (Schauder *et al.*, 1976) and diazoxide (Samols *et al.*, 1977) inhibit both insulin and somatostatin. This parallelism between the somatostatin and insulin responses to nutrients and to insulin-stimulating hormones raises the possibility that the two islet hormones may have a common function, one involving nutrient flux.

Somatostatin administered in pharmacologic doses profoundly influences functions of the gastrointestinal tract, gall bladder, and the exocrine pancreas. Evidence of an inhibitory influence on HCl and pepsin secretion (Bloom *et al.*, 1974), gastrin release (Bloom *et al.*, 1974), gastrin-stimulated HCl secretion (Bloom *et al.*, 1974), gastric emptying (Bloom *et al.*, 1975), duodenal motility (Boden *et al.*, 1976), release of secretin (Boden *et al.*, 1975) and GLI (Sakurai *et al.*, 1975a), gall bladder contraction (Creutzfeldt *et al.*, 1975), pancreatic exocrine function (Creutzfeldt *et al.*, 1975; Boden *et al.*, 1975), motilin secretion (Bloom *et al.*, 1975), and glucose and xylose absorption (Wahren and Felig, 1976) have been reported. While these effects have been considered pharmacologic, it has been suggested more recently that they may reflect the physiologic role of the polypeptide (Schusdziarra *et al.*, 1977). In dogs, the intraportal infusion of somatostatin at a physiologic rate also reduces the rate of xylose absorption after a xylose meal (Schusdziarra *et al.*, 1977). This could mean that somatostatin is the third islet-cell hormone that controls nutrient flux—influx of nutrients from the gut. This would provide the islets of Langerhans with influence over every avenue of nutrient flux into and out of the extracellular space (Fig. 2). It also raises a question of the role of D-cell dysfunction in certain forms of diabetes and related disorders. For example, in diabetes characterized by extensive destruction of the B-cells by streptozotocin-diabetic rats, and in juvenile-type diabetics, Orci *et al.* (1976) report immunocytochemical evidence of within-islet hyperplasia of D-cells, confirming an earlier observation of Petersson and Hellman (1963) in alloxan-diabetic guinea pigs. In the obese hyperglycemic mouse, a form of diabetes in which insulin-containing cells are abundant, a marked deficiency of somatostatin (Patel *et al.,* 1976) and of somatostatin-containing cells within the islets (Baetens *et al.,* 1976a) has been reported.

The role of the pancreatic and gastrointestinal D-cells remains to be clearly defined. Nevertheless, their discovery constitutes an exciting new area of future study. It is not clear whether somatostatin's inhibition of insulin and glucagon secretion is a purely local paracrine effect or whether circulating somatostatin also controls insulin and glucagon secretion (Porte *et al.,* 1975). Nakabayashi *et al.* (1976) observed inhibition of IRI and IRG secretion during the perfusion of 1.25 ng/min into the pancreatic artery of dogs, and in man, 1-ng pulses of somatostatin were reported by Leblanc *et al.* (1975) to inhibit insulin and glucagon. Samols and Harrison (1976) observed inhibition of glucagon secretion by the perfused pancreas by somatostatin concentrations of as little as 5 pg/ml, well below levels in the arterial plasma.

3.10.1.3. Mechanism of Action on Islet Cells

Calcium in concentrations of 15.2 mEq/liter reverses somatostatin-induced inhibition of IRG and IRI during arginine perfusion of the isolated pancreas, while potassium reverses somatostatin-induced inhibition of IRI but does not effect IRG inhibition (Bhathena *et al.,* 1976). Somatostatin inhibits calcium uptake of islets, suggesting that somatostatin's effects on the islets of Langerhans involve an action on calcium uptake.

3.11. Morphofunctional Interrelationships of the Endocrine Pancreas: Microanatomic Organization of the Islets of Langerhans

Our knowledge of the relationship of the four major islet-cell types (A-, B-, D-, and the pancreatic polypeptide-secreting cells) to one another and of their subcellular specializations of islet cells has been advanced through the recent application of powerful morphological technology.

3.11.1. Organization of Islet Cells

Immunofluorescent studies reveal that in man and in the rat, the A-cells are situated in the outer rim of the islet and constitute approximately 25% of the total islet-cell population (Orci *et al.,* 1976) (Fig. 3). In man, the A-cells may also be seen in the more central portions of the islet, aligning themselves in proximity to the vascular elements. In certain islets, however, A-cells seem to be replaced by pancreatic polypeptide-containing cells, probably F-cells. In the rat, such islets are located near the duodenum (Orci, 1977), while in the dog, they are most abundant in the uncinate process (Orci, 1977). The central mass of endocrine cells is insulin-containing B-cells, constituting approximately 60% of the endocrine cell population. Between the A- and B-cells are the somatostatin-containing D-cells, which make up approximately 10% of the total. The possible paracrine roles of islet cells on their neighboring cells have already been discussed (Fig. 3), and the heterocellular regions, in which local contacts between heterologous cells are maximal, are the very areas that receive afferent nerves and blood vessels, suggesting their possible "pacemaker role" (Meissner, 1976) in islet function.

The fact that the islets are dispersed into discrete microorgans of relatively homogeneous size may also have functional importance, since it makes possible a given ratio of cellular elements within a certain radius.

3.11.2. Subcellular Specialization of Islet Cells

Two types of subcellular specializations could play a functional role in this type of system. First, tight junctions (Orci *et al.,* 1973, 1975b,c), linear sites of fusion between the outer leaflets of the plasma membranes of adjacent cells, may form constantly changing compartments within the intercellular space (Orci, 1976). This extensive network forms a barrier to diffusion of secretory product released into the intercellular space (Orci *et al.,* 1973) and could have the function of directing secreted material toward the effluent capillaries or to or away from adjacent cells, thus permitting intended contacts with adjacent target cells and preventing unintended interactions with adjacent cells.

Gap junctions are low-resistance pathways through which electrical and metabolic coupling of adjacent cells may occur (for a review, see Staehelin, 1974), enabling molecules of less than 500 daltons to pass from the cytosol of one cell to that of another cell without entering the intercellular space. They were first discovered between islet cells of the same and different types by Orci *et al.* (1973, 1975b,c). Such contacts between

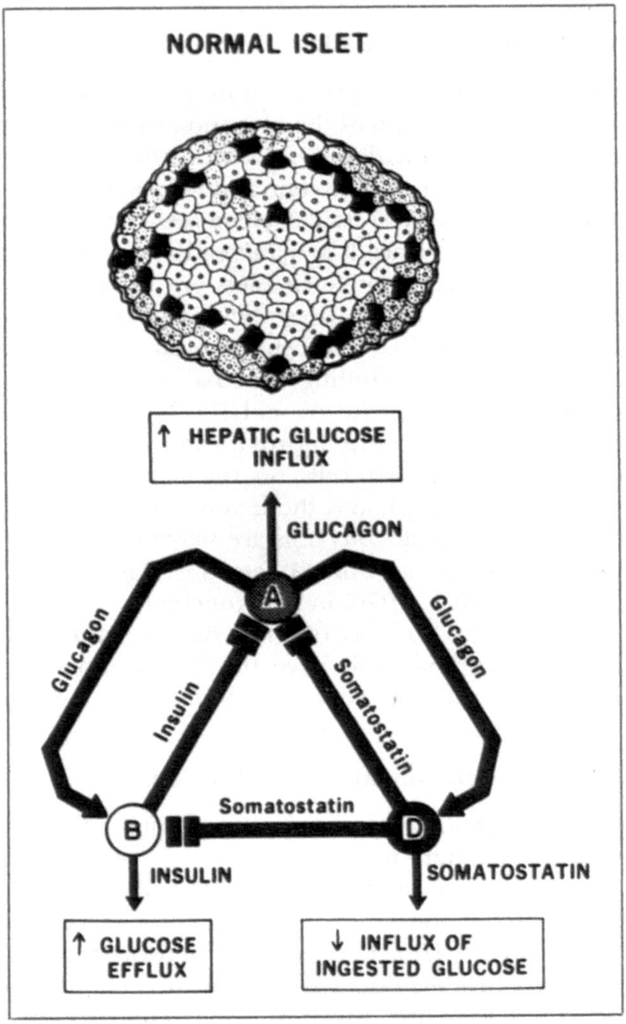

Fig. 3. Schematic representation of the distribution of A-, D-, and B-cells of the rat islet. Reprinted from Orci and Unger (1975) with permission of *Lancet*. Below are depicted possible local or "paracrine" actions of insulin, glucagon, and somatostatin on other islet cells, together with their established, or in the case of somatostatin, postulated endocrine actions. Reprinted from Unger (1977) with permission of the *New England Journal of Medicine*.

heterologous cells of other peptide-secreting endocrine glands have not been observed, raising the question of a specialized need for the islet cells to form a functional syncytium, perhaps to provide the means for coordinated secretion of its principal hormones. These intercellular communications could perhaps be involved in the reciprocal high-frequency oscillations in insulin and glucagon secretion (Goodner *et al.*, 1976).

In summary, the topographical relationships and ultrastructural specializations of the islets of Langerhans may be essential for their normal function, the regulation of nutrient flux. The obvious disruption of certain of these relationships in islet-cell diseases may prove to be of pathophysiologic significance.

3.12. Importance of Glucagon in Clinical Medicine—Diabetes Mellitus

3.12.1. A-Cell Function in Human Diabetes

It is generally agreed that absolute or relative hyperglucagonemia is uniformly present in diabetes (Aguilar-Parada *et al.*, 1969; Unger *et al.*, 1970). In poorly controlled diabetes mellitus, whether the metabolic picture is one of ketoacidosis (Assan *et al.*, 1969; Unger, 1971a; Müller *et al.*, 1973) or nonketotic hyperglycemia (Lindsey *et al.*, 1974b), plasma IRG levels are high. The hyperglucagonemia is the result of increased IRG secretion, but may be exaggerated by decreased renal clearance of glucagon in markedly dehydrated, volume-contracted patients. Nevertheless, even in relatively well controlled insulin-requiring diabetic subjects (Müller *et al.*, 1970; Raskin *et al.*, 1975) and animals (Müller *et al.*, 1971) and in insulin-independent subjects with high insulin levels (Müller *et al.*, 1970; Aronoff *et al.*, 1976a), the pattern of A-cell secretion is distinctly abnormal. The abnormalities include hyperresponsiveness to stimuli such as arginine (Unger *et al.*, 1970) and alanine (Felig *et al.*, 1974) and A-cell insensitivity to glycemic change; hyperglycemia fails to elicit the decline in plasma IRG that characterizes the nondiabetic subject (Unger *et al.*, 1970; Müller *et al.*, 1970), and hypoglycemia fails to stimulate the normal increase in glucagon secretion (Gerich *et al.*, 1973). It is accurate to say that in all forms of overt diabetes, the A-cell is autonomous of glycemic control.

The etiology of the hyperresponsiveness to stimulation and the loss of glucose-sensing that characterize the diabetic state is uncertain. The view that it might constitute a primary lesion of the A-cell is possible, but Aronoff *et al.* (1976b) were unable to detect arginine-induced hyperglucagonemia in presumably "prediabetic" Pima Indians. However, the fact that insulin reduces or corrects the hyperglucagonemia of juvenile-type diabetics (Gerich *et al.,* 1975c), in whom a within-islet deficiency of insulin exists, and that insulin suppresses glucagon secretion by A-cell tumors (Tiengo *et al.,* 1976) and by gastric A-cells (Blazquez *et al.,* 1976) suggests that when they lack contacts with B-cells and insulin, the A-cells lack glucose-sensing capability. Somatostatin, which is also stimulated by a rising glucose concentration (Schauder *et al.,* 1976; Ipp *et al.,* 1977), could also play a role in the glucose-related response of the A-cell. It is noteworthy that in those forms of diabetes characterized by an abundance of insulin-secreting cells, the abnormal A-cell function appears not to respond to supraphysiologic doses of insulin (Unger *et al.,* 1972; Raskin *et al.,* 1975), as does diabetes characterized by insulin deficiency (Gerich *et al.,* 1976b; Raskin *et al.,* 1976). Possibly the normal response of the A-cell to changes in glycemia may require the local presence of both glucagon-suppressing polypeptides, insulin and somatostatin. A-cell hyperresponsiveness to stimulation may reflect lack of restraint by insulin or somatostatin or both; in the insulin-deficient diabetic, this abnormality is readily restored to normal by modest doses of insulin (Gerich *et al.,* 1975c; Raskin *et al.,* 1976), but in the adult-type diabetic, in whom islet insulin is not lacking, even large doses are ineffective (Raskin *et al.,* 1976).

3.12.2. The Bihormonal Abnormality Hypothesis

It was recently proposed (Unger and Orci, 1975) that the complete metabolic syndrome of uncontrolled diabetes is not the result of insulin lack alone, but is the consequence of *both* insulin lack (or insulin insensitivity) and relative or absolute excess of glucagon. Deficiency of insulin or of insulin action is unquestionably the *sine qua non* of diabetes, without which few if any of the metabolic aberrations of the diabetic state occur. According to this bihormonal abnormality hypothesis (Table II), the absence of insulin by itself will result in defective glucose utilization, modest glucose overproduction by the liver, and increased lipolysis, but not in the marked hepatic overproduction of glucose and ketones that characterizes the clinically decompensated diabetic; these require the combination of insulin deficiency and a relative excess of glucagon.

The evidence in support of this concept is as follows: Gerich *et al.* (1975b) demonstrated that in human juvenile-type diabetics made acutely insulin-deficient by abrupt termination of a continuing insulin infusion, endogenous hyperglycemia in excess of 170 mg/dl and β-hydroxybutyrate levels above 1 mM do not occur when glucagon is suppressed to 40 pg/ml or below by somatostatin infusion; only when endogenous or exogenous glucagon is present does marked endogenous hyperglycemia appear

Table II. Contribution of Islet-Cell Abnormalities to the Metabolic Abnormalities of Diabetes Mellitus

Abnormalities	Insulin deficiency	Relative IRG excess
↓ Glucose utilization	++++	0
↑ Hepatic glucose production	+	++++
↑ Lipolysis	++++	+(?)
↑ Ketogenic capacity of liver	+(?)	++++

(Gerich *et al.*, 1976c). Also, in hyperglycemic alloxan-diabetic dogs, suppression of hyperglucagonemia to levels of 50 pg/ml or below results in a gradual decline in their hyperglycemia (Sakurai *et al.*, 1975b). Following insulin withdrawal in totally depancreatized dogs, suppression of extrapancreatic glucagon secretion by somatostatin similarly limits endogenous hyperglycemia to the 150–170 mg/dl range (Sakurai *et al.*, 1975b). And Sherwin *et al.* (1977) demonstrated in intact humans that during the suppression of both insulin and glucagon by somatostatin, glucose concentration rises only to between 135 and 150 mg/dl, very modest endogenous hyperglycemia compared with that produced by insulin deficiency in the presence of glucagon (Sherwin *et al.*, 1976). These findings indicate that at least in the short time frame of the foregoing experiments, lack of insulin does not lead to severe endogenous hyperglycemia in the absence of glucagon, in contrast to the massive hyperglycemia induced wthin hours by insulin deprivation plus hyperglucagonemia. A similar conclusion can be drawn with respect to the ketoacidosis of uncontrolled diabetes.

On the other hand, it is equally clear that when insulin is deficient, marked *exogenous* hyperglycemia (hyperglycemia derived from the diet rather than from hepatic glucose production) can occur whether or not glucagon is present. When glucose efflux is reduced by insulin deficiency, if ingested glucose enters the circulation at a rate exceeding its removal via insulin-independent avenues of glucose clearance, severe hyperglycemia and glycosuria will eventuate, even in the absence of glucagon. However, the rare circumstance of diabetes without glucagon, reported in the somatostatinoma syndrome (Ganda *et al.*, 1977; Larsson *et al.*, 1977), is characterized by only modest endogenous hyperglycemia, marked improvement of exogenous hyperglycemia by carbohydrate restriction, and absence of ketoacidosis.

Another controversial issue concerns the consequence of an increase in glucagon secretion, such as might be induced by infection (Rocha *et al.*, 1973) or any type of stress (Lindsey *et al.*, 1974a; Wilmore *et al.*, 1974), on hyperglycemia and ketonemia in diabetic patients receiving insulin. Sherwin *et al.* (1976) observed no deterioration in the hyperglycemia of two insulin-treated juvenile-type diabetics when glucagon was infused and IRG levels raised to as high as 750 pg/ml; they concluded that glucagon has no deleterious effect on diabetic control as long as insulin is present. Raskin and Unger (1977), however, infused precisely the same amount of glucagon as Sherwin to a group of four diabetics, all receiving constant intravenous insulin, and all four developed a statistically significant increase in glycemia, glycosuria, urea nitrogen, and ketone excretion while receiving glucagon, even though all had been well controlled prior to the day of glucagon infusion. All the adverse metabolic effects of glucagon receded promptly on its being discontinued. Raskin and Unger concluded, therefore, that hyperglucagonemia of relatively modest degree, such as may occur in infection and other stressful events, may result in deterioration of diabetic control despite the continued administration of insulin.

3.12.3. Glucagon Suppression as a Therapeutic Adjunct in Juvenile Diabetes

Another controversial issue concerns the potential value of glucagon suppression in the treatment of diabetic patients in the hyperglycemia in juvenile diabetic patients. It is clear that when glycemia is measured many times per day (Service *et al.,* 1970), even large doses of insulin do not eliminate postprandial hyperglycemia. Juvenile diabetics are hyperglycemic for about 16 hr per day, even though their plasma glucose levels are normal in the early morning hours (Unger *et al.,* 1977). Much of this hyperglycemia is the result of dietary carbohydrate, but some of it may be of endogenous origin, a consequence of the effect of exaggerated hyperglucagonemia that accompanies a meal on hepatic glucose production. The demonstration by Gerich *et al.* (1975a) that somatostatin blocks both postprandial hyperglucagonemia and postprandial hyperglycemia was initially interpreted as evidence of a role of inappropriate glucagon secretion. Wahren and Felig (1976), however, reported that doses of somatostatin comparable to those employed by Gerich blocked the absorption of xylose and glucose and argued that the effect of somatostatin on postprandial hyperglycemia could therefore be attributed to reduced absorption of glucose. It is indeed true that somatostatin has a profound effect on gastrointestinal function and that the frequently gratifying effects of high-dose somatostatin infusion in juvenile-type diabetics may be the consequence of a delay in the rate of glucose entry. However, reduction of hyperglucagonemia during meals may also help reduce hyperglycemia, and in fact reduces the hyperglycemic effects of intravenously administered alanine (Sakurai *et al.,* 1974). In addition, there is preliminary evidence of a direct inhibitory effect of somatostatin on glucagon-mediated glucose production (Sacks *et al.,* 1977).

The inadequacy of conventional therapy in maintaining euglycemia in diabetic patients has led to examination of the possibility that a glucagon suppressant such as somatostatin might improve the therapeutic results. Because of its very short biological half-life, somatostatin must be given by continuous intravenous infusion. Therapeutic trials of somatostatin have been conducted in selected patients with juvenile-type diabetes for up to 5 days at a dose of 2.0–2.4 mg/day (Gerich, 1976). The results have been remarkable in some patients (Fig. 4). In juvenile diabetics with fasting normoglycemia but extremely high postprandial blood sugars between breakfast time and after midnight, the infusion of somatostatin significantly lowered plasma glucagon and glucose levels, maintaining normoglycemia around the clock, something that could not be achieved by any previous schedule of insulin dosage. As Wahren and Felig (1976) have maintained, this effect may be due in large part to reduced entry of carbohydrate; however, no clinical or laboratory evidence of malabsorption occurred in 5 days of therapy, and weight was maintained. Conceivably, the rate at which glucose enters the circulation is reduced by the somatostatin to one closer to the rate of glucose disposal.

Efforts to dissociate some of somatostatin's effects (Rivier *et al.,* 1976; Brown *et al.,* 1976b) are now being made. Des-Asn^{5}-somatostatin inhibits insulin but not glucagon secretion, while [D-Trp^{8}]somatostatin is several times as potent as somatostatin in inhibiting growth hormone, insulin, and glucagon. [D-Cys^{14}]somatostatin is more potent than insulin in inhibiting glucagon, and [D-Trp^{8}-D-Cys^{14}]somatostatin is extremely potent in inhibiting both. When administered to diabetic dogs (Dobbs *et al.,* 1977), [D-Trp^{8}],[D-Cys^{14}]somatostatin and [D-Trp^{8}-D-Cys^{14}]somatostatin are more effective glucagon suppressants than somatostatin when injected subcutaneously, their effects lasting for more than 150 min. In fasted insulin-deprived dogs, both a glucose-lowering and a triglyceride-lowering effect were observed (Dobbs *et al.,* 1977). Their possible role in the future treatment of diabetes mellitus remains to be evaluated.

3.12.4. Glucagonoma

The glucagonoma syndrome has been well described clinically (McGavran *et al.,* 1966; Mallinson *et al.* 1974). There is now increasing evidence (Valverde *et al.,* 1976) that the high IRG levels in patients with glucagonoma syndrome may be the consequence not only of an increase in true glucagon but also of a prominent increase in IRG$^{\sim 9000}$, considered to be a glucagon precursor. In the case reported by Valverde *et al.* (1976),

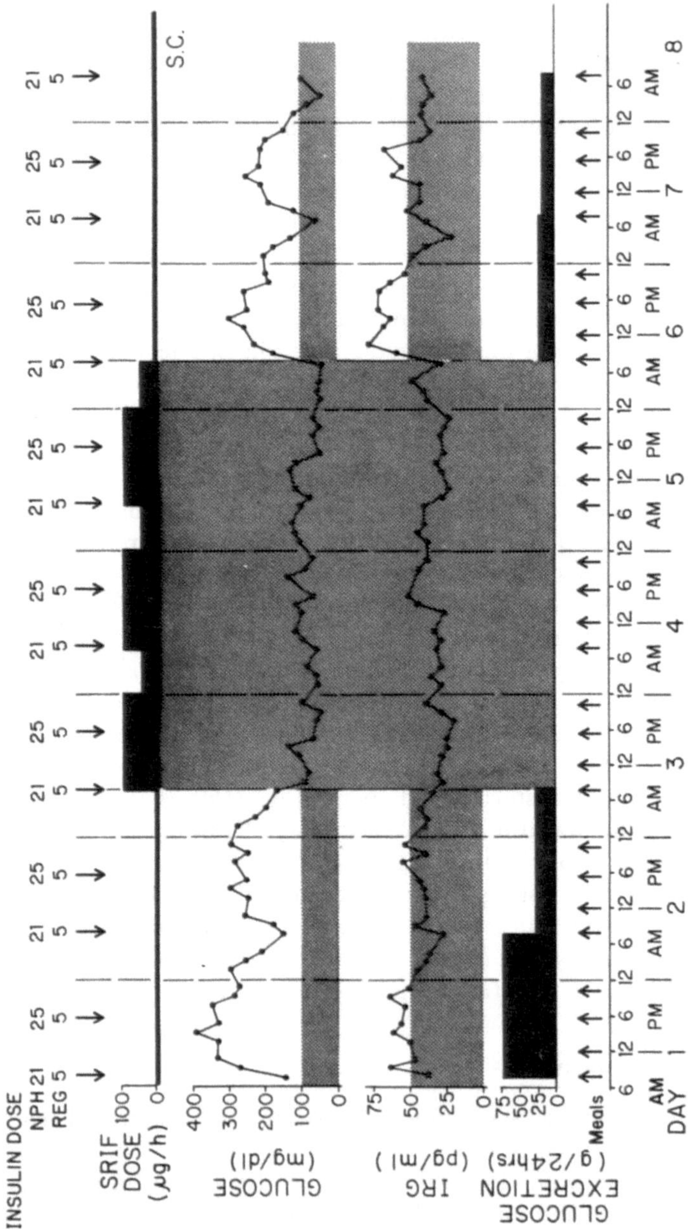

Fig. 4. Effect of continuous intravenous infusion of somatostatin on plasma glucose and IRG levels and glycosuria in a juvenile diabetic.

the total IRG of 2600 pg/ml included 1435 pg true glucagon/ml, the normal average being 31 pg/ml, and about 625 pg $IRG^{\sim 9000}$/ml, the normal average being 11, while BPG, which normally averages 113±79 pg/ml, was 190. Recant *et al.* (1976) reported four new cases of glucagonoma syndrome and suggested the diagnostic importance of a high $IRG^{\sim 9000}$ level in glucagonoma syndrome. Perhaps this is analogous to the high proinsulin levels that characterize insulinomas. As for the glucagonoma syndrome itself, the etiology of frequently associated skin disease remains unknown.

References

Aguilar-Parada, E., Eisentraut, A. M., and Unger, R. H., 1969, Pancreatic glucagon secretion in normal and diabetic subjects, *Amer. J. Med. Sci.* **257**:415.

Arimura, A., Sato, H., Dupont, A., Nishi, N., and Schally, A. V., 1975, Somatostatin: Abundance of immunoreactive hormone in rat stomach and pancreas, *Science* **189**:1007.

Aronoff, S. L., Bennett, P. H., Rushforth, N. B., Miller, M., and Unger, R. H., 1976a, Arginine stimulated hyperglucagonemia in diabetic Pima Indians, *Diabetes* **25**:404.

Aronoff, S. L., Bennett, P. H., Rushforth, N. B., Miller, M., and Unger, R. H., 1976b, Normal glucagon response to arginine infusion in "prediabetic" Pima Indians, *J. Clin. Endocrinol. Metab.* **43**:279.

Ashby, J. P., and Speake, R. N., 1975, Insulin and glucagon secretion from isolated islets of Langerhans. The effects of calcium ionophores, *Biochem. J.* **150**:89.

Assan, R., 1972, *In vivo* metabolism of glucagon, in: *Glucagon: Molecular Physiology, Clinical and Therapeutic Implications* (P. J. Lefebvre and R. H. Unger, eds.), pp. 47–59, Pergamon Press, Oxford.

Assan, R., and Slusher, N., 1972, Structure/function and structure/immunoreactivity relationships of the glucagon molecule and related synthetic peptides, *Diabetes* **21**:843.

Assan, R., Hautecouverture, G., Guillemant, S., Douchy, F., Protin, P., and Derot, M., 1969, Evolution de parametres hormonaux (glucagon, cortisol, hormone somatotrope) et energetiques (glucose, acides gras glycerol libre) dans dix acido-cetoses diabetiques graves traitees, *Pathol. Biol.* **17**:1095.

Baetens, D., Coleman, D. L., and Orci, L., 1976a, Islet cell population in ob/ob and db/db mice, *Diabetes* **25**:344.

Baetens, D., Rufener, C., Srikant, C. B., Dobbs, R., Unger, R., and Orci, L., 1976b, Identification of glucagon-producing cells (A-cells) in dog gastric mucosa, *J. Cell Biol.* **69**:455.

Barden, N., Lavoie, M., Alvarado-Urbina, G., Cote, J.-P., and Dupont, A., 1977, A physiologic role of somatostatin in the control of insulin and glucagon secretion, *Fed. Proc. Fed. Amer. Soc. Exp. Biol.* **36**:298.

Barnes, A. J., and Bloom, S. R., 1976, Pancreatectomized man: A model for diabetes without glucagon, *Lancet* **1**:219.

Bhathena, S. J., Perrino, P. V., Voyles, N. R., Smith, S. S., Wilkins, S. D., Coy, D.

H., Schally, A. V., and Recant, L., 1976, Reversal of somatostatin inhibition of insulin and glucagon secretion, *Diabetes* **25**:1031.

Bilbrey, G. L., Faloona, G. R., White, M. C., and Knochel, J. P., 1974, Hyperglucagonemia of renal failure, *J. Clin, Invest.* **53**:841.

Bilheimer, D. W., Goldstein, J. L., Grundy, S. M., and Brown, M. S., 1975, Reduction in cholesterol and low density lipoprotein synthesis after portacaval shunt surgery in a patient with homozygous familial hypercholesterolemia, *J. Clin. Invest.* **56**:1420.

Blackard, W. G., Nelson, N. C., and Andrews, S. S., 1974, Portal and peripheral vein immunoreactive glucagon concentrations after arginine or glucose infusions, *Diabetes* **23**:199.

Blair, J. B., Cimbala, M. A., Foster, J. L., and Morgan, R. A., 1976, Hepatic pyruvate kinase. Regulation by glucagon, cyclic adenosine 3′-5′-monophosphate, and insulin in the perfused rat liver, *J. Biol. Chem.* **251**:3756.

Blazquez, E., Muñoz-Barragan, L., Patton, G. S., Orci, L., Dobbs, R. E., and Unger, R. H., 1976, Gastric A-cell function in insulin-deprived depancreatized dogs, *Endocrinology* **99**:1182.

Blazquez, E., Muñoz-Barragan, L., Patton, G. S., Dobbs, R. E., and Unger, R. H., 1977, Demonstration of gastric glucagon hypersecretion in insulin-deprived alloxan diabetic dogs, *J. Lab. Clin. Med.* **89**:971.

Bloom, S. R., Mortimer, C. H., Thorner, M. O., Besser, G. M., Hall, R., Gomez-Pan, A., Roy, V. M., Russell, R. C. G., Coy, D. H., Kastin, A. J., and Schally, A. V., 1974, Inhibition of gastrin and gastric acid secretion by growth-hormone release-inhibiting hormone, *Lancet* **2**:1106.

Bloom, S. R., Ralphs, D. N., Besser, G. M., Hall, R., Coy, D. H., Kastin, A. J., and Schally, A. V., 1975, Effect of somatostatin on motilin levels and gastric emptying, *Gut* **16**:834.

Blundell, T. L., Dockerill, S., Sasaki, K., Tickle, I. J., and Wood, S. P., 1976, The relation of structure to storage and receptor binding of glucagon, *Metabolism* **25**(Suppl.):1331.

Boden, G., Sivitz, M. C., Owen, O. E., Essakoumar, N., and Lauder, J. H., 1975, Somatostatin suppresses secretin and pancreatic exocrine secretion, *Science* **190**:163.

Boden, G., Jacoby, H. I., and Staus, A., 1976, Somatostatin interacts with basal and carbachol stimulated antral and duodenal motility, *Gastroenterology* **70**:961.

Böttger, L., Schlein, E., Faloona, G. R., Knochel, J. P., and Unger, R. H., 1972, The effect of exercise on glucagon secretion, *J. Clin. Endocrinol. Metab.* **35**:117.

Braaten, J. T., Faloona, G. R., and Unger, R. H., 1974, The effect of insulin on the alpha-cell response to hyperglycemia in long-standing alloxan diabetes, *J. Clin. Invest.* **53**:1017.

Brazeau, P., Vale, W., Burgus, R., Ling, N., Butcher, M., Rivier, J., and Guillemin, R., 1973, Hypothalamic polypeptide that inhibits the secretion of immunoreactive pituitary growth hormone, *Science* **179**:77.

Brockman, R. P., Bergman, E. N., Joo, P. K., and Manns, J. G., 1975, Effects of glucagon and insulin on net hepatic metabolism of glucose precursors in sheep, *Amer. J. Physiol.* **229**:1344.

Bromer, W. W., 1976, Studies with glucagon analogs, *Metabolism* **25**(Suppl.):1315.

Bromer, W. W., Sinn, L. G., and Behrens, O. K., 1957, The amino acid sequence of glucagon. V. Location of amide groups, acid degradation studies, and summary of sequential evidence, *J. Amer. Chem. Soc.* **79**:2807.

Bromer, W. W., Boucher, M. E., and Koffenberger, J. E., Jr., 1971, Amino acid sequence of bovine glucagon, *J. Biol. Chem.* **246**:2822.

Brown, M., and Vale, W., 1976, Effects of neurotensin and substance P on plasma insulin, glucagon and glucose levels, *Endocrinology* **98**:819.

Brown, M., Villarreal, J., and Vale, W., 1976a, Neurotensin and substance P. Effects on plasma insulin and glucagon levels, *Metabolism* **25**(Suppl.):1459.

Brown, M., Rivier, J., and Vale, W., 1976b, Somatostatin analogs with selected biologic activities, *Metabolism* **25**(Suppl.):1501.

Buchanan, K. D., and McCarroll, A. M., 1972, Abnormalities of glucagon metabolism in untreated diabetes mellitus, *Lancet* **2**:1394.

Cahill, G. F., Jr., 1971, Physiology of insulin in man (Banting Memorial Lecture), *Diabetes* **20**:785.

Cherrington, A. D., and Exton, J. H., 1976, Studies on the role of cAMP-dependent protein kinase in the actions of glucagon and catecholamines on liver glycogen metabolism, *Metabolism* **25**(Suppl.):1351.

Cherrington, A., and Vranic, M., 1974, Effect of interaction between insulin and glucagon on glucose turnover and FFA concentration in normal and depancreatized dogs, *Metabolism* **23**:729.

Chiasson, J. L., Liljenquist, J. E., Sinclair-Smith, B. C., and Lacy, W. W., 1975, Gluconeogenesis from alanine in normal postabsorptive man. Intrahepatic stimulatory effect of glucagon, *Diabetes* **24**:574.

Creutzfeldt, W., Raubisch, P. G., and Folsch, U. R., 1975, Hemmung der Sekretin- und Cholezystokinin-pankreozymin induzieken Saft- und Enzymsekretin des Pankreas und der gallenblasen Kontraktion beim Menschen durch Somatostatin, *Dtsch. Med. Wochenschr.* **100**:1135.

Danforth, D. N., Jr., Triche, T., Doppman, J. L., Beazley, R. M., Perrino, P. V., and Recant, L., 1976, Elevated plasma proglucagon-like component with a glucagon-secreting tumor. Effect of streptozotocin, *N. Engl. J. Med.* **295**:242.

Dencker, H., Hedner, P., Holst, J., and Tranberg, K. G., 1975, Pancreatic glucagon response to an ordinary meal, *Scand. J. Gastroenterol.* **10**:471.

Dich, J., and Gluud, C. N., 1976, Effect of glucagon on cyclic AMP, albumin, metabolism and incorporation of ^{14}C-leucine into proteins in isolated parenchymal rat liver cells, *Acta Physiol. Scand.* **97**:457.

Dobbs, R. E., Sakurai, H., Sasaki, H., Faloona, G. R., Valverde, I., Baetens, D., Orci, L., and Unger, R. H., 1975, Glucagon: Role in the hyperglycemia of diabetes mellitus, *Science* **187**:544.

Dobbs, R., Schusdziarra, V., Rivier, J., and Brown, M., 1977, Somatostatin analogs as glucagon suppressants in diabetes, *Diabetes* **26**(Suppl.):360.

Dubois, M. P., 1975, Immunoreactive somatostatin is present in discrete cells of the endocrine pancreas, *Proc. Natl. Acad. Sci. U.S.A.* **72**:1340.

Duckworth, W. C., and Kitabchi, A. E., 1974, Insulin and glucagon degradation by the same enzyme, *Diabetes* **23**:536.

Eisenstein, A. B., and Strack, I., 1976, A nonsuppressible increase of glucagon secretion by isolated islets of high-protein-fed rats, *Diabetes* **25**:51.

Ensinck, J. W., and Palmer, J. P., 1976, Dominant inheritance of large molecular weight species of glucagon, *Metabolism* **25**(Suppl.):1409.

Epand, R. M., Cote, T. E., Hui Bon Hoa, D., Rosselin, G., and Schreier, S., 1976, Biologic activity and conformational properties of glucagon and glucagon analogs, *Metabolism* **25**(Suppl.):1317.

Exton, J. H., and Park, C. R., 1969, Control of gluconeogenesis in liver. III. Effects of L-lactate, pyruvate, fructose, glucagon, epinephrine, and adenosine 3′,5′-monophosphate on gluconeogenic intermediates in the perfused rat liver, *J. Biol. Chem.* **244**:1424.

Faloona, G. R., 1972, The structure–function relationships of pancreatic glucagon, in: *Glucagon: Molecular Physiology, Clinical and Therapeutic Implications* (P. J. Lefebvre and R. H. Unger, eds.), pp. 201–204, Pergamon Press, Oxford.

Felig, P., Gusberg, R., Hendler, R., Gump, F. E., and Kinney, J. M., 1974, Concentrations of glucagon and the insulin:glucagon ratio in the portal and peripheral circulation (38286), *Proc. Soc. Exp. Biol. Med.* **147**:88.

Felig, P., Wahren, J., and Hendler, R., 1976, Influence of physiologic hyperglucagonemia on basal and insulin-inhibited splanchnic glucose output in normal man, *J. Clin. Invest.* **58**:761.

Feliu, J. E., Hue, L., and Hers, H. G., 1976, Hormonal control of pyruvate kinase activity and of gluconeogenesis in isolated hepatocytes, *Proc. Natl. Acad. Sci. U.S.A.* **73**:2762.

Ferner, H., 1953, The A- and B-cells of the pancreatic islets as sources of the antagonistic hormones glucagon and insulin. The shift of the AB-relation in diabetes mellitus, *Amer. J. Dig. Dis.* **20**:301.

Fisher, M., Sherwin, R. S., Hendler, R., and Felig, P., 1976, Kinetics of glucagon in man: Effects of starvation, *Proc. Natl. Acad. Sci. U.S.A.* **73**:1735.

Frame, C. M., Davidson, M. B., and Sturdevant, R. A. L., 1975, Effects of the octapeptide of cholecystokinin on insulin and glucagon secretion in the dog, *Endocrinology* **97**:549.

Freinkel, N., and Goodner, C. J., 1960, Carbohydrate metabolism in pregnancy. I. The metabolism of insulin by human placental tissue, *J. Clin. Invest.* **39**:116.

Gabbay, K. H., DeLuca, K., Fisher, J. N., Jr., Mako, M. E., and Rubenstein, A. H., 1976, Familial hyperproinsulinemia: An autosomal dominant defect, *N. Engl. J. Med.* **294**:911.

Galbo, H., and Holst, J. J., 1976, The influence of glucagon on hepatic glycogen mobilization in exercising rats, *Pfluegers Arch.* **363**:49.

Galbo, H., Holst J. J., Christensen, N. J., and Hilsted, J., 1976, Glucagon and plasma catecholamines during beta-receptor blockade in exercising man, *J. Appl. Physiol.* **40**:855.

Ganda, O. P., Weir, G. C., Soeldner, J. S., Legg, M. A., Chick, W. L., Patel, Y. C., Ebeid, A. M., Gabbay, K. H., and Reichlin, S., 1977, Somatostatinoma: A somatostatin containing tumor of the endocrine pancreas, *N. Engl. J. Med.* **296**:963.

Gerich, J. E., 1976, Metabolic effects of longterm somatostatin infusion in man, *Metabolism* **25**(Suppl.):1505.

Gerich, J. E., Langlois, M., Noacco, C., Karam, J. H., and Forsham, P. H., 1973, Lack of glucagon response to hypoglycemia in diabetes: Evidence for an intrinsic pancreatic alpha cell defect, *Science* **182**:171.

Gerich, J. E., Lorenzi, M., Karam, J. H., Schneider, V., and Forsham, P. H., 1975a, Abnormal pancreatic glucagon secretion and postprandial hyperglycemia in diabetes mellitus, *J. Amer. Med. Assoc.* **234**:159.

Gerich, J. E., Lorenzi, M., Bier, D. M., Schneider, V., Tsalikian, E., Karam, J. H., and Forsham, P. H., 1975b, Prevention of human diabetic ketoacidosis by somatostatin: Evidence for an essential role of glucagon, *N. Engl. J. Med.* **292**:985.

Gerich, J. E., Tsalikian, E., Lorenzi, M., Karam, J. H., Schneider, V., Gustafson, G., and Bohannon, N. V., 1975c, Normalization of fasting hyperglucagonemia and excessive glucagon responses to intravenous arginine in human diabetes mellitus by prolonged infusion of insulin, *J. Clin. Endocrinol. Metab.* **41**:1178.

Gerich, J. E., Lorenzi, M., Tsalikian, E., and Karam, J. H., 1976a, Studies on the mechanism of epinephrine-induced hyperglycemia in man. Evidence for participation of pancreatic glucagon secretion, *Diabetes* **25**:65.

Gerich, J. E., Langlois, M., Noacco, C., Lorenzi, M., Karam, J. H., and Forsham, P. H., 1976b, Comparison of the suppressive effects of elevated plasma glucose and free fatty acid levels on glucagon secretion in normal and insulin-dependent diabetic subjects. Evidence for selective alpha-cell insensitivity to glucose in diabetes mellitus, *J. Clin. Invest.* **58**:320.

Gerich, J. E., Lorenzi, M., Bier, D. M., Tsalikian, E., Schneider, V., Karam, J. H., and Forsham, P. H., 1976c, Effects of physiologic levels of glucagon and growth hormone of human carbohydrate and lipid metabolism: Studies involving administration of exogenous hormone during suppression of endogenous hormone secretion with somatostatin, *J. Clin. Invest.* **57**:875.

Girard, J. R., Guillet, I., Marty, J., Assan, R., and Marliss, E. B., 1976, Effects of exogenous hormones and glucose on plasma levels and hepatic metabolism of amino acids in the fetus and in the newborn rat, *Diabetologia* **12**:327.

Girardier, L., Seydoux, J., and Campfield, L. A., 1976, Control of A and B cells *in vivo* by sympathetic nervous input and selective hyper- or hypoglycemia in dog pancreas, *J. Physiol. (Paris)* **72**:801.

Goldfine, I. D., and Smith, G. J., 1976, Binding of insulin to isolated nuclei, *Proc. Natl. Acad. Sci. U.S.A.* **73**:1427.

Goodner, C. J., Walike, B. C., Koerker, D. J., Brown, A. C., Ensinck, J. W., Chideckel, E. W., Palmer, J., and Kalnasy, L. W., 1976, Insulin, glucagon and glucose: Synchronous, stable oscillations in the Rhesus monkey, *Diabetes* **25**(Suppl.):340.

Hammes, G. G., and Rodbell, M., 1976, Simple model for hormone-activated adenylate cyclase systems, *Proc. Natl. Acad. Sci. U.S.A.* **73**:1189.

Harvey, W. D., Faloona, G. R., and Unger, R. H., 1974, The effect of adrenergic blockade on exercise-induced hyperglucagonemia, *Endocrinology* **94**:1254.

Heding, L. G., Frandsen, E. K., and Jacobsen, H., 1976, Structure–function relationship: Immunologic, *Metabolism* **25**(Suppl.):1327.

Hruby, V. J., Wright, D. E., Lin, M. C., and Rodbell, M., 1976, Semisynthetic glucagon derivatives for structure–function studies, *Metabolism* **25**(Suppl.):1323.

Hutson, N. J., Brumley, F. T., Assimacopoulos, F. D., Harper, S. C., and Exton, J. H., 1976, Studies on the alpha-adrenergic activation of hepatic glucose output. I. Studies on the alpha-adrenergic activation of phosphorylase and gluconeogenesis and inactivation of glycogen synthase in isolated rat liver parenchymal cells, *J. Biol. Chem.* **251**:5200.

Ipp, E., Patton, G., Dobbs, R., Harris, V., Vale, W., and Unger, R. H., 1977, Endogenous immunoreactive somatostatin (IRS) secretion by the pancreas, *Diabetes* **26**:359.

Ishida, T., Kawamura, K., Goto, A., Nishina, Y., Takahara, J., Yamamoto, S., Kawanishi, K., and Ofjui, T., 1976, Comparison studies of neurotensin and xenopsin upon pancreatic secretion in dog, *Metabolism* **25**(Suppl.):1467.

Ito, S., and Kobayashi, S., 1976, Immunohistochemical demonstration of glucagon- and GLI-containing cells in the canine gut and pancreas, *Arch. Histol. Jpn.* **39**:193.

Jaspan, J. B., Kuku, S. F., Locker, J. D., Huen, A. H.-J., Emmanouel, D. S., Katz, A. I., and Rubenstein, A. H., 1976, Heterogeneity of plasma glucagon in man, *Metabolism* **25**(Suppl.):1397.

Johnson, D. G., and Ensinck, J. W., 1976, Stimulation of glucagon secretion by scorpion toxin in the perfused rat pancreas, *Diabetes* **25**:645.

Kakiuchi, S., and Tomizawa, H. H., 1964, Properties of a glucagon-degrading enzyme of beef liver, *J. Biol. Chem.* **239**:2160.

Koerker, D. J., Ruch, W., Chideckel, E., Palmer, J., Goodner, C. J., Ensinck, J., and Gale, C. C., 1974, Somatostatin: Hypothalamic inhibitor of the endocrine pancreas, *Science* **184**:482.

Kuku, S. F., Jaspan, J. B., Emmanouel, D. S., Zeidler, A., Katz, A. I., and Rubenstein, A. H., 1976, Heterogeneity of plasma glucagon, circulating components in normal subjects and patients with chronic renal failure, *J. Clin. Invest.* **58**:742.

Larsson, L.-I., Holst, J., Häkanson, R., and Sundler, F., 1975, Distribution and properties of glucagon immunoreactivity in the digestive tract of various mammals: An immunohistochemical and immunochemical study, *Histochemistry* **44**:281.

Larsson, L.-I., Hirsch, M. A., Holst, J. J., Ingemansson, S., Kuhl, C., Lindkaer Jensen, S., Lundqvist, G., Rehfeld, J. F., and Schwartz, T. W., 1977, Pancreatic somatostatinoma: Clinical features and physiological implications, *Lancet* **1**:666.

Lawrence, A. M., Tan, S., Hojvat, S., Kirsteins, L., and Mitton, J., 1976, Salivary gland glucagon in man and animals, *Metabolism* **25**(Suppl.):1405.

Leblanc, H., Rigg, L. A., and Yen, S. S., 1975, The response of pancreatic and pituitary hormones to pulses and constant infusion of somatostatin, *J. Clin. Endocrinol. Metab.* **41**:1105.

Leclercq-Meyer, V., Rebolledo, O., Marchano, J., and Malaisse, W., 1975, Glucagon release: Paradoxical stimulation by glucose during calcium deprivation, *Science* **189**:897.

Lefebvre, P. J., and Luyckx, A. S., 1972, Glucagon and catecholamines, in: *Glucagon: Molecular Physiology, Clinical and Therapeutic Implications* (P. J. Lefebvre and R. H. Unger, eds.), pp. 175–180, Pergamon Press, Oxford.

Lefebvre, P. J., and Luyckx, A. S., 1975, Effect of acute kidney exclusion by ligation of renal arteries on peripheral plasma glucagon levels and pancreatic glucagon production in the anesthetized dog, *Metabolism* **24**:1169.

Lefebvre, P. J., and Luyckx, A. S., 1976, Plasma glucagon after kidney exclusion: Experiments in somatostatin-infused and in eviscerated dogs, *Metabolism* **25**:761.

Liljenquist, J. E., Chiasson, J. L., Cherrington, A. D., Keller, U., Jennings, A. S., Bomboy, J. D., and Lacy, W. W., 1976, An important role for glucagon in the regulation of glucose production *in vivo, Metabolism* **25**(Suppl.):1371.

Lin, M. C., Nicosia, S., and Rodbell, M., 1976, Effects of iodination of tyrosyl residues on the binding and action of glucagon and its receptor, *Biochemistry* **15**:4537.

Lindsey, C. A., Santeusanio, F., Braaten, J., Faloona, G. R., and Unger, R. H., 1974a, Pancreatic alpha-cell function in trauma, *J. Amer. Med. Assoc.* **227**:757.

Lindsey, C. A., Faloona, G. R., and Unger, R. H., 1974b, Plasma glucagon in nonketotic hyperosmolar coma, *J. Amer. Med. Assoc.* **229**:1771.

Luft, R., Efendic, S., Hökfelt, T., Johansson, O., and Arimura, A., 1974, Immunohistochemical evidence for the localization of somatostatin-like immunoreactivity in a cell population of the pancreatic islets, *Med. Biol.* **52**:428.

Lundquist, I., Fanska, R., and Grodsky, G. M., 1976a, Direct calcium-stimulated release of glucagon from the isolated perfused rat pancreas and the effect of chemical sympathectomy, *Endocrinology* **98**:815.

Lundquist, I., Fanska, R., and Grodsky, G., 1976b, Interaction of calcium and glucose on glucagon secretion, *Endocrinology* **99**:1304.

Luyckx, A. S., and Lefebvre, P. J., 1972, Role of catecholamines in exercise-induced glucagon secretion in rats, *Diabetes* **21**(Suppl.):334.

Mackrell, D. J., and Sokal, J. E., 1969, Antagonism between the effects of insulin and glucagon on the isolated liver, *Diabetes* **18**:724.

Madison, L. L., Seyffert, W. A., Jr., Unger, R. H., and Baker, B., 1968, Effect of plasma free fatty acids on plasma glucagon and serum insulin concentrations, *Metabolism* **17**:301.

Mallinson, C. N., Bloom, S. R., Warin, A. P., Salmon, P. R., and Cox, B., 1974, A glucagonoma syndrome, *Lancet* **2**:1.

Marco, J., Calle, C., Roman, D., Diaz-Fierros, M., Villanueva, M. L., and Valverde, I., 1973, Hyperglucagonism induced by glucocorticoid treatment in man, *N. Engl. J. Med.* **288**:128.

Marco, J., Calle, C., Hedo, J. A., and Villanueva, M. L., 1976, Enhanced glucagon secretion by pancreatic islets from prednisolone-treated mice, *Diabetologia* **12**:307.

Markussen, J., Frandsen, E., Heding, L. G., and Sundby, F., 1972, Turkey glucagon: Crystallization, amino acid composition, and immunology, *Horm. Metab. Res.* **4**:360.

Marliss, E. B., Girardier, L., Seydoux, J., Wollheim, C. B., Kanazawa, Y., Orci, L., Renold, A. E., and Porte, D., Jr., 1973, Glucagon release induced by pancreatic nerve stimulation in the dog, *J. Clin. Invest.* **52**:1246.

Mashiter, K., Harding, P. E., Chou, M., Mashiter, G. D., Stout, J., Diamond, D., and Field, J. B., 1975, Persistent pancreatic glucagon but not insulin response to arginine in pancreatectomized dogs, *Endocrinology* **96**:678.

Matschinsky, F. M., Pagliara, A. S., Hover, B. A., Haymond, M. W., and Stillings, S. N., 1975, Differential effects of alpha- and beta-D-glucose on insulin and glucagon secretion from the isolated perfused rat pancreas, *Diabetes* **24**:369.

Matschinsky, F. M., Pagliara, A. S., Stillings, S. N., and Hover, B. A., 1976, Glucose and ATP levels in pancreatic islet tissue of normal and diabetic rats, *J. Clin. Invest.* **58**:1193.

Matsuyama, T., and Foa, P. P., 1975, Plasma glucose, insulin, pancreatic and enteroglucagon levels in normal and depancreatized dogs (38288), *Proc. Soc. Exp. Biol. Med.* **147**:97.

McGarry, J. D., Robles-Valdes, C., and Foster, D. W., 1976, Glucagon and ketogenesis, *Metabolism* **25**(Suppl.):1387.

McGavran, M. H., Unger, R. H., Recant, L., Polk, H. C., Kilo, C., and Levin, M. E., 1966, A glucagon-secreting alpha cell carcinoma of the pancreas, *N. Engl. J. Med.* **274**:1408.

Meissner, H. P., 1976, Electrophysiological evidence for coupling between B-cells of pancreatic islets, *Nature (London)* **262**:502.

Metzger, B. E., Unger, R. H., and Freinkel, N., 1977, Carbohydrate metabolism in pregnancy. XVI. Relationships between circulating glucagon, insulin, glucose and amino acids in response to a "mixed meal" in late pregnancy, *Metabolism* **26**:151.

Miller, L. L., 1976, Direct effects of glucagon on protein and amino acid metabolism in the isolated perfused rat liver. Interactions with insulin and dexamethasone in net synthesis of albumin and acute-phase proteins, *Diabetes* **25**(Suppl.):865.

Miyata, M., Yamamoyo, T., Yamaguchi, M., Nakao, K., and Yoshida, T., 1976, Plasma glucagon after total resection of the pancreas in man (39435), *Proc. Soc. Exp. Biol. Med.* **152**:510.

Moody, A. J., Frandsen, E. K., Jacobsen, H., Sundby, F., and Orci, L., 1976, Discussion, *Metabolism* **25**(Suppl.):1336.

Mortimer, C. H., Turnbridge, W. M. G., Carr, D., Yeomans, L., Lind, T., Coy, D. H., Bloom, S. R., Kastin, A., Mallinson, C. N., Besser, G. M., Schally, A. V., and Hall, R., 1974, Effects of growth hormone release-inhibiting hormone on circulating glucagon, insulin and growth hormone in normal, diabetic, acromegalic and hypopituitary patients, *Lancet* **1**:697.

Müller, W. A., Faloona, G. R., Unger, R. H., and Aguilar-Parada, E., 1970, Abnormal alpha cell function in diabetes. Response to carbohydrate and protein ingestion, *N. Engl. J. Med.* **283**:109.

Müller, W. A., Faloona, G. R., and Unger, R. H., 1971, The effect of experimental insulin deficiency on glucagon secretion, *J. Clin. Invest.* **50**:1992.

Müller, W. A., Faloona, G. R., and Unger, R. H., 1973, Hyperglucagonemia in diabetic ketoacidosis: Its prevalence and significance, *Amer. J. Med.* **54**:52.

Muñoz-Barragan, L., Rufener, C., Srikant, C. B., Dobbs, R. E., Shannon, W. A., Baetens, D., and Unger, R. H., 1977, Immunocytochemical evidence for glucagon-containing cells in the human stomach, *Horm. Metab. Res.* **9**:37.

Nagai, K., and Frohman, L. A., 1976, Hyperglycemia and hyperglucagonemia following neurotensin administration, *Life Sci.* **19**:273.

Nakabayashi, H., Yoshimitsu, K., Kishitani, M., Ueda, M., and Kawato, M., 1976, Effect of somatostatin on pancreatic endocrine—Experiment by somatostatin infusion into the pancreaticoduodenal artery in dogs, *Folia Endocrinol. Jpn.* **52**:218.

Noe, B. D., 1976, Biosynthesis of glucagon, *Metabolism* **25**(Suppl.):1339.

Noe, B. D., and Bauer, G. E., 1971, Evidence for glucagon biosynthesis involving a protein intermediate in islets of the anglerfish *(Lophius americanus), Endocrinology* **89**:642.

Noe, B. D., Bauer, G. E., Steffes, M. W., Sutherland, D. E. R., and Najarian, J. S., 1975, Glucagon biosynthesis in human pancreatic islets: Preliminary evidence for a biosynthetic intermediate, *Horm. Metab. Res.* **7**:314.

O'Connor, K. J., and Lazarus, N. R., 1976, Studies on the biosynthesis of pancreatic glucagon in the pigeon *(Columba livia), Biochem. J.* **156**:279.

Orci, L., 1976, The microanatomy of the islets of Langerhans, *Metabolism* **25**(Suppl.):1303.

Orci, L., 1977, Discussion, in: *Recent Progress in Hormone Research,* Vol. 33 (R. O. Greep, ed.), Academic Press, New York.

Orci, L., and Unger, R. H., 1975, Functional subdivision of islets of Langerhans and possible role of D-cells, *Lancet* **2**:1243.

Orci, L., Pictet, R., Forssmann, W. G., Renold, A. E., and Rouiller, C., 1968, Structural evidence for glucagon producing cells in the intestinal mucosa of the rat, *Diabetologia* **4**:56.

Orci, L., Unger, R. H., and Renold, A. E., 1973, Structural coupling between pancreatic islet cells, *Experientia* **29**:1015.

Orci, L., Baetens, D., Dubois, M. P., and Rufener, C., 1975a, Evidence for the D-cell of the pancreas secreting somatostatin, *Horm. Metab. Res.* **7**:400.

Orci, L., Malaisse-Lagae, F., Amherdt, M., Ravazzola, M., Weisswange, A., Dobbs, R., Perrelet, A., and Unger, R., 1975b, Cell contacts in human islets of Langerhans, *J. Clin. Endocrinol. Metab.* **41**:841.

Orci, L., Malaisse-Lagae, F., Ravazzola, M., Rouiller, D., Renold, A. E., Perrelet, A., and Unger, R. H., 1975c, A morphological basis for intercellular communication between A- and B-cells in the endocrine pancreas, *J. Clin. Invest.* **56**:1066.

Orci, L., Baetens, D., Rufener, C., Amherdt, M., Ravazzola, M., Studer, P., Malaisse-Lagae, F., and Unger, R. H., 1976, Hypertrophy and hyperplasia of somatostatin-containing D-cells in diabetes, *Proc. Natl. Acad. Sci. U.S.A.* **73**:1338.

Palmer, J. P., Werner, P. L., Benson, J. W., and Ensinck, J. W., 1976, Immunoreactive glucagon responses to arginine in three pancreatectomized humans, *Metabolism* **25**(Suppl.):1483.

Parrilla, R., Jimenez, I., and Ayuso-Parrilla, M. S., 1975, Glucagon and insulin control in gluconeogenesis in the perfused isolated rat liver. Effects on cellular metabolite distribution, *Eur. J. Biochem.* **56**:375.

Park, C. R., and Exton, J. H., 1972, Glucagon and the metabolism of glucose, in: *Glucagon: Molecular Physiology, Clinical and Therapeutic Implications* (P. J. Lefebvre and R. H., Unger, eds.), pp. 77–108, Pergamon Press, Oxford.

Patel, Y. C., Orci, L., Bankier, A., and Cameron, D. P., 1976, Decreased pancreatic somatostatin (SRIF) concentration in spontaneously diabetic mice, *Endocrinology* **99**:1415.

Patton, G., Brown, M., Dobbs, R., Vale, W., and Unger, R. H., 1976a, Effects of neurotensin and substance P on insulin and glucagon release by the perfused dog pancreas, *Metabolism* **25**(Suppl.):1465.

Patton, G. S., Dobbs, R., Orci, L., Vale, W., and Unger, R. H., 1976b, Stimulation of pancreatic immunoreactive somatostatin (IRS) release by glucagon, *Metabolism* **25**(Suppl.):1499.

Patton, G. S., Ipp, E., Dobbs, R. E., Vale, W., Orci, L., and Unger, R. H., 1976c, Response of pancreatic immunoreactive somatostatin to arginine, *Life Sci.* **19**:1957.

Patton, G. S., Ipp, E., Dobbs, R. E., Orci, L., Vale, W., and Unger, R. H., 1977, Pancreatic immunoreactive somatostatin release, *Proc. Natl. Acad. Sci. U.S.A.* **74**:2140.

Pek, S., Tai, T. Y., Elster, A., and Fajans, S. S., 1975, Stimulation by prostaglandin E_2 of glucagon and insulin release from isolated rat pancreas, *Prostaglandins* **10**:493.

Pelletier, G., Leclerc, R., Arimura, A., and Schally, A. V., 1975, Immunohistochemical localization of somatostatin in the rat pancreas, *J. Histochem. Cytochem.* **23**:699.

Penhos, J. C., Ezequiel, M., Lepp, A., and Ramey, E. R., 1975, Plasma immunoreactive insulin (IRI) and immunoreactive glucagon (IRG) after evisceration with and without a functional liver, *Diabetes* **24**:637.

Permutt, M. A., Delmez, J., and Stenson, W., 1976, Effects of carbohydrate restriction on the hypoglycemic phase of the glucose tolerance test, *J. Clin. Endocrinol. Metab.* **43**:1088.

Petersson, B., and Hellman, B., 1963, Effects of long-term administration of glucagon on the pancreatic islet tissue of rats and guinea pigs, *Acta Endocrinol.* **44**:139.

Pilkis, S. J., Claus, T. H., Riou, J. P., and Park, C. R., 1976, Possible role of pyruvate kinase in the hormonal control of dihydroxyacetone gluconeogenesis in isolated hepatocytes, *Metabolism* **25**(Suppl.):1355.

Polak, J. M., Pearse, A. G. E., Grimelius, L., Bloom, S. R., and Arimura, A., 1975, Growth-hormone release-inhibiting hormone in gastrointestinal and pancreatic D-cells, *Lancet* **1**:1220.

Pollock, H. G., and Kimmel, J. R., 1975, Chicken glucagon: Isolation and amino acid sequence studies, *J. Biol. Chem.* **250**:9377.

Porte, D., Jr., Woods, S. C., Chen, M., Smith, P. H., and Ensinck, J. W., 1975, Central factors in the control of insulin and glucagon secretion, *Pharmacol. Biochem. Behav.* **3**:127.

Rabinovitch, A., and Dupre, J., 1974, Effects of gastric inhibitory polypeptide present in impure pancreozymin-cholecystokinin on plasma insulin and glucagon in the rat, *Endocrinology* **94**:1139.

Raskin, P., and Unger, R. H., 1977, Effects of hyperglucagonemia in well controlled insulin-treated diabetics *Diabetes* (in press).

Raskin, P., Fujita, Y., and Unger, R. H., 1975, Effect of insulin–glucose infusions on plasma glucagon levels in fasting diabetics and nondiabetics, *J. Clin. Invest.* **56**:1132.

Raskin, P., Aydin, I., and Unger, R. H., 1976, The effect of insulin on the exaggerated glucagon response to arginine stimulation in diabetes mellitus, *Diabetes* **25**:227.

Recant, L., Perrino, P. V., Bhathena, S. J., Danfort, D. N., Jr., and Levine, R. L., 1976, Plasma immunoreactive glucagon fractions in four cases of glucagonoma: Increased "large glucagon immunoreactivity," *Diabetologia* **12**:319.

Rigopoulou, D., Valverde, I., Marco, J., Faloona, G., and Unger, R. H., 1970, Large glucagon immunoreactivity in extracts of pancreas, *J. Biol. Chem.* **245**:496.

Rivier, J. E., Brown, M. R., and Vale, W. W., 1976, Tyrosylated analogues of somatostatin, *J. Med. Chem.* **19**:1010.

Rocha, D. M., Faloona, G. R., and Unger, R. H., 1972, Glucagon stimulating activity of twenty amino acids in dogs, *J. Clin. Invest.* **51**:2346.

Rocha, D. M., Santeusanio, F., Faloona, G. R., and Unger, R. H., 1973, Abnormal pancreatic alpha-cell function in bacterial infections, *N. Engl. J. Med.* **288**:700.

Rodbell, M., and Londos, C., 1976, Regulation of hepatic adenylate cyclase by glucagon, GTP, divalent cations, ana adenosine, *Metabolism* **25**(Suppl.): 1347.

Sacks, H., Waligora, K., Matthews, J., and Pimstone, B., 1977, Inhibition by somatostatin of glucagon-induced glucose release from the isolated perfused rat liver, *Diabetes* **26**:358.

Sakurai, H., Dobbs, R., and Unger, R. H., 1974, Somatostatin-induced changes in insulin and glucagon secretion in normal and diabetic dogs, *J. Clin. Invest.* **54**:1395.

Sakurai, H., Dobbs, R. E., and Unger, R. H., 1975a, The effect of somatostatin on the response of GLI to the intraduodenal administration of glucose, protein and fat, *Diabetologia* **11**:427.

Sakurai, H., Dobbs, R. E., and Unger, R. H., 1975b, The role of glucagon in the pathogenesis of the endogenous hyperglycemia of diabetes mellitus, *Metabolism* **24**:1287.

Samols, E., and Harrison, J., 1976, Remarkable potency of somatostatin as a glucagon suppressant, *Metabolism* **25**(Suppl.):1495.

Samols, E., Marri, G., and Marks, V., 1965, Promotion of insulin secretion by glucagon, *Lancet* **2**:415.

Samols, E., Tyler, J., and Marks, V., 1972, Glucagon–insulin interrelationships, in: *Glucagon: Molecular Physiology, Clinical and Therapeutic Implications* (P. J. Lefebvre and R. H. Unger, eds.), pp. 151–174, Pergamon Press, Oxford.

Samols, E., Weir, G. C., Patel, Y. C., Fernandez-Durango, R., Arimura, A., and Loo, S. W., 1977, Suppression of canine pancreatic A, B, D and PP cell secretion bv diazoxide, *Diabetes* **26**(Suppl.):375.

Sasagawa, T., Kobayashi, S., and Fujita, T., 1973, Electron microscopy studies on the GEP endocrine cells of the human gut and pancreas, in: *Gastro–Entero–Pancreatic Endocrine System* (T. Fujita, ed.), pp. 17–38, Igaku Shoin, Tokyo.

Sasaki, H., Rubalcava, B., Baetens, D., Blazquez, E., Srikant, C. B., Orci, L., and Unger, R. H., 1975a, Identification of glucagon in the gastrointestinal tract, *J. Clin. Invest.* **56**:135.

Sasaki, H., Rubalcava, B., Srikant, C. B., Baetens, D., Orci, L., and Unger, R. H., 1975b, Gut glucagonoid (GLI) and gut glucagon, in: *Gastrointestinal Hormones* (J. C. Thompsen, ed.), pp. 519–528, University of Texas Press, Austin.

Schauder, P., McIntosh, C., Arends, J., Arnold, R., Frerichs, H., and Creutzfeldt, W., 1976, Somatostatin and insulin release from isolated rat pancreatic islets stimulated by glucose, *FEBS Lett.* **68**:225.

Schebalin, M., Said, S. I., and Makhlouf, G. M., 1977, Stimulation of insulin and glucagon secretion by vasoactive intestinal peptide, *Amer. J. Physiol.* **232**: E197.

Schusdziarra, V., Ipp, E., and Unger, R. H., 1977, Somatostatin, a physiologic regulator of nutrient influx, *Diabetes* **26**(Suppl.):359.

Seitz, H. J., Muller, M. J., Nordmeyer, P., Krone, W., and Tarnowski, W., 1976,

Concentration of cyclic AMP in rat liver as a function of the insulin/glucagon ratio in blood under standardized physiological conditions, *Endocrinology* **99**:1313.

Service, F. J., Molnar, G. D., Rosevear, J. W., Ackerman, E., Gatewood, L. C., and Taylor, W. F., 1970, Mean amplitude of glycemic excursions, a measure of diabetic instability, *Diabetes* **19**:644.

Sherwin, R. S., Fisher, M., Hendler, R., and Felig, P., 1976, Hyperglucagonemia and blood glucose regulation in normal, obese, and diabetic subjects, *N. Engl. J. Med* **294**:455.

Sherwin, R. S., Hendler, R., Defronzo, R., Wahren, J., and Felig, P., 1977, Glucose homeostasis during prolonged suppression of glucagon and insulin secretion by somatostatin, *Proc. Natl. Acad. Sci. U.S.A.* **74**:348.

Soeters, P. B., and Fischer, J. E., 1976, Insulin, glucagon, amino acid imbalance, and hepatic encephalopathy, *Lancet* **2**:880.

Sperling, M. A., Grajwer, L. A., Leake, R., and Fisher, D. A., 1976, Role of glucagon in perinatal glucose homeostasis, *Metabolism* **25**(Suppl.):1385.

Srikant, C. B., and Unger, R. H., 1976, Evidence for the presence of glucagon-like immunoreactivity (GLI) in the pancreas, *Endocrinology* **99**:1655.

Srikant, C. B., McCorkle, K., and Unger, R. H., 1977, Properties of immunoreactive glucagon fractions of canine stomach and pancreas, *J. Biol. Chem.* **252**: 1847.

Staehelin, L. A., 1974, Structure and function of intercellular junctions, *Int. Rev. Cytol.* **39**:191.

Sundby, F., 1976, Species variations in the primary structure of glucagon, *Metabolism* **25**(Suppl.):1319.

Sundby, F., and Markussen, J., 1971, Isolation, crystallization, and amino acid composition of rat glucagon, *Horm. Metab. Res.* **3**:184.

Sundby, F., and Markussen, J., 1972, Rabbit glucagon: Isolation, crystallization, and amino acid composition, *Horm. Metab. Res.* **4**:56.

Sundby, F., Frandsen, E. K., Thomsen, J., Kristiansen, K., and Brundfeldt, K., 1972, Crystallization and amino acid sequence of duck glucagon, *FEBS Lett.* **26**:289.

Sundby, F., Jacobsen, H., and Moody, A. J., 1976, Purification and characterization of a protein from porcine gut with glucagon-like immunoreactivity, *Horm. Metab. Res.* **8**:366.

Sutherland, E. W., and DeDuve, C., 1948, Origin and distribution of the hyperglycemic–glycogenolytic factor of the pancreas, *J. Biol. Chem.* **175**:663.

Tager, H. S., and Markese, J., 1976, Immunoreactive glucagon in pancreatic islets, *Metabolism* **25**(Suppl.):1343.

Tager, H. S., and Steiner, D. F., 1973, Isolation of a glucagon-containing peptide: Primary structure of a possible fragment of proglucagon, *Proc. Natl. Acad. Sci. U.S.A.* **70**:2321.

Tai, T. Y., and Pek, S., 1976, Direct stimulation by growth hormone of glucagon and insulin release from isolated rat pancreas, *Endocrinology* **99**:669.

Thomsen, J., Kristiansen, K., Brunfeldt, K., and Sundby, F., 1972, The amino acid sequence of human glucagon, *FEBS Lett.* **21**:315.

Tiengo, A., Fedele, D., Marchiori, E., Nosadini, R., and Muggeo, M., 1976,

Suppression and stimulation mechanisms controlling glucagon secretion in a case of islet-cell tumor producing glucagon, insulin and gastrin, *Diabetes* **25**:408.

Unger, R. H., 1971a, Glucagon physiology and pathophysiology, *N. Engl. J. Med.* **285**:443.

Unger, R. H., 1971b, Glucagon and the insulin:glucagon ratio in diabetes and other catabolic illnesses, *Diabetes* **20**:834.

Unger, R. H., 1976, Diabetes and the alpha cell (Banting Memorial Lecture), *Diabetes* **25**:136.

Unger, R. H., 1977, Editorial: Somatostatinoma, *N. Engl. J. Med.* **296**:998.

Unger, R. H., and Orci, L., 1975, The essential role of glucagon in the pathogenesis of diabetes mellitus, *Lancet* **1**:14.

Unger, R. H., and Orci, L., 1977, Possible roles of the pancreatic D-cell in the normal and diabetic states, *Diabetes* **26**:241.

Unger, R. H., Ketterer, H., Dupre, J., and Eisentraut, A. M., 1967, The effects of secretin, pancreozymin, and gastrin on insulin and glucagon secretion in anesthetized dogs, *J. Clin. Invest.* **46**:630.

Unger, R. H., Ohneda, A., Valverde, I., Eisentraut, A. M., and Exton, J., 1968, Characterization of the responses of circulating glucagon-like immunoreactivity to intraduodenal and intravenous administration of glucose, *J. Clin. Invest.* **47**:48.

Unger, R. H., Ohneda, A., Aguilar-Parada, E., and Eisentraut, A. M., 1969, The role of aminogenic glucagon secretion in blood glucose homeostasis, *J. Clin. Invest.* **48**:810.

Unger, R. H., Aguilar-Parada, E., Müller, W. A., and Eisentraut, A. M., 1970, Studies of pancreatic alpha cell function in normal and diabetic subjects, *J. Clin. Invest.* **49**:837.

Unger, R. H., Madison, L. L., and Müller, W. A., 1972, Abnormal alpha cell function in diabetics: Response to insulin, *Diabetes* **21**:301.

Unger, R. H., Aydin, I., Nakabayashi, H., Srikant, C. B., and Raskin, P., 1976, The effects of glucagon administration to nondiabetics and diabetics, *Metabolism* **25**(Suppl.):1523.

Unger, R. H., Raskin, P., Srikant, C. B., and Orci, L., 1977, Glucagon and the A-cells, in: *Recent Progress in Hormone Research,* Vol. 33 (R. O. Greep, ed.), pp. 477–517, Academic Press, New York.

Vale, W., Ling, N., Rivier, J., Villarreal, J., Rivier, C., Brown, M., and Douglas, C., 1976, Anatomic and phylogenetic distribution of somatostatin, *Metabolism* **25**(Suppl.):1491.

Valverde, I., Rigopoulou, D., Marco, J., Faloona, G. R., and Unger, R. H., 1970, Molecular size of extractable glucagon and glucagon-like immunoreactivity (GLI) in plasma, *Diabetes* **19**:624.

Valverde, I., Villanueva, M. L., Lozano, I., and Marco, J., 1974, Presence of glucagon immunoreactivity in the globulin fraction of human plasma ("big plasma glucagon"). *J. Clin. Endocrinol. Metab.* **39**:1090.

Valverde, L., Dobbs, R., and Unger, R. H., 1975, Heterogeneity of plasma glucagon immunoreactivity in normal, depancreatized, and alloxan diabetic dogs, *Metabolism* **24**:1021.

Valverde, L., Lemon, H. M., Kessinger, A., and Unger, R. H., 1976, Distribution of plasma glucagon immunoreactivity in a patient with a suspected glucagonoma, *J. Clin. Endocrinol. Metab.* **42**:804.

Veneziale, C. M., Deering, N. G., and Thompsen, H. J., 1976, Gluconeogenesis in isolated rat hepatic parenchymal cells. IX. Differential effects of glucagon and epinephrine on phosphofructokinase and pyruvate kinase, *Mayo Clin. Proc.* **51**:624.

Vranic, M., Pek, S., and Kawamori, R., 1974, Increased "glucagon immunoreactivity" in plasma of totally depancreatized dogs, *Diabetes* **23**:905.

Vranic, M., Engerman, R., Doi, K., Morita, S., and Yip, C. C., 1976, Extrapancreatic glucagon in the dog, *Metabolism* **25**(Suppl.):1469.

Wahren, J., and Felig, P., 1976, Influence of somatostatin on carbohydrate disposal and absorption in diabetes mellitus, *Lancet* **2**:1213.

Wahren, J., Felig, P., and Hagenfeldt, L., 1976, Effect of protein ingestion on splanchnic and leg metabolism in normal man and in patients with diabetes mellitus, *J. Clin. Invest.* **57**:987.

Weir, G. C., Turner, R. C., and Martin, D. B., 1973, Glucagon radioimmunoassay using antiserum 30K: Interference by plasma, *Horm. Metab. Res.* **5**:241.

Weir, G. C., Knowlton, S. D., Atkins, R. F., McKennan, K. X., and Martin, D. B., 1976, Glucagon secretion from the perfused pancreas of streptozotocin-treated rats, *Diabetes* **25**:275.

Weir, G. C., Samols, E., Ramseur, R., Day, J. A., Jr., and Patel, Y. C., 1977, Influence of glucose and glucagon upon somatostatin secretion from the isolated perfused canine pancreas, *Clin. Res.* **25**:403A.

Werner, P., and Palmer, J., 1977, The role of immunoreactive glucagon (IRG) in the control of plasma glucose in pancreatectomized (Px) man, *Diabetes* **26**(Suppl.):383.

Wilmore, D. W., Lindsey, C. A., Moylan, J. A., Faloona, G. R., Pruitt, B. A., and Unger, R. H., 1974, Hyperglucagonemia after burns, *Lancet* **1**:73.

Wise, J. K., Hendler, R., and Felig, P., 1973, Influence of glucocorticoids on glucagon secretion and plasma amino acid concentrations in man, *J. Clin. Invest.* **52**:2774.

Wollheim, C. B., Blondel, B., Renold, A. E., and Sharp, G. W., 1976a, Stimulatory and inhibitory effects of cyclic AMP on pancreatic glucagon release from monolayer cultures and the controlling role of calcium, *Diabetologia* **12**:269.

Wollheim, C. B., Blondel, B., Renold, A. E., and Sharp, G. W., 1976b, Calcium induced glucagon release in monolayer culture of the endocrine pancreas. Studies with ionophore A23187, *Diabetologia* **12**:287.

4

Body Fuel Metabolism

Philip Felig and Veikko Koivisto

4.1. Introduction

Fuel homeostasis in normal man involves the assimilation, storage, and utilization primarily of glucose, fat (triglyceride, free fatty acids, and glycerol), and protein (amino acids and peptides). Body fuel metabolism is of particular importance in such conditions as starvation and exercise and in disease states such as diabetes. This review will focus primarily on normal physiology, with some discussion of the abnormalities observed in diabetes.

4.2. Glucose Metabolism

4.2.1. Glucose Absorption: Effects of Somatostatin

New understanding regarding the interaction of insulin and glucagon in glucose homeostasis is derived from recent studies with somatosta-

PHILIP FELIG • Professor and Vice Chairman, Department of Internal Medicine; Chief, Section of Endocrinology, Yale University School of Medicine, New Haven, Connecticut 06510. VEIKKO KOIVISTO • Visiting Research Fellow, Section of Endocrinology, Department of Internal Medicine, Yale University School of Medicine, New Haven, Connecticut 06510.

tin (Gerich, 1977). Somatostatin is a tetradecapeptide isolated from the hypothalamus and demonstrated to inhibit the secretion of growth hormone (Brazeau *et al.,* 1973), insulin (Siler *et al.,* 1973), and glucagon (Koerker *et al.,* 1974). In diabetic subjects, somatostatin was demonstrated to markedly decrease the blood glucose rise that follows carbohydrate-containing meals (Gerich *et al.,* 1974). Those observations suggested a major role for glucagon in postprandial hyperglycemia in diabetes (Gerich *et al.,* 1974). In contrast, the work of Sherwin *et al.* (1976b), in which hyperglucagonemia was induced by infusion, suggested that glucagon elevations in the absence of insulin deficiency could not substantially alter glucose metabolism in man. The seeming contradiction between the salutary effect of isolated removal of glucagon in diabetic patients and the lack of an aggravating effect of addition of glucagon in diabetic patients raised the possibility that somatostatin might have effects on blood glucose levels by mechanisms other than tissue disposal of ingested glucose. Accordingly, Wahren and Felig (1976) compared the effects of somatostatin on oral and intravenous glucose tolerance and on xylose tolerance in insulin-dependent diabetic subjects. Their data demonstrated that while somatostatin markedly lowered the glucose response to oral glucose ingestion, there was no effect observed on the disposal of intravenous glucose. This dissociation between the response to oral and intravenous glucose raised the possibility that somatostatin altered glucose absorption. Supporting the latter possibility was the demonstration that somatostatin markedly blunted the blood xylose elevation following ingestion of that pentose (Wahren and Felig, 1976). Furthermore, the addition of glucagon to somatostatin failed to improve the rise in blood xylose (Felig *et al.,* 1976b) (Fig. 1). Interestingly, somatostatin was demonstrated to induce a prompt, 30–40% decline in splanchnic blood flow, providing a possible mechanism for its effects on blood xylose (Wahren and Felig, 1976). Subsequent studies in the dog also showed that endoportal infusion of somatostatin diminishes carbohydrate absorption (Patton *et al.,* 1977).

In addition to these effects of somatostatin on blood xylose, somatostatin has been demonstrated to have suppressive effects on a variety of endocrine as well as nonendocrine functions of the GI tract. Specifically, decreased secretion of gastrin (Bloom *et al.,* 1974) and secretin (Bonden *et al.,* 1975), and diminished gastric acid secretion in response to gastrin administration (Gomez-Pan *et al.,* 1975) were observed in association with administration of somatostatin. In addition, somatostatin was reported to delay gastric emptying by 70% (Bloom *et al.,* 1975).

The available data would thus suggest that somatostatin has a variety of effects on GI function. Specifically, the dissociation between the effects of somatostatin on intravenous and oral glucose tolerance and its marked blunting of the rise in blood xylose following administration of this pentose strongly suggest that this agent inhibits carbohydrate absorption.

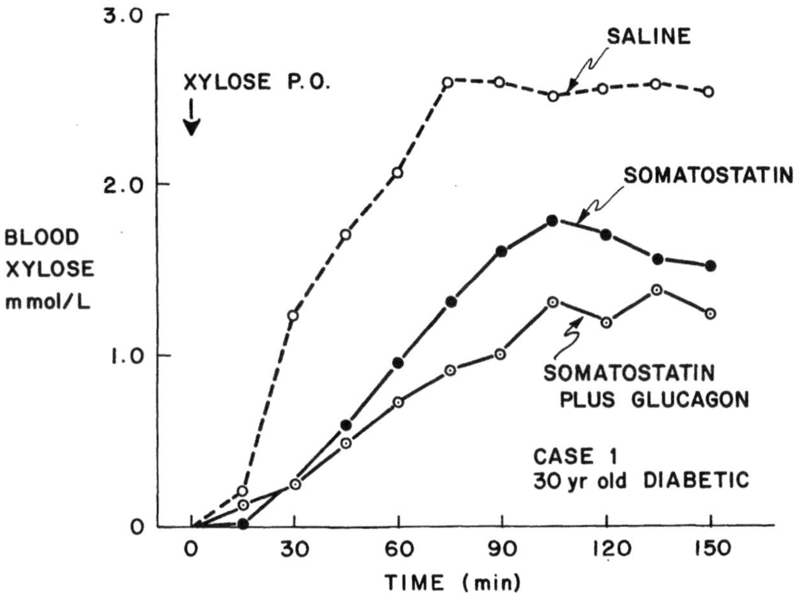

Fig. 1. Influence of somatostatin on blood xylose after oral administration of 25 g xylose in a diabetic subject. Administration of glucagon (3 ng/kg per min) failed to reverse the inhibitory effect of somatostatin on xylose absorption. Based on the data of Wahren and Felig (1976).

Whether this effect of somatostatin is due primarily to altered splanchnic blood flow, decreased gastric emptying, or other effects on GI function remains to be established. Nevertheless, these findings indicate the need for caution in attributing the hypoglycemic effects of somatostatin in the postprandial state to glucagon suppression. In addition, these findings raise the strong possibility that the diminution in insulin requirements demonstrated in diabetic patients treated with somatostatin for several days (Gerich, 1977) may be due to decreased carbohydrate absorption, rather than altered glucagon availability.

4.2.2. Glucose Production

4.2.2.1. Protein Ingestion

It has been recognized since the work of Floyd *et al.* (1966) that ingestion of protein is a stimulus of insulin secretion. Nevertheless, protein feeding does not result in hypoglycemia. The initial studies of Unger, in which protein-stimulated glucagon secretion was demonstrated, suggested that glucagon allowed for an increase in glucose production following protein feeding so as to counterbalance the increase in glucose utilization engendered by insulin secretion (Unger *et al.*, 1969). More recently, the splanchnic glucose response to protein feeding has been directly examined. In normal subjects, following a protein meal, there is neither an increase nor a decrease in splanchnic glucose production (Wahren *et al.*, 1976). The question thus arises whether the increment in glucagon that follows a protein meal does in fact counteract the inhibitory effect on hepatic glucose production that would otherwise accompany an increase in insulin secretion (Felig *et al.*, 1976a). This hypothesis was directly examined by evaluating the effects of physiologic increments in glucagon secretion on insulin-inhibited splanchnic glucose production. In these studies, glucose was infused at a rate of 2 mg/kg per min so as to induce a rise in peripheral insulin levels (60–80%) that simulates the insulin rise accompanying a protein meal (Felig *et al.*, 1976a). This rise in insulin was associated with virtually complete cessation of hepatic glucose production. The glucagon increment accompanying protein feeding was then simulated by adding an infusion of glucagon at a concentration of 3 ng/kg per min. With the addition of the glucagon infusion, a rise in plasma glucagon simulating that observed following a protein meal was induced. Particularly noteworthy was the prompt increase in splanchnic glucose production to basal or slightly above basal levels (Felig *et al.*, 1976a). Thus, administration of physiologic amounts of glucagon was directly demonstrated to be capable of reversing insulin-inhibited splanchnic glucose production. These findings provide strong evidence in support of the hypothesis first advanced by Unger *et al.* (1969) that hyperglucagonemia accompanying protein ingestion is of major importance in preventing the hypoglycemia that would otherwise accompany the increase in insulin secretion that accompanies protein feeding.

Wahren *et al.* (1976) also compared normal and diabetic subjects with respect to the splanchnic glucose response to protein feeding. In these studies, protein meals (3 g lean cooked beef/kg body wt.) were fed to healthy subjects and to insulin-withdrawn diabetic subjects after an overnight fast. In contrast to the normal group, in whom splanchnic glucose output remained at basal levels, in the diabetics, splanchnic glucose production rose two- to four-fold, and gradually returned to base line. This greater glycemic effect of protein feeding in diabetes appeared to represent the effects of hyperglucagonemia in the absence of an accompanying rise in insulin secretion. Thus, in the insulin-deficient diabetic, protein feeding may be viewed as a hyperglycemic stimulus resulting from glucagon-mediated overproduction of glucose.

4.2.2.2. Starvation

The maintenance of normal blood glucose levels during starvation is dependent on ongoing glucose release from the liver. In the postabsorptive state and for the first 24 hr of fasting, glucose release from the liver is primarily a result of glycogen breakdown (Felig, 1973). The demonstration that somatostatin lowers blood glucose levels and decreases glucose output in the postabsorptive state provided evidence that glucagon is necessary for glycogenolysis during starvation (Alford *et al.,* 1974). Of additional interest is the question whether glucagon plays a role in gluconeogenesis in starvation. Inasmuch as glycogen stores in the liver amount to no more than generally 70–90 g in postabsorptive subjects, liver glycogen stores are generally dissipated within 48–72 hr of starvation (Hultman and Nillsson, 1971). Thus, in subjects fasted for 72 hr or longer, splanchnic glucose output consists virtually entirely of gluconeogenesis. To examine the role of somatostatin in gluconeogenesis, the effects of this agent on splanchnic glucose output and substrate utilization in 3-day-fasted subjects were examined (Wahren *et al.,* 1977). After a 3-day fast, somatostatin-mediated inhibition of insulin and glucagon secretion was followed by a 70% decrease in glucose production. Splanchnic uptake of lactate and pyruvate fell by 30–40%, while amino acid uptake remained unchanged. Interestingly, splanchnic uptake of free fatty acids rose fourfold during somatostatin infusion, while production of β-hydroxybutyrate increased by 75%. These findings indicating that somatostatin-induced hypoglucagonemia results in decreased hepatic glucose production in glycogen-depleted subjects indicate a role for glucagon in hepatic gluconeogenesis as well as glycogenolysis. In addition, inasmuch as hepatic uptake of gluconeogenic substrates persists despite an inhibition in splanchnic glucose output, the data suggest that the glucagon-sensitive steps in gluconeogenesis affected by somatostatin involve primarily intrahepatic disposal, rather than net hepatic uptake of glucose precursors. Finally, the findings that splanchnic uptake of fatty acids and ketone output are increased in the face of combined insulin and glucagon deficiency indicate the primary role of hypoinsulinemia, rather than hyperglucagonemia, in starvation-mediated ketogenesis.

In addition to the importance of hepatic glycogenolysis and gluconeogenesis in maintenance of blood glucose homeostasis during starvation, Sugden *et al.* (1976) recently called attention to the potential role of muscle glycogen as a source of glucose during short-term starvation. Studying fasted rats, the authors demonstrated that 35–40% of the total body glycogenolysis occurring during 1- to 2-day fasts in the rats represented breakdown of carcass glycogen, while the remaining 60–65% represented breakdown of liver glycogen. Carcass glycogen could thus potentially serve as a source of blood glucose during short-term starvation, provided the glycogen is muscle is not broken down beyond the level of lactate or pyruvate and is then released into the bloodstream. However, data are not available as to the proportion of muscle glycogen that is terminally oxidized to CO_2 and the proportion that undergoes glycolysis and is released into the bloodstream as lactate and pyruvate. Until such data are available, the contribution of muscle to glucose recycling and hepatic glucose output remains conjectural.

4.2.2.3. Evanescent Effects of Hyperglucagonemia

As noted above, studies involving physiologic infusions of glucagon and studies in which glucagon secretion was suppressed by somatostatin suggest that glucagon secretion is necessary for the maintenance of basal rates of hepatic glucose production during protein feeding (Felig *et al.*, 1976a) and during brief or prolonged starvation (Wahren *et al.*, 1977). These ongoing effects of glucagon in maintaining basal glucose production contrast with the evanescent effect of glucagon in increasing glucose production above basal levels. When physiologic hyperglucagonemia is induced by infusion of this hormone in doses of 3 ng/kg per min, splanchnic glucose output shows a prompt rise within 7 min to levels twice the basal rate of glucose output (Felig *et al.*, 1976a). However, this increase in glucose output persists for less than 30 min. By 30 min after the infusion of glucagon, splanchnic glucose output has returned to base line despite ongoing hyperglucagonemia in the range of 300–400 pg/ml (Felig *et al.*, 1976a). This fall in splanchnic glucose output cannot be ascribed to hyperinsulinemia, inasmuch as it occurs in the face of plasma insulin concentrations that are no higher than those observed in the initial 15–20 min of the glucagon infusion. Furthermore, in insulin-dependent diabetic patients, a similar evanescence in the response to glucagon is observed (Bomboy *et al.*, 1977a).

The very transient nature of the stimulatory action of glucagon on hepatic glucose output has implications for a variety of pathophysiological conditions. Persistent hyperglucagonemia has been demonstrated in a number of clinical conditions, including severe infection (Rocha *et al.*, 1973), trauma (Lindsey *et al.*, 1974), cirrhosis (Sherwin *et al.*, 1974), and uremia (Sherwin *et al.*, 1976a). In the case of uremia, increased tissue sensitivity to the hyperglycemic effects of glucagon was demonstrated (Sherwin *et al.*, 1976a). On the other hand, in the remaining conditions in which altered sensitivity to glucagon was not demonstrated, in view of the evanescent nature of this hormone, it is unlikely that persistent hyperglucagonemia has an ongoing effect on hepatic mechanisms of glucose production. In the case of the diabetic, in whom the hyperglycemic effects of glucagon are exaggerated (Sherwin *et al.*, 1976b), glucagon is as evanescent in its effect as in normal individuals (Bomboy *et al.*, 1977a). Thus, it is likely that the greater glycemic response to glucagon in diabetes is a consequence of ongoing inability to metabolize the increased amounts of glucose transiently released by the liver in response to an increase in glucagon (Felig *et al.*, 1976b).

4.2.2.4. Evanescent Effects of Hypoglucagonemia: Prolonged Infusion of Somatostatin

Short-term studies involving infusions of somatostatin for 60–120 min suggested an essential role for glucagon in the maintainence of diabetic hyperglycemia (Gerich *et al.*, 1974; Dobbs *et al.*, 1975). In these studies in human and experimental diabetes, hyperglycemia was demonstrated to be reduced in association with a fall of plasma glucagon. In addition, in normal subjects, somatostatin-induced reductions in plasma glucagon and insulin lasting for 60–120 min resulted in a fall rather than a rise in plasma glucose (Alford *et al.*, 1974). Interestingly, in studies in normal, conscious dogs involving 2-hr infusions of somatostatin, Altszuler *et al.* (1976) demonstrated that prior to termination of 90-min infusions of somatostatin, splanchnic glucose production had returned to base line despite ongoing suppression of plasma glucagon. More recently, Sherwin *et al.* (1977) examined the effects of 6- to 8-hr infusions of somatostatin on glucose kinetics in normal, conscious dogs and in healthy humans. In these studies, somatostatin resulted in a persistent decline in plasma glucagon (50–60%) and insulin (40%). Plasma glucose fell during the initial hour of the infusion. Beyond 2 hr, however, the hypoglycemic effect waned and hyperglycemia invariably occurred, reaching levels of 150 mg/100 ml at 6–7 hr (Fig. 2). This delayed hyperglycemia occurred despite ongoing suppression of glucagon and insulin. To exclude the possibility that the delayed hyperglycemia is a nonspecific response to early hypoglycemia, a variable glucose infusion was given for the initial 3 hr to prevent hypoglycemia. Despite the prevention of early hypoglycemia, a comparable delayed rise in fasting blood glucose levels occurred. Furthermore, when insulin was infused in physiologic amounts (0.15 mU/kg per min) so as to restore plasma insulin to preinfusion values, plasma glucose promptly fell to basal levels despite continued somatostatin infusion.

Studies of glucose kinetics in subjects given prolonged infusions of somatostatin demonstrated that endogenous glucose production initially declined by 40–50% but subsequently increased to levels that were 15–20% above base line. In addition, glucose utilization rates also declined during the latter part of the somatostatin infusions. In human subjects studied by catheterization, an increase in splanchnic glucose output was also demonstrable (Sherwin *et al.*, 1977).

These observations indicate that during prolonged suppression of insulin as well as glucagon secretion, the effect of insulin deficiency predominates. Thus, fasting hyperglycemia and absolute glucose overproduction occur despite ongoing hypoglucagonemia. That insulin deficiency appears to be the primary factor responsible for these changes in blood glucose and glucose production is indicated by the prompt decline

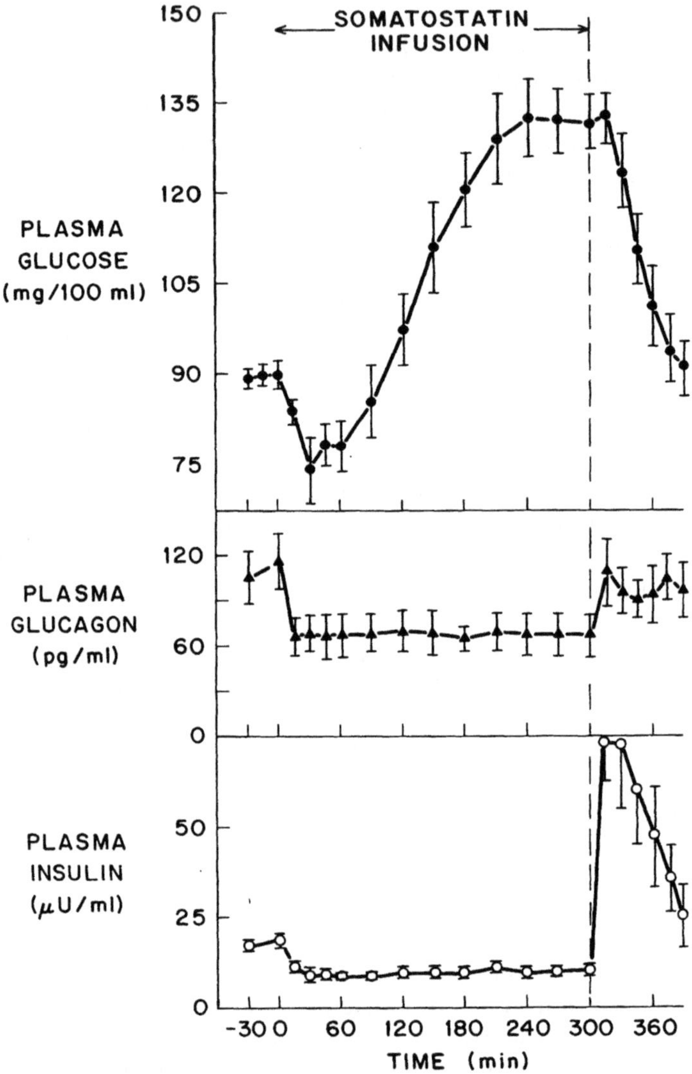

Fig. 2. Effect of prolonged infusion of somatostatin on plasma glucose, insulin, and glucagon levels in normal subjects. Following an initial, transient hypoglycemic response, fasting hyperglycemia develops despite ongoing suppression of glucagon. Reproduced from Sherwin *et al.* (1977), by permission, from the *Proceedings of the National Academy of Sciences.*

in blood glucose in association with restoration of insulin levels either by cessation of somatostatin or by infusion of physiologic replacement doses of insulin. These findings provide evidence that basal secretion of glucagon is not essential for the development of fasting hyperglycemia, but underscore the necessary role of insulin deficiency in the pathogenesis of the diabetic syndrome (Felig *et al.,* 1976b).

4.2.3. Insulin and Hepatic Glucose Output

It has long been recognized that the liver plays an essential role in glucose homeostasis (Mann and McGath, 1922; Bondy *et al.,* 1949; Madison, 1969). Felig and Wahren (1971a) demonstrated that glucose-induced increments of plasma insulin amounting to 60–100% of basal levels result in an 85% inhibition of splanchnic glucose output. These decrements in splanchnic glucose output occurred in the absence of an increase in peripheral glucose utilization, indicating that the liver is a more sensitive site of insulin action than peripheral tissues. In addition, despite the reduction in splanchnic glucose output, uptake of glucose precursors such as lactate, alanine, and pyruvate was unaffected by the small increments in plasma insulin. In contrast, when glucose was infused at a rate of 25 mg/kg per min, resulting in fivefold increments in plasma insulin, splanchnic glucose balance reverted from a net output to a net uptake, and splanchnic uptake of gluconeogenic precursors was completely inhibited; in the case of lactate, a net splanchnic uptake was observed. These observations demonstrating that gluconeogenic substrate uptake was inhibited only at higher levels of plasma insulin suggested that glycogenolysis was more sensitive to inhibition by insulin than was gluconeogenesis (Felig and Wahren, 1971a). More recently, Chiasson *et al.* (1976) examined the differential sensitivity of glycogenolysis and gluconeogenesis to insulin by employing the hepatic venous catheter technique and infusions of alanine-U[^{14}C] in fasted, anesthetized dogs. In these studies, insulin was infused at doses of 1 or 5 mU/kg per min in association with a variable glucose infusion so as to maintain euglycemia. When insulin was infused at 1 mU/kg per min, plasma insulin rose by 50 μU/ml, while splanchnic glucose production was completely suppressed. However, neither the uptake of alanine by the splanchnic bed nor the conversion of [^{14}C]alanine to glucose was affected. In contrast, when insulin was infused at 5 mU/kg per min, causing increments in plasma insulin of 200 μU/ml, conversion of plasma alanine to glucose was inhibited by 90%. These data provide isotopic confirmation of the earlier observations suggesting that small increments in insulin that are capable of inhibiting glycogenolysis may nevertheless fail to inhibit gluconeogenesis.

4.2.4. Counterregulation during Insulin Hypoglycemia

As noted above, the hypoglycemic effects of insulin involve an inhibition of hepatic glucose production as well as increased peripheral glucose utilization. Garber *et al.* (1976a) examined the effects of insulin-induced hypoglycemia on glucose kinetics and on plasma levels of counterregulatory hormones (epinephrine, norepinephrine, cortisol, glucagon, and growth hormone). Within 15 min after the intravenous injection of insulin (0.15 U/kg), glucose production is diminished by 75%, gluconeogenesis from alanine being reduced by 55%. By 20–25 minutes after insulin injection, however, glucose production rapidly increases, reaching twice the basal rate at 50 min. This initial increase results principally from accelerated glycogenolysis. Gluconeogenesis from alanine returns to basal levels at 30 min, and by 2 hr after insulin administration, gluconeogenesis from alanine increases to 250% of the preinjection rate.

The hormonal regulation of glucose production in response to insulin hypoglycemia involves several factors. During insulin-induced hypoglycemia, the most rapid rise is observed in the level of plasma catecholamines. The rise in epinephrine is demonstrable in the peripheral blood within 20 min of insulin injection, reaching a peak at 60 min. In contrast, significant increments in cortisol and glucagon are not observed until 30 min and in growth hormone at 40 min. The time course of the hormonal response to insulin-induced hypoglycemia thus suggests that augmented secretion of epinephrine and perhaps norepinephrine may initiate the secondary increase in glucose production (Garber *et al.,* 1976a).

It is noteworthy that the increase in glucose production following insulin hypoglycemia occurs in the face of plasma insulin levels of 100–200 μU/ml, or 10–20 times the basal concentration (Garber *et al.,* 1976a). Previous studies have shown that physiologic hyperglucagonemia fails to interfere with insulin-mediated alterations in hepatic glucose output or disposal (Sherwin *et al.,* 1976b; Bomboy *et al.,* 1977b). It is thus unlikely that glucagon of itself is a major counterregulatory factor in the response to insulin hypoglycemia. Similarly, the adrenergic response to hyperglycemia plays a central role in the rat. In sympathectomized rats, insulin-induced hyperglycemia is more severe and the rate of glucose production in response to hyperglycemia is smaller than in normal animals, despite identical glucagon responses in both groups of animals (Sacca *et al.,* 1977).

In addition to the secondary rise in glucose production, insulin-induced hypoglycemia is accompanied by biphasic changes in glucose utilization. Glucose utilization initially rises, reaching values three times the basal rate at 15–25 min, but abruptly falls to base-line levels at 30–40 min. As noted above, the fall in glucose utilization (as well as the rise in glucose production) occurs in the face of ongoing hyperinsulinemia (Garber *et al.,* 1976a). Recent observations have emphasized the role of β-

receptor-mediated effects of epinephrine in inhibiting peripheral glucose utilization (Shikama and Ui, 1975). Thus, it is likely that catecholamines contribute to restoration of euglycemia by inhibiting insulin-stimulated glucose utilization as well as by reversing insulin inhibition of glucose production.

4.2.5. Neonatal Hypoglycemia

A fall in blood glucose characterizes the immediate postnatal period. Although there is some dispute as to the lower limits of blood glucose in the normal neonate, there is universal agreement that neonatal hypoglycemia is a frequent complication of maternal diabetes (Felig, 1977). Maternal hyperglycemia resulting in fetal and subsequently neonatal hyperinsulinemia has been implicated as the mechanism of this hypoglycemia (Pederson *et al.*, 1954). In addition to fetal hyperinsulinemia, decreased secretion of glucagon (Bloom and Johnston, 1972) and reduced levels of epinephrine (Stern *et al.*, 1968) have been implicated in the pathogenesis of neonatal hypoglycemia. Less clear has been the relative contribution of decreased hepatic glucose production and increased peripheral glucose utilization to the development of hypoglycemia in the infant of the diabetic mother. This question was evaluated by Kalhan *et al.* (1977), using the continous infusion of glucose-1[^{13}C]. With this technique, Kalhan and co-workers demonstrated glucose production rates of 4.2 mg/kg per min in normal infants. In contrast, in infants of diabetic mothers, the glucose production rate was reduced by 35–40%.

It was of interest that no correlation was observed between antenatal management of diabetes and the rate of glucose production. In addition, in other studies, neonatal hypoglycemia was observed in the offspring of mothers whose diabetes had been under strict metabolic control with virtually no maternal hyperglycemia during pregnancy (Persson *et al.*, 1973). Thus, the hypothesis first suggested by Pederson, in which maternal hyperglycemia leads to fetal hyperinsulinemia, may not be the sole explanation of neonatal hypoglycemia in infants of diabetic mothers. Regardless of the mechanism involved, the recent work by Kalhan and co-workers provides evidence that inhibition of neonatal glucose production is the major factor responsible for hypoglycemia in this syndrome.

4.3. Amino Acid Metabolism

4.3.1. Alanine Synthesis in Muscle

It is now well established that the release of alanine and glutamine from muscle tissue exceeds that of all other amino acids (Felig, 1975).

Evidence supporting the primacy of alanine in amino acid transfer from muscle to liver derives from studies using arterial and venous catheterizations in humans (Pozefsky *et al.*, 1969; Felig *et al.*, 1970; Felig and Wahren, 1971b) and in rats (Aikawa *et al.*, 1973), as well as *in vitro* studies employing the isolated rat diaphragm (Goldberg and Odessey, 1972; Odessey *et al.*, 1974; Palaiologos and Felig, 1976), the perfused rat hindlimb (Ruderman and Berger, 1974), and the isolated rat epitrochlearis muscle (Garber *et al.*, 1976b). Inasmuch as alanine comprises only 7% of the amino acid residues in muscle protein but accounts for 30–40% of muscle amino acid output, *de novo* synthesis of alanine in muscle tissue by transamination of glucose-derived pyruvate was suggested by Felig *et al.*, (1970). In addition, since alanine is a major precursor in glucose formation in the liver, the glucose–alanine cycle was proposed (Mallette *et al.*, 1969; Felig *et al.*, 1970; Felig, 1973). By this formulation, alanine is synthesized in muscle by transamination of glucose-derived pyruvate. The alanine is then released from muscle and taken up by the liver, where its carbon skeleton is reconverted to glucose.

Since the original formulation of the glucose–alanine cycle, a variety of studies have provided confirmation of alanine synthesis in muscle by transamination of pyruvate. Observations have been made with dichloracetate, an agent that depletes tissue pyruvate by stimulating oxidation of this substrate. Addition of dichloracetate markedly decreases *in vitro* synthesis and release of alanine from the isolated diaphragm (Snell and Duff, 1977). A similar *in vivo* effect was observed in hepatectomized rats (Blackshear *et al.*, 1975). Furthermore, the administration of inhibitors of transamination of pyruvate (alanine aminotransferase) such as cycloserine or aminooxyacetate results in a marked diminution in alanine release in the hepatectomized rat (Blackshear *et al.*, 1975) and in various muscle preparations, including incubated diaphragm (Snell and Duff, 1977), the isolated perfused hindlimb (Ruderman and Berger, 1974), and the isolated epitrochlearis (Garber *et al.*, 1976b).

Despite the unanimity regarding the regulatory role of pyruvate in muscle alanine formation, controversy exists as to the quantitative importance of glucose vs. muscle amino acids (particularly valine and isoleucine) as precursors for the pyruvate employed in alanine synthesis. Felig (1973) emphasized the importance of glucose-derived pyruvate on the basis of a variety of observations in intact man: (1) In healthy, resting subjects, a direct correlation is observed between blood pyruvate (which is known to be glucose-derived) and blood alanine (Felig and Wahren, 1971b). (2) In exercise, a circumstance in which muscle glucose uptake increases in proportion to the intensity of the exercise, a similar increase in muscle alanine release is observed (Felig and Wahren, 1971b). (3) In circumstances of augmented pyruvate and lactate accumulation such as systemic lactic acidosis (Marliss *et al.*, 1972), marked increases in blood alanine are noted. (4) In a like manner, in patients with a hereditary myopathy characterized by augmented pyruvate formation in exercise, muscle alanine synthesis is enhanced (Wahren, Linderholm, and Felig, unpublished). (5) In McArdle's syndrome, in which myophosphorylase is decreased, glucose-derived pyruvate availability is diminished and exercise fails to cause an increase in muscle output of alanine (Wahren *et al.*, 1973).

On the basis of the findings described above, the arteriovenous differences of alanine and lysine (an amino acid that is not metabolized in muscle and is present in amounts similar to alanine) were employed to estimate the proportion of muscle alanine release that is glucose-derived (Felig, 1973). The estimates for "glucose-derived alanine" as a proportion of total alanine release were remarkably similar in the forearm (65%) and in the leg (72%) (Felig, 1973).

Subsequent *in vitro* studies have provided confirmation of these *in vivo* findings, while other *in vitro* studies have suggested that muscle amino acids, rather than glucose, are important sources of pyruvate for alanine synthesis. Using the isolated rat diaphragm, Odessey *et al.* (1974) demonstrated that addition of glucose stimulates alanine formation, an observation that was confirmed in other laboratories (Palaiologos and Felig, 1976; Snell and Duff, 1977). More important, using isotopically labeled glucose, Odessey *et al.* (1974) demonstrated that 60% of alanine is formed by transamination of glucose-derived pyruvate. The latter observation is remarkably close to the *in vivo* estimates of 66–70% (Felig, 1973).

In contrast to the findings described above, other workers have suggested that the carbon skeletons of valine and isoleucine are converted to pyruvate and subsequently transaminated. With the use of inhibitors of glycolysis such as NaF, an increase rather than a decrease in alanine synthesis was reported (Goldstein and Newsholme, 1976; Garber, *et al.*, 1976b). Furthermore, inhibitors of decarboxylation (a necessary step in the formation of pyruvate from valine or isoleucine) have been demonstrated to reduce alanine output (Snell, 1976; Garber *et al.*, 1976b; Snell and Duff, 1977). It should be noted, however, that direct effects of these enzyme inhibitors on protein synthesis or catabolism or both have not been excluded. For example, there is at least indirect evidence that NaF is a proteolytic agent (Goldstein and Newsholme, 1976), which could explain enhanced alanine availability in the face of diminished glycolysis. Furthermore, inhibitors of decarboxylation fail to interfere with alanine formation in diaphragm from fed rats and cause no more than a 40–60% reduction in valine- or isoleucine-stimulated alanine formation in fasted rats (Snell and Duff, 1977).

Taken together, the *in vivo* human data and *in vitro* rat data suggest that so long as muscle glycogen is available (i.e., in the fed or postabsorptive state), the pyruvate used in the formation of alanine in resting or exercising muscle is largely (at least 60–70%) glucose-derived. In the fasted animal, the findings also suggest that at least 40–50% (Snell and Duff 1977) or as much as 60–70% (Felig, 1973; Odessey *et al.*, 1974) of alanine is synthesized from glucose-derived pyruvate.

4.3.2. Metabolism of Branched-Chain Amino Acids in Normal and Diabetic Subjects

As noted above, controversy exists as to the relative importance of glucose and amino acids as precursors for the carbon skeletons of alanine synthesis in muscle. In contrast, the evidence is uniform in its support of the branched-chain amino acids as the nitrogen donors for alanine synthesis. As first demonstrated in the isolated diaphragm by Buse *et al.* (1972) and by Odessey and Goldberg (1972), branched-chain amino acids are rapidly oxidized by muscle tissues. Subsequent studies have demonstrated the unique role of branched-chain amino acids in stimulating alanine release from muscle tissue (Odessey *et al.*, 1974; Palaiologos and Felig, 1976; Goldstein and Newsholme, 1976). Complementing these *in vitro* studies are observations in intact humans emphasizing the role of branched-chain amino acids in nitrogen repletion in muscle. Following the ingestion of a protein meal, branched-chain amino acids account for 60–90% of the total amino acid residues released by the splanchnic bed and for a similar proportion of the amino acid residues taken up by the leg (Wahren *et al.*, 1976). Interestingly, during protein feeding, alanine continues to be released from muscle, albeit at a transiently reduced rate. Thus, it is clear that the branched-chain amino acids represent the major form of repletion of nitrogen in muscle tissue that is continuously releasing alanine and glutamine in the fed as well as the fasted state. Inasmuch as the uptake of branched-chain amino acids far exceeds their potential contribution to muscle protein synthesis, it is likely that the major fate of these amino acids is oxidation in muscle and thus availability of their amino groups for alanine formation (Wahren *et al.*, 1976; Felig *et al.*, 1977). The branched-chain amino acids also become important fuels for muscle in prolonged exercise. In that circumstance, a net flow of amino acids from liver to muscle tissue is observed (Ahlborg *et al.*, 1974).

In diabetic subjects, abnormalities in muscle metabolism of branched-chain amino acids have been demonstrated. The nature of these abnormalities in isolated muscle tissue and in the intact human does, however, appear to be at variance. Specifically, in diabetic patients, protein feeding is followed by an increased accumulation of branched-chain amino acids in arterial blood and a diminished uptake of these amino acids by leg muscle tissue (Wahren *et al.,* 1976). In contrast, studies with the isolated rat diaphragm have demonstrated that the oxidation of branched-chain amino acids is increased in diaphragms from diabetic rats (Buse *et al.,* 1976). In addition, the stimulating effect of diabetes on leucine oxidation *in vitro* is reversible by insulin therapy prior to sacrifice (Buse *et al.,* 1976). Subsequent studies involving infusions of leucine in intact diabetics indicate that the overall metabolic clearance of intravenously administered leucine is reduced in diabetes, and that the clearance rate is augmented by insulin administration (Sherwin *et al.,* 1976d). The overall data thus suggest that while intramuscular oxidation of branched-chain amino acids may be increased in the diabetic state, uptake and net disposal of these amino acids is reduced. A number of factors may account for the seeming discrepancy between the human and *in vitro* rat data. First, the rate-limiting step in overall leucine disposal may be at the site of transport into the muscle cell, rather than oxidation. Second, nonoxidative metabolism of leucine (e.g., protein synthesis) may be of greater importance in the overall disposal of leucine. Accordingly, uptake and disposal of leucine could be reduced as a consequence of decreased transport or utilization for protein synthesis despite augmented rates of intracellular oxidation.

4.4. Ketone and Fatty Acid Metabolism

4.4.1. Hormonal Regulation of Ketogenesis

Administration of pharmacologic amounts of glucagon (50 ug/kg per min) has been demonstrated to stimulate lipolysis and ketogenesis in normal man (Liljenquist *et al.,* 1974). In contrast, physiologic doses of glucagon (3 ng/kg per min) causing hyperglucagonemia comparable to that observed in fasting or diabetes fail to induce hyperketonemia (Schade and Eaton, 1976). Furthermore, when substrate availability is markedly enhanced by a fat meal and heparin injection, activating FFA generation, glucagon infusion still fails to induce ketosis (Schade and Eaton, 1976). It should be noted that during such infusions of glucagon, plasma insulin levels vary from base line by no more than 2–3 μU/ml. Similarly, when glucagon is infused along with insulin replacement doses to juvenile diabetics to produce physiologic hyperglucagonemia (200–250 pg/ml), the level of plasma ketone bodies remains unchanged (Gerich *et al.,* 1976). In contrast, if insulin is withdrawn and glucagon is infused along with somatostatin, circulating β-hydroxybutyrate and FFA increase to a higher level than when insulin withdrawal is accompanied by somatostatin-induced suppression of glucagon secretion (Gerich *et al.,* 1976). These findings indicate that physiologic hyperglucagonemia is not of itself ketogenic in normal man or in diabetics when physiologic amounts of insulin are available. The data thus suggest the essential role of absolute insulin deficiency in the ketogenic effects of hyperglucagonemia.

Observations with physiologic increments in growth hormone are similar to those with glucagon. In juvenile diabetics, physiologic increments of circulating growth hormone have no effect on lipid mobilization or ketogenesis as long as growth hormone is infused along with insulin. In contrast, when growth hormone is administered during insulin withdrawal, the levels of circulating glycerol, FFA, and β-hydroxybutyrate all rise markedly (Gerich *et al.*, 1976). This increment exceeds that observed with growth hormone suppression by somatostatin. These findings indicate that as in the case of glucagon, physiologic amounts of insulin can overcome the hyperketonemic effect of growth hormone (see above). Experiments using perfused liver failed to demonstrate any direct stimulation of ketone production by growth hormone (Chernick *et al.*, 1972). It is therefore likely that growth-hormone-induced hyperketonemia during insulin deficiency results from augmented lipid mobilization.

4.4.2. Substrate Regulation of Ketogenesis

The rate of ketogenesis increases rapidly during the first 3 days of starvation, but shows no further increase thereafter (Garber *et al.*, 1974). This finding raises questions about the regulatory mechanism of ketogenesis during prolonged fasting. To determine whether the increased levels of circulating ketones during fasting have any influence on ketone production, Balasse and Neef (1975) infused acetoacetate to obese subjects after 2- to 23-day fast. The infusion achieved a 47–92% increase in total ketone body levels. During the infusions, the endogenous ketone production fell by 15–30%. Simultaneous with the fall in ketone production, the level of plasma FFA and glycerol decreased by 14–17%, whereas the level of plasma insulin remained unchanged.

The data indicate that during fasting, hyperketonemia may exert an inhibitory effect on ketogenesis. This mechanism, which seems to be related to the diminished lipolysis caused by ketone bodies, might play an important role in preventing uncontrolled hyperketonemia during starvation (Balasse and Neef, 1975).

4.4.3. Role of Ketone Disposal in Hyperketonemia

The rapid development of uncontrolled hyperketonemia in insulin-deficient diabetes raises the question whether ketone disposal is also impaired in insulin deficiency. This was recently studied by Sherwin *et al.* (1976c). They infused β-hydroxybutyrate to juvenile diabetics with mild

(0.5 mM) hyperketonemia. Following an equimolar ketone infusion, total blood ketone levels rose twofold greater in diabetics than in controls. The metabolic clearance rate of ketone bodies was reduced by 42% in diabetics, whereas the calculated production rate did not differ from that in controls. This finding suggests that the rate of ketone utilization is impaired and may be a more sensitive index of insulin deficiency than is ketone production (Sherwin *et al.,* 1976c). The fall in ketone disposal was also confirmed in juvenile diabetics with more severe hyperketonemia (2 mM) as well as in nonobese adult-onset diabetics with a moderate hyperketonemia (0.7 mM) (Wildenhof, 1976).

The role of insulin in altering ketone utilization rates is evident from studies in normal as well as diabetic subjects. In normals, infusion of glucose and insulin results in an acceleration in ketone utilization above that observed in the basal state (Sherwin *et al.,* 1976c). In diabetics, insulin administration normalizes the defect in ketone utilization (Wildenhof, 1976). In both groups, hyperinsulinemia lowered β-hydroxybutyrate levels without influencing the concentration of acetoacetate. These findings of selective enhancement of β-hydroxybutyrate uptake provide an explanation for the fall in the β-hydroxybutyrate/acetoacetate ratio that is observed after insulin administration (Stephens *et al.,* 1971). The data also agree with earlier work in experimental animals (Balasse and Havel, 1971).

Regardless of the mechanism whereby insulin alters ketone disposal, it is apparent that the pathogenesis of hyperketonemia in diabetes involves underutilization as well as overproduction of ketones. Hyperketonemia thus may be viewed as the sum of alterations in three processes at three target tissues (Fig. 3): (1) lipolysis at adipose tissue, (2) fatty acid oxidation and ketone formation in liver, and (3) ketone oxidation in muscle.

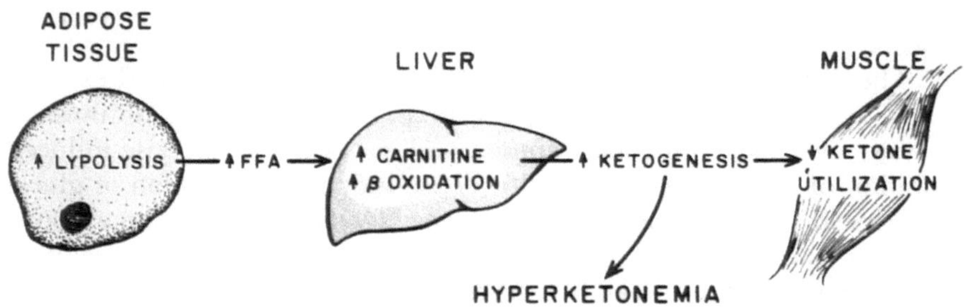

Fig. 3. Pathogenesis of hyperketonemia in diabetes. Hyperketonemia is the net result of alterations in three insulin-dependent processes: (1) augmented lipolysis in adipose tissue, (2) increased β-oxidation of fatty acids (consequent to elevated carnitine levels) in liver, and (3) decreased ketone utilization in muscle.

4.5. Fuel Metabolism in Exercise

The pattern of fuel utilization during brief and prolonged exercise in normal and diabetic subjects has recently been reviewed (Felig and Wahren, 1975; Felig, 1976). In the past year, a number of studies have been reported that demonstrate the effects of altered availability of glucose, fatty acids, and insulin on the fuel–hormone response to exercise.

4.5.1. Influence of Glucose Ingestion

Prolonged exercise in nonfed subjects leads to the mobilization of hepatic glycogen stores, augmented hepatic gluconeogenesis, and accelerated lipolysis. These changes are primarily related to the fall in plasma insulin and, possibly, to the rise in plasma glucagon (Ahlborg *et al.,* 1974). The effect of ingestion of glucose during exercise on the response to prolonged work was examined by Ahlborg and Felig (1976). Normal subjects performed bicycle exercise at 30% of maximal capacity for 90 min, and were then fed 200 g glucose. Exercise was then continued for an additional 2½ hr. The response was compared with that of controls in whom no glucose was ingested during a comparable 4-hr period of exercise. Following the ingestion of glucose, arterial glucose rose by 35%, splanchnic glucose output rose to values twice those observed in controls, and glucose uptake by the exercising legs was twofold greater than controls, accounting for 60% of leg oxygen consumption. The total splanchnic glucose escape after glucose ingestion was 84 ± 5 g, representing 42% of the ingested load. Despite the increase in splanchnic glucose output, splanchnic uptake of gluconeogenic precursors (lactate, pyruvate, and glycerol) fell by 70–100%. In association with the rise in arterial glucose, the plasma insulin levels rose two- to threefold, while arterial free fatty acids and glycerol fell by 60–70%. In addition, plasma glucagon, which rose fourfold in controls, failed to rise in the glucose-fed subjects.

These data indicate that glucose feeding during prolonged exercise results in increased glucose delivery to peripheral tissues, diminished lipolysis, decreased gluconeogenesis, and reversal of exercise-induced inhibition of insulin secretion and exercise-induced stimulation of glucagon secretion. The overall effect of glucose feeding is thus to spare body fat stores and utilization of gluconeogenic substrate while promoting glucose delivery and uptake by exercising muscle.

4.5.2. Glucose-Sparing Effect of Free Fatty Acids

The glucose–fatty acid cycle proposed by Randle *et al.* (1963) provides a mechanism whereby the increased availability of fatty acids decreases carbohydrate utilization in heart muscle. However, studies on voluntary muscle fibers *in vitro* (Beatty and Bocek, 1971) and on rat hindquarter preparations (Berger *et al.*, 1976) have not uniformly shown an inhibitory effect of fatty acids on glucose utilization.

Recently, Rennie *et al.* (1976) demonstrated that increased availability of FFA may have a glucose-sparing effect in exercising rats. Elevations in plasma FFA were induced by feeding corn oil and injecting heparin. In these animals, the degree of glycogen depletion during 40 min of exercise was markedly diminished. Liver glycogen decreased by only 23% in animals with increased FFA, as compared with 83% in control rats. In red muscle fibers, glycogen depletion during exercise was also reduced in animals with high FFA levels. However, in white muscle fibers, the capacity of which to oxidize FFA is very low, no difference was observed in glycogen depletion. The blood glucose level was also higher at the end of exercise in the rats with the high FFA levels. The total estimated glucose utilization during exercise was 50% lower in the rats with elevated FFA levels as compared with controls. It was of interest that elevating the plasma FFA concentration resulted in a rise in plasma insulin and blunted the exercise-induced rise in plasma glucagon (Rennie *et al.*, 1976). Taken together with the previously discussed response to glucose ingestion (Ahlborg and Felig, 1976), the data suggest that increased delivery of either glucose or fat results in sparing of the other fuel (fat or glucose) during exercise.

4.5.3. Interaction of Exercise and Insulin in Diabetes

Previous studies have demonatrated that diabetic humans studied 24 hr after administration of intermediate-acting insulin demonstrate an accelerated fuel response to exercise (Wahren *et al.*, 1975; Felig and Wahren, 1975). In such patients, glucose utilization is comparable to that in healthy controls. However, the gluconeogenic and lipolytic response to exercise is accelerated. In addition, utilization of branched-chain amino acids by exercising muscle occurs more rapidly in the diabetic as compared with controls (Wahren *et al.*, 1975). These studies indicated that an increase in insulin secretion is unnecessary for augmented glucose utilization during exercise (Sanders *et al.*, 1964). The question whether insulin exerts a permissive action on glucose uptake during exercise remains unanswered. *In vitro* studies by Berger *et al.* (1975, 1976) suggested that the totally insulin-deprived muscle has a diminshed increase in glucose utilization in response to contraction. Studies in intact, depancreatized dogs by Vranic *et al.* (1976) also emphasized an "essential" role for insulin in glucose utilization during exercise.

In the studies by Vranic *et al.* (1976), glucose production and utilization were compared in normal dogs, depancreatized dogs infused with intraportal insulin, and insulin-withdrawn depancreatized dogs. Glucose utilization and production during exercise were comparable in normal and depancreatized insulin-infused dogs. In the insulin-withdrawn dogs, a comparable increase in blood glucose and glucose utilization rate occurred. Consequently, glucose clearance remained unchanged. This suggested to the authors that exercise failed to have the stimulatory effect on glucose utilization observed in normal animals or in insulin-infused diabetic animals (Vranic *et al.,* 1976). It is noteworthy, however, that in the insulin-deprived animals, the rate of glucose utilization during exercise (4–6 mg/kg per min) was no different than that observed in controls or insulin-treated diabetic animals. Furthermore, while the glucose metabolic clearance rate was progressively falling when insulin was withdrawn in the resting state, this fall in glucose clearance was rapidly reversed by exercise in these animals. Thus, the data of Vranic *et al.* (1976) may be interpreted as demonstrating that during exercise, the markedly insulin-deprived dog is in fact capable of stimulating glucose utilization in a manner comparable to controls, and that exercise has the effect of reversing the progressive fall in glucose metabolic clearance that would otherwise accompany insulin deprivation.

As noted, the insulin-deprived diabetic dogs demonstrated an augmented hyperglycemic response to exercise. This appears to be a consequence of the exaggerated increment in glucose production that accompanies exercise in these animals (Vranic *et al.,* 1976). The exaggerated hyperglycemic response to diabetes has previously been noted in diabetic humans. Wahren *et al.* (1975) demonstrated that the effect of exercise on plasma glucose and ketone levels is dependent in part on the basal concentration of these substrates prior to exercise. Thus, in subjects with basal glucose levels in excess of 300–400 mg/100 ml and plasma ketone levels in excess of 2 mM/liter, exercise had a hyperglycemic effect and increased ketogenesis. In contrast, in individuals with lower basal glucose and ketone levels, exercise failed to raise glucose levels or stimulate ketone production. Thus, the effect of exercise in exaggerating glucose and ketone production during exercise is probably dependent on the extent of insulin depletion at the time exercise is initiated.

In addition to the variable effect of exercise on fuel homeostasis in insulin-withdrawn diabetics, exercise is known to induce hypoglycemia in insulin-treated diabetic patients. Recent studies by Kawamori and Vranic (1977) provide new insights regarding the mechanism of this hypoglycemia. Kawamori and Vranic investigated the response to exercise in depancreatized dogs injected with protamine zinc and crystalline insulin 8 hr before exercise. In these animals, glucose utilization increased in amounts comparable to controls. Glucose production increased only marginally, however, resulting in a fall in plasma glucose. Of interest was the observation that serum immunoreactive insulin levels increased in the insulin-treated animals during exercise. These findings indicate that exercise has the effect of increasing the availability of subcutaneously injected insulin during exercise. Exercise-induced hyperinsulinemia thus may account for the diminution in glucose production and resultant hypoglycemia that may complicate exercise. The relative importance of increased absorption of insulin from injection sites vs. diminished degradation of insulin in the pathogenesis of exercise-induced hyperinsulinemia in insulin-treated diabetics has not been established. Recent studies suggest, however, that augmented insulin delivery from the injection site in the exercising limb may be the major factor that increased insulin availability during exercise (Koivisto and Felig, 1977).

References

Ahlborg, G., and Felig, P., 1976, Influence of glucose ingestion on fuel-hormone response during prolonged exercise, *J. Appl. Physiol.* **41**:683.

Ahlborg, G., Felig, P., Hagenfeldt, L., Hendler, R., and Wahren, J., 1974, Substrate turnover during prolonged exercise in man: Splanchnic and leg metabolism of glucose, free fatty acids and amino acids, *J. Clin. Invest.* **53**:1080.

Aikawa, T., Matsutaka, H., Yamamoto, H., Okuda, T., Ishikawa, E., Kawano, T., and Matsumura, E., 1973, Gluconeogenesis and amino acid metabolism. II. Interorganal relations and roles of glutamine and alanine in the amino acid metabolism of fasted rats, *J. Biochem. (Tokyo)* **74**:1003.

Alford, F., Bloom, S., Nabarro, J., Hall, R., Besser, G., Coy, D., Kastin, A., and Schally, A. V., 1974, Glucagon control of fasting glucose in man, *Lancet* **2**:974.

Altszuler, N., Gottlieb, B., and Hampshire, J., 1976, Interaction of somatostatin, glucagon and insulin on hepatic glucose output in the normal dog, *Diabetes* **25**:116.

Balasse, E. O., and Havel, R. J., 1971, Evidence for an effect of insulin on the peripheral utilization of ketone bodies in dogs, *J. Clin. Invest.* **50**:801.

Balasse, E. O., and Neef, M. A., 1975, Inhibition of ketogenesis by ketone bodies in fasting humans, *Metabolism* **24**:999.

Beatty, C. H., and Bocek, R. M., 1971, Interrelation of carbohydrate and palmitate metabolism in skeletal muscle, *Amer. J. Physiol.* **220**:1928.

Berger, M., Hagg, S., and Ruderman, N. B., 1975, Glucose metabolism in perfused skeletal muscle; interaction of insulin and exercise on glucose uptake, *Biochem. J.* **146**:231.

Berger, M., Hagg, S. A., Goodman, M. N., and Ruderman, N. B., 1976, Glucose metabolism in perfused skeleton muscle. Effects of starvation, diabetes, fatty acids, acetoacetate, insulin and exercise on glucose uptake and disposition, *Biochem. J.* **158**:191.

Blackshear, P. J., Holloway, P. A. H., and Alberti, K. G. M. M., 1975, Factors regulating amino acid release from extrasplanchnic tissues in the rat. Interactions of alanine and glutamine, *Biochem. J.* **150**:379.

Bloom, S. R., and Johnston, D. I., 1972, Failure of glucagon release in infants of diabetic mothers, *Br. Med. J.* **4**:453.
Bloom, S. R., Mortimer, C. H., Thorner, M. O., Besser, G. M., Hall, R., Gomez-Pan, A., Roy, V. M., Russel, R. C. G., Coy, D. H., Kastin, A. J., and Schally, A. V., 1974, Inhibition of gastrin and gastric acid secretion by growth hormone release-inhibiting hormone, *Lancet* **2**:1106.
Bloom, S. R., Ralphs, D. W., Besser, G. M., Hall, R., Coy, D. H., Kastin, A. J., and Schally, A. V., 1975, Effect of somatostatin on motillin levels and gastric emptying, *Gut* **16**:834 (abstract).
Boden, G., Sivitz, M. C., Owen, O. E., Essa-Koumar, N., and Landor, J. H., 1975, Somatostatin suppresses secretion and pancreatic exocrine secretion, *Science* **190**:163.
Bomboy, J. D., Jr., Lewis, S. B., Lacy, W. W., Sinclair-Smith, B. C., and Liljenquist, J. E., 1977a, Transient stimulatory effect of sustained hyperglucagonemia on splanchnic glucose production in normal and diabetic man, *Diabetes* **26**: 177.
Bomboy, J. D., Jr., Lewis, S. B., Sinclair-Smith, B. C., Lacy, W. W., and Liljenquist, J. E., 1977b, Insulin–glucagon interaction in controlling splanchnic glucose production in normal man, *J. Clin. Endocrinol. Metab.* **44**:474.
Bondy, P. K., James, D. F., and Farrar, B. W., 1949, Studies of the role of liver in human carbohydrate metabolism by the venous catheter technic. I. Normal subjects under fasting conditions and following the injection of glucose, *J. Clin. Invest.* **28**:238.
Brazeau, P., Vale, W., Burgus, R., Ling, N., Butcher, M., Rivier, J., and Guillemin, R., 1973, Hypothalamic polypeptide that inhibits the secretion of immunoreactive growth hormone, *Science* **179**:77.
Buse, M. G., Biggers, J. F., Friderici, K. H., and Buse, J. F., 1972, Oxidation of branched chain amino acids by isolated hearts and diaphragms of the rat: The effect of fatty acids, glucose, and pyruvate respiration, *J. Biol. Chem.* **247**:8085.
Buse, M. G., Herlong, H. G., and Weigand, D. A., 1976, The effect of diabetes, insulin, and the redox potential on leucine metabolism by isolated rat hemidiaphragm, *Endocrinology* **98**:1166.
Chernick, S. S., Clark, C. M., Jr., Gardiner, R. J., and Scow, R. O., 1972, Role of lipolytic and glucocorticoid hormones in the development of diabetic ketosis, *Diabetes* **21**:946.
Chiasson, J. L., Liljenquist, J. E., Finger, F. E., and Lacy, W. W., 1976, Differential sensitivity of glycogenolysis and gluconeogenesis to insulin infusions in dogs, *Diabetes* **25**:283.
Dobbs, R., Sakurai, H., Sasaki, H., Faloona, G., Valverde, I., Baetens, D., Orci, L., and Unger, R., 1975, Glucagon: Role in the hyperglycemia of diabetes mellitus, *Science* **187**:544.
Felig, P., 1973, The glucose–alanine cycle, *Metabolism* **22**:179.
Felig, P., 1975, Amino acid metabolism in man, *Annu. Rev. Biochem.* **44**:933.
Felig, P., 1976, Recent developments in body fuel metabolism, in: *The Year in Metabolism 1975–76* (N. Freinkel, ed.), p. 113–136, Plenum Press, New York.
Felig, P., 1977, Body fuel metabolism and diabetes mellitus in pregnancy, *Med. Clin. North Amer.* **61**:43.
Felig, P., and Wahren, J., 1971a, Influence of endogenous insulin secretion on

splanchnic glucose and amino acid metabolism in man, *J. Clin. Invest.* **50**:1702.

Felig, P., and Wahren, J., 1971b, Amino acid metabolism in exercising man, *J. Clin. Invest.* **50**:2703.

Felig, P., and Wahren, J., 1975, Fuel homeostasis in exercise (Seminars of the Beth Israel Hospital), *N. Engl. J. Med.* **293**:1078.

Felig, P., Pozefsky, T., Marliss, E., and Cahill, G. F. Jr., 1970, Alanine: Key role in gluconeogenesis, *Science* **167**:1003.

Felig, P., Wahren, J., and Hendler, R., 1976a, Influence of physiologic hyperglucagonemia on basal and insulin-inhibited splanchnic glucose output in normal man, *J. Clin. Invest.* **58**:761.

Felig, P., Wahren, J., Sherwin, R., and Hendler, R., 1976b, Insulin, glucagon and somatostatin in normal physiology and diabetes mellitus, *Diabetes* **25**:1091.

Felig, P., Wahren, J., Sherwin, R., and Palaiologos, G., 1977, Amino acid and protein metabolism in diabetes mellitus, *Arch. Intern. Med.* **137**:507.

Floyd, J. C., Jr., Fajans, S. S., Conn, J. W., Knopf, R. F., and Rull, J., 1966, Insulin secretion in response to protein ingestion, *J. Clin. Invest.* **45**:1479.

Garber, A. J., Menzel, P. H., Boden, G., and Owen, O. E., 1974, Hepatic ketogenesis and gluconeogenesis in humans, *J. Clin. Invest.* **54**:981.

Garber, A. J., Cryer, P. E., Santiago, J. V., Haymond, M. W., Pagliara, A. S., and Kipnis, D. M., 1976a, The role of adrenergic mechanism in the substrate and hormonal response to insulin-induced hypoglycemia in man, *J. Clin. Invest.* **58**:7.

Garber, A. J., Karl, I. E., and Kipnis, D. M., 1976b, Alanine and glutamine synthesis and release from skeletal muscle. II. The precursor role of amino acids in alanine and glutamine synthesis, *J. Biol. Chem.* **251**:836.

Gerich, J. E., 1977, Somatostatin: Its possible role in carbohydrate homeostasis and the treatment of diabetes mellitus, *Arch. Intern. Med.* (in press).

Gerich, J. E., Lorenzi, M., Schneider, V., Karam, J. H., Rivier, J., Guillemin, R., and Forsham, P. H., 1974, Effects of somatostatin on plasma glucose and glucagon levels in human diabetes mellitus, *N. Engl. J. Med.* **291**:544.

Gerich, J. E., Lorenzi, M., Bier, D. M., Tsalikian, E., Schneider, V., Karam, J. H., and Forsham, P. H., 1976, Effects of physiologic levels of glucagon and growth hormone on human carbohydrate and lipid metabolism, *J. Clin. Invest.* **57**:875.

Goldberg, A. L., and Odessey, R., 1972, Oxidation of amino acids by diaphragms from fed and fasted rats, *Amer. J. Physiol.* **223**:1384.

Goldstein, L., and Newsholme, E. A., 1976, The formation of alanine from amino acids in diaphragm muscle of the rat, *Biochem. J.* **154**:555.

Gomez-Pan, A., Reed, J. D., Albinus, M., Shaw, B., Hall, R., Besser, G. M., Coy, D. H., Kastin, A. J., and Schally, A. V., 1975, Direct inhibition of gastric acid and pepsin secretion by growth hormone release-inhibiting hormone in cats, *Lancet* **1**:888.

Hultman, E., and Nillsson, L. H., 1971, Liver glycogen in man. Effect of different diets and muscular exercise, *Adv. Exp. Med. Biol.* **11**:143.

Kalhan, S. C., Savin, S. M., and Adam, P. A. J., 1977, Attenuated glucose production rate in newborn infants of insulin-dependent diabetic mothers, *N. Engl. J. Med.* **296**:375.

Kawamori, R., and Vranic, M., 1977, Mechanism of exercise-induced hypoglycemia in depancreatized dogs maintained on long-acting insulin, *J. Clin. Invest.* **59**:331.

Koerker, D. L., Ruch, W., Chideckel, E., Palmer, J., Goodner, C. J., Ensinck, J., and Gale, C. C., 1974, Somatostatin: Hypothalamic inhibitor of the endocrine pancreas, *Science* **184**:482.

Koivisto, V. A., and Felig, P., 1977, Effects of exercise on insulin release from injection sites in diabetic man, *Diabetes* **26** (Suppl. 1):357.

Liljenquist, J. E., Bomboy, J. D., Lewis, S. B., Sinclair-Smith, B. C., Felts, P. W., Lacy, W. W., Crofford, O. B., and Liddle, G. W., 1974, Effects of glucagon on lipolysis and ketogenesis in normal and diabetic man, *J. Clin. Invest.* **53**:190.

Lindsey, A., Santeusanio, F., Braaten, J., Faloona, G. F., and Unger, R. H., 1974, Pancreatic alpha cell function in trauma, *J. Amer. Med. Assoc.* **227**:757.

Madison, L. L., 1969, Role of insulin in the hepatic handling of glucose, *Arch. Intern. Med.* **123**:284.

Mallette, L. E., Exton, J. H., and Park, C. R., 1969, Control of gluconeogenesis from amino acids in the perfused rat liver, *J. Biol. Chem.* **244**:5713.

Mann, F. S., and MaGath, T. B., 1922, Studies on the physiology of the liver. II. The effect of the removal of the liver on the blood sugar level, *Arch. Intern. Med.* **30**:73.

Marliss, E. B., Aoki, T. T., Toews, C. J., Felig, P., Connon, J. J., Kyner, J., Huckabee, W. E., and Cahill, G. F., Jr., 1972, Amino acid metabolism in lactic acidosis, *Amer. J. Med.* **52**:474.

Odessey, R., and Goldberg, A. L., 1972, Oxidation of leucine by rat skeletal muscle, *Amer. J. Physiol.* **223**:1376.

Odessey, R., Khairallah, E. A., and Goldberg, A. L., 1974, Origin and possible significance of alanine production by skeletal muscle, *J. Biol. Chem.* **249**:7623.

Palaiologos, G., and Felig, P., 1976, Effects of ketone bodies on amino acid metabolism in isolated rat diaphragm, *Biochem. J.* **154**:709.

Patton, G., Ipp, E., Schusdziarra, V., Dobbs, R., Orci, L., Vale, W., and Unger, R., 1977, Studies of pancreatic somatostatin secretion, *Clin. Res.* **25**:523A.

Pederson, J., Boljsen-Moller, B., and Poulsen, H., 1954, Blood sugar in newborn infants of diabetic mothers, *Acta Endocrinol. (Copenhagen)* **15**:33.

Persson, B., Gentz, J., and Kellum, M., 1973, Metabolic observations in infants of strictly controlled diabetic mothers; plasma levels of glucose, FFA, glycerol and D-beta-hydroxybutyrate during the first two hours after birth, *Acta Paediatr. Scand.* **62**:465.

Pozefsky, T., Felig, P., Tobin, J., Soeldner, J. S., and Cahill, G. F., Jr., 1969, Amino acid balance across tissues of the forearm in postabsorptive man: Effects of insulin at two dose levels, *J. Clin. Invest.* **48**:2273.

Randle, P. J., Garland, P. B., Hales, C. N., and Newsholme, E. A., 1963, The glucose fatty acid cycle. Its role in insulin sensitivity and the metabolic disturbances of diabetes mellitus, *Lancet* **1**:785.

Rennie, M. J., Winder, W. W., and Holloszy, J. O., 1976, A sparing effect of increased plasma fatty acids on muscle and liver glycogen content in the exercising rat, *Biochem. J.* **156**:647.

Rocha, D. M., Santeusanio, F., Faloona, G. R., and Unger, R. H., 1973, Abnormal pancreatic alpha cell function in bacterial infections, *N. Engl. J. Med.* **288**:700.

Ruderman, N. B., and Berger, M., 1974, The formation of glutamine and alanine in skeletal muscle, *J. Biol. Chem.* **249**:5500.

Sacca, L., Perez, G., Carteni, G., and Frengo, F., 1977, Evaluation of the role of the sympathetic nervous system in the glucoregulatory response to insulin-induced hypoglycemia in the rat, *Endocrinology* (in press).

Sanders, C. A., Levinson, G. E., Abelman, W. H., and Freinkel, N., 1964, Effect of exercise on peripheral utilization of glucose in man, *N. Engl. J. Med.* **271**:220.

Schade, D. S., and Eaton, R. P., 1976, Modulation of fatty acid metabolism by glucagon in man. IV. Effects of physiologic hormone infusion in normal man, *Diabetes* **25**:978.

Sherwin, R., Joshi, P., Hendler, R., Felig, P., and Conn, H. O., 1974, Hyperglucagonemia in Laennec's cirrhosis. The role of portal–systemic shunting, *N. Engl. J. Med.* **290**:239.

Sherwin, R. S., Bastl, C., Finkelstein, F. O., Fisher, M., Black, H., Hendler, R., and Felig, P., 1976a, Influence of uremia and hemodialysis on the turnover and metabolic effects of glucagon, *J. Clin. Invest.* **57**:722.

Sherwin, R. S., Fisher, M., Hendler, R., and Felig, P., 1976b, Hyperglucagonemia and blood glucose regulation in normal, obese and diabetic subjects, *N. Engl. J. Med.* **294**:455.

Sherwin, R. S., Hendler, R., and Felig, P., 1976c, Effect of diabetes mellitus and insulin on the turnover and metabolic response to ketones in man, *Diabetes* **25**:776.

Sherwin, R., Rosenzweig, J., Soman, V., Hendler, R., and Felig, P., 1976d, Effect of insulin and diabetes on protein and branched chain amino acid utilization, *Diabetes* **25** (Suppl. 1):332.

Sherwin, R. S., Hendler, R., DeFronzo, R. A., Wahren, J., and Felig, P., 1977, Glucose homeostatis during prolonged suppression of glucagon and insulin secretion by somatostatin, *Proc. Natl. Acad. Sci. U.S.A.* **74**:348.

Shikama, H., and Ui, M., 1975, Adrenergic receptor and epinephrine-induced hyperglycemia and glucose tolerance, *Amer. J. Physiol.* **229**:962.

Siler, T. M., Vandenberg, G., and Yen, S. S. C., 1973, Inhibition of growth hormone release in humans by somatostatin, *J. Clin Endocrinol. Metab.* **37**:632.

Snell, K., 1976, Alanine release by rat hemidiaphragm muscle *in vitro, Biochem. Soc. Trans.* **4**:287.

Snell, K., and Duff, D. A., 1977, The release of alanine by rat diaphragm muscle *in vitro, Biochem. J.* **162**:399.

Stephens, J. M., Sulway, M. J., and Watkins, P. J., 1971, Relationship of blood acetoacetate and 3-beta-hydroxybutyrate in diabetes, *Diabetes* **20**:485.

Stern, L., Ramos, A., and Leduc, J., 1968, Urinary catecholamine excretion in infants of diabetic mothers, *Pediatrics* **42**:598.

Sugden, M. C., Sharples, S. C., and Randle, P., 1976, Carcass glycogen as a potential source of glucose during short-term starvation, *Biochem. J.* **160**:817.

Unger, R. H., Ohneda, A., Aquilar-Parada, E., and Eisentraut, A. M., 1969, The role of aminogenic glucagon secretion in blood glucose homeostatis, *J. Clin. Invest.* **48**:810.

Vranic, M., Kawamori, R., Pek, S., Kovacevic, N., and Wrenshall, G. A., 1976, The essentiality of insulin and the role of glucagon in regulating glucose utilization and production during strenous exercise in dogs, *J. Clin. Invest.* **57**:245.

Wahren, J., and Felig, P., 1976, Influence of somatostatin on carbohydrate disposal and absorption in diabetes mellitus, *Lancet* **2**:1213.

Wahren, J., Felig, P., Havel, R. J., Jorfeldt, L., Pernow, B., and Saltin, B., 1973, Amino acid metabolism in McArdle's syndrome, *N. Engl. J. Med.* **288**:774.

Wahren, J., Hagenfeldt, L., and Felig, P., 1975, Splanchnic and leg exchange of glucose, amino acids, and free fatty acids during exercise in diabetes mellitus, *J. Clin. Invest.* **55**:1303.

Wahren, J., Felig, P., and Hangefeldt, L., 1976, Effect of protein ingestion on splanchnic and leg metabolism in normal man and in patients with diabetes mellitus, *J. Clin. Invest.* **57**:987.

Wahren, J., Efendic, S., Luft, R., Hagenfeldt, L., Bjorkman, O., and Felig, P., 1977, Influence of somatostatin on splanchnic glucose metabolism in postabsorptive and 60-hour fasted humans, *J. Clin. Invest.* **59**:299.

Wildenhof, K. E., 1976, Blood ketone body disappearance rate in diabetics and normals after rapid infusion of DL-3-hydroxybutyrate. Studies before and after diabetic treatment, *Acta Med. Scand.* **200**:79.

5

What's New in the Treatment of Obesity?

Jules Hirsch

5.1. Introduction

There has been mounting pressure to translate research findings into useful information for the medical community in its quest for the prevention and treatment of disease. Research in disorders such as obesity, which are of clear relevance to public health, must be translated periodically into brief reviews that bear directly on therapy. Recently, laboratories of endocrinology and metabolism, as well as of sociology, psychology, and physiology, have studied a variety of approaches to the treatment of obesity. It is with these considerations in mind that this chapter on obesity for *The Year in Metabolism 1976–1977* is concerned exclusively with the question "what's new in the treatment of obesity?" The most concise answer to this question is: Nothing of low risk and proven lasting benefit.

It might be judicious to end discussion at this point, were it not for

Jules Hirsch • The Rockefeller University, New York, New York 10021.

two considerations: (1) It is worthwhile to examine in a general way those basic problems that prevent treatment success. (2) It is timely to examine more specifically those treatments currently receiving most attention and notoriety. Untested or unproved as these treatments may be, a closer evaluation may point the way for better treatments yet to come.

During the past year, three treatments have been widely discussed: dietary, by the use of a low-calorie, high-protein diet, the so-called "protein-sparing modified fast"; psychological, by the methods of behavior modification; and surgical, by the creation of a permanent jejunoileal shunt. This essay will examine problems that make all treatment of obesity a difficult and largely unsuccessful endeavor and then examine the three newer treatments in the light of basic information as to why treatments fail.

5.2. The Core Problem of Treatment

Simple or so-called "exogenous" obesity is an excessive accumulation of body fat in adipose tissue in the absence of any neural or endocrine abnormalities known to affect food intake or fat storage. In this circumstance, the obesity appears to be "defended" by the afflicted subject. The defense is manifested by a return to the obese state following weight reduction or the necessity for continuous treatment as a counterforce to the defense. Implicating a "defense" may seem to be no more than a tautological restatement of the fact that relapse after treatment is exceedingly common, yet considering obesity as a defended state such as the level of serum osmolarity or systolic blood pressure can be of conceptual help. The nature of such defense and the consequences or risks of establishing counterposing forces are key to any evaluation of the efficacy and hazards of treatment.

5.3. Hypothetical Defended Variables in Obesity

5.3.1. Hyperphagia

An excess of food intake has been primary in many considerations of the pathogenesis as well as the treatment of obesity. The concept that a need for hyperphagia, or defense of excess food intake, could be the primary etiology of obesity has led to the proposition that obesity, which is a necessary consequence of this need, can be considered an addictive disorder. The need for hyperphagia has been dealt with in terms of psychoanalytic reasoning, hypothesizing that hyperphagia is related to disturbed orality (Bychowski, 1950). The feeding disturbance of the obese has been further delineated into specific syndromes of binge eating or night eating (Stunkard, 1950). The concept that hyperphagia is a prime defended variable is given force by the rare situation in which a brain neoplasm or other pathological state in or near the hypothalamus provokes sudden and uncontrolled increase in food intake. It is evident, however, that in the majority of obese patients, most of whom have only moderate obesity, the acquisition of excess weight is gradual, and thus the increase in food intake must have of necessity been small. The bizarre eating patterns of some obese patients may in fact be the result of dieting with intermittent brief weight loss followed by transient hyperphagia, rather than any primary disturbances of food intake. Furthermore, it has been shown that some obese individuals have developed obesity while on "normal" food intake, undoubtedly as a consequence of diminished activity (Johnson *et al.*, 1956).

5.3.2. Symbolic Meaning of Obesity

The physical appearance of obesity has been symbolically equated with feelings of power or of protection from injury and illness, with femaleness, or with a covering of sexuality and protection from sexual attractiveness. Bruch (1973) speculated on the strength of these symbolic aspects of obesity, and it can be asked whether these meanings of obesity are in some way specifically needed by the affected subject and thus constitute defended variables that resist treatment and weight loss. Clearly, there is great variation in the degree to which these symbolic aspects are of consequence to the obese. In many instances, there is a strongly felt loathing of the obese state; indeed, the continuous quest of the obese for new methods of weight reduction would appear to indicate their strong desire to be rid of any symbolic advantages. Yet, the relationship between obesity and personality disorders or intrapsychic conflict cannot be so readily dismissed. In a study by Rand and Stunkard (1977), psychoanalysts of 84 patients were asked to complete an extensive questionnaire concerning obese patients receiving intensive psychoanalytic treatment. Only 6% of the patients sought treatment for obesity. Depression, anxiety, or other problems were the more usual reasons for seeking therapy. Interestingly, 19% of the patients lost 40 pounds or more and 54% lost 20 pounds or more. The mean weight loss was 21 pounds over an average treatment time of roughly 4 years. Exactly what had happened during psychoanalysis to ameliorate obesity is not clear, yet the degree of treatment success is impressive.

5.3.3. A Life Style

The life style of the affluent Western world is surely conducive to the production of obesity. The ready availability of a variety of enticing foods and their conspicuous consumption are marks of success in our culture. A growing interest in gourmet dining and the use of specially prepared foods to enhance social encounters are increasingly in evidence. Simultaneously, the use of labor-saving devices such as electrically driven window openers and a variety of pushbutton devices, used as evidence of plentitude and the good life, all operate to reduce caloric output and hence to produce obesity. It is reasonable to suggest that these new and enjoyable ways of life are not only readily assumed but also in fact defended as highly desirable aspects of modern life. To the extent that this is true, obesity may be the consequence of the defense of a highly desired, much-sought-after and advertised way of life.

A subtle and more-argued question is whether or not early life alterations can lead to lasting changes in life style. The most attractive form in which this hypothesis has been put forward is the notion that inappropriate use of food early in childhood may lead to patterns of eating for inappropriate and unphysiological reasons. Schachter (see Schachter and Rodin, 1974) has been a student and proponent of such concepts. He and his colleagues have shown that under some experimental circumstances, obese individuals tend to ignore internal cues such as gastric filling and eat more readily in response to such external cues as the mode of food presentation, the time of day, or the circumstances under which food is made available. An underlying premise is that some infants or children can develop compliance with the new life style of abundance. A mother who overfeeds or feeds in response to needs other than hunger could be the essential vector. Compliance develops and is manifest as a heightened ability to eat when it is socially appropriate and, at the same time, a developed ability to ignore or suppress physiological signals of satiety. Rodin *et al.* (1974) amassed evidence of heightened external sensitivity in some obese. Coddington and Bruch (1970) suggested that the obese have lessened sensitivity to the signals of gastric filling, although in a detailed and critical study by Stunkard and Koch (1964), the nature of this lessened sensitivity was shown to be more of a denial than a true difference in sensitivity to internal cues.

The subject of internality vs. externality in the obese remains *sub judice.* In a recent comprehensive review of this matter, Leon and Roth (1977) commented that "the support for Schachter's externality theory of obesity appears to be equivocal at best." Thus, obesity in defense of life style, although significant and perhaps even commonplace in adults, has not yet been proved to have made lasting impacts on the psychology of children so as to provoke adult obesity. An even more difficult possibility to evaluate is whether childhood feeding practices have created cellular or biochemical changes leading to a defense of increased adipose mass.

5.3.4. Adipose Mass

During growth and development, roughly 10–20% of ingested calories are held as stored triglyceride, of obvious utility to the organism in the event of food deprivation. Fat storage behaves like a defended variable. Thus, over- or underfed aminals will eat appropriately when returned to *ad libitum* feeding to restore the previous adipose mass (Cohn and Joseph, 1962). That obese persons are primarily defending an obese level of fat storage and achieving this end by appropriate food intake and activity remains an unproved contention.

The finding that obese subjects, particularly those with massive obesity and with onset early in life, have an excessive and fixed number of adipocytes (Hirsch and Batchelor, 1976) is certainly suggestive that adipose mass is in someway involved in the perpetuation of the obese state and hence the resistance to treatment. A recent study (Faust *et al.*, 1977) showing that fat-cell size has a marked influence on the food intake of lipectomized rodents lends support to a fat-cell–food-intake relationship, but still does not give any quantitative notion of the role of adipose mass itself in defense of the obese state. It is possible that early childhood feeding practices dictated by life style or cultural patterns may leave an impact on the organism in terms of adipose cellularity that in later life is manifest as hypercellular obesity. The evidence for such a possiblity is more readily found in the rat (Knittle and Hirsch, 1968) than it is in man.

5.4. Implications for Treatment

If none of the defenses discussed above was present, it could be assumed that therapy for obesity would be a simple matter. Merely advising a patient that obesity is present and prescribing an appropriate diet, low in calories, would be uniformly successful. The almost universal failure of this approach attests to the power of defense against treatment. One might suppose that defended hyperphagia or a defense of the symbolic value of the obese state would be best treated by intensive psychotherapy. Although psychotherapy or psychoanalysis can be helpful, as described above, there is no evidence that psychotherapy can so remove either the symptoms of hyperphagia or a detrimental symbolization of the obese state as to eradicate obesity without simultaneous intensive dieting.

Likewise, the adherence to a particular life style would appear to be so deeply ingrained that simple advice or even warning has little lasting effect. All considerations converge on the fact that whatever is defended is defended in a peculiarly tenacious way; hence, therapy must be equally intensive and protracted.

The therapeutic counterforce should probably not be the same for all patients. The adult-onset, moderate, or minimally obese subject can be treated by changes in diet and activity in a variety of outpatient settings. Whatever defenses of obesity are present in these subjects can be overcome in roughly one-third of cases. The more markedly obese individual with childhood onset will require more drastic intervention, and success is an unlikely outcome however intensive the efforts.

5.5. Current New Approaches to Treatment

5.5.1. The Protein-Sparing Modified Fast

A diet composed of 1–1.5 g protein/kg per day, in the form of lean meat or protein hydrolysates, supplemented with potassium, calcium, iron, and vitamins, has been termed a protein-sparing modified fast (PSMF). Bistrian *et al.* (1977) used lean meat as the source of protein, but recently there has been a great deal of publicity given to the use of special protein preparations with or without small amounts of carbohydrate. This diet has been popularized by Robert Linn (1977) an osteopathic physician in Philadelphia, in a book entitled, *The Last Chance Diet.* The diet is apparently being so commonly used that the Department of Foods and Nutrition of The American Medical Association has expressed concern in the form of a special warning in the *American Medical News* (1977), noting that this diet should not be used without proper medical supervision, since it may lead to "nausea, vomiting, constipation, electrolyte imbalance, dehydration, hyperuricemia, and postural hypotension."

The rationale for this diet and its special advantage as compared with any other mixture of foods, similarly reduced in total caloric intake, was best stated by Bistrian *et al.* (1976). These investigators feel that the advantage rests in the fact that PSMF markedly lowers serum insulin levels. Since it is known that insulin has an antilipolytic effect on adipose tissue, this hormone will favor the uptake and storage of triglyceride by adipose tissue, thus opposing the effects of treatment. These investigators reason that the administration of carbohydrate-containing foods, rather than the PSMF diet, would increase insulin levels, thereby reducing lipolysis. The ketosis that occurs with carbohydrate-restricted feeding is thought to be advantageous in sparing protein loss and also in lessening hunger. If all these contentions were totally correct, then a total fast would be the optimal method of weight reduction. It is realized, however, that total fasting will have a variety of adverse effects including the loss of lean body mass and possibly hepatic and renal dysfunction. Hence, a lean-body-mass-sparing fast with enough protein to reverse the loss of nitrogen, but no carbohydrate to elevate insulin levels, is thought to be an optimal method for weight reduction. Bistrian *et al.* (1976, 1977) reported on the use of a PSMF diet in diabetics and in four young subjects with the Prader–Willi syndrome. In these reports, the diets led to weight loss with maintenance of nitrogen balance. Indeed, there is no reason adherence to such a diet should not lead to continuous weight loss. If, however, this particular diet is considered to be a specific treatment for obesity, which corrects some metabolic disturbance found in the obese state, then several issues must be examined more carefully.

The idea that high insulin levels in obesity promote fat storage runs counter to the fact that obesity is a state in which marked resistance to insulin action is found. It is difficult if not impossible to compare the effects of insulin in normal subjects and in the obese, who are relatively resistant to insulin action, and then determine whether endogenously produced insulin in the obese is in fact a significant antilipolytic force. What speaks against the notion of insulin as an impediment to weight loss is that weight loss in the long run is proportionate to caloric deficit, whether these calories are from protein or carbohydate foods. Thus, in a study by Yang and Van Itallie (1976), it could be shown that regardless of the nature of fed calories, fat loss due to a hypocaloric diet is strictly proportional to the caloric deficit. If carbohydrate calories had some specific antilipolytic effect, one might have supposed that fat loss would diminish during carbohydrate feeding. This was not the case. Of course, a carbohydrate-restricted diet will lead to loss of calories as urinary or expired ketones, but such caloric wastage is small, only 16–32 kcal/day (Yang and Van Itallie, 1976). Water and electrolyte loss in acidosis will lead to prompt decline in body weight, but fat loss, the desired effect, is no greater than is found with any other hypocaloric diet. It must be concluded, then, that any biochemical theory used as a basis for advocating a ketogenic diet is found lacking in practice. Indeed, it is difficult to conceive of any other result if ordinary thermodynamic or caloric balance considerations are not to be radically altered. This leaves open the question whether a ketogenic diet or PSMF may not have some special advantage other than the rate of fat loss.

It has been claimed that ketosis is anorexigenic and hence can be a valuable counterforce to the hunger that is expected on any weight-reducing regimen. An early report of the effect of total starvation (Bloom, 1959) stated that starving obese subjects did not frequently complain of hunger. This study was of brief fasting (4–9 days) of nine obese subjects. The author also noted that "an unexpected result of the study was the patient's satisfaction with a 600–800 calorie diet following the completion of the fast, whereas prior to the fast this type of diet had been very unsatisfactory." Some years later, Silverstone *et al.* (1966) made quantitative evaluations of hunger during total starvation. They found "no evidence that hunger diminished during starvation." Since mild nausea may occur with ketosis, this may have been a confounding factor in evaluating hunger, but clearly the quantitative measures of Silverstone and his colleagues establish that the clinical impression of diminished hunger during starvation is not borne out. Both Bloom (1959) and Silverstone *et al.* (1966) wondered whether hunger might not be diminished on a hypocaloric diet following starvation and thus whether starvation or perhaps PSMF might be considered a good introduction to a weight-reducing regimen. The data of Drenick (1973) seem to demolish this argument effectively. Prolonged starvation leads to weight loss, but Drenick's subjects regained the lost weight afterward. There was no reason to believe that any hypothetical "appestat" had been reset by starvation or that ketosis had removed the defenses for the maintenance of obesity.

Thus, one must conclude that there is neither a valid theoretical basis nor any quantitative empirical observations to support the use of PSMF for weight reduction. The successes that have been reported with PSMF may relate to the predicted success of any method that is novel and highly publicized, and also to the fact that some obese subjects may respond better to a precise, simple formulation of dietary ingredients than the more difficult matter of "counting calories" and using various exchange lists. An appropriate control for evaluating the effects of PSMF would be an equally simple formula diet or diet composed of only one or two foods. However useful a simple diet of this type may be, it will not prepare the obese subject for the lifelong period of weight maintenance following weight reduction. Presumably, a diet using the more usually consumed foodstuffs is a better one for learning those principles of nutrition that will have to be closely followed after weight reduction. The unusual nature of "last-chance" diets using formula mixtures is hardly a preparation for lifelong care in food intake, which remains the only known nutritional therapy for obesity.

5.5.2. Behavior Modification

If obesity were the result of a life style that is so deeply committed to practice as to be defended, it might be expected that brief or few interventions by a physician would not constitute a sufficient counterforce. Thus, Penick and Stunkard (1970), commenting on the value of sustained influences conducive to weight reduction, note that the medical model may be inappropriate for the treatment of obesity. They state that the medical model "defines an authoritarian role for the physician, who prescribes a diet and appetite-suppressing medication. The patient loses weight, if at all, in large part to please the doctor and to meet his expectations. When the relationship is terminated or attenuated, the patient discontinues the diet and regains weight." A variety of other models have been developed that can be administered by nonmedical personnel and that involve a longer contact of the patient and therapist than is customarily the case in the medical model. These methods of behavior modification are based on such premises as the following:

1. Hyperphagia and underactivity are to some degree learned behaviors. What is learned can be relearned in a way that is more conducive to the maintenance of normal weight.
2. Regardless of what the etiology of obesity may be, ultimately its symptomatic expression is through hyperphagia with or without underactivity. Treatment should therefore be directed to these two symptoms.

More specifically, behavior modification involves an analysis of the setting and circumstances in which eating occurs. Usually a careful day-to-day record of eating is kept. An effort is then made to dissociate eating from causes that are "nonphysiological." For example, the advice to eat only after setting the table, following planning of the meal, and then with frequent pauses between bites is a set of suggestions designed to dissociate eating from sudden impulses for uncontrolled hyperphagia that might result from feelings of anger, depression, or boredom. Similarly, the systematic evaluation and understanding of stimuli for eating is introduced so as to remove excess eating in response to the presence of food in social settings in which overeating has become a usual or characteristic response.

A variety of programmed instructions have been developed, some of which can be administered by therapists with very little training or even self-administered. A text by Stuart and Davis (1972) reviews the basic strategems and methods for the behavioral control of food intake and physical activity. There are a number of obvious advantages to this approach. To begin with, the aim of treatment is to establish new, lifelong habits. Given the known chronicity and tendency to relapse, this approach is far more sensible than crash diets or other fads that, by their nature, cannot be followed for long periods of time. Furthermore, behavior modification can be done in groups and is thus not likely to be as expensive as repeated visits to the physician's office or to such commercial enterprises as spas or weight-reducing salons. Finally, the treatment appears sensible to most sufferers from obesity, since it focuses directly on the symptom that most troubles them, namely, an inability to control their own behavior.

It is still too early to evaluate the long-term results of treatment. In general, the results show moderate weight loss and a tendency for this loss to be more lasting than that found with more medically oriented approaches. Leon (1977) recently reviewed 11 studies. Eliminating one study in which only a single patient was treated and an unusually large weight loss of 102 pounds was achieved, the other 10 studies involved a total of 450 patients. Treatment was from 4 to 18 weeks and follow-up from 4 to 52 weeks. The average weight loss was roughly 16 pounds, and in 7 of the 10 studies, significant weight loss was maintained at follow-up times. Unfortunately, most follow-ups of these studies have not been for sufficiently long periods to ascertain the lasting impact of behavior modification. In one study (Penick and Stunkard, 1977) in which a group of patients were treated weekly for 3 months, an unusually long, 5-year follow-up was obtained, and the results were exceedingly disappointing. Clearly, more experience with these methods and longer follow-ups will be needed before any final evaluations can be made.

Most programs of behavior modification have been administered by psychologists, social workers, or nutritionists. In recent years, community self-help groups of different types have developed. These are not, strictly speaking, formal efforts at behavior modification, although at times the same principles have been used by these groups. One of the first groups to develop was TOPS (Take off Pounds Sensibly), which was founded roughly 30 years ago. It sponsors small community meetings in homes or other meeting places during which members have a form of group therapy, which is often continued informally by contacts outside the group meetings. A diet prescribed by each client's own physician is used, and competition for weight loss among members is stressed. Another group, Overeaters Anonymous (OA), stresses a buddy system similar to that used by Alcoholics Anonymous. Perhaps the most widely known community self-help group for obesity is Weight Watchers. A specific Weight Watchers diet composed of mixed foods is taught. Members attend meetings weekly for a fee of roughly $3 per session. A group leader or lecturer discusses techniques for following the diet, sometimes with an emphasis on behavior-modification techniques. Awards are presented to those who have attained their desired weight or otherwise complied with the program. A comparison study of this method (Williams and Duncan, 1976) and a hospital-based weight-reduction program found the Weight Watcher's approach to be more successful in pounds lost.

It seems reasonable that behavior-modification programs, whether administered in a formal way by a professional or as a less well structured self-help type community group, could be useful, particularly for modest weight reduction, in those of moderate obesity of adult onset. It is this type of obesity that is most likely to be involved in life-style problems and is thus more likely to be amenable to changes in food intake behavior and its relationship to life styles. Certainly behavior modification is of low medical risk and relatively low cost. At younger ages, when patterns of life style are more flexible, the best results might be expected to occur; thus, one might hope that programs of this type would be devised for school children. Physicians should be aware of these programs, and familiarize themselves with resources available in their own communities.

5.5.3. Jejunoileal Shunt

A symposium held in 1976 and published in January 1977 in the *American Journal of Clinical Nutrition* contains a comprehensive review of this subject. Iber and Cooper (1977) estimate that by the end of 1975, between 12,000 and 20,000 such operations had been performed in this country. End-to-end anastomosis of roughly 12 inches of proximal jejunum to a smaller segment of distal ileum (Scott procedure) is a common method, although a similar end-to-side anastomosis (Payne procedure) has also been widely performed. In both instances, a major portion of the small intestinal absorptive bed is bypassed. Rapid weight loss ensues. Eventually, patients come into a new balance between food intake and caloric need with a stabilization of weight at 150–225 pounds, or roughly 60% of the initial, obese weight.

This approach to the treatment of obesity is conceptually sound in that it has as an underlying premise the idea that obesity is fundamentally a chronic, incurable disorder, all too well defended from readily available therapeutic techniques and thus in need of a potent, lasting counterforce to food intake. In some respects, it partakes of the same therapeutic philosophy as jaw-wiring to prevent food intake or the use of digitalis intoxication to induce anorexia. The counterforce of jejunoileal shunting is, to be sure, more hidden than is jaw-wiring and, it is to be hoped, less hazardous than digitalis intoxication. When considered in this way, the central concern is the degree of hazard of the procedure.

The complications of jejunoileal shunt are numerous; an incomplete list including wound infection, dehiscence, intussusception, intractable diarrhea with hypocalcemia and hypomagnesemia, hepatic steatosis progressing to cirrhosis and liver failure, renal and biliary stones, arthritis, a peculiar bypass enteropathy, and psychiatric disorders. Since reestablishment of intestinal continuity leads to regain of the lost weight, the shunt is meant to be a permanent anatomical change. Whether long-term complications such as immunological disorders, bowel neoplasms, osteoporosis, or other unwanted surprises are in store 10 or more years after shunting awaits the judgment of time. A general estimate of the more immediate hazard would suggest that there is roughly a 5% mortality. About half the patients will have complications severe enough to require periodic hospitalization, and roughly one-fifth will require reestablishment of normal intestinal continuity because of progressive, life-menacing complications.

These conclusions are drawn from a broad overview of many studies. Undoubtedly, the statistics are more favorable if the shunt is performed in an institution with experience and with aggressive follow-up care. Undoubtedly, too, the statistics are much less favorable if the procedure is performed without meticulous attention to pre- and postoperative care and diligent medical follow-up. Obviously, unless an obese patient has a 5% likelihood of death from obesity in the immediate future, as is the case with massively obese subjects with the Pickwickian syndrome or with progressive heart failure due to hypoventilation, the shunt cannot be justified in terms of balancing benefit and hazard.

The cost of a surgical procedure of this magnitude is high, and the cost of postoperative care is also considerable. One wonders what results might be achieved by equivalent expenditure for in-hospital weight reduction with psychiatric assistance, vocational rehabilitation, and other needed help for the obese. The results would be less dramatic and less predictable than shunting, but surely less hazardous as well. The funding apparatus for medical care, via third-party payment, has usually accepted surgical treatment of obesity as fundable therapy, but often has not accepted the costs for other in-hospital treatment for the obese. It may be that this unfortunate pattern of payment has been an occasional inducement to shunting. To be sure, the juvenile-onset, massively obese individual requires expensive and chronic care, but the decision as to the mode of care should be one to be made freely by the patient and physician, not one made on the basis of decisions by third-party payers.

5.6. Conclusion

Treatment of obesity remains at best a difficult and not frequently successful undertaking. Of the three newer treatments most discussed in 1977, the surgical approach is the most likely to effect weight reduction. It remains hazardous and to be used only when obesity threatens life and all other measures have failed. The use of the surgical approach is a clear acknowledgment that the cause for obesity cannot be ascertained and only a countermeasure will be effective in reducing body weight. The techniques of behavior modification attempt to reshape life style and should be most effective when obesity is moderate and can be related to adverse nutritional practices—practices that, it is to be hoped, are not of too long standing, so as to still be modifiable. The protein-sparing modified fast is most likely to be yet another of the innumerable new diets that have no lasting effect. To the extent that it is simple to administer, it may have some advantages over more complex diets of mixed foods, yet without retraining or behavior modification, it is difficult to see why it should be more effective than any other liquid formula or equally simple diet.

What is still missing is some better understanding of the normal operation of caloric balance and the pathophysiology of the disturbances of energy regulation that lead to a chronic excess of stored calories in adipose tissue. Progress in this area has been all too slow. It remains a hope that the nature of the defense of the obese individual to weight loss will in the future be sufficiently understood to make the correction of obesity a less hazardous and more successful endeavor than is now possible. Until that time, the endocrinologist or internist may not be able to provide specific therápy, but he can continue to be helpful to the obese patient. He can direct the patient to appropriate resources for nutritional, behavioral, or psychiatric help, counsel against useless drug or hormone therapies, treat complications such as hypertension or hyperlipidemia when these arise, and not reject or castigate the patient who finds weight loss a difficult or impossible objective to achieve.

References

American Medical News, 1977, AMA advises caution on diet, May 23, p. 9.

Bistrian, B. R., Blackburn, G. L., Flatt, J. P., Sizer, J., Scrimshaw, N. S., and Sherman, M., 1976, Nitrogen metabolism and insulin requirements in obese diabetic adults on a protein-sparing modified fast, *Diabetes* **25**:494–504.

Bistrian, B. R., Blackburn, G. L., and Stanbury, J. B., 1977, Metabolic aspects of a protein-sparing modified fast in the dietary management of Prader–Willi obesity, *N. Engl. J. Med.* **296**:774–779.

Bloom, W. L., 1959, Fasting as an introduction to the treatment of obesity, *Metabolism* **8**:214–220.

Bruch, H., 1973, *Eating Disorders: Obesity, Anorexia Nervosa and the Person Within,* p. 396, Basic Books, New York.

Bychowski, G., 1950, On neurotic obesity, *Psychoanal. Rev.* **37**:301–319.

Coddington, R. D., and Bruch, H., 1970, Gastric perceptivity in normal, obese and schizophrenic subjects, *Psychosomatics* **11**:571–579.

Cohn, C., and Joseph, D., 1962, Influence of body weight and body fat on appetite of "normal" lean and obese rats, *Yale J. Biol. Med.* **34**:598.

Drenick, E. J., 1973, Weight reduction by prolonged fasting in obesity in perspective, DHEW Publication No. (NIH) 75-708, Stock No. 017-053-00046-9, pp. 341–360, U.S. Goverment Printing Office, Washington, D.C.

Faust, I. M., Johnson, P. R., and Hirsch, J., 1977, Surgical removal of adipose tissue alters feeding behavior and the development of obesity in rats, *Science* **197**:393–396.

Hirsch, J., and Batchelor, B. R., 1976, Adipose tissue cellularity in human obesity, *Clin. Endocrinol. Metab.* **5**:299–311.

Iber, F. L., and Cooper, M., 1977, Jejunoileal bypass for the treatment of massive obesity: Prevalence, morbidity, and short- and long-term consequences, *Am. J. Clin. Nutr.* **30**:4–15.

Johnson, M. L., Burke, B. S., and Mayer, J., 1956, Relative importance of inactivity and overeating in the energy balance of obese high school girls, *Am. J. Clin. Nutr.* **4**:37.

Knittle, J. L., and Hirsch, J., 1968, Effect of early nutrition on the development of rat epididymal fat pads: Cellularity and metabolism, *J. Clin. Invest.* **47**:2091–2098.

Leon, G. R., 1977, A behavioral approach to obesity, *Am. J. Clin. Nutr.* **30**:785–789.

Leon, G. R., and Roth, L., 1977, Obesity: Psychological causes, correlations and speculations, *Psychol. Bull.* **84**:117–139.

Linn, R., 1977, *The Last Chance Diet,* Bantam Books, New York.

Penick, S. B., and Stunkard, A. J., 1970, Newer concepts of obesity, *Med. Clin. North Am.* **54**:745.

Penick, S. B., and Stunkard, A. J., 1977 (personal communication).

Rand, C. S. W., and Stunkard, A. J., 1977, Obesity and psychoanalysis, *Arch. Gen. Psychiatry* (in press).

Rodin, J., Herman, C. P., and Schachter, S., 1974, Obesity and various tests of external sensitivity, *in: Obese Humans and Rats* (S. Schachter and J. Rodin, eds.), pp. 89–96, Erlbaum, Potomac, Maryland.

Schachter, S., and Rodin, J. (eds.), 1974, *Obese Humans and Rats,* p. 182, Erlbaum, Potomac, Maryland.

Silverstone, J. T., Stark, J. E., and Buckle, R. M., 1966, Hunger during total starvation, *Lancet* **1**:1343–1344.

Stuart, R. B., and Davis, B., 1972, *Slim Chance in a Fat World,* p. 240, Research Press, Champaign, Illinois.

Stunkard, A. J., 1950, Eating patterns of obesity, *Psychiatr. Q.* **33**:284–295.

Stunkard, A. J., and Koch, C., 1964, The interpretation of gastric motility. 1. Apparent bias in the reports of hunger by obese persons, *Arch. Gen. Psychiatry* **11**:74–81.

Williams, A. E., and Duncan, B., 1976, Comparative results of an obesity clinic and a commercial weight reducing organization, *Med. J. Aust.* **1**:800–802.

Yang, M., and Van Itallie, T. B., 1976, Composition of weight loss during short term weight reduction: Metabolic responses of obese subjects to starvation and low-calorie ketogenic and nonketogenic diets, *J. Clin. Invest.* **58**:722–730.

6

Disorders of Lipid and Lipoprotein Metabolism

DeWitt S. Goodman

6.1. Introduction

It is the aim of this chapter to review the major advances that occurred during 1976 with regard to our knowledge about the metabolism of the major plasma lipids and lipoproteins and about clinical abnormalities in lipid transport, with particular emphasis on the hyperlipidemias. The chapter will build on, and in part briefly summarize, the information and ideas reviewed last year (Goodman, 1976), and will also review briefly some other major developments that occurred before 1976 in order to provide important background information.

DeWITT S. GOODMAN • Department of Medicine, College of Physicians and Surgeons, Columbia University, New York, New York 10032.

6.2. Lipoprotein Structure and Metabolism

6.2.1. General Review

Lipids are not soluble in water and circulate in plasma in association with certain specific proteins in the form of plasma lipoproteins. Four classes of specific lipoproteins circulate in plasma, and the characteristics of these classes were reviewed last year (Goodman, 1976). Two of these, chylomicrons and very-low-density lipoproteins (VLDL), are composed primarily of triglyceride and represent, respectively, the transport form of exogenous (dietary) and of endogenous triglyceride. Chylomicrons are normally not present in postabsorptive plasma after an overnight fast. Low-density lipoproteins (LDL) contain cholesterol as their major component and normally represent the circulating form of most of the plasma cholesterol. High-density lipoproteins (HDL) are comprised of approximately half protein and half lipid, and will be discussed in more detail later in this chapter.

Each lipoprotein class is heterogeneous with respect to its protein constituents. At least eight distinct lipoprotein proteins (apolipoproteins) have been described (Jackson *et al.,* 1976; Eisenberg and Levy, 1975). Although there is no universally accepted system of nomenclature of the apolipoproteins at present, most investigators group the apolipoproteins into five families (generally designated apoA, apoB, apoC, apoD, and apoE) on the basis of their chemical, immunologic, and metabolic characteristics. ApoA refers to the apolipoproteins (apoA-I and apoA-II) that are primarily, but not exclusively, found in HDL. ApoB is the major apoprotein of LDL, but also comprises about 35% of VLDL protein. ApoC represents a group of proteins (apoC-I, apoC-II, and apoC-III) that were originally described as major components of VLDL, but that are also present (as minor components) in HDL. ApoD refers to a protein present as a quantitatively minor lipoprotein component that has also been referred to as the "thin-line" protein. Recent studies have shown that this apolipoprotein has a molecular weight of approximately 22,100 and is unusual in having a high content of sugar constituents, which account for approximately 18% of its dry weight (McConathy and Alaupovic, 1976). ApoE, also known as the "arginine-rich" protein, occurs as a major component in VLDL, and as a minor one in HDL. ApoE has a molecular weight of approximately 33,000. It has been of particular, recent interest because it is found in elevated concentrations in several hypercholesterolemic atherogenic states, both in man (i.e., in Type III hyperlipoproteinemia) (Ganesan *et al.,* 1976) and in experimental animals (cholesterol-fed rabbits, swine, dogs, and monkeys) (Mahley *et al.,* 1975, 1976). The prominence of apoE in these human and animal hypercholesterolemic states has prompted the suggestion that this apolipoprotein may be of importance in cholesterol transport and in atherogenesis.

The total chemical synthesis of apoC-I was recently accomplished by solid-phase techniques (Sigler *et al.,* 1976). The synthetic apoprotein, comprising a single chain of 57 amino acids, was shown to activate lecithin:cholesterol acyltransferase (LCAT) to the same extent as the native protein. The synthetic and native apoproteins had comparable phospholipid-binding properties as well.

Considerable information is now available about the metabolism of the different lipoproteins and apoproteins. Both VLDL and HDL are synthesized in the liver; the intestine also participates in VLDL and HDL production, and is the site of chylomicron formation. In man, LDL is largely a catabolic product resulting from VLDL degradation. In the process of VLDL catabolism, VLDL triglyceride is largely removed from the blood by a lipolytic process, mainly involving the enzyme lipoprotein lipase. During this process, the bulk of the apoC proteins are removed, mainly by transfer to HDL. This leads to the formation of a lipoprotein of intermediate density (intermediate lipoprotein or IDL, density 1.006–1.019, S_f 12–60), which in turn is further catabolized to LDL. Thus, current evidence strongly suggests that, in man, most, if not all, of LDL apoB is normally derived from VLDL apoB.

In a recent report, the metabolism of VLDL apoB was studied in 19 patients with endogenous hypertriglyceridemia, 3 patients with heterozygous familial hypercholesterolemia, and 8 normal subjects (Sigurdsson *et al.,* 1976). The mean turnover rate of VLDL apoB was significantly higher in the hypertriglyceridemia group than in the controls, but a considerable overlap in turnover rate was found between these groups. It was concluded that the underlying defect in endogenous hypertriglyceridemia is heterogeneous; overproduction of VLDL is a major determining factor in some patients, whereas a reduced clearance is probably the determining factor in others.

An excellent review on lipoprotein structure and metabolism appeared in 1976 (Jackson *et al.,* 1976); this review complements and extends the extensive review of lipoprotein structure, function, and metabolism by Eisenberg and Levy (1975).

6.2.2. The Lp(a) Lipoprotein

The Lp(a) lipoprotein represents a different and additional lipoprotein class found in human plasma in low and varying concentrations. This lipoprotein was originally discovered because of its distinct immunologic properties (distinct from the other plasma lipoproteins), and was studied as a possible human genetic marker. In early studies, Lp(a) was detected in about 30–40% of persons tested. In recent reports, however, using more sensitive and quantitative immunologic methods, the Lp(a) lipoprotein was found to be detectable in 75% of a random British population (Walton *et al.,* 1974), and in 89% of 485 persons tested in Seattle (Albers *et al.,* 1975). It now seems clear that the frequency of Lp(a)-positive reactivity found in a given population depends on the sensitivity of the technique used and on the potency of the antiserum used in immunologic methods.

The Lp(a) lipoprotein is found in the density range 1.05–1.09, has pre-β mobility on electrophoresis, and is composed of 27% protein, 65% lipid (mainly esterified cholesterol), and 8% carbohydrate. Its protein has been found to contain 65% apoB, 15% albumin, and 20% of a unique apoprotein called apo-Lp(a). Lp(a) lipoprotein appears to be identical to lipoproteins referred to in the literature as the "sinking pre-β lipoprotein" (one that would sediment—i.e., "sink"—at density 1.006) and as the slowly migrating or pre-β_1 lipoprotein. These latter, operationally defined lipoproteins were apparently detected only in persons with high levels of Lp(a) because of the relative insensitivity of the detection methods used.

The distribution of Lp(a) concentration in the general population is highly skewed. In the recent Seattle study (Albers *et al.,* 1975), the median Lp(a) level was 7.6 mg/dl, and the 95th percentile value was 51.2 mg/dl. Lp(a) levels appeared independent of total plasma apoB levels, as assessed by radioimmunoassay. Furthermore, changes in apoB levels in response to dietary or drug manipulations or both were not accompanied by changes in Lp(a) levels. In addition, the concentration of Lp(a) was not correlated with plasma net cholesterol [total cholesterol minus Lp(a) cholesterol], triglyceride, or age. Thus, Lp(a) appears to be metabolically independent of LDL, even though it shares the same structural protein, apoB. The origin, metabolic characteristics, and function of Lp(a) are not known. It has been suggested, however, that there might be a relationship between the presence of higher levels of Lp(a) lipoprotein and coronary artery atherosclerotic disease. Thus, in a group of Finnish patients with coronary heart disease undergoing coronary arteriography, a highly significant association was found between an increased degree of obstructive disease (as graded by a "coronary score") and the presence of a strongly positive pre-β_1 lipoprotein zone in electrophoresis (Dahlén *et al.,* 1976). The latter finding presumably reflects the presence of higher levels of Lp(a) lipoprotein in those particular patients. In addition, Lp(a) was demonstrated, along with LDL, in human atherosclerotic lesions (Walton *et al.,* 1974). Further information is needed about the metabolic and genetic control of Lp(a) and about its possible participation in the atherosclerotic process.

6.2.3. Lipoprotein-X and Liver Disease

It is now well recognized that the characteristic elevation of free (unesterified) cholesterol and phospholipid in patients with cholestasis is due to the presence of an abnormal lipoprotein in the LDL density range (density 1.006–1.063). This lipoprotein, designated "lipoprotein-X" or "LP-X," contains about 65% lecithin, 25–30% free cholesterol, and 5% protein. Studies on the protein moiety have revealed that it is composed mainly of albumin (20–40% of total protein) and apoC. In the electron microscope, LP-X particles appear as disk-shaped rouleaux structures. Similar particles are found in the plasma LDL class in patients with familial LCAT deficiency (see Goodman, 1976).

In a recent study on the formation of LP-X (Manzato *et al.*, 1976), it was demonstrated that in native bile, lipids are organized in the form of a lipoprotein (bile LP) with a lipid composition almost identical to that of LP-X. The bile LP contained albumin as its major or only protein and had a lower protein/lipid ratio than that of LP-X. Bile LP could be converted to LP-X by adding serum to native bile. It was suggested that bile LP is a precursor lipoprotein for LP-X, and that it refluxes into the plasma pool under cholestatic conditions.

Several studies have demonstrated the usefulness of a qualitative test for the detection of LP-X in the diagnosis and study of patients with obstructive jaundice. Recently, the results of quantitative determinations of LP-X levels in 81 LP-X positive patients with different liver disorders were reported (Ritland, 1975). The plasma concentrations of LP-X in patients with extrahepatic cholestasis (median 158 mg/dl) were significantly higher than in patients with intrahepatic cholestasis. Plasma LP-X levels were significantly correlated with the plasma levels of alkaline phosphatase and of bilirubin, but were thought to be superior to these two parameters in the differentiation between intrahepatic and extrahepatic cholestasis.

6.3. Hyperlipidemias

6.3.1. Definition and Classification

The definition and classification of the hyperlipidemias was reviewed last year (Goodman, 1976). Hyperlipidemia is usually defined arbitrarily as being present when the plasma cholesterol or triglyceride level or both are above the 95th percentile value (for a given age, sex, race, and community). Patients with hyperlipidemia can be classified by: (1) lipid elevation (hypercholesterolemia, hypertriglyceridemia, or mixed hyperlipidemia, i.e., hypercholesterolemia and -triglyceridemia); (2) type of hyperlipoproteinemia (type I, IIa, IIb, III, IV, or V, depending on which lipoproteins are elevated); and (3) genetic categories. An excellent review of the classification and the characteristics, including the frequencies, of the genetic hyperlipidemias was reported recently by Motulsky (1976). A valuable review of the genetic hyperlipidemias and their relationships to coronary heart disease was also presented by Slack (1975).

6.3.2. Epidemiology

A number of reports have appeared during the past two years, providing additional epidemiologic information about serum lipids or lipoproteins or both in several populations that have been participating in epidemiologic studies of coronary risk factors or cardiovascular disease or both. These reports include information from the Honolulu Heart Study (Rhoads *et al.*, 1976), the Tecumseh Study (Sing *et al.*, 1975), the Evans County Cardiovascular Study (Tyroler *et al.*, 1975), the Stockholm–Edinburgh comparison study (Oliver *et al.*, 1975), and the Chicago Peoples Gas Company Study (Dyer, 1975). The findings of these studies, together with those of the Framingham Study (Kannel *et al.*, 1971; Dawber, 1973), the Stockholm Study (Carlson and Böttiger, 1972), and others, provide a wealth of detailed epidemiologic information about coronary risk factors and about the well-established association between the presence of hyperlipidemia and an increased risk of the development of coronary heart disease. In addition, an extensive review of the world epidemiology of coronary heart disease was published by Keys (1975).

Two recent reports of epidemiologic studies in children warrant more extended comment. One report was from the Bogalusa Heart Study, which is an epidemiologic study of risk factor variables in some 5000 children in the biracial community of Bogalusa, Louisiana. Serum cholesterol and triglyceride levels of 3446 children ages 5–14 (91% of the population in this age range) were reported (Frerichs *et al.*, 1976). Black children had significantly higher mean levels of serum cholesterol than white children (170 vs. 162 mg/dl, $p<0.0001$). On the other hand, significantly lower levels of triglycerides were found in blacks than in whites (means of 61 vs. 73 mg/dl). Girls had higher levels of triglycerides than boys in both races. The racial differences in serum cholesterol and triglyceride levels were even more apparent at the 95% percentile. The serum cholesterol level remained relatively constant in all children until ages 11–12, after which a slight reduction occurred. In contrast, a significant increase in the level of triglyceride with age was observed in all children except black girls. This study is continuing, with cross-sectional and longitudinal observations, to obtain more extensive data on serum lipids and other risk factor variables in children ages 0–17.

Similar observations were reported from the Muscatine Study in 1975 (Lauer *et al.,* 1975). In this report, the frequency of coronary risk factors was documented in 4829 school children in Muscatine, Iowa, over a 14-month period. Serum cholesterol levels were similar for children of all ages studied. The mean serum cholesterol level was 182 mg/dl (S.D. ± 29); 24% had levels ≥200 mg/dl, 9% were ≥220 mg/dl, 3% were ≥240 mg/dl, and 1% were ≥260 mg/dl. Casual levels of serum triglyceride increased with age; the mean level was 71 mg/dl (S.D. ± 36) at age 6 years and 108 mg/dl (S.D. ± 45) at age 18 years. Only 15% of the children had serum triglyceride levels of 140 mg/dl or more. Detailed information about blood pressure and obesity (body weight) was also reported. It was concluded that a considerable number of school-age children have risk factors that in adults are predictive of coronary heart disease. It was felt that the identification of such children (by school survey programs), in addition to leading to benefits for the children themselves, may also allow the discovery of other family members with high coronary risk because of the known clustering of several risk factors within family members. Such persons could then be enrolled in preventive treatment programs directed at the risk factors, in the hope of reducing their coronary risk.

6.4. High-Density-Lipoprotein Levels and Coronary Heart Disease

6.4.1. Epidemiologic Studies

Considerable evidence has accumulated recently indicating that in addition to the concentration of plasma total cholesterol, the manner in which cholesterol is distributed among the plasma lipoproteins bears an important relationship to the risk of developing coronary heart disease. In particular, it has been shown that the correlation between HDL concentration and coronary risk is a negative one, in contrast to the positive correlation found between coronary risk and LDL concentration. In other words, raised concentrations of plasma HDL appear to exert a protective, preventive effect, whereas raised concentrations of LDL increase the risk of coronary disease.

Quantitative information about the relationships between lipoprotein levels and coronary heart disease was reported recently from the Honolulu Heart Study (Rhoads *et al.,* 1976). This is a prospective study that is following a cohort of men of Japanese ancestry born in the years 1900–

1919 and living on the Hawaiian island of Oahu in 1965. Serum lipid (cholesterol and triglyceride) and lipoprotein levels were determined on a large subsample of the entire study population, comprising 264 men who had developed coronary heart disease, and 1755 men without coronary disease. As expected, a highly significant correlation was found between the prevalence of coronary heart disease and the level of serum total cholesterol or beta (LDL) cholesterol. Since about two-thirds of the total serum cholesterol is found in the beta (LDL) fraction, the correlation of beta cholesterol with total cholesterol was high ($r = 0.78$). In contrast, a highly significant inverse relationship was found between the prevalence of coronary heart disease and the level of alpha (HDL) cholesterol. Thus, men in the highest quartile by total or by LDL cholesterol were 1.8 times as likely to have coronary heart disease as men in the lowest quartile. In contrast, the relative risk for coronary disease between the highest and lowest quartiles for HDL cholesterol was 0.46. The inverse relationship of alpha (HDL) cholesterol to prevalence of coronary disease was independent of total or beta (LDL) cholesterol, blood pressure, obesity, and other factors.

Other recent studies have shown a significantly lower level of serum HDL in men with coronary heart disease, compared with age-matched, healthy men. Using an immunoassay for apoA-I, Berg *et al.* (1976) determined serum HDL concentrations in 49 men who had had a myocardial infarction and in 102 healthy, middle-aged men, all from northern Sweden. The mean HDL concentration was significantly lower in the men with coronary heart disease than in the controls. Similarly, Albers *et al.* (1976), in studies measuring both apoA-I levels by immunoassay and HDL cholesterol levels, observed that HDL levels were significantly lower among a group of American myocardial infarction survivors as compared with controls.

ApoA-I levels were found to be higher in women than in men and to be increased by estrogen (Albers *et al.*, 1976). Furthermore, as discussed by Miller and Miller (1975), plasma HDL appears to be reduced in several conditions associated with an increased risk of developing ischemic heart disease. All these observations support the conclusion that low levels of HDL may accelerate, and high levels of HDL may protect against, the development of atherosclerotic coronary artery disease.

Stimulated by the evidence of an inverse relationship between HDL levels and coronary risk, Wood *et al.* (1976) determined the concentrations of fasting plasma lipids and lipoproteins in 41 middle-aged male runners (running more than 15 miles per week for the previous year) and in a randomly selected comparison group of men of similar age. The runners had significantly lower mean levels of plasma total cholesterol, total triglyceride, and LDL cholesterol, and a significantly higher mean level of HDL cholesterol, compared with the comparison group. In fact, these very active men exhibited a plasma lipoprotein profile resembling that of younger women, rather than of sedentary, middle-aged men. Although it cannot be concluded that this pattern results from running *per se*, it is clear that the runners had all the lipoprotein characteristics associated with a low risk of developing coronary heart disease.

6.4.2. Familial Hyperalpha and Familial Hypobeta Lipoproteinemia

These two familial conditions have recently been shown to be associated with both increased life expectancy and decreased prevalence of coronary heart disease. In the newly recognized familial hyperalpha lipoproteinemia, affected probands and relatives had distinctive elevations of HDL cholesterol, slight elevations of total serum cholesterol, and normal levels of LDL cholesterol and serum total triglyceride (Glueck *et al.*, 1975). Longevity analysis demonstrated elongation of life expectancy for kindred members, and there was an apparent rarity of premature cardiac events. Genetic analysis in 18 kindreds failed to fully clarify the mode of inheritance, and suggested that environmental factors may also play a role. The mean ratio of LDL to HDL cholesterol levels in 67 affected subjects was found to be 1.21, compared with 2.41 for 124 normal controls (Glueck *et al.*, 1976b).

Familial hypobeta lipoproteinemia is a condition that appears to be transmitted as an autosomal dominant trait and is characterized by the presence of very low levels of plasma total and LDL cholesterol. There are generally few or no associated clinical symptoms or physical findings, although the condition is also sometimes associated with neurological disease. The diagnosis is often made by chance observation of a low total or LDL cholesterol level, and most kindreds probably go unrecognized. In 31 affected subjects, the mean ratio of LDL to HDL cholesterol was found to be 0.79 (Glueck *et al.*, 1976b).

Glueck *et al.* (1976b) recently examined morbidity and death from ischemic heart disease in 8 kindreds with familial hypobeta lipoproteinemia and compared the findings with data in 18 kindreds with familial hyperalpha lipoproteinemia. Expectation of life for males and females from kindreds with hypobeta lipoproteinemia was 9 and 12 years longer ($p < 0.01$) than that indicated by population statistics for United States white populations, whereas expectation of life for males and females from kindreds with hyperalpha lipoproteinemia was 5 and 7 years longer ($p < 0.02$). In addition, the frequency of myocardial infarction in living adult first-degree relatives of hypobeta and hyperalpha kindred members as a group was considerably less than that of a normal control population. Combined morbidity and mortality rates from myocardial infarction were lower for grouped hypobeta and hyperalpha kindred members than for normolipidemic spouse control kindreds. It was pointed out that subjects with familial hypobeta and hyperalpha lipoproteinemia share one common characteristic, namely, a ratio of LDL to HDL cholesterol of approximately 1:1. The ratio is considerably lower than the usual 2.5:1 level observed in the population. It was concluded that "if HDL confer protection against development of atherosclerosis, whereas LDL have opposite effects, then . . . the low ratio of LDL to HDL cholesterol may be related to prolonged longevity and decreased morbidity from myocardial infarction in familial hypobeta and hyperalpha lipoproteinemias" (Glueck *et al.*, 1976b).

6.4.3. Possible Mechanisms

A possible mechanism whereby HDL may exert a protective role toward the development of atherosclerosis was proposed by Carew *et al.* (1976), who investigated the interaction between porcine lipoproteins and cultured smooth muscle cells derived from the arterial wall. Arterial smooth muscle cells have specific surface receptors for LDL and regulate cellular cholesterol metabolism in a manner very similar to fibroblasts (see the discussion in Section 6.6.2). Arterial smooth muscle cells were studied because these cells have been shown to play a key role in the atherogenic process (Ross and Glomset, 1976). It was found that the extent to which these cells accumulated cholesterol when incubated with LDL could be greatly decreased by simultaneous addition of HDL to the incubation medium. The presence of HDL in the medium also partially inhibited uptake and degradation of LDL by the cells. These effects appeared to be due to a reduction in the amount of LDL bound to smooth muscle cells, possibly owing to competition between HDL and LDL for lipoprotein receptors on the cell surface. In contrast to LDL, HDL binding to the surface receptor was not followed by lipoprotein uptake and metabolism by the cell. These findings imply that HDL may play a role in limiting the rate of cholesterol uptake and accumulation in the arterial intima.

Evidence has also been presented that an interaction between HDL and LDL may occur in passage through the arterial endothelial layer. Thus, Stein and Stein (1976) found that cultured human umbilical vein endothelial cells bound and took up LDL in preference to HDL. When HDL was added to the medium, however, the cellular uptake of LDL was markedly reduced. The results suggested that different levels of HDL encountered in plasma could modulate the transendothelial transport of LDL and provide a possible explanation for the protective effect of HDL on atherosclerotic disease.

An additional mechanism for the effect of HDL may relate to its functional role in the transport of cholesterol from peripheral tissues to the liver (Miller and Miller, 1975; Glomset, 1968). Thus, removal of cholesterol from the arterial wall might be facilitated in the presence of higher levels of HDL.

6.4.4. Implications

A number of implications arise from these various findings on the relationship between HDL and atherosclerotic coronary heart disease. Clinically, it might be quite desirable to determine HDL levels in patients with marginally high levels of serum cholesterol, to help decide whether the patient's coronary risk status warrants therapeutic intervention beyond diet. Certainly, in clinical trials and other research studies, it will be important to measure HDL levels and use these levels along with data on serum lipids and other lipoproteins in final data analysis. At present, measurements of HDL are available only in a limited number of research laboratories and clinics, for research purposes. HDL is usually quantitated as HDL cholesterol by measurement of the residual cholesterol in plasma after removal of VLDL and LDL by precipitation with a polyanion–divalent cation mixture. Immunochemical methods for quantitating either apoA-I or apoA-II look promising, however, especially if used in conjunction with immunochemical measurement of apoB.

A final implication in regard to therapy: In view of the findings with HDL, it would seem worthwhile to encourage measures that increase the concentration of HDL in plasma and avoid those that have the opposite effect. In this regard, the findings with exercise (running) discussed above are of interest. In addition, efforts are being developed in the pharmaceutical industry and elsewhere to look for drugs that might raise HDL levels, or raise the HDL/LDL ratio. An agent that could both raise HDL and lower LDL levels, if such an agent could be developed, would have considerable potential as preventive therapy for atherosclerotic vascular disease.

6.5. Type III Hyperlipoproteinemia

The characteristics of this disorder, which is also referred to as "broad-beta disease" and "dysbetalipoproteinemia," were reviewed last year (Goodman, 1976). Patients with type III hyperlipoproteinemia have been of special interest because of a high incidence of premature vascular disease and because of a good response of their hyperlipidemia to diet and clofibrate therapy.

Familial type III hyperlipoproteinemia is an abnormality generally first diagnosed in adults. A recent report described the diagnosis of familial type III hyperlipoproteinemia in a 16-year-old girl and in a 16-

year-old boy with palmar xanthomas (Glueck *et al.*, 1976a). The hyperlipidemia characteristics of the two kindreds of these two children were described. It was pointed out that it is important to consider the diagnosis of type III hyperlipoproteinemia in the pediatric age group, particularly in evaluating children from families with type III or with admixtures of types III and IV hyperlipoproteinemia.

Evidence was summarized last year (Goodman, 1976) that the unusual floating-beta VLDL that is found in type III hyperlipoproteinemia represents the abnormal accumulation of normal intermediates in the metabolism of triglyceride-rich lipoproteins (chylomicrons and VLDL). More recent studies by Hazzard and Bierman (1976) further support this hypothesis. Patients with type III hyperlipoproteinemia and with endogenous hypertriglyceridemia (and a type IV pattern) were fed an oral fat load together with labeled vitamin A. Vitamin A was used as a marker for lipid particles of exogenous origin because, like cholesterol, it is absorbed (as an ester) with triglyceride in the chylomicron core. Unlike cholesterol, however, after removal by the liver, vitamin A cannot be recycled into VLDL but circulates bound to its specific (and density >1.21) transport protein, retinol-binding protein (Goodman, 1974). Thus, following its ingestion, all vitamin A in S_f >20 lipoproteins represents that en route in a one-way transit between gut and liver.

In subjects with moderate endogenous hypertriglyceridemia, the data showed the rapid passage of vitamin A through the chylomicron and VLDL compartments to a smaller particle ("remnant") of S_f 20–30 by 24 hr after the oral fat load. In contrast, in the type III patients, an increasing vitamin A/triglyceride ratio was observed between 6 and 24 hr in both the chylomicron and in various VLDL subclasses, and a high vitamin A/triglyceride ratio was found in the abnormal beta-VLDL in these patients. The findings suggest that chylomicron (and exogenously derived VLDL) remnants accumulate in the plasma of subjects with type III hyperlipoproteinemia because of a defect in their removal (or further catabolism or both) that may be specific to this disorder.

6.6. Cholesterol Metabolism and Its Regulation

6.6.1. In Intact Humans

During the past decade, a great deal of information has been obtained about total body cholesterol metabolism *in vivo* in normal humans and in patients with various types of lipid disorders. One or both of two major methods have been used in most research clinics for these studies. One approach, the sterol balance method, involves the measurement of the excretion of all steroids derived from cholesterol under steady-state conditions (Grundy and Ahrens, 1969). The other, kinetic approach involves studies of the turnover of plasma cholesterol after pulse-labeling with isotopic cholesterol (Goodman *et al.*, 1973). The agreement between the two methods for measurement of body cholesterol turnover rate is quite good (Grundy and Ahrens, 1969).

Long-term studies of the turnover of plasma cholesterol were recently reported in 24 normal and hyperlipidemic subjects (Smith *et al.*, 1976). Many of the hyperlipidemic patients had a definite familial disorder. In all subjects, a simple three-pool compartmental model provided the best description of total body cholesterol turnover. The parameters of this three-pool model found in normal subjects were compared with those found in patients with different kinds of hyperlipidemia. The cholesterol production rate (total body turnover rate) in normal subjects (1.14 ± 0.19 g/day, mean ± S.D.) was not significantly different from that found in patients with hypercholesterolemia, with or without hypertriglyceridemia. The major determinant of cholesterol production rate was overall body size, expressed either as total body weight or as surface area. In fact, differences in total body size accounted for 64% of the observed differences in cholesterol production rate in this series. Other studies from several laboratories showed that obese subjects have increased body cholesterol synthesis and turnover rates both by sterol balance and by kinetic methods. It is thus clear that total body cholesterol turnover in man is highly regulated, and that overall body size is its major determinant.

After adjustment for body-size variation, the cholesterol production (turnover) rate was not correlated with the serum cholesterol concentration (Smith *et al.*, 1976). Other studies also showed similar turnover rates of cholesterol in patients with hypercholesterolemia (including familial hypercholesterolemia, FH) and in normal subjects. Thus, hypercholesterolemia (both familial and nonfamilial) is not associated with abnormal rates of total body cholesterol formation or excretion, but rather with some impediment to the "clearance" or removal of cholesterol from the plasma pool. This conclusion is consistent with the observed decreased fractional rate of LDL degradation in patients with FH (Langer *et al.*, 1972). The mechanism responsible for the decreased fractional rate of LDL degradation in FH has been elucidated by the studies with cultured fibroblasts discussed below. The abnormality in hypercholesterolemia (particularly FH) thus appears to be mainly an abnormality in the metabolism of plasma lipoproteins (and hence of lipoprotein cholesterol), rather than an abnormality in the major parameters (e.g., synthesis, excretion) of total body cholesterol metabolism *per se*. Of note, however, was the finding that the size of pool 3, the most slowly exchanging compartment of body cholesterol, was highly correlated with the serum cholesterol level (Smith *et al.*, 1976). This finding suggests that the amounts of cholesterol in slowly equilibrating tissue sites (including arteries) increase in relation to elevations in the serum cholesterol level. The accumulation of cholesterol in atherosclerotic arteries in patients with hypercholesterolemia may represent one aspect of this phenomenon.

The effect of hypertriglyceridemia on the turnover rate of cholesterol is not comparably clear. Several recent studies have reported increased rates of cholesterol turnover in patients with elevated serum triglyceride (and VLDL) levels (Sodhi and Kudchodkar, 1973; Miller, N. E., *et al.*, 1976; Kudchodkar and Sodhi, 1976). On the other hand, other studies have reported results that do not support this conclusion (Smith *et al.*, 1976; Grundy, 1975). The apparent conflict can be resolved by the interpretation that hypertriglyceridemic patients represent a heterogeneous population and that there are subsets of such patients who manifest increased synthesis and turnover of cholesterol, whereas others do not. This interpretation is consistent with the conclusion discussed above, from studies on the metabolism of VLDL apoB, that the underlying defect in endogenous hypertriglyceridemia is heterogeneous. It is hoped that future research will lead to effective methods for segregating and classifying hypertriglyceridemic patients according to the pathogenetic mechanisms involved in their hyperlipidemia, and that this will in turn lead to more specific therapy for each individual patient.

6.6.2. In Cultured Cells

Cholesterol metabolism in fibroblasts and certain other cells in culture *in vitro* has been shown to be a highly regulated process. Similar regulatory mechanisms presumably also operate in these kinds of cells *in vivo.* It was pointed out by Brown and Goldstein (1976a) that cholesterol, a major component of all mammalian plasma membranes, is vital to cell growth and survival. On the other hand, excessive amounts of this sterol can also be lethal, as is evidenced by the cholesterol deposition in arterial cells that potentiates the development of atherosclerosis. "Thus, mammalian cells are faced wih the dual problem of providing sufficient cholesterol for membrane growth and replenishment and, at the same time, of avoiding excessive accumulation of this insoluble substance."

The mechanisms whereby cells resolve this problem have recently been elucidated by the elegant studies of Brown and Goldstein, and other investigators. As discussed last year (Goodman, 1976), cholesterol metabolism in fibroblasts appears to be mainly controlled by a pathway involving specific cell-surface receptors for LDL. This LDL pathway constitutes a mechanism by which fibroblasts take up plasma LDL and consequently regulate their cellular cholesterol metabolism. The critical feature of the LDL pathway is a cell-surface receptor, termed the "LDL receptor," that binds the lipoprotein at the plasma membrane. The surface-bound LDL is then internalized by endocytosis and delivered to lysosomes. Within the lysosome, the protein component of the LDL is rapidly degraded to free amino acids that are then released into the culture medium. The cholesteryl ester component of LDL is hydrolyzed by a lysosomal acid lipase, and the resultant unesterified cholesterol is transferred to the cellular compartment, where it is found largely associated with cell membranes and, in turn, regulates three events in cellular cholesterol metabolism. First, it suppresses the activity of the enzyme HMG CoA reductase, causing a reduction of cholesterol synthesis. Second, it activates a fatty acyl-CoA:cholesterol acyltransferase (ACAT) enzyme that catalyzes the esterification of excess incoming cholesterol so that it can be stored within the cell as cholesteryl esters. Third, it exerts a feedback suppression on the activity of the LDL receptor itself, thereby limiting the further cellular uptake of LDL.

In addition to the regulation mediated by LDL-derived cholesterol, suppression of cholesterol synthesis (of HMG CoA reductase activity), activation of cholesterol esterification (of ACAT activity), and suppression of LDL receptor activity in human fibroblasts can also be achieved by addition to the culture medium of either purified cholesterol or one of its oxygenated derivatives (such as 7-ketocholesterol or 25-hydroxycholesterol). In contrast to the LDL-receptor-mediated pathway, this latter form of regulation does not require either the LDL receptor or lysosomal action.

Fibroblasts derived from patients with homozygous FH have as their primary genetic defect a deficiency in functional LDL receptors. As a result of their failure to bind LDL at this specific surface receptor, these FH homozygote cells fail to take up LDL with high affinity, and therefore fail to hydrolyze its protein or cholesteryl ester components. As a consequence, LDL neither suppresses cholesterol synthesis nor activates cholesterol esterification in these cells.

The LDL receptor pathway, the regulation of cholesterol metabolism in cultured cells, and the biochemical defects in FH cells were extensively and effectively reviewed in 1976 (Brown and Goldstein, 1976a,b; Brown *et al.*, 1976a; Goldstein and Brown, 1976).

A good deal of new information about these phenomena was reported in 1976. Detailed studies of the binding of human radioiodinated LDL to its receptor (on fibroblasts) showed that the binding appears to involve an ionic interaction between positive charges on the protein component of the LDL particle and negative charges on the LDL receptor (Goldstein *et al.*, 1976a). Thus, certain negatively charged glycosaminoglycans, such as heparin, can release labeled LDL from the LDL receptor. Accordingly, separate measurements could be made of the initial binding of labeled LDL to its receptor and of its subsequent cellular uptake. These studies clarified the kinetics of LDL uptake in human fibroblasts and established the system as an example of receptor-mediated adsorptive endocytosis.

Information about the sites on the cell surface at which initial binding takes place was obtained by electron-microscopic studies using ferritin-labeled LDL (Anderson, R. G. W., *et al.,* 1976). The ferritin-labeled LDL was found to bind preferentially to localized regions of the plasma membrane that had an appearance similar to the "coated regions" or "coated pits" described by other workers in other cell types. These regions appeared indented and thickened, with fuzzy coats. These regions are thought to be specialized sites on the cell surface where adsorptive endocytosis of proteins and colloidal particles is initiated, i.e., where endocytotic vesicles are formed. A variety of data were obtained suggesting that the LDL receptor is localized to these indented, coated regions of the plasma membrane. In addition, it was found that fibroblasts from a patient with homozygous FH contained normal numbers of indented, coated membrane regions, but that no LDL-ferritin was observed to bind to the cell membrane in these mutant cells.

The LDL receptor can be bypassed by chemically modifying LDL with the addition of a large number of positive charges to the molecule. Such "cationized LDL" was found to be taken up and degraded by FH homozygote cells and to effectively regulate cholesterol metabolism in such cells (Basu *et al.,* 1976).

The important role of the lysosome in the LDL pathway was dramatically illustrated by studies on fibroblasts from patients with Wolman syndrome or with cholesteryl ester storage disease. The genetic defect in these disorders involves a lysosomal acid lipase that is responsible for cholesteryl ester hydrolysis in lysosomes. When fibroblasts from patients with these disorders were incubated with LDL, the binding, uptake, and proteolytic degradation of the LDL proceeded normally, but the defective lysosomal enzyme caused an accumulation of unhydrolyzed LDL-derived cholesteryl ester within lysosomes. This in turn led to impaired suppression of cholesterol synthesis and impaired activation of cholesterol esterification. When, however, these cells were cultured in a single dish together with homozygous FH cells, the biochemical defects in the Wolman syndrome and cholesteryl ester storage disease cells were reversed (Brown *et al.,* 1976b). This effect was shown to result from the release of lysosomal acid lipase from the FH cells into the culture medium and its subsequent uptake by the acid-lipase-deficient cells. The data thus emphasize the importance of the lysosomal acid lipase in the cellular metabolism of LDL cholesteryl esters and, in addition, demonstrate that delivery of this enzyme to genetically deficient cells can enhance the regulatory response to the lipoprotein.

Evidence exists that the LDL pathway and the LDL-receptor-mediated regulation of cholesterol metabolism operate in a variety of mammalian cells maintained in tissue culture, in addition to fibroblasts. The cells that have been studied in some detail include arterial smooth muscle cells, long-term human lymphoid cell lines, and freshly isolated human lymphocytes (Goldstein and Brown, 1976; Ho *et al.,* 1976a,b). In addition, studies in the rat have suggested that *in vivo,* a large number of extrahepatic tissues are regulated by similar mechanisms, and that the low levels of cholesterol synthesis normally observed in many nonhepatic tissues in the rat (and presumably in man, as well) are due to an active form of feedback regulation mediated by cholesterol carried in plasma lipoproteins (Balasubramaniam *et al.,* 1976; Andersen and Dietschy, 1976).

6.7. Familial Hypercholesterolemia

FH, a single-gene disorder that produces hypercholesterolemia, xanthomatosis, and premature atherosclerosis, was discussed in some detail last year (Goodman, 1976). This section will review briefly the major developments that were reported in 1976.

6.7.1. Genetics

It is well established that FH is transmitted as an autosomal dominant trait in humans. The prevalence of the disorder is approximately 1 in 500 persons in the general American population.

In an extensive study of xanthomatosis in Norway, 132 affected kindreds were investigated in detail (Heiberg and Berg, 1976). Of the probands, 20% belonged to 7 large kindreds (Heiberg, 1976). Hyperlipidemia (values above the 95th percentile) was found in 40.8% of 554 first-degree relatives of probands with xanthomatosis. The distribution curve was bimodal for total and LDL cholesterol concentrations, but not for triglyceride levels. The prevalence of FH with xanthomatosis was estimated to be 2.2 per 1000.

6.7.2. Pathogenesis

As discussed above, the pathogenetic defect in FH has been shown to be a defect in LDL-receptor activity. This defect leads to hyperbeta lipoproteinemia (and hypercholesterolemia), which then, in turn, leads to accelerated atherosclerosis via mechanisms involving excessive proliferation of arterial smooth muscle cells (Ross and Glomset, 1976; Ross and Harker, 1976). This defect in the LDL-receptor pathway has been extensively examined in fibroblasts from patients with FH, and has also been shown to be present in other cells as well (Ho *et al.,* 1976a,b).

Fibroblasts from patients with the clinical phenotype of homozygous FH can be divided into two classes. One class of mutant cells, termed "receptor-negative," completely lacks the cell-surface LDL receptor. The second class, termed "receptor-defective," exhibits a low but detectable ability to bind LDL at the receptor site; in these cells, the functional receptor activity is reduced to 5–20% of normal. Since in both types of mutant cells, LDL binds in markedly subnormal amounts to the cell surface, the subsequent internalization of the LDL cannot occur at normal rates, and defective regulation of cholesterol metabolism ensues. As discussed last year (Goodman, 1976), patients with receptor-negative homozygous FH are apparently resistant to therapy, whereas those with the receptor-defective mutation were found to show some response.

Brown and Goldstein (1976c) recently reported findings with 22 strains of fibroblasts derived from subjects with the clinical phenotype of homozygous FH. Of these strains, 12 were receptor-negative, and 9 were receptor-defective. In one strain, however, a new type of mutation that appeared to affect the internalization (adsorptive endocytosis) process was identified. In this unique mutant strain, the cell-surface LDL receptor was able to bind labeled LDL normally, but internalization of the receptor-bound lipoprotein failed to occur. As a result, lysosomal degradation of the LDL did not occur, nor did the subsequent metabolic regulatory processes. Thus, at least three types of mutations can produce the clinical phenotype of homozygous FH, and this raises the possibility of extensive genetic heterogeneity among phenotypic homozygotes as well as heterozygotes with this syndrome. The clinical implications of these new observations remain to be explored.

The finding that the LDL surface receptor is itself under feedback regulation raises interesting questions regarding such regulation in FH heterozygotes. Studies were therefore carried out to determine the receptor activity of fibroblasts from patients with heterozygous FH, as compared with normals, when grown in the presence of increasing amounts of exogenous cholesterol (Goldstein *et al.,* 1976b). Over a wide range of LDL-receptor activities, at each level of cellular esterified cholesterol, the FH heterozygote cells expressed about one-half as many LDL receptors as did the normal cells. This relationship persisted even in the range of LDL-receptor activity in which the heterozygote cells clearly had the capacity to produce as many LDL receptors as did the normal cells. The data thus demonstrate that the two alleles at the LDL-receptor locus are regulated independently, and that there appears to be no compensatory mechanism that senses when one of the two alleles is failing to produce a functional gene product.

The findings with FH heterozygote cells are consistent with the *in vivo* observations (discussed above) that total body cholesterol synthesis (turnover) rates are not increased in heterozygous FH patients. FH heterozygote cells will display normal suppression of cholesterol synthesis and normal absolute rates of LDL degradation when the LDL concentration in the culture medium is much higher than (approximately double) normal. Thus, one would anticipate that in a heterozygous FH patient, elevated LDL levels would be associated with normal absolute (and low fractional) catabolic rates of LDL and normal rates of cholesterol synthesis, and these are indeed the findings in such patients.

Evidence that the LDL in FH is structurally not abnormal was obtained by studies of the metabolism of LDL isolated from a patient with FH, as compared with that of LDL from a normal subject (Myant *et al.*, 1976). The two LDL preparations were labeled, respectively, with ^{125}I and ^{131}I, and were injected together into a normal subject. The turnover rates of the two apolipoproteins were identical. Moreover, the uptake and catabolism of the two types of LDL by normal lymphocytes *in vitro* were similar. Since this study involved LDL from a single FH patient, further studies, particularly with LDL preparations from many different FH homozygote patients, would be of interest to try to determine whether any phenotypic FH patients might have a structurally abnormal LDL as their basic defect.

Studies on the turnover of the apoprotein of LDL were carried out in two FH homozygotes and in one control subject after plasma exchange (Thompson and Myant, 1976). The use of plasma exchange in the management of homozygous FH by these investigators was discussed last year (Goodman, 1976). One patient with a type IIa lipoprotein pattern (and later shown to have the receptor-negative mutation) had a markedly reduced fractional catabolic rate over a wide range of cholesterol levels and a moderate increase in synthesis of apoLDL. The second patient, with a type IIb pattern (and later shown to have the receptor-defective mutation), had a normal or slightly subnormal fractional catabolic rate, but a marked increase in apoLDL synthesis. Combined therapy with cholestyramine and clofibrate increased the fractional catabolic rate and decreased the synthesis of apoLDL in both patients. It was concluded that both decreased catabolism and increased synthesis of apoLDL occur in homozygous FH, but to a different extent in individual patients. These findings and conclusions are consistent with earlier reports on the turnover of apoLDL in patients with homozygous FH discussed last year.

6.7.3. Therapy

The recent interest in, and experience with, portacaval shunt surgery in patients with homozygous FH, together with the results seen in 7 patients (mostly children) subjected to this procedure and reported in the literature, were discussed last year (Goodman, 1976). The results observed in 4 additional patients have also been reported. In 2 infants reported from France (Farriaux *et al.*, 1976), the results were considered to be excellent in the first patient and partially successful in the second. In 2 other young children reported from South Africa (Cywes *et al.*, 1976), an excellent result was seen in one. This patient, a 4-year-old girl, showed a steady fall in plasma cholesterol level from 681 to 435 mg/dl during an

8-month postoperative interval, together with reduction in xanthomas and relief of her preoperative angina pectoris. As discussed last year, the mechanism whereby portacaval shunt surgery leads to these changes is not known; since the procedure is not without risks, it should be viewed with great caution before being recommended for any given patient. The National Heart, Lung, and Blood Institute in Bethesda, Maryland, has been acting as a registry for information exchange and planning in this subject.

A new approach to the management of FH involving the use of an extravascular technique for removal of LDL and based on the principle of affinity chromatography was described by Lupien *et al.* (1976). LDL were removed from blood by interaction with heparin linked to agarose beads in the presence of calcium ions; no effects on the concentrations of HDL were seen. Reductions of plasma cholesterol levels of 16 and 19% were obtained with two heterozygous FH patients and of 5% in a normal volunteer. The technique was described as being relatively simple and well tolerated by all three subjects.

The results of a moderately long-term period of treatment with diet and cholestyramine resin in a group of heterozygous FH patients were reported recently (Witters *et al.*, 1976). In this study, 34 patients who had previously participated in a short-term, double-blind trial of cholestyramine plus diet (low cholesterol, high polyunsaturated/saturated fat ratio diet) were maintained on the same treatment regimen for 2–5 years. During the previous trial, a mean decrease of cholesterol of 20% was seen in the drug-treated group (compared with the diet-alone base line). This therapeutic response was maintained during the ensuing 36 months. In the fourth year of follow-up, however, a progressive rise in total and LDL cholesterol was noted, so that by 48 months, a mean decrease of cholesterol of only 5% (not statistically significant) was present. Outpatient and inpatient studies in a subset of these patients demonstrated that the secondary therapeutic failure was due mainly to patient noncompliance, particularly with the dietary regimen. It was concluded that cholestyramine together with a low cholesterol (and relatively high polyunsaturated fat) diet can be an effective treatment for FH, but that a comprehensive program of outpatient follow-up with continued emphasis on dietary principles and drug adherence is critical for the continued success of this treatment program.

A review of experience during an 8-year period in the management of 45 children, ages 1–16 years, with heterozygous FH was reported in 1975 (West *et al.*, 1975). Three different treatment regimens had been employed: diet alone (17 children), diet plus clofibrate (9 children), and cholestyramine resin (36 children). Several of the children were managed sequentially by more than one regimen. The diet (low saturated fat, less than 20 g/day, together with polyunsaturated fat) provided a mean reduction in serum cholesterol of about 20%, and no advantage was found by increasing total intake of polyunsaturated fat to high levels. Adherence to the diet was poor, however, with only 3 of 17 children remaining satisfactorily controlled after 2 years. Addition of clofibrate to diet provided a further 10% reduction in serum cholesterol, but adherence was again poor, and by 2 years, the results were unsatisfactory. Cholestyramine in a mean dose of 0.6 mg/kg body wt. per day in two divided doses lowered cholesterol levels by a mean of 36%. It proved effective, moreover, without the need for dietary restriction (in contrast to the results in adults reported above). Adherence over a 3-year period was only moderately good (57% maintaining satisfactory adherence and control). All children continued to grow normally. Folate deficiency was observed as a side effect, and it was recommended that folic acid supplements should be given to all patients receiving cholestyramine.

6.8. β-Sitosterolemia and Cerebrotendinous Xanthomatosis

β-Sitosterolemia is a rare disorder recently described in 3 young adult females (Bhattacharyya and Connor, 1974; Shulman *et al.,* 1976). The clinical features in 2 of the patients who are sisters (Bhattacharyya and Connor, 1974) included extensive tendon and tuberous xanthomata, with normal plasma cholesterol levels and with high concentrations of β-sitosterol (and of the other common plant sterols, campesterol and stigmasterol) in the plasma, lipoproteins, red blood cells, xanthomas, adipose tissue, and skin surface lipids. Besides β-sitosterolemia and xanthomatosis, no other physical, mental, or biochemical abnormalities were detected. Plant sterols constituted approximately 10–15% of the total plasma sterols, and were present at a similar order of magnitude in the other tissues studied. The intestinal absorption of β-sitosterol was greatly increased in both patients (24–28% absorbed, normal being less than 5%). More recently, a similar disorder was reported in a 31-year-old woman with mild hypercholesterolemia unrelated to the two sisters (Shulman *et al.,* 1976). No other family members were affected in either instance, although it was pointed out that the occurrence of the disorder in two sisters with unaffected parents suggests an inherited recessive trait.

Cerebrotendinous xanthomatosis (CTX) is a rare lipid disorder inherited as a recessive disease that has been more extensively studied and defined than has β-sitosterolemia. The major clinical manifestations of CTX include progressive neurological dysfunction (spinal cord paresis, dementia), tuberous and tendon xanthomas, premature atherosclerosis, pulmonary insufficiency, cataracts, and endocrine hypofunction. Although tissue sterol concentrations are abnormally high, as manifested by the brain and tendon xanthomas, plasma cholesterol levels are low.

Biochemically, greatly increased concentrations of cholestanol, the 5α-dihydro derivative of cholesterol, have been found in all tissues, notably in the xanthomas, and this disorder is now considered a systemic cholestanolosis. It has also been reported that total bile acid production is abnormally low in CTX patients, and that, in particular, the production and the biliary pool of the bile acid chenodeoxycholic acid are exceedingly low in these patients (Salen and Grundy, 1973). These abnormalities in bile acid metabolism were found associated with large amounts of bile alcohols in the bile and the feces. In view of these observations, studies were undertaken in which exogenous chenodeoxycholic acid is being administered to CTX patients, in the hope of correcting their abnormal hepatic sterol metabolism (Salen *et al.,* 1975). It has been proposed that the abnormal neutral sterol metabolism seen in CTX may be secondary to abnormal bile acid synthesis and metabolism, including impairment in side-chain oxidation on the path of cholesterol to bile acid and the accumulation of bile alcohols (Salen *et al.,* 1977).

A common feature of these two rare disorders is the occurrence of xanthomas associated with the accumulation in tissues (and plasma) of sterols other than cholesterol, despite the presence of normal or low levels of plasma cholesterol itself. In CTX, sterols (both cholesterol and cholestanol) accumulate in many tissues, including arteries, in which premature atherosclerosis is found. In β-sitosterolemia, there is, as yet, no evidence for increased sterol accumulation in arteries and other tissues (other than sites of xanthomas). The mechanism of xanthoma (and atheroma, in CTX) formation in these diseases is not known. The diseases do, however, provide models for study that may lead to insights about the mechanisms involved in xanthoma and atheroma formation in hyperlipidemic and other patients.

6.9. Hypertriglyceridemia

6.9.1. Pathophysiology and Other Features

It is generally thought that lipoprotein lipase plays a key role in the removal and utilization of circulating chylomicron and VLDL triglyceride. The site of action of this enzyme is at the capillary endothelium; it is present in several extrahepatic tissues, and is released by heparin into the bloodstream. The lipolytic activity of postheparin plasma (postheparin lipolytic activity, PHLA) has been widely used in the past as a measure of tissue lipoprotein lipase activity. More recently, however, it has become clear that heparin is able to liberate several lipases from tissues. Thus, a triglyceride lipase released from liver is now known to contribute significantly to the PHLA.

In a recent study, Huttunen *et al.* (1976) used a selective immunochemical method to measure postheparin plasma lipoprotein lipase and hepatic lipase activity in 82 normal subjects and in 20 patients with type IIb, IV, or V hypertriglyceridemia. In 26 normal subjects, the activity of postheparin plasma lipases was compared with the kinetic parameters of endogenous plasma triglyceride metabolism. The activity of postheparin lipoprotein lipase was significantly higher in normal females than in males, whereas the activity of hepatic lipase showed an opposite sex ratio. The activity of lipoprotein lipase decreased with age in both males and females, whereas no significant age variation was seen in hepatic lipase activity.

In normal subjects, a highly significant negative correlation was present between the activity of postheparin lipoprotein lipase and fasting serum triglyceride concentration, but not between the activity of postheparin hepatic lipase and serum triglycerides. Moreover, the fractional removal rate of endogenous triglyceride was positively correlated with the activity of lipoprotein lipase, but not with that of hepatic lipase. These findings demonstrate that the activity of lipoprotein lipase is an important factor in determining the efficiency of removal of triglycerides from the circulation, and suggest that the removal rate plays a major role in regulating the plasma triglyceride level within physiologic range.

The average lipoprotein lipase activity of postheparin plasma was reduced in the hypertriglyceridemic patients, whereas the activity of hepatic lipase was normal or increased. Many hypertriglyceridemic patients had lipoprotein lipase within the normal range, however, and there was no correlation between serum triglyceride concentration and the activity of postheparin lipases. All 3 patients with fasting chylomicronemia (type V) had low postheparin lipoprotein lipase activity. These findings are consistent with the interpretation (discussed earlier in this chapter) from other studies that hypertriglyceridemic patients represent a heterogeneous population in which either overproduction or defective removal may be the major determining factor.

The role of insulin in the pathophysiology of endogenous hypertriglyceridemia has been studied extensively in the past, but remains rather controversial. In a recent report by Glueck *et al.* (1977), 16 children with primary familial hypertriglyceridemia were studied to explore whether there were any distinctive relationships among insulin, triglyceride levels, and obesity in such a pediatric population. Most of the children were obese (11 of 16 were >97th percentile for fat mass). Plasma triglycerides did not correlate significantly with measurements of insulin or obesity in these hypertriglyceridemic children. It was concluded that within the limits of a small sample size and in the presence of obesity, insulin does not appear to play a predominant role in the genesis of hypertriglyceridemia in children with familial hypertriglyceridemia. It was also noted, however, that since the study was in children (many of whom were obese), this conclusion might not be generalizable to nonobese normotriglyceridemic or moderately hypertriglyceridemic adults.

A study of the characteristics of type V hyperlipoproteinemia was reported from the same clinic (Fallat and Glueck, 1976). Of 29 adults presenting with the type V lipoprotein pattern, 23 had various metabolic perturbations (diabetes out of control, estrogenic agents, pancreatitis, ethanolism) superimposed on their acute hypertriglyceridemia. After metabolic stabilization, 17 of the 29 subjects were shown to have familial hypertriglyceridemia. In each of these 17 kindreds, at least one other family member could be shown to have primary hypertriglyceridemia with either a type IV or type V pattern. Nearly 50% of the 33 siblings of the 17 propositi had primary hypertriglyceridemia, 10 with a type IV and 5 with a type V pattern. It was pointed out that the lack of a specific distinctive marker for either the type V or type IV presumed genotypes limits interpretation of kindred data.

6.9.2. Hypertriglyceridemia and Coronary Heart Disease

An important study of the risk of myocardial infarction in persons with familial combined hyperlipidemia and with familial hypertriglyceridemia was reported recently by Brunzell *et al.* (1976). Risk was assessed by examination of relatives of patients referred for evaluation of hypertriglyceridemia. Among 74 such hypertriglyceridemic patients, family studies detected 19 with familial hypertriglyceridemia and 24 with familial combined hyperlipidemia. The frequency of myocardial infarction among adult living hyperlipidemic relatives of patients with familial combined hyperlipidemia was 17.5% (10 of 57). Of these relatives, 5 had their infarcts between the ages of 40 and 50, and 5 before the age of 40. In contrast, the frequency of myocardial infarction in living hyperlipidemic relatives with familial hypertriglyceridemia was 4.7%, and was similar to the frequency of myocardial infarction found among normolipidemic relatives (4.5%) or among spouse controls (5.2%). Mortality data due to myocardial infarction among relatives of index patients failed to contribute meaningful information. These findings strongly suggest that the entity of familial combined hyperlipidemia represents a more significant risk factor for premature coronary artery disease than does familial hypertriglyceridemia. Further studies are needed to clarify the extent to which familial or sporadic hypertriglyceridemia may be associated with an increased risk of coronary heart disease. The results underscore the importance of performing family studies in all hyperlipidemic patients to more effectively assess risk status and develop plans for clinical management.

A comparison was made of the coronary arteriographic findings in 24 patients with type II hyperlipoproteinemia and in 22 patients with the type IV pattern (Bloch *et al.,* 1976). The patients had clinical ischemic heart disease and familial forms of hyperlipidemia (including 3 type II patients with homozygous FH); patients with familial combined hyperlipidemia were specifically excluded. The type II patients had a high prevalence of main left coronary disease, multiple vessel stenosis, and distal vessel disease. The type IV patients usually had disease localized to proximal arteries, and only infrequently (3 of 22 patients) had three- or four-vessel disease. Since the clinical data and the prevalence of other risk factors were similar for the two groups of patients, it was suggested that the observed differences in distribution of lesions might be secondary to the different kinds of lipoprotein disorders present. This study extends previous studies from several laboratories (e.g., Heinle *et al.,* 1969; Salel *et al.,* 1974; Murray *et al.,* 1975) that have shown a high prevalence of hyperlipidemia (with both type II and type IV patterns, i.e., with either or both hypercholesterolemia or hypertriglyceridemia) in patients with angiographically proved coronary artery disease.

6.10. Chronic Renal Failure and Hyperlipidemia

It is now well established that hyperlipidemia is present in the majority of patients who are uremic or on maintenance hemodialysis and is also very common following successful renal transplantation. As discussed last year (Goodman, 1976), it has also been shown that patients receiving long-term dialysis manifest accelerated atherosclerosis and a high risk of premature cardiovascular disease. Since hyperlipidemia may be importantly involved in the genesis of the atherosclerotic disease in these patients, there is considerable interest in trying to develop better understanding and management of this problem.

A number of studies of hyperlipidemia in patients with chronic renal failure were reported in 1976. In general, these and other studies have consistently found that hypertriglyceridemia (usually with the type IV lipoprotein pattern) is present in a large proportion of patients with chronic uremia and in renal failure patients being maintained on hemodialysis programs (Ibels *et al.,* 1975, 1976a; Daubresse *et al.,* 1976; Norbeck *et al.,* 1976; Cattran *et al.,* 1976). The mechanism of hypertriglyceridemia in these patients appears to be defective triglyceride removal (clearance) from plasma (Ibels *et al.,* 1976a; Cattran *et al.,* 1976). Renal failure patients receiving chronic peritoneal dialysis have also been reported to show hyperlipidemia and impaired triglyceride removal from plasma (Cattran *et al.,* 1976).

Hyperlipidemia is also common in patients who have undergone renal transplantation. In these patients, however, hypertriglyceridemia appears to be less common, and hypercholesterolemia more common, than in uremic or chronic dialysis groups of patients (Ibels *et al.,* 1975, 1976a,b; Pennisi *et al.,* 1976). The possible relationship between hyperlipidemia and corticosteroid therapy in renal transplant patients has been commented on repeatedly by workers in this field. Thus, in one study (Ibels *et al.,* 1976b), in a series of 175 adult renal transplant patients, 59% had hyperlipidemia, characterized by either or both hypercholesterolemia and hypertriglyceridemia, with types IIa, IIb, and IV patterns on lipoprotein electrophoresis. Serum cholesterol and triglyceride levels could both be related to the dosage of prednisone these patients received. Serum triglyceride levels could further be correlated with obesity and negatively with duration of graft function (thought to reflect the lower dose of steroids administered the longer the duration of graft function).

Hyperlipidemia is also commonly found in children treated with maintenance hemodialysis or renal transplantation for chronic renal failure. As in adults, hypertriglyceridemia alone appears to be most common in children on maintenance dialysis, whereas renal transplant patients show both (or either) hypertriglyceridemia and hypercholesterolemia (Pennisi *et al.,* 1976). Because of the high risk of premature coronary artery disease in such children, it was suggested by Pennisi *et al.* (1976) that efforts should be made to control the hyperlipidemia, as well as to reduce immunosuppressive doses of corticosteroid in such children. A similar approach to the treatment of adults would also seem in order.

6.11. Treatment of Hyperlipidemia

6.11.1. Diet

As discussed last year (Goodman, 1976), treatment of hyperlipidemia is based on the assumption that the lowering of the coronary risk factor (hyperlipidemia) will result in a commensurate lowering of coronary risk itself. Definitive evidence that lowering serum lipids will reduce coronary risk is not yet available. Large-scale clinical trials designed to test this assumption, using hyperlipidemic subjects treated with lipid-lowering drugs, are in progress.

Management of hyperlipidemia first involves modifying the diet so as to lower serum cholesterol or triglyceride level or both. Definitive testing of the hypothesis that dietary intervention to lower serum lipid levels will reduce coronary risk would require mass field trials using a relatively young, healthy population of from 8,000 to 219,000 subjects, depending on the design of the study (Ahrens, 1969). Such an extensive diet–heart study has not been undertaken, largely because of the enormous costs involved, but smaller studies testing the diet hypothesis have been undertaken. Experimental subjects on a low-cholesterol, low-saturated-fat, higher-polyunsaturated-fat diet have been compared with control subjects by Dayton *et al.* (1969) over 8 years using domiciled veterans, by Leren (1970) over 11 years using men in Oslo after an initial myocardial infarction, and by Miettinen *et al.* (1972) over 12 years using a crossover design involving the inhabitants of two mental hospitals in Helsinki. The results of these studies, together with epidemiological considerations (Connor and Connor, 1972), suggest that lowering the serum cholesterol concentration by dietary means will lower the incidence of new events of coronary heart disease.

The most generally recommended diet is the American Heart Association fat-controlled diet, limited in cholesterol and saturated animal fat, with caloric intake appropriate for the patient to achieve and maintain an ideal body weight. Weight reduction is stressed in overweight patients, particularly in those with hypertriglyceridemia. Dietary cholesterol is limited to less than 300 mg per day, the fat content to 35% of total calories, and the saturated fat to less than 10% of calories. With such a diet, one can anticipate a 10–20% reduction in serum cholesterol concentration and significant reductions in serum triglyceride levels (particularly in patients who are both hypertriglyceridemic and overweight).

Evidence for the independence of the effects of cholesterol and of degree of saturation of the fat in the diet on serum cholesterol level was reported recently by J. T. Anderson *et al.* (1976). In this study, 12 young men were fed very-low-cholesterol diets containing 97 g of either saturated or polyunsaturated fat per day, with or without the addition of 291 mg cholesterol per day. Addition of cholesterol produced statistically significant elevations of serum cholesterol of 9 ± 2.1 mg/dl (mean ± S.E.M.) on the saturated diet and of 8 ± 1.6 mg/dl on the polyunsaturated diet. Substitution of the saturated diet for the polyunsaturated diet caused a significant elevation of serum cholesterol that was the same when the substitution was made in the presence or in the absence of added dietary cholesterol. These findings underscore the importance of restricting both cholesterol and saturated fat in the dietary treatment of hyperlipidemia.

In treating patients with diet, caution should be exercised with regard to the extent of restriction of the total fat content of the diet. Thus, it has been reported recently that low-fat, high-carbohydrate diets very often lead to elevations in the plasma triglyceride level, in both normal and hypertriglyceridemic subjects (Ginsberg *et al.*, 1976; Olefsky *et al.*, 1976). Accordingly, it is probably advisable to emphasize the restriction of saturated, rather than of total, fat in dietary intervention. It also seems clear that plasma lipid responses to diet should be monitored carefully in patients under treatment to determine in each patient whether an appropriate and effective response is being obtained.

6.11.2. Drugs

Many patients will remain hyperlipidemic despite dietary therapy, and in these patients, the question of the desirability of drug treatment to lower serum lipid levels must then be considered. As discussed last year (Goodman, 1976), it is often difficult to decide whether a given patient warrants treatment with lipid-lowering drugs. Many experts in this field currently believe that the benefit/risk ratio is high enough in the high-risk patients (lipid values above the 95th percentile) to warrant such treatment. This is particularly true for those patients who manifest other risk factors or who have a familial form of hyperlipidemia.

Only a very limited number of lipid-lowering drugs are currently available for general medical practice in the United States. The most widely used drug during 1975 and 1976 was clofibrate, which is currently considered the drug of choice for patients with hypertriglyceridemia, with or without hypercholesterolemia. A great deal of information about clofibrate was obtained during the Coronary Drug Project, discussed in detail last year.

Cholestyramine resin, a nonabsorbable bile acid sequestrant, is considered by many clinical investigators in this field to be the drug of choice for patients with hypercholesterolemia alone, particularly for patients with familial disease. Cholestyramine has some theoretical advantages, deriving from the fact that this drug produces a high fecal output of sterol derivatives (bile acids) without itself being absorbed by the body. Thus, it seems unlikely that unforeseen long-term toxic side effects will appear after many years of therapy due to a slow cumulative effect of some sort. Another bile acid-binding resin, colestipol hydrochloride, has been under clinical investigation for many years, and is expected to be approved for general use before mid-1977 by the Food and Drug Administration. A number of studies (e.g., Ryan *et al.*, 1975; Harvengt and Desager, 1976) have shown that this drug is usually highly effective in the treatment of hypercholesterolemia.

Nicotinic acid (niacin) in large doses (3–6 g/day) will lower serum lipid levels. At this dose, unpleasant side effects are extremely common and limit the patient acceptance and potential usefulness of this drug. Although the Coronary Drug Project (see Goodman, 1976) did not show prolongation of life in patients taking niacin, niacin did appear to be slightly, but significantly, beneficial in reducing the incidence of definite, nonfatal recurrent myocardial infarction.

A new drug, probucol, was very recently (early 1977) approved by the

FDA. It appears to lower serum cholesterol levels, with variable or slight effects on the triglyceride levels. More experience is needed to evaluate the potential of this agent.

Other drugs available that have been used (mainly in research clinics) as lipid-lowering agents include *p*-amino salicylic acid and sitosterol. As a result of the experience of the Coronary Drug Project, estrogen derivatives and D-thyroxine are no longer considered as appropriate agents to use for lipid-lowering purposes.

An unusual, new agent that has been studied experimentally as a potential cholesterol-lowering agent is sucrose polyester (SPE) (Fallat *et al.*, 1976). SPE is a fatlike material with the appearance and physical properties of the usual dietary fats that is neither digested nor absorbed. Addition or substitution of SPE for dietary fat in 13 normal subjects produced a significant 14% mean reduction in plasma cholesterol. A similar effect was not seen in 7 patients with FH. SPE was recovered quantitatively in the stools, but was not associated with clinical or chemical steatorrhea. The agent was easily incorporated into routine foodstuffs in addition to or in substitution for conventional dietary fats. It was pointed out that the ability to incorporate an inert, nonabsorbable, cholesterol-lowering fat substitute into the diet might provide a new approach to improved patient adherence and better treatment results in patients with hyperlipidemia.

6.11.3. Partial Ileal Bypass Surgery

Partial ileal bypass surgery represents another approach that has been used in the treatment of hyperlipidemia. The results of 10 years of clinical experience with this approach were reported in 1974 (Buchwald *et al.*, 1974a,b). As reported, 126 hyperlipidemic patients had been operated on and followed for more than 3 months. Surgery resulted in a lowering of plasma cholesterol levels an average of 41% from the preoperative, but postdietary, base line, with an average 53% reduction achieved with diet plus surgery. Plasma triglycerides were reduced in type IV patients an average of 53% beyond effects of diet alone. The complications and side effects of the procedure were felt to be acceptable and manageable. The effectiveness and potential of this procedure are currently under more extended investigation.

6.11.4. Primary Prevention of Ischemic Heart Disease

As discussed last year (Goodman, 1976), the question whether treatment of hyperlipidemia with lipid-lowering drugs can prevent the development of ischemic heart disease is being addressed by major collaborative clinical trials. One of these, a cooperative trial conducted in Edinburgh, Prague, and Budapest, and sponsored by the World Health Organization, represents a primary prevention trial using clofibrate to lower hyperlipidemia in healthy men aged 30–59. This trial has been completed, and it is anticipated that the results of this study will be reported some time during 1977. Another major trial that will continue for several more years is the Lipid Research Clinics' primary prevention trial of cholestyramine resin in type II hyperlipoproteinemic men, sponsored by the National Heart, Lung, and Blood Institute. A related clinical trial is the Multiple Risk Factor Intervention Trial, designed to assess the effectiveness of measures to reduce elevated serum cholesterol (by diet), high blood pressure (by diet and drugs), and cigarette smoking. As pointed out last year, it is hoped that these studies will, in time, provide definitive evidence that intervention programs directed at known coronary risk factors, and specifically at hyperlipidemia, can indeed prevent coronary disease.

References

Ahrens, E. H., Jr., 1969, Mass field trials of the diet–heart question: Their significance, timeliness, feasibility, and applicability, Report of the Diet–Heart Panel of the National Heart Institute, *Amer. Heart Assoc. Monogr. No. 28,* American Heart Association, New York (now Dallas, Texas).

Albers, J. J., Cabana, V. G., Warnick, G. R., and Hazzard, W. R., 1975, Lp(a) lipoprotein: Relationship to sinking pre-β lipoprotein, hyperlipoproteinemia, and apolipoprotein B, *Metabolism* **24**:1047–1054.

Albers, J. J., Wahl, P. W., Cabana, V. G., Hazzard, W. R., and Hoover, J. J., 1976, Quantitation of apolipoprotein A-I of human plasma high density lipoprotein, *Metabolism* **25**:633–644.

Andersen, J. M., and Dietschy, J. M., 1976, Cholesterogenesis: Derepression in extrahepatic tissues with 4-aminopyrazolo[3,4-d]pyrimidine, *Science* **193**:903–905.

Anderson, J. T., Grande, F., and Keys, A., 1976, Independence of the effects of cholesterol and degree of saturation of the fat in the diet on serum cholesterol in man, *Amer. J. Clin. Nutr.* **29**:1184–1189.

Anderson, R. G. W., Goldstein, J. L., and Brown, M. S., 1976, Localization of low density lipoprotein receptors on plasma membrane of normal human fibroblasts and their absence in cells from a familial hypercholesterolemia homozygote, *Proc. Natl. Acad. Sci. U.S.A.* **73**:2434–2438.

Balasubramaniam, S., Goldstein, J. L., Faust, J. R., and Brown, M. S., 1976, Evidence for regulation of 3-hydroxy-3-methylglutaryl coenzyme A reductase activity and cholesterol synthesis in nonhepatic tissues of rat, *Proc. Natl. Acad. Sci. U.S.A.* **73**:2564–2568.

Basu, S. K., Goldstein, J. L., Anderson, R. G. W., and Brown, M. S., 1976, Degradation of cationized low density lipoprotein and regulation of cholesterol metabolism in homozygous familial hypercholesterolemia fibroblasts, *Proc. Natl. Acad. Sci. U.S.A.* **73**:3178–3182.

Berg, K., Børresen, A.-L., and Dahlén, G., 1976, Serum-high-density-lipoprotein and atherosclerotic heart-disease, *Lancet* **1**:499–501.

Bhattacharyya, A. K., and Connor, W. E., 1974, β-Sitosterolemia and xanthomatosis: A newly described lipid storage disease in two sisters, *J. Clin. Invest.* **53**:1033–1043.

Bloch, A., Dinsmore, R. E., and Lees, R. S., 1976, Coronary arteriographic findings in type-II and type-IV hyperlipoproteinaemia, *Lancet* **1**:928–930.

Brown, M. S., and Goldstein, J. L., 1976a, Receptor-mediated control of cholesterol metabolism: Study of human mutants has disclosed how cells regulate a substance that is both vital and lethal, *Science* **191**:150–154.

Brown, M. S., and Goldstein, J. L., 1976b, Familial hypercholesterolemia: A genetic defect in the low-density lipoprotein receptor, *N. Engl. J. Med.* **294**:1386–1390.

Brown, M. S., and Goldstein, J. L., 1976c, Analysis of a mutant strain of human fibroblasts with a defect in the internalization of receptor-bound low density lipoprotein, *Cell* **9**:663–674.

Brown, M. S., Ho, Y. K., and Goldstein, J. L., 1976a, The low-density lipoprotein pathway in human fibroblasts: Relation between cell surface receptor binding and endocytosis of low-density lipoprotein, *Ann. N.Y. Acad. Sci.* **275**:244–257.

Brown, M. S., Sobhani, M. K., Brunschede, G. Y., and Goldstein, J. L., 1976b, Restoration of a regulatory response to low density lipoprotein in acid lipase-deficient human fibroblasts, *J. Biol. Chem.* **251**:3277–3286.

Brunzell, J. D., Schrott, H. C., Motulsky, A. G., and Bierman, E. L., 1976, Myocardial infarction in the familial forms of hypertriglyceridemia, *Metabolism* **25**:313–320.

Buchwald, H., Moore, R. B., and Varco, R. L., 1974a, Ten years clinical experience with partial ileal bypass in management of the hyperlipidemias, *Ann. Surg.* **180**:384–392.

Buchwald, H., Moore, R. B., and Varco, R. L., 1974b, Surgical treatment of hyperlipidemia, *Circulation* **49**(Suppl. I):1–37.

Carew, T. E., Hayes, S. B., Koschinsky, T., and Steinberg, D., 1976, A mechanism by which high-density lipoproteins may slow the atherogenic process, *Lancet* **1**:1315–1317.

Carlson, L. A., and Böttiger, L. E., 1972, Ischemic heart disease in relation to fasting values of plasma triglycerides and cholesterol, *Lancet* **1**:865–868.

Cattran, D. C., Fenton, S. S. A., Wilson, D. R., and Steiner, G., 1976, Defective triglyceride removal in lipemia associated with peritoneal dialysis and haemodialysis, *Ann. Intern. Med.* **85**:29–33.

Connor, W. E., and Connor, S. L., 1972, The key role of nutritional factors in the prevention of coronary heart disease, *Prev. Med.* **1**:49–83.

Cywes, S., Davies, M. R. Q., Louw, J. H., Berger, G. M. B., Bonnici, F., and Joffe, H. S., 1976, Portacaval shunt in two patients with homozygous type II hyperlipoproteinaemia, *S. Afr. Med. J.* **50**:239–243.

Dahlén, G., Berg, K., and Frick, M. H., 1976, Lp(a) lipoprotein, pre-β_1-lipoprotein, serum lipids and atherosclerotic disease, *Clin. Genet.* **9**:558–566.

Daubresse, J. C., Lerson, G., Plomteux, G., Rorive, G., Luyckx, A. S., and Lefebvre, P. J., 1976, Lipids and lipoproteins in chronic uraemia: A study of the influence of regular haemodialysis, *Eur. J. Clin. Invest.* **6**:159–166.

Dawber, T. R., 1973, Risk factors in young adults: The lessons from epidemiologic studies of cardiovascular disease—Framingham, Tecumseh, and Evans County, *J. Amer. Coll. Health Assoc.* **22**:84–95.

Dayton, S., Pearce, M. L., Hashimoto, S., Dixon, W. V., and Tomiyasu, V., 1969, A controlled clinical trial of a diet high in unsaturated fat in preventing complications of atherosclerosis, *Circulation* **40**(Suppl. II):1–63.

Dyer, A. R., 1975, An analysis of the relationship of systolic blood pressure, serum cholesterol, and smoking to 14-year mortality in the Chicago Peoples Gas Company study. I. Total mortality in exponential–Weibull model, *J. Chron. Dis.* **28**:565–570.

Eisenberg, S., and Levy, R. I., 1975, Lipoprotein metabolism, in: *Advances in Lipid Research,* Vol. 13 (R. Paoletti and D. Kritchevsky, eds.) pp. 1–89, Academic Press, New York.

Fallat, R. W., and Glueck, C. J., 1976, Familial and acquired type V hyperlipoproteinemia, *Atherosclerosis* **23**:41–62.

Fallat, R. W., Glueck, C. J., Lutmer, R., and Mattson, F. H., 1976, Short term study of sucrose polyester, a nonabsorbable fat-like material, as a dietary agent for lowering plasma cholesterol, *Amer. J. Clin. Nutr.* **29**:1204–1215.

Farriaux, J.-P., Ribet, M., Bertrand, M., Higgins, M., Mazzuca, M., and Luyckx, A., 1976, Traitement de l'hypercholésterolémie familiale de type II par shunt porto-cave, *Arch. Fr. Pediatr.* **33**:745–759.

Frerichs, R. R., Srinivasan, S. R., Webber, L. S., and Berenson, G. S., 1976, Serum cholesterol and triglyceride levels in 3,446 children from a biracial community: The Bogalusa heart study, *Circulation* **54**:302–309.

Ganesan, D., Bass, H. B., McConathy, W. J., and Alaupovic, P., 1976, Is decreased activity of C-II activated lipoprotein lipase in type III hyperlipoproteinemia (broad-β-disease) a cause or an effect of increased apolipoprotein E levels?, *Metabolism* **25**:1189–1195.

Ginsberg, H., Olefsky, J. M., Kimmerling, G., Crapo, P., and Reaven, G. M., 1976, Induction of hypertriglyceridemia by a low-fat diet, *J. Clin. Endocrinol. Metab.* **42**:729–735.

Glomset, J. A., 1968, The plasma lecithin:cholesterol acyltransferase reaction, *J. Lipid Res.* **9**:155–167.

Glueck, C. J., Fallat, R. W., Millett, F., Gartside, P., Elston, R. C., and Go, R. C. P., 1975, Familial hyper-alpha-lipoproteinemia: Studies in eighteen kindreds, *Metabolism* **24**:1243–1265.

Glueck, C. J., Fallat, R. W., Mellies, M. J., and Steiner, P. M., 1976a, Pediatric familial type III hyperlipoproteinemia, *Metabolism* **25**:1269–1274.

Glueck, C. J., Gartside, P., Fallat, R. W., Sielski, J., and Steiner, P. M., 1976b, Longevity syndromes: Familial hypobeta and familial hyperalpha lipoproteinemia, *J. Lab. Clin. Med.* **88**:941–957.

Glueck, C. J., Mellies, M. J., Srivastava, L., Knowles, H. C., Jr., Fallat, R. W., Tsang, R. C., Wacholder, S., and Buncher, C. R., 1977, Insulin, obesity, and triglyceride interrelationships in sixteen children with familial hypertriglyceridemia, *Pediatr. Res.* **11**:13–18.

Goldstein, J. L., and Brown, M. S., 1976, The LDL pathway in human fibroblasts: A receptor-mediated mechanism for the regulation of cholesterol metabolism, in: *Current Topics in Cellular Regulation,* Vol. II (B. L. Horecker and E. R. Stadtman, eds.) pp. 147–178, Academic Press, New York.

Goldstein, J. L., Basu, S. K., Brunschede, G. Y., and Brown, M. S., 1976a, Release of low density lipoprotein from its cell surface receptor by sulfated glycosaminoglycans, *Cell* **7**:85–95.

Goldstein, J. L., Sobhani, M. K., Faust, J. R., and Brown, M. S., 1976b, Heterozygous familial hypercholesterolemia: Failure of normal allele to compensate for mutant allele at a regulated genetic locus, *Cell* **9**:195–203.

Goodman, DeW. S., 1974, Vitamin A transport and retinol-binding protein metabolism, *Vitam. Horm.* **32**:167–180.

Goodman, DeW. S., 1976, Disorders of lipid and lipoprotein metabolism, in: *The Year in Metabolism 1975–1976* (N. Freinkel, ed.), pp. 153–180, Plenum Press, New York.

Goodman, DeW. S., Noble, R. P., and Dell, R. B., 1973, Three-pool model of the long-term turnover of plasma cholesterol in man, *J. Lipid Res.* **14**:178–188.

Grundy, S. M., 1975, Effects of polyunsaturated fats on lipid metabolism in patients with hypertriglyceridemia, *J. Clin. Invest.* **55**:269–282.

Grundy, S. M., and Ahrens, E. H., Jr., 1969, Measurements of cholesterol turnover, synthesis, and absorption in man, carried out by isotopic kinetic and sterol balance methods, *J. Lipid Res.* **10**:91–107.

Harvengt, C., and Desager, J.-P., 1976, Colestipol in familial type II hyperlipoproteinemia: A three-year trial, *Clin. Pharmacol. Ther.* **20**:310–314.

Hazzard, W. R., and Bierman, E. L., 1976, Delayed clearance of chylomicron remnants following vitamin-A-containing oral fat loads in broad-β disease (type III hyperlipoproteinemia), *Metabolism* **25**:777–801.

Heiberg, A., 1976, Inheritance of xanthomatosis and hyper-β-lipoproteinaemia: A study of 7 large kindreds, *Clin. Genet.* **9**:92–111.

Heiberg, A., and Berg, K., 1976, The inheritance of hyperlipoproteinaemia with xanthomatosis: A study of 132 kindreds, *Clin. Genet.* **9**:203–233.

Heinle, R. A., Levy, R. I., Fredrickson, D. S., and Gorlin, R., 1969, Lipid and carbohydrate abnormalities in patients with angiographically documented coronary artery disease, *Amer. J. Cardiol.* **24**:178–186.

Ho, Y. K., Brown, M. S., Bilheimer, D. W., and Goldstein, J. L., 1976a, Regulation of low density lipoprotein receptor activity in freshly isolated human lymphocytes, *J. Clin. Invest.* **58**:1465–1474.

Ho, Y. K., Brown, M. S., Kayden, H. J., and Goldstein, J. L., 1976b, Binding, internalization, and hydrolysis of low density lipoprotein in long-term lymphoid cell lines from a normal subject and a patient with homozygous familial hypercholesterolemia, *J. Exp. Med.* **144**:444–455.

Huttunen, J. K., Ehnholm, C., Kekki, M., and Nikkilä, E. A., 1976, Postheparin plasma lipoprotein lipase and hepatic lipase in normal subjects and in patients with hypertriglyceridaemia: Correlations to sex, age and various parameters of triglyceride metabolism, *Clin. Sci. Mol. Med.* **50**:249–260.

Ibels, L. S., Simons, L. A., King, J. O., Williams, P. F., Neale, F. C., and Stewart, J. H., 1975, Studies on the nature and causes of hyperlipidaemia in uraemia, maintenance dialysis and renal transplantation, *Q. J. Med. N.S.* **44**:601–614.

Ibels, L. S., Reardon, M. F., and Nestel, P. J., 1976a, Plasma post-heparin lipolytic activity and triglyceride clearance in uremic and hemodialysis patients and renal allograft recipients, *J. Lab. Clin. Med.* **87**:648–658.

Ibels, L. S., Alfrey, A. C., Subryan, V., and Weil, R., III, 1976b, Hyperlipidemia following renal transplantation, *Trans. Amer. Soc. Artif. Intern. Organs* **22**:46–53.

Jackson, R. L., Morrisett, J. D., and Gotto, A. M., Jr., 1976, Lipoprotein structure and metabolism, *Physiol. Rev.* **56**:259–316.

Kannel, W. B., Castelli, W. P., Gordon, T., and McNamara, P. M., 1971, Serum cholesterol, lipoproteins, and the risk of coronary heart disease, *Ann. Intern. Med.* **74**:1–12.

Keys, A., 1975, Coronary heart disease: The global picture, *Atherosclerosis* **22**:149–192.

Kudchodkar, B. J., and Sodhi, H. S., 1976, Turnover of plasma cholesteryl esters and its relationship to other parameters of lipid metabolism in man, *Eur. J. Clin. Invest.* **6**:285–298.

Langer, T., Strober, W., and Levy, R. I., 1972, The metabolism of low density lipoprotein in familial type II hyperlipoproteinemia, *J. Clin. Invest.* **51**:1528–1536.

Lauer, R. M., Connor, W. E., Leaverton, P. E., Reiter, M. A., and Clarke, W. R., 1975, Coronary heart disease risk factors in school children: The Muscatine study, *J. Pediatr.* **86**:697–706.

Leren, P., 1970, The Oslo diet–heart study: Eleven year report, *Circulation* **42**:935–942.

Lupien, P.-J., Moorjani, S., and Awad, J., 1976, A new approach to the management of familial hypercholesterolaemia: Removal of plasma-cholesterol based on the principle of affinity chromatography, *Lancet* **1**:1261–1265.

Mahley, R. W., Weisgraber, K. H., Innerarity, T., and Brewer, H. B., 1975, Swine lipoproteins and atherosclerosis: Changes in the plasma lipoproteins and apoproteins induced by cholesterol feeding, *Biochemistry* **14**:2817–2823.

Mahley, R. W., Weisgraber, K. H., and Innerarity, T., 1976, Atherogenic hyperlipoproteinemia induced by cholesterol feeding in the Patas monkey, *Biochemistry* **15**:2979–2985.

Manzato, E., Fellin, R., Baggio, G., Walch, S., Neubeck, W., and Seidel, D., 1976, Formation of lipoprotein-X: Its relationship to bile compounds, *J. Clin. Invest.* **57**:1248–1260.

McConathy, W. J., and Alaupovic, P., 1976, Studies on the isolation and partial characterization of apolipoprotein D and lipoprotein D of human plasma, *Biochemistry* **15**:515–520.

Miettinen, M., Turpeinen, O., Karvonen, M. J., Elosuo, R., and Paavilainen, E., 1972, Effect of cholesterol-lowering diet on mortality from coronary heart disease and other causes: A twelve year clinical trial in men and women, *Lancet* **2**:835–838.

Miller, G. J., and Miller, N. E., 1975, Plasma-high-density-lipoprotein concentration and development of ischaemic heart-disease, *Lancet* **1**:16–19.

Miller, N. E., Nestel, P. J., and Clifton-Bligh, P., 1976, Relationships between plasma lipoprotein cholesterol concentrations and the pool size and metabolism of cholesterol in man, *Atherosclerosis* **23**:535–547.

Motulsky, A. G., 1976, Current concepts in genetics: The genetic hyperlipidemias, *N. Engl. J. Med.* **294**:823–827.

Murray, R. G., Tweddel, A., Third, J. L. H. C., Hutton, I., Hillis, W. S., Lorimer, A. R., and Lawrie, T. D. V., 1975, Relation between extent of coronary artery disease and severity of hyperlipoproteinaemia, *Br. Heart J.* **37**:1205–1209.

Myant, N. B., Reichl, D., Thompson, G. R., Higgins, M. J. P., and Galton, D. J., 1976, The metabolism *in vivo* and *in vitro* of plasma low-density lipoprotein from a subject with inherited hypercholesterolaemia, *Clin. Sci. Mol. Med.* **51**:463–465.

Norbeck, H.-E., Orö, L., and Carlson, L. A., 1976, Serum lipid and lipoprotein concentrations in chronic uremia, *Acta Med. Scand.* **200**:487–492.

Olefsky, J. M., Crapo, P., and Reaven, G. M., 1976, Postprandial plasma triglyceride and cholesterol responses to a low-fat meal, *Amer. J. Clin. Nutr.* **29**:535–539.

Oliver, M. F., Nimmo, I. A., Cooke, M., Carlson, L. A., and Olsson, A. G., 1975, Ischaemic heart disease and associated risk factors in 40 year old men in Edinburgh and Stockholm, *Eur. J. Clin. Invest.* **5**:507–514.

Pennisi, A. J., Heuser, E. T., Mickey, M. R., Lipsey, A., Malekzadeh, M. H., and Fine, R. N., 1976, Hyperlipidemia in pediatric hemodialysis and renal transplant patients, *Amer. J. Dis. Child.* **130**:957–961.

Rhoads, G. G., Gulbrandsen, C. L., and Kagan, A., 1976, Serum lipoproteins and coronary heart disease in a population study of Hawaii Japanese men, *N. Engl. J. Med.* **294**:293–298.

Ritland, S., 1975, Quantitative determination of the abnormal lipoprotein of cholestasis, LP-X, in liver disease, *Scand. J. Gastroenterol.* **10**:5–15.

Ross, R., and Glomset, J. A., 1976, The pathogenesis of atherosclerosis, *N. Engl. J. Med.* **295**:369–377, 420–425.

Ross, R., and Harker, L., 1976, Hyperlipidemia and atherosclerosis: Chronic hyperlipidemia initiates and maintains lesions by endothelial cell desquamation and lipid accumulation, *Science* **193**:1094–1100.

Ryan, J. R., Jain, A. K., and McMahon, F. G., 1975, Long-term treatment of hypercholesterolemia with colestipol hydrochloride, *Clin. Pharmacol. Ther.* **17**:83–87.

Salel, A. F., Riggs, K., Mason, D. T., Amsterdam, E. A., and Zelis, R., 1974, The importance of type IV hyperlipoproteinemia as a predisposing factor in coronary artery disease, *Amer. J. Med.* **57**:897–903.

Salen, G., and Grundy, S. M., 1973, The metabolism of cholestanol, cholesterol, and bile acids in cerebrotendinous xanthomatosis, *J. Clin. Invest.* **52**:2822–2835.

Salen, G., Meriwether, T. W., and Nicolau, G., 1975, Chenodeoxycholic acid inhibits increased cholesterol and cholestanol synthesis in patients wtih cerebrotendinous xanthomatosis, *Biochem. Med.* **14**:57–74.

Salen, G., Shefer, S., Zaki, F. G., and Mosbach, E. H., 1977, Inborn errors of bile acid synthesis, *Clin. Gastroenterol.* **6**:91–101.

Shulman, R. S., Bhattacharyya, A. K., Connor, W. E., and Fredrickson, D. S., 1976, β-Sitosterolemia and xanthomatosis, *N. Engl. J. Med.* **294**:482–483.

Sigler, G. F., Soutar, A. K., Smith, L. C., Gotto, A. M., Jr., and Sparrow, J. T., 1976, The solid phase synthesis of a protein activator for lecithin-cholesterol acyltransferase corresponding to human plasma apoC-I, *Proc. Natl. Acad. Sci. U.S.A.* **73**:1422–1426.

Sigurdsson, G., Nicoll, A., and Lewis, B., 1976, Metabolism of very low density lipoproteins in hyperlipidaemia: Studies of apolipoprotein B kinetics in man, *Eur. J. Clin. Invest.* **6**:167–177.

Sing, C. F., Chamberlain, M. A., Block, W. D., and Feiler, S., 1975, Analysis of genetic and environmental sources of variation in serum cholesterol in Tecumseh, Michigan. I. Analysis of the frequency distribution for evidence of a genetic polymorphism, *Amer. J. Hum. Genet.* **27**:333–347.

Slack, J., 1975, The genetic contribution to coronary heart disease through lipoprotein concentrations, *Postgrad. Med. J.* **51**(Suppl. 8):27–32.

Smith, F. R., Dell, R. B., Noble, R. P., and Goodman, DeW. S., 1976, Parameters of the three-pool model of the turnover of plasma cholesterol in normal and hyperlipidemic humans, *J. Clin. Invest.* **57**:137–148.

Sodhi, H. S., and Kudchodkar, B. J., 1973, Synthesis of cholesterol in hypercholesterolemia and its relationship to plasma triglycerides, *Metab. (Clin. Exp.)* **22**:895–912.

Stein, O., and Stein, Y., 1976, High density lipoproteins reduce the uptake of low density lipoproteins by human endothelial cells in culture, *Biochim. Biophys. Acta* **431**:363–368.

Thompson, G. R., and Myant, N. B., 1976, Low density lipoprotein turnover in familial hypercholesterolaemia after plasma exchange, *Atherosclerosis* **23**:371–377.

Tyroler, H. A., Hames, C. G., Krishan, I., Heyden, S., Cooper, G., and Cassel, J. C., 1975, Black–white differences in serum lipids and lipoproteins in Evans county, *Prev. Med.* **4**:541–549.

Walton, K. W., Hitchens, J., Magnani, H. N., and Khan, M., 1974, A study of methods of identification and estimation of LP(a) lipoprotein and of its significance in health, hyperlipidaemia and atherosclerosis, *Atherosclerosis* **20**:323–346.

West, R. J., Fosbrooke, A. S., and Lloyd, J. K., 1975, Treatment of children with familial hypercholesterolemia, *Postgrad. Med. J.* **51**(Suppl. 8):82–86.

Witters, L. A., Herbert, P. N., Shulman, R. S., Krauss, R. M., and Levy, R. I., 1976, Therapeutic failure in familial type II hyperlipoproteinemia, *Metabolism* **25**:1017–1026.

Wood, P. D., Haskell, W., Klein, H., Lewis, S., Stern, M. P., and Farquhar, J. W., 1976, The distribution of plasma lipoproteins in middle-aged male runners, *Metabolism* **25**:1249–1257.

7

Metabolism of Amino Acids and Organic Acids

Leon E. Rosenberg and Kay Tanaka

7.1. Introduction

In last year's introductory volume to this series, we indicated that our strategy in these annual surveys of amino acid and organic acid metabolism would involve detailed discussion of a few topics rather than cursory treatment of many. We have maintained that posture this year. Three topics have been chosen for discussion: phenylketonuria and its variants, the γ-glutamyl cycle and 5-oxoprolinuria, and Jamaican vomiting sickness and glutaric aciduria. These areas concern "old" (phenylketonuria) and "new" (5-oxoprolinuria) diseases, common (Jamaican vomiting sickness) and rare (glutaric aciduria) ones. Although the metabolic pathways chosen for discussion are widely different, the scientific and clinical signposts are familiar. They include considerations of biochemical and genetic heterogeneity, evaluation of diagnostic and therapeutic modalities, the convergence of information gained from related acquired and inherited abnor-

LEON E. ROSENBERG and KAY TANAKA • Department of Human Genetics, Yale University School of Medicine, New Haven, Connecticut 06510.

malities, and, in all instances, the existence of important, unanswered questions. We have attempted to cite only major, recent references individually, and have depended on reviews in each section to provide the interested reader with older but clearly not lesser works. In this way, we hope that involved workers and serious readers will gain the flavor of the field without much in the way of a bitter or sour aftertaste.

7.2. Phenylketonuria and Its Variants

Phenylketonuria (PKU) rightly deserves to be regarded as the classic inherited disorder of amino acid metabolism (Knox, 1972; Scriver and Rosenberg, 1973). It has earned this distinction because of its many "firsts" among the inborn errors: first shown to result in mental retardation, first demonstrated to be due to a specific enzyme defect, first successfully treated by dietary restriction, and first amenable to mass neonatal screening. "But," the reader may say, "this volume is not intended to hail the icons of its contributors' faiths. Its purpose is to focus on new information, and surely there can be nothing new about PKU." In the next few pages, we hope to convince you that such an assessment is incorrect.

It is, in a very real sense, sobering to realize how incomplete our understanding of this condition still is. It is more than 40 years since Fölling, in 1934, described blond, microcephalic, severely retarded children with phenylpyruvate in their urine and increased phenylalanine in their blood; yet we still do not know either the chemical(s) responsible for the observed intellectual impairment or the biochemical mechanism of the nervous system dysfunction. It is 25 years since Jervis and Udenfriend demonstrated independently that liver tissue from patients with PKU failed to convert phenylalanine to tyrosine; yet this phenylalanine-hydroxylating system is only now being understood in molecular terms and continues to surprise us with its intricacies (Kaufman, 1976). It is more than 20 years since Bickel showed that feeding children with PKU a protein hydrolysate from which phenylalanine had been removed resulted in distinct reduction in plasma and urinary concentrations of phenylalanine and its by-products; yet we do not know precisely how good such dietary treatment is or how long to employ it (Koch *et al.,* 1974). Finally, it is more than 10 years since Guthrie developed his reknowned bacterial inhibition assay for phenylalanine content that led to the mass screening of neonates; yet we know little about why PKU occurs so much more commonly (about 1/10,000 births) than most other inborn errors, and we continue to be frustrated by children who slip through the screening system and suffer thereby. Answers to some of these questions are emerging, however, and the recent literature contains several new insights, to which we shall now turn.

7.2.1. Phenylalanine Hydroxylation: Enzymes and Coenzymes

7.2.1.1. The Hydroxylation System

Phenylalanine is an essential amino acid for humans and has only two major fates: incorporation into protein and hydroxylation to tyrosine. Tyrosine, unessential in the dietary sense, is metabolically far more versatile than phenylalanine, since it is the precursor of such important products as thyroxine, catecholamines, and melanin. Thus, phenylalanine hydroxylase (now officially designated phenylalanine 4-monooxygenase) is the gateway to several critical metabolic pathways. From comparison of the structural formulas for phenylalanine and tyrosine, the reaction looks simple—addition of an OH radical to the aromatic ring. Yet, as shown in Fig. 1, this hydroxylation requires at least three specific proteins and two cofactors. One protein, designated phenylalanine hydroxylase, has three substrates: phenylalanine, molecular oxygen, and a reduced pteridine cofactor, tetrahydrobiopterin (XH_4). The hydroxylase catalyzes the formation of tyrosine, water, and a quinonoid form of dihydrobiopterin (XH_2). Two other proteins are responsible for maintaining the necessary intracellular concentration of tetrahydrobiopterin: dihydropteridine reductase is the catalyst for the interaction between quinonoid XH_2 and

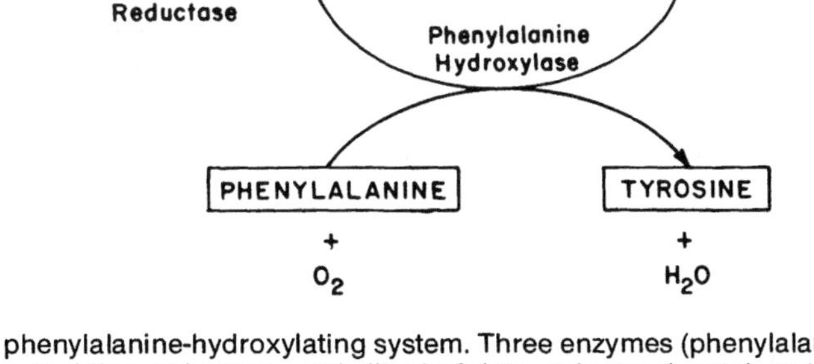

Fig. 1. The phenylalanine-hydroxylating system. Three enzymes (phenylalanine hydroxylase, dihydropteridine reductase, and dihydrofolate reductase) catalyze this process, which also depends on the availability of nicotinamide adenine dicleotide (NADP and NADPH) and biopterin (XH_2, XH_4, quinonoid XH_2) cofactors.

NADPH; dihydrofolate reductase enzymatically converts nonquinonoid XH_2 to XH_4, again using NADPH as the electron donor.

Each of these proteins has been purified from animal tissues to homogeneity or near homogeneity (Kaufman, 1976). Only the properties of the hydroxylase will be discussed here. It is probably composed of two nonidentical subunits, each with a molecular weight of 50,000–55,000. The active enzyme exists as a dimer or possibly even a tetramer. It is found in largest amounts in the liver, but also exists in the kidney, gut, and pancreas. Trace activity has been reported recently in cultured fibroblasts, but this finding remains controversial (Hoffbauer and Schrempf, 1976). The reductases, on the other hand, appear to be widely distributed in virtually all animal tissues.

7.2.1.2. The Defect in Classic Phenylketonuria

A series of elegant experiments in Kaufman's laboratory have led to our current understanding of the biochemical basis for classic PKU, as distinguished from variants to be discussed subsequently. In brief, they showed first that hydroxylating activity was virtually absent in the liver of affected patients, that tetrahydrobiopterin concentrations in the liver were normal, and that reconstitution of hydroxylating activity could be achieved by addition of pure hydroxylase protein, but not by addition of cofactors or cofactor-regenerating enzymes (Kaufman, 1976). Thus, the defect resides in the hydroxylase protein *per se.* Then, they developed a very sensitive radioisotopic assay for hydroxylating activity and showed conclusively that trace activity (~0.27% of normal) was present in liver tissue from a PKU patient (Friedman *et al.,* 1973). This observation excluded the possibility that the entire gene for one or both of the hydroxylase polypeptides was deleted, and left these workers with two other possible explanations: presence of minute amounts of normal protein, or presence of normal or abnormal amounts of a catalytically defective molecule. To distinguish between these possibilities, they carried out additional immunochemical and enzymologic studies (Kaufman, 1976). They raised an antibody in sheep to rat liver hydroxylase and showed that the antibody cross-reacted extensively with the human enzyme. Then they carried out double-diffusion experiments capable of detecting as little as 5% residual cross-reacting material (CRM), but found no precipitin arc with liver from the PKU patient. This excluded the notion that the mutant enzyme contained normal antigenic deteriminants in normal amounts. Next, they showed that the antihydroxylase antibody inhibited normal human hydroxylase activity by as much as 60% but observed only 18% inhibition of activity with PKU liver. This observation, coupled with the findings that hydroxylase activity in PKU liver was activated to a much smaller degree by lysolecithin than observed with normal liver and that substrate inhibition of the mutant enzyme was not observed, led Kaufman to propose that the underlying defect in PKU resides with a mutation of a structural gene locus for a hydroxylase polypeptide that leads to the synthesis of a protein with altered antigenic and catalytic activity and that may be present in minute amounts.

7.2.1.3. 'Benign' Hyperphenylalaninemia

Data obtained from newborn screening studies demonstrated in the 1960's that all hyperphenylalaninemia is not PKU, i.e., that some children with abnormal blood phenylalanine concentrations at birth have transient or milder manifestations than those noted in typical PKU patients (Scriver and Rosenberg, 1973). In some of these patients, the blood phenylalanine returns to normal within a few months, suggesting delayed maturation of some component of the hydroxylating system. In others, the elevated blood phenylalanine persists, but dietary control is easier and blood phenylalanine levels tend to be less elevated than in classic PKU. It is from this group of patients with "atypical PKU" or "benign hyperphenylalaninemia" that some interesting biochemical and genetic data have recently been obtained. Liver biopsies from several individuals with "benign" hyperphenylalaninemia showed between 2 and 10% of residual hydroxylating activity (Kaufman *et al.*, 1975b; Bartholomé *et al.*, 1975). Once again, reconstitution experiments point to the hydroxylase protein, and kinetic analyses suggested an altered affinity of the mutant enzyme for phenylalanine (Kaufman, 1976). A recent family study, however, yielded interesting and perplexing results (Kaufman *et al.*, 1975b). As noted in Table I, hydroxylase activity in the liver of three probands with hyperphenylalaninemia averaged 4.9% of control. Surprisingly, activity in the livers of the six parents of these three patients averaged only 13% of control, with a range of 5.8–30%. Since none of these parents had hyperphenylalaninemia, it seems likely that they are, as suspected, heterozygous for a mutant allele of the hydroxylase protein. Why, then, are their hydroxylase activities so much less that 50% of normal? The answer probably lies in the phenomenon of negative interallelic complementation, which may occur in enzymes composed of nonidentical subunits. If we propose that phenylalanine hydroxylase is a dimer of two nonidentical subunits (α and β) and that the α subunit is defective (α') in the probands with hyperphenylalaninemia, then their hydroxylase can be denoted $\alpha'\beta$. Their parents' cells should contain both normal α and mutant α' subunits, as well as normal β subunits. In the event that the α' subunits are synthesized more rapidly than the wild-type polypeptide, or turn over more slowly, or have a competitive advantage over the normal α subunit for interacting with β polypeptide, then more defective α' enzyme molecules may exist intracellularly than normal α ones. In the event that the

Table I. Hepatic Phenylalanine Hydroxylase Activity in Families with Hyperphenylalaninemia[a]

Subjects	Hydroxylase activity (units)[b]	Percentage of mean control activity
Controls		
1	96	
2	59	
3	71	
4	49	
5	95	
6	83	
	$\bar{x}$ = 75.5	
Patients		
1	4.7	6.2
2	3.8	5.0
3	2.7	3.6
	$\bar{x}$ = 3.7	$\bar{x}$ = 4.9
Patients' parents[c]		
1M	7.2	9.5
1F	23.0	30.9
2M	7.7	10.2
2F	4.4	5.8
3M	11.4	15.1
3F	5.8	7.7
	$\bar{x}$ = 9.9	$\bar{x}$ = 13.0

[a]From Kaufman *et al.* (1975b).
[b]Units defined as μmol tyrosine formed/g protein per hr.
[c]1M refers to mother of patient 1, 1F to the father of patient 1, etc.

enzyme exists as a tetramer, such theoretical considerations could lead to an even greater negative distortion of expected activity than that just proposed. These results, then, lend considerable support to the concept that phenylalanine hydroxylase is a multimeric enzyme and indicate the need for still additional purification and enzymologic reconstitution studies.

7.2.1.4. Dihydropteridine Reductase Deficiency

Since 1975, four children (3 males, 1 female) with a most unusual and important variant of PKU have been described. Three infants, two of them sibs (1 male, 1 female) were reported by Smith *et al.* (1975). The clinical histories in these children were remarkably similar. Each had a diagnosis of PKU made soon after birth because of a positive Guthrie test. Each responded to a low-phenylalanine diet promptly and tolerated considerably more phenylalanine in their feeds than usual PKU patients.

Most dramatically, each developed progressive neurologic dysfunction despite adequate biochemical control. The dysfunction began at age 2 months with difficulty swallowing, and proceeded to seizures and developmental delay by 5–7 months of age and to progressive cerebral and basal ganglia symptoms thereafter (rigidity, chorea, oculomotor spasms, hypotonia). All died of secondary infection, one at 22 months, the others at 6 and 7 years. Significantly, hepatic phenylalanine hydroxylation activity in the one child in whom it was measured was within the normal range. This led the authors to postulate a defect in biopterin metabolism, but no experimental proof was sought.

The fourth child, a male, was described independently but coincidentally by Kaufman *et al.* (1975a). The clinical picture was strikingly similar to that just described: positive Guthrie test and good dietary control from birth, onset of convulsions at age 7½ months, progressive deterioration thereafter. A liver biopsy at age 14 months provided much useful information. Hydroxylating activity was present at 20% of normal (distinctly higher than that observed in classic PKU or its "benign" variants). Two observations demonstrated defective biopterin metabolism: absence of detectable tetrahydrobiopterin in the patient's liver, and absence of dihydropteridine reductase activity in his liver, brain, or cultured fibroblasts. Immunochemical characterization (Milstien and Kaufman, 1975) using anti-sheep liver dihydropteridine reductase raised in rabbits showed that normal human liver has significant CRM in this heterologous system, but the patient's liver had none (with an assay sensitivity of <5% of normal).

These results demonstrate convincingly that hydroxylation of phenylalanine can be imparied by interfering with cofactor availability as well as by the more usual alteration of the hydroxylase protein. The observed deficiency of dihydropteridine reductase has many implications. First, since tetrahydrobiopterin and its regenerating systems are required for normal hydroxylation of tyrosine to DOPA and of tryptophan to 5-OH-tryptophan (a serotinin precursor) as well as for conversion of phenylalanine to tyrosine, it seems very likely that the profound neurologic impairment observed in these children reflects a generalized defect in neurotransmitter metabolism not found in classic PKU. Second, the observation that the reductase is normally expressed in cultured fibroblasts (and therefore probably in cultured amniotic fluid cells as well) indicates that prenatal diagnosis of affected fetuses with this variant of PKU may be feasible and raises a question about the advisability of measuring reductase activity in the fibroblasts of all infants diagnosed as having PKU. This would unquestionably be a formidable undertaking technically, but could identify those children destined to do badly on dietary phenylalanine restriction. Third, we must ask whether there is any way that this defect can be treated effectively. At first glance, one is attracted to supplying the tetrahydrobiopterin exogenously. Kaufman *et al.* (1975a) pointed out two important theoretical objections to this notion: without a regenerating system for the biopterin cofactor, they estimate that one would have to give 100 mg tetrahydrobiopterin/kg body weight per day just to keep pace with stoichiometric phenylalanine hydroxylation; furthermore, tetrahydrobiopterin apparently enters the brain very poorly, and may therefore not reach the tissue in which aromatic amino acid hydroxylation is most critical. Nonetheless, it would appear that biopterin derivatives of some sort should be administered to such children early in their course, since the untreated disorder appears to have such a dismal prognosis.

7.2.2. Clinical Phenylketonuria: Incidence and Outcome

7.2.2.1. Phenylketonuria as a Balanced Polymorphism

A genetic locus may be defined as polymorphic if two different alleles each occur with a gene frequency greater than 1%. It is becoming apparent that such genetic polymorphism is very common—occurring at perhaps one-third of all loci (Harris, 1975). In the main, such polymorphisms have been reported for loci unassociated with significant human disease (i.e., peptidases, phosphoglucomatase). This is, of course, not absolute, since such important recessively inherited disorders as sickle cell anemia, Tay–Sachs disease, and cystic fibrosis are each reported in selected populations with incidences greater than 1/10,000, meaning that the gene frequency is greater than 1/100 (i.e., >1%) and that the locus in question is polymorphic. For such loci, an intriguing question concerns the means by which the gene frequency is maintained at such a high level. Surely gene frequencies of greater than 1% cannot be accounted for by new mutations, and the evidence for genetic drift or founder effects is lacking. Hence, it has long been proposed that some advantage accrues to the heterozygote that balances the obvious disadvantage to the affected homozygote. The term *balanced polymorphism* is used to describe this situation, and it is best typified in man by the increased resistance of heterozygotes for hemoglobin S to falciparum malaria.

PKU occurs with a frequency of greater than 1/10,000 in numerous populations (Irish, Scottish, Yemenite Jews, Poles, and Germans). Thus, the gene (and heterozygote) frequency in these populations must be greater than 1%, meaning that at least one of the loci coding for hydroxylase polypeptides is polymorphic. No suggestion of advantage to the heterozygote had been reported prior to 1975. In that year, Woolf *et al.* (1975) carried out a study in Scotland and Ireland on 57 families containing at least one PKU proband and on 412 matched controls. To test the hypothesis, that the slightly higher blood phenylalanine concentrations found in PKU heterozygotes might be advantageous to non-PKU fetuses carried by PKU heterozygote mothers, they examined fecundity, fetal salvage, and live births in the two populations. No distinct difference in number of pregnancies per family was found between the two groups, thereby excluding a source of ascertainment bias. PKU families, however, had a statistically significant higher incidence of live births (89.2%) than did controls (80.9%) and a much reduced incidence of early spontaneous abortions (8.6% PKU; 17.2% control). The authors suggest that the PKU gene is, in some way, protective against fetal death early in gestation, and thereby constitutes a heterozygote advantage. It is not at all clear how this advantage comes about or whether it is related to the modestly increased blood phenylalanine content observed in PKU heterozygotes. Follow-up of this intriguing hypothesis should prove interesting.

7.2.2.2. Dietary Treatment of Phenylketonuria

It is abundantly clear that early institution of a phenylalanine-restricted diet is of enormous benefit in classic PKU. Whereas most such children had IQ scores of less than 40 in the pretreatment era and languished in hospitals for the severely retarded, the vast majority of early and effectively treated children now grow and develop normally or near-normally. Outcome is related to age of diagnosis and institution of dietary treatment: the earlier the regimen is begun, the better the result. The "fine-tuning" of this therapeutic instrument is not at all simple, and questions remain. Since early diagnosis is important, how early is early enough? How long need dietary restriction be continued? What happens to PKU children when they grow up and have families of their own? Answers to these questions are emerging.

Since 1967, a collaborative study of PKU children treated dietarily has been ongoing in 15 centers in the United States. The primary objective of this study is to ascertain the physical, cognitive, and psychosocial consequences of dietary therapy for PKU children identified in newborn-screening programs. Systematic study of affected children and their sibs and parents has been undertaken, and results are now beginning to appear. In 1976, Dobson *et al.* (1976) reported the preliminary findings of the collaborative group with regard to intellectual performance of 36 PKU children treated at or before 4 months of age. When such children were between 4 and 6 years of age, their intellectual attainment, assessed by Stanford–Binet testing, was compared with that of their own non-PKU sibs matched carefully for age. The mean IQ of the PKU group was 94; that of their sib controls was 99 ($p<0.02$). In 24 of the 36 sib pairs, the test score of the PKU child was below that of the sib control. Since the only feature that appeared to distinguish the patients from the controls was the presence of PKU in one of each pair of sibs but not the other, these data suggest that there is a small degree of intellectual impairment in the treated PKU group—even when diet is instituted within the first 4 months. The explanation for this impairment is not at all clear. *In utero* damage, or subtle dietary indiscretions, or the necessity to begin treatment by 60 days of life rather than 120 days could all be playing a part. If these results are borne out by findings in the total patient group under investigation, they may show that early treatment can allow nearly but not absolutely maximal attainment of developmental potential—no small achievement indeed when one considers the status of such patients prior to the era of diet therapy.

Whereas there is no longer much disagreement about the efficacy of diet therapy for classic PKU, there is considerable controversy about how long such treatment should be continued. Some investigators argue that the disease exists for life, and that treatment should therefore be continued for life. Others say that brain development is essentially completed by 2–3 years of age, and that treatment can be discontinued thereafter with no significant deleterious consequences. Neither side has the data to support its position, and it will take many years before the matter is clarified. In this setting, it is gratifying to see the first randomized, control study of the effect of termination of the phenylalanine-restricted diet (Holtzman *et al.*, 1975). Ten PKU children, all treated from 1 month of age or less to 4 years of age, were randomized into two groups: those in whom dietary treatment would be continued and those in whom it would be terminated. The five children in each group were then followed serially for two additional years. As expected, the children in whom dietary restriction was terminated had far higher plasma phenylalanine concentrations at age 6 than did those in whom treatment was continued. No statistically significant differences between the groups in head circumference, height, or IQ were noted at age 6 years. It should be noted, however, that the mean IQ in the terminated group at age 6 was 99.8, compared with 103.6 in the treated group. At age 4, both groups had virtually identical means (102.6, terminated; 103, treated). Though the observed difference at age 6 years was not *statistically* significant, it is far too early to be sure that it is not *biologically* significant. Only more time and more such studies will resolve this vital question. We remain concerned that clinics throughout the United States are terminating diet therapy at 4–6 years of age *before* proof of the harmlessness of such a course has been presented. It would be unfortunate if the great advances in dietary management of PKU in the past 20 years were mitigated by impatient and imprudent dietary termination during the next 20 years.

7.2.2.3. Maternal Phenylketonuria

Although most untreated patients with classic PKU are profoundly retarded and fail to reproduce, it has been known for many years that occasional women with the disorder will reproduce (Scriver and Rosenberg, 1973). The non-PKU progeny of such affected women have done badly. One-fourth of the reported offspring had significant congenital anomalies involving many different systems. All have manifested some degree of intrauterine growth retardation, and more than 90% are distinctly retarded even though they are not themselves homozygous for the mutant gene. Perry *et al.* (1973) called attention to this problem most recently. They described a family in which four adult siblings had previously unrecognized and untreated PKU. Three were of normal intelligence; one was a college graduate. Two of these adults suffered major psychotic illnesses resulting in admission to mental hospitals. The three adult sibs who were females had given birth to nine non-PKU offspring, all of whom had variable but distinct intellectual impairment. These authors suggested that PKU should be excluded in all pregnant women by doing a blood or urine test. The implications of this situation go further, however. As more and more female patients with PKU diagnosed early and treated effectively reach adulthood, we must face the question of their reproductive potential. Should such women be placed on a phenylalanine-restricted diet before considering pregnancy or at least as soon as pregnancy is documented? Does the disturbing report of major psychiatric illness in those patients reported by Perry and co-workers who never received treatment mean that the risk of psychiatric problems may also be increased in PKU individuals treated early but not permanently? Answers to these questions are important if we are to assess the societal impact of this well-known disease and its now well-known treatment accurately, ethically, and humanely.

7.3. The γ-Glutamyl Cycle and 5-Oxoprolinuria

7.3.1. 5-Oxoprolinuria

5-Oxoprolinuria (pyroglutamic aciduria) was first described by Jellum *et al.* (1970) in a Norwegian male. Since then, six additional cases have been reported (Larsson and Mattson, 1976). When first described, this disease seemed most unusual in that its biochemical basis could not be explained by a block of any known metabolic pathway.

The first reported patient was a 19-year-old male. His major clinical findings were spastic tetraparesis, mental retardation (an IQ of 57), and metabolic acidosis. Additional neurologic abnormalities included such cerebellar dysfunctions as an intention tremor and an ataxic gait. During the neonatal period, he developed jaundice of unknown degree and was seriously ill for 2 weeks. Evidence of developmental retardation and neurologic deficit became apparent at 1–2 years of age. At 16 years of age, he began to have almost daily episodes of violent vomiting and developed hematemesis. Examination revealed a large esophageal hiatus hernia. After a successful operation, the vomiting lessened but did not disappear. Because of a prominent metabolic acidosis noted in this period, the patient's urine was analyzed for organic acids. A large amount of an unusual metabolite was detected and was identified by gas chromatography–mass spectrometry (GC-MS) as 5-oxoproline (pyroglutamic acid, pyrrolidonecarboxylic acid). The amount of 5-oxoproline excreted in the urine was enormously large, ranging from 24 to 35 g/day. Its concentration in cerebrospinal fluid was 30 mg/dl. Serum concentration of 5-oxoproline was initially calculated to be in the range of 5 mg/dl (Eldjarn *et al.*, 1972), but this was later shown to be erroneously low due to a calculation error, and the actual value was 50 mg/dl (Eldjarn *et al.*, 1972, 1973). Unfortunately, this calculation error and its attendant underestimation of the total body pool of 5-oxoproline misdirected early efforts at understanding this condition.

Clinical manifestations in the other reported patients have differed considerably. Three of seven patients have presented with neurologic symptoms. Chronic metabolic acidosis and an increased rate of hemolysis have been observed in most of the cases. Free amino acid concentrations in urine and blood are normal except for slight elevations of plasma aspartate, serine, glutamate, citrulline, glycine, and leucine. These increases are only up to 1.5 times the upper range of normal values.

5-Oxoproline (Fig. 2), is a ninhydrin-negative, acidic lactam of glutamic acid. It is known that 5-oxoproline is found at the N-terminus of several peptides and proteins, such as the H chain of γ-globulins, collagen, and TSH-releasing factor. Breakdown of these peptides, however, could not possibly account for the enormous amount of 5-oxoproline found in the urine of patients with 5-oxoprolinuria.

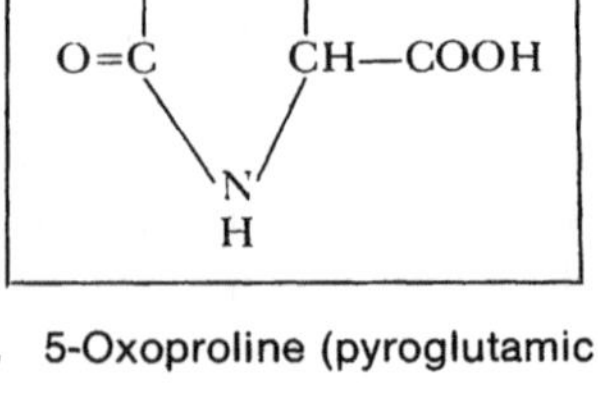

Fig. 2. 5-Oxoproline (pyroglutamic acid).

7.3.2. The γ-Glutamyl Cycle

At about this same time, Orlowski and Meister (1970) proposed independently a cycle consisting of five enzymatically catalyzed reactions that concern the transpeptidation of the γ-glutamyl moiety of glutathione (GSH) and its resynthesis. As shown in Fig. 3, the cycle was initially proposed as a possible enzymatic mechanism for the active transport of amino acids in several tissues, including kidney. γ-Glutamyltranspeptidase (GGTP) catalyzes the transfer of the γ-glutamyl moiety of glutathione to a wide spectrum of amino acids, resulting in the formation of γ-glutamyl dipeptides (Fig. 3, step 1). This enzyme is known to be distributed widely in many tissues, but kidney cortex has by far the highest specific activity. GGTP is localized in brush border membranes of kidney tubular cells (Albert *et al.*, 1961; Glenner and Folk, 1961; Booth and Kenney, 1974) and that of intestinal mucosa (Garvey *et al.*, 1976). Partial digestion of membrane vesicles prepared from pig, rat, and rabbit jejunal brush border with papain showed that GGTP resides on the luminal side of the

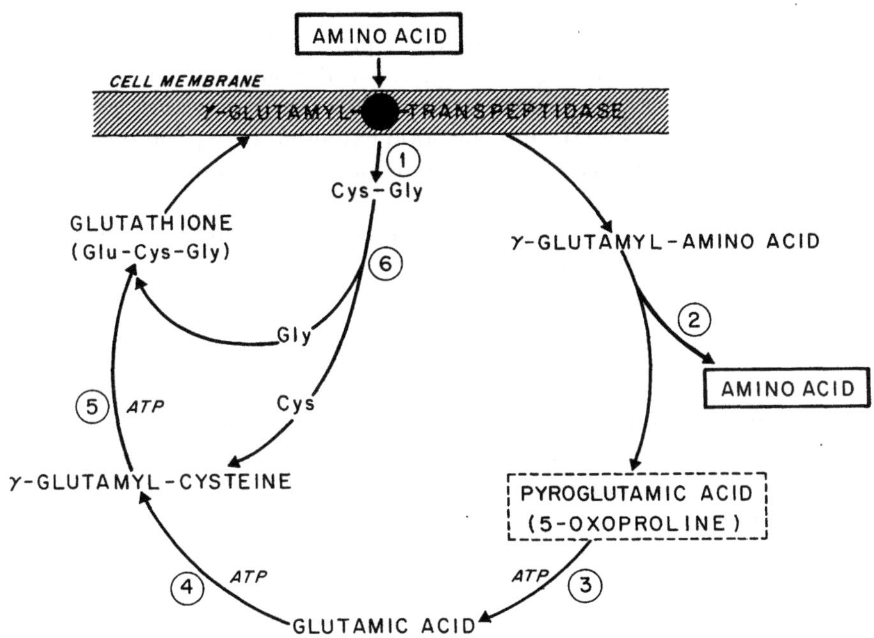

Fig. 3. The γ-glutamyl cycle, drawn to emphasize its possible involvement in transmembrane transport of amino acids. The circled numbers refer to the five enzymes that catalyze the depicted reactions: (1) γ-glutamyltranspeptidase (GGTP); (2) γ-glutamylcyclotransferase; (3) 5-oxoprolinase; (4) γ-glutamylcysteine synthetase; (5) glutathione synthetase.

membrane (Louvard *et al.,* 1975). γ-Glutamyl cyclotransferase, which catalyzes the release of an amino acid from γ-glutamyl dipeptides with the concomitant formation of 5-oxoproline (step 2), was already well characterized, as were γ-glutamylcysteine synthetase (step 4) and GSH synthetase (step 5). Each of the last three enzymes is found in the cytosol. Orlowski and Meister (1970) hypothesized that these four enzymatic reactions would form a cycle if one added a step in which 5-oxoproline was converted to glutamate (step 3). Soon thereafter, 5-oxoprolinase was demonstrated and purified from the soluble fraction of rat kidney, and was shown to catalyze formation of glutamate from 5-oxoproline (Van Der Werf *et al.,* 1971). Orlowski and Meister reasoned that if extracellular amino acids acted as the γ-glutamyl acceptor of the first reaction, the overall sequence of these five reactions could account for the stoichiometric transfer of amino acid from the outside of cells to the inside. They proposed further that GGTP was the long-sought "carrier" molecule (Meister, 1973). The requirement for ATP (3 molecules/cycle) seemed to account for the energy required for active transport. It is important to note that GSH is not a substrate for γ-glutamylcyclotransferase and was believed not to permeate cell membranes. Since the activities of GGTP and of the other enzymes are particularly great in kidney, they proposed that this cycle, named the *γ-glutamyl cycle,* was the biochemical mechanism by which kidney tubular cells reabsorb amino acids so effectively from glomerular filtrate. This concept was soon extended to explain the mechanism of amino acid transport in other tissues such as jejunal villous cells (Garvey *et al.,* 1976; Cornell and Meister, 1976), retina (Tate *et al.,* 1975), ciliary body and lens (Ross *et al.,* 1973), red cells (Palekar *et al.,* 1974), and seminal vesicle (DeLap *et al.,* 1975).

7.3.3. Biochemical Basis of 5-Oxoprolinuria

The interesting hypothesis just described was not received enthusiastically by other students of amino acid transport, since it does not explain, in and of itself, certain important features of amino acid transport in mammals such as sodium dependency and structural specificity. Nonetheless, the very existence of the cycle is important, since, from the time Meister's hypothesis was first published, it appeared likely that a dysfunction of such an active cyclic event would account for the enormous amounts of 5-oxoproline excreted in the urine of patients with 5-oxoprolinuria.

Based on the existence of a γ-glutamyl cycle, Eldjarn *et al.* (1972) carried out a series of extensive studies on the formation of 5-oxoproline in their patient with 5-oxoprolinuria. First, they measured urinary 5-oxoproline and other nitrogen-containing compounds (including ammonia, urea, uric acid, and creatinine) during several periods in which ammonium bicarbonate, a low-protein diet, or oral glutamate was given. Changes in the amount of administered nitrogen-containing compounds were reflected mostly by large changes in urea excretion, indicating that ureagenesis was intact. The amount of urinary 5-oxoproline excreted remained constant despite considerable variation in total ntirogen excretion. The excretion of a large amount of 5-oxoproline, even during a low-protein diet, excluded the possibility that exogenous glutamic acid or glutamine is the direct precursor of 5-oxoproline.

Eldjarn *et al.* (1972) also injected [^{14}C]5-oxoproline, L-[U-^{14}C]glutamate and L-[U-^{14}C]glutamine into the patient. The oxidation of [^{14}C]5-oxoproline to labeled CO_2 was very slow in the patient compared with that in controls, and 65% of the injected [^{14}C]5-oxoproline was excreted in his urine during the first 24 hr. In contrast, the patient oxidized [^{14}C]glutamate at a normal rate. These results seemed to suggest that the hydrolysis of 5-oxoproline to glutamate was defective in the patient. Unfortunately, this initial conclusion was wrong because of the gross underestimation of the total body pool of 5-oxoproline discussed earlier. After learning that the second reported patient with 5-oxoprolinuria from Sweden had 10 times more 5-oxoproline in serum than they had found, Eldjarn *et al.* (1973) reexamined their earlier data and found that in fact their patient, too, had a very high serum 5-oxoproline concentration, ranging from 50 to 65 mg/dl. With these new, correct values and with knowledge of the half-time of [^{14}C]5-oxoproline disappearance from plasma, they reestimated "the total extracellular 5-oxoproline pool" as well as the rate of synthesis. They found that the rate of synthesis in their patient was as much as 85 g/day, of which 35 g is daily excreted in urine. From further studies on the patient as well as controls, they concluded that the patient, like normal controls, was able to degrade 5-oxoproline to glutamate, and proposed that the 5-oxoprolinuria reflected an enormous overproduction of 5-oxoproline. A similar conclusion was reached the following year in the second reported patient from Sweden (Hagenfeldt *et al.*, 1974). Normal 5-oxoprolinase activity in fibroblast extracts from the first patient (Strömme and Eldjarn, 1972) was also in agreement with the overproduction hypothesis, but the biochemical basis for such exaggerated synthesis remained obscure.

The breakthrough came in 1974 as a result of a study by Wellner *et al.* (1974), who assayed four enzymes of the γ-glutamyl cycle (GSH synthetase, γ-glutamylcysteine synthetase, γ-glutamylcyclotransferase, and 5-oxoprolinase) in fibroblasts and placenta of the affected newborn sister of the second patient and in erythrocytes of both affected sibs. GSH synthetase activity was only 2–10% of that in controls, whereas activities of the other three enzymes were normal. GSH concentration in the patients' erythrocytes was less than 1% of normal. They suggested that the γ-glutamyl cycle in these patients continued to function with only four enzymes because γ-glutamylcysteine is also a good substrate for γ-glutamyltranspeptidase. They also speculated that γ-glutamylcysteine is normally protected from the action of γ-glutamylcyclotransferase either by compartmentalization within the cells or by a close spatial linkage between the two synthetases. With the marked deficiency of GSH synthetase, however, unprotected γ-glutamylcysteine would be subject to the action of γ-glutamylcyclotransferase. This would lead to a futile cycle of γ-glutamylcysteine synthesis followed by its breakdown to 5-oxoproline and cysteine. They also speculated that GSH normally exerts feedback inhibition on the rate of γ-glutamylcysteine synthesis (Jackson, 1969; Richman and Meister, 1975).

Larsson *et al.* (1976) also studied GSH synthetase in erythrocytes from these two patients and confirmed that their activities were 1–2% of normal. The values for their parents were approximately 50% of the mean of 20 normal controls. The mutant enzyme did not differ significantly from normal enzyme in its affinity for substrates or in its Mg^{2+} requirement. Larsson and Mattson (1976) further pursued the mechanism of 5-oxoproline overproduction in this disease. They assayed 5-oxoproline production from glutamate using cell-free extracts of erythrocytes as an enzyme source. Addition of ATP, Mg^{2+}, and α-aminobutyrate was necessary for this activity. α-Aminobutyrate and γ-glutamyl-α-aminobutyrate had been shown to be good substrates for γ-glutamylcysteine synthetase and GSH synthetase, respectively (Meister, 1974). Therefore, these stable artificial substrates were used in place of cysteine and γ-glutamylcysteine in assays of these enzymes. The conversion of glutamate to 5-oxoproline occurred in two steps: γ-glutamyl-γ-aminobutyrate formation, and its hydrolysis. This was evidenced by identification of the γ-glutamyldipeptide as an intermediate in the reaction mixture. These steps are presumably catalyzed by γ-glutamylcysteine synthetase and 5-oxoprolinase, respectively. Since glycine was omitted in this system, γ-glutamyl-α-aminobutyryl-glycine, a tripeptide equivalent to GSH, was not synthesized, but rather the γ-glutamyl-α-aminobutyrate was subject to the action of γ-glutamylcyclotransferase. They found that extracts of erythrocytes from controls and patients with 5-oxoprolinuria had a similar activity of 5-oxoproline production. When glycine (5–20 mM) was added to the system with dialyzed extracts of control erythrocytes, 5-oxoproline formation was inhibited by as much as 80%. This inhibition by glycine was not observed with similar tissue preparations from patients with 5-oxoprolinuria. This difference is presumably due to the diversion of γ-glutamyl-α-aminobutyrate from γ-glutamylcyclotransferase action to that of GSH synthetase.

The lack of this inhibition in the patients' tissues is in accord with the documented deficiency of GSH synthetase activity.

The formation of 5-oxoproline was also inhibited about 50% by 5 mM GSH, a concentration similar to its intracellular value. The inhibition by GSH was greatly augmented by keeping GSH in a reduced form with addition of NADH and GSH reductase, or with dithiothreitol. The addition of dithiothreitol alone or NADH plus GSH reductase alone to crude homogenates of control cells also resulted in a small but significant inhibition of the 5-oxoproline formation. This inhibition by the reducing agents alone is presumably due to the reduction of a small amount of GSH naturally present in the enzyme source. Such inhibition was not observed with crude homogenates of the patient's erythrocytes.

Thus, the studies by Wellner and co-workers and Larsson and co-workers convincingly demonstrated that patients with 5-oxoprolinuria have a deficiency of GSH synthetase, and that the urinary excretion of an enormous amount of 5-oxoproline in these patients is due to its overproduction through a futile cycle of synthesis and breakdown of γ-glutamylcysteine. The futile cycle is initiated by a lack of feedback inhibition of γ-glutamylcysteine synthesis by GSH.

These findings in patients with 5-oxoprolinuria seem to give strong support to the sequential functional relationship (Fig. 3) from γ-glutamylcyclotransferase (step 2) to 5-oxoprolinase (step 3), γ-glutamylcysteine synthetase (step 4), and GSH synthetase (step 5), but they do not necessarily confirm the entire concept of the γ-glutamyl cycle as proposed by Meister. Specifically, the functional role of the only membrane-bound enzyme, GGTP, and its relationship to the other enzymes *in situ* are neither supported nor denied by the evidence from these studies. As discussed previously, there is no evidence of abnormal amino acid transport in any one of the patients with 5-oxoprolinuria (Jellum *et al.,* 1970; Larsson *et al.,* 1974). If the γ-glutamyl cycle is a major means of amino acid transport, one would expect to see an inhibition of amino acid transport in these patients, since GSH is not available for the transpeptidation reaction noted in step 1. Wellner *et al.* (1974) offered an explanation for the lack of abnormal amino acid transport by proposing that γ-glutamylcysteine is a good substrate for GGTP and could serve as a γ-glutamyl donor in place of GSH in this reation.

7.3.4. Evidence For and Against the Role of the γ-Glutamyl Cycle in Amino Acid Transport

In regard to the possible role of the γ-glutamyl cycle in amino acid transport, Meister and associates presented a number of kinds of experimental evidence that, they believe, support their hypothesis. These include the turnover rate of GSH in mouse kidney (Sekura and Meister, 1974), the finding of a significant amount of labeled 5-oxoproline in kidney and liver after administration of labeled L-glutamate to rats (Meister and Tate, 1976; Orlowski and Wilk, 1975), and the 5-oxoproline accumulation in mice treated with 2-imidazolidone-4-carboxylate, an effective competitive inhibitor of 5-oxoprolinase (Van Der Werf *et al.*, 1974). These mice accumulated several times more 5-oxoproline when amino acids were given with the inhibitor than when they were given the inhibitor alone. Topological distribution of GGTP in jejunal mucosa is also consistent with a transport role. A high activity in villus tip (the site for amino acid absorption) and a low activity in the crypt region are noteworthy (Cornell and Meister, 1976; Garvey *et al.*, 1976). All this evidence is circumstantial, however, and there is still a total lack of direct evidence to support the role of the γ-glutamyl cycle in amino acid transport.

On the other hand, there are a number of observations that do not support the role of the cycle in amino acid transport. First, there are observations on a patient with glutathionuria who is deficient in GGTP activity in fibroblasts and in serum. The GSH concentrations in his serum and urine were 4 and 1000 times normal, respectively (Goodman *et al.*, 1971; Schulman *et al.*, 1975). Schulman and co-workers measured amino acid concentrations in serum and urine and calculated percentage tubular reabsorption of individual amino acids. These clearance parameters all fell within or very close to the normal range. They also showed that the uptake of amino acids by fibroblasts of this patient was normal (Pellefigue *et al.*, 1976). They argued from their data that GGTP is not likely to be a mediator of amino acid transport in man.

Young *et al.* (1975a, 1976) studied amino acid transport in red cells from two mutant sheep of two different breeds (Merino and Finnish Landrace), both of which have congenital erythrocyte GSH deficiency. The GSH concentrations in erythrocytes were 27 and 42% of controls, respectively. The low GSH concentration in the mutant Merino sheep is caused by a deficiency of γ-glutamylcysteine synthetase, but amino acid concentrations and the uptake of glycine and cysteine in erythrocytes were normal in this mutant. In the mutant Finnish sheep, γ-glutamylcysteine synthetase and GSH synthetase were both normal, but the uptake of a number of amino acids such as L-alanine, cysteine, α-aminobutyrate, serine, and lysine was low. Since α-aminobutyrate and alanine inhibited lysine uptake in normal Finnish sheep, they concluded that only one transport system is deficient in the Finnish mutant, and that the diminished GSH concentration is probably due to the diminished availability of cysteine. They also studied the change of GSH concentrations during amino acid uptake in rabbit erythrocytes thought to have a high activity of

GGTP (Young *et al.*, 1975b). GSH concentration did not significantly change during amino acid uptake. From these studies on red cells of mutant sheep and those of the rabbit, they concluded that the γ-glutamyl cycle does not participate in amino acid transport in these cells.

It should be noted, however, that evidence from studies on fibroblasts of the glutathionuria patient and also those on erythrocytes of mutant sheep and normal rabbit does not constitute direct evidence against the γ-glutamyl cycle hypothesis. This cycle was initially proposed specifically as a mechanism for active amino acid transport in kidney and several other tissues that have high GGTP activity, not as a universal mechanism for all tissues (Meister, 1973). The diminished GSH concentration in erythrocytes of the mutant sheep are also not as low as those observed in patients with 5-oxoprolinuria. It must also be pointed out that GGTP activity in kidney was not measured in the patient with glutathionuria.

More recently, very striking but puzzling data have been reported by the Norwegian group. They confirmed that erythrocytes from their first case of 5-oxoprolinuria also contained no detectable amount of GSH. GSH synthetase activity was 1.5% of control. His erythrocytes, however, are loaded with extremely large amounts of free amino acids, most of them in concentrations 5–100 times normal (Marstein *et al.*, 1976). In contrast, there was no amino acid accumulation in skeletal muscle, in which GSH was reduced to 3% of normal. They attributed the extraordinary loading of free amino acids in red cells of their patient to a possible absence of substrate inhibition of GGTP activity and to excessive production of γ-glutamylcysteine as an alternate substrate. They took this observation as strong evidence for a role of the γ-glutamyl cycle in amino acid transport. They attributed the lack of amino acid accumulation in muscle to the small but significant amount of GSH present, which might have exerted sufficient substrate inhibition. Unfortunately, GGTP activity was not measured to support their contention. Beutler (1976) argued, however, that the conclusion of the Norwegian workers was unlikely, since erythrocytes (human, rabbit) had no detectable GGTP activity when leukocytes were completely removed from the preparation (Srivastava *et al.*, 1976).

In summary, it may be resonable to conclude at present that there is a cycle of several enzymatic reactions in tissues that are concerned with the synthesis and breakdown of GSH. It appears very likely that inherited deficiency of GSH synthetase causes 5-oxoprolinuria by formation of a futile cycle of γ-glutamylcysteine synthesis and breakdown due to a lack of feedback inhibition of γ-glutamylcysteine synthetase by GSH. No clear conclusion can yet be drawn about the role of the γ-glutamyl cycle in amino acid transport. Strong direct evidence for or against this hypothesis is needed to end the controversy. Finally, a role of GSH and GGTP in secretory processes was recently proposed (Binkley and Wiesemann, 1975). They claim that the secretory component of secretory IgA is identical with GGTP. This new hypothesis must now be tested rigorously.

7.4. Jamaican Vomiting Sickness and Glutaric Aciduria Type II: Similar Organic Acidurias with Different Etiologies

7.4.1. Jamaican Vomiting Sickness

Jamaican vomiting sickness has been known to occur endemically in Jamaica since as early as 1875 (Bressler *et al.*, 1969). Ingestion of the arillus of unripe ackee, a local fruit, had been identified since early in this century as a source of this disease. Cooked ripe ackee fruit, on the other hand, is a staple in the Jamaicans' diet and is believed to be nontoxic. The disease occurs prominently in children from 1 to 6 years of age, but it may also occur in adults. It is characterized by a sudden onset of violent vomiting and retching accompanied by a feeling of intense weakness. These symptoms appear from 2 hr to 3 days after the ingestion of unripe ackee. The patient later becomes prostrate, and body temperature may fall to subnormal values. After some period of prostration followed by apparent improvement, a second bout of vomiting occurs, and this is usually followed by convulsions, lethargy, coma, and death. Mortality rates reached 80% in the past. At necropsy, extensive diffuse fatty degeneration of liver and kidneys is invariably found. The lipid accumulation in the liver is of a specific type. Small fat droplets, which occur without zonal predilection, are characteristic, and necrotic foci are not found. Glycogen granules in hepatic parenchymal cells are depleted. These histological findings are very similar to those later described in patients with Reye's syndrome.

In 1953, Jelliffe and Stuart (1954) made an important observation. In five patients with this disease, blood glucose concentrations were invariably low, with values ranging from 3 to 19 mg/dl. Infusion of glucose was effective, however, in only three of them. The clinical response in the other two patients was minimal, and both died. Jelliffe and Stuart attributed the poor response to glucose infusion to the time elapsed before the institution of therapy, during which irreversible changes might have occurred in the brain due to hypoglycemia. They also suggested that there might be other, as yet undiscovered, biochemical derangements. Another important laboratory observation was that these patients were acidotic but not ketotic (Hill, 1952). In retrospect, this finding was suggestive of severe organic acidemia. Liver function tests, such as serum bilirubin and serum albumin, were normal, but measurements of blood ammonia and serum transaminases were not reported.

Although it was long suspected, the association of unripe ackee with this disease was not scientifically substantiated until the isolation of two toxins, hypoglycins A and B, from arilli and seeds of unripe ackee by Hassal and Reyle (1955). Hypoglycin A in a single dose induces acute symptoms such as severe hypoglycemia, vomiting, prostration, coma, and death in laboratory animals. Severe histologic changes such as depletion of hepatic glycogen and fatty infiltration of viscera, very much like the changes seen in patients with Jamaican vomiting sickness, are also observed.

7.4.1.1. Metabolic Effects of Hypoglycin

The chemistry and biochemistry of hypoglycins were pursued vigorously in the late 1950's (Bressler *et al.,* 1969). It was soon established that hypoglycin A (now referred to simply as *hypoglycin*) is an unusual amino acid, L-α-amino-methylene-cyclopropylpropionic acid, that is metabolized to its toxic form, methylenecyclopropylacetic acid (MCPA), in tissues (Fig. 4). Hypoglycin B is the γ-glutamyl conjugate of hypoglycin, and is believed to be less toxic than the nonconjugated moiety.

During the early biochemical investigations of the mode of action of hypoglycin, efforts were directed toward elucidating its effects on intermediary metabolism of carbohydrate, fatty acids, and amino acids. Particular emphasis was placed on the mechanism of its potent hypoglycemic effect. Results from these investigations indicated that glycolysis was somewhat enhanced, whereas gluconeogenesis and fatty acid oxidation

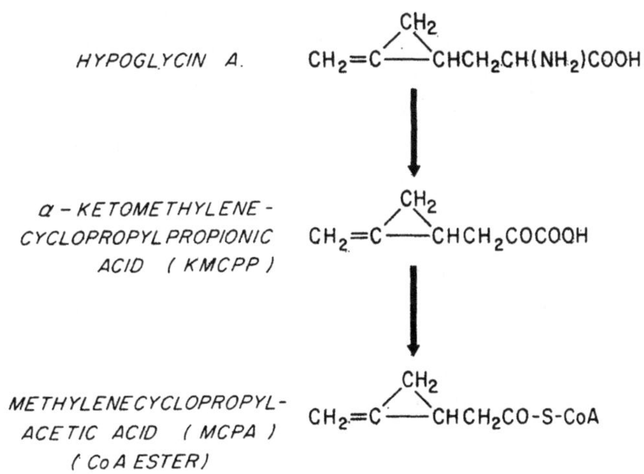

Fig. 4. Structure and metabolism of hypoglycin A. The parent amino acid, containing methylene and cyclopropyl groups, is catabolized successively to its keto analogue and CoA ester.

were severely inhibited. The hypoglycemic action was not mediated by increased insulin secretion.

In the 1960's, major efforts were made to elucidate the mechanisms by which hypoglycin inhibited fatty acid oxidation (Bressler *et al.,* 1969). von Holt and Benedict (1959) observed that the oxidation *in vivo* of [1-^{14}C]palmitate was inhibited in hypoglycin-treated rats, whereas that of [1-^{14}C]octanoate was not inhibited. In 1967, Enteman and Bressler (1967) reported that myocardial homogenates from hypoglycin-treated mice had an impaired capacity to oxidize palmitate, while their ability to oxidize hexanoate was normal. von Holt *et al.* (1966) showed that MCPA inhibited oxidation of [1-^{14}C]myristate (14 carbons), palmitate (16 carbons), and stearate (18 carbons) by rat liver mitochondria by 30–45% but did not inhibit the oxidation of fatty acids with shorter chain lengths (4 to 10 carbons). These data were in sharp contrast to the observation by McKerns *et al.* (1960) that [1-^{14}C]butyrate and [1-^{14}C]palmitate oxidation *in vivo* were both inhibited in hypoglycin-treated rats to about 40% of control values. It is still not clear why these three groups obtained such discrepant results from similar studies, but as will be shown later, the differences are of crucial importance in view of recent data.

von Holt and Bressler explored the mechanism of hypoglycin action by contrasting its effects on fatty acids of different chain length. There are several discrete steps in fatty acid oxidation at which fatty acids with different chain lengths are handled by different enzymes or totally different mechanisms. These include mechanisms of uptake by mitochondria; action of thiokinases, which convert free fatty acids to the corresponding acyl-CoAs; and activity of acyl-CoA dehydrogenases. von Holt *et al.* (1966) proposed that acyl-CoA dehydrogenase is the likely site of hypoglycin action. They observed a specific effect of riboflavin in preventing the development of hypoglycin poisoning in rats and mice. Since there are three acyl-CoA dehydrogenases, G (green), Y_1, and Y_2, which are known to catalyze dehydrogenation of acyl-CoAs with 4–8 carbons, those with 8–12 carbons, and those with 8–16 carbons, respectively (Green and Allman, 1968), and since each of these acyl-CoA dehydrogenases is a flavin-dependent enzyme, von Holt *et al.* deduced that the protection afforded by riboflavin pointed to the dehydrogenases.

Bressler and associates took a different view. They hypothesized that MCPA inhibits carnitine-dependent transport of long-chain fatty acids into mitochondria. It had earlier been established that (−)carnitine is required for the uptake of long-chain fatty acids by mitochondria, but not for that of short-chain fatty acids. Enteman and Bressler (1967) added (−)carnitine to incubation media containing [^{14}C]palmitate and myocardial homogenates from hypoglycin-treated mice and noted full restoration of palmitate oxidation. Corredor *et al.* (1967) observed that the effects of 4-pentenoic acid, a synthetic, biologically active analogue of

MCPA that lacks the cyclopropyl structure, could be reversed by the additon of (−)carnitine. They also showed that inhibition of gluconeogenesis in pigeon liver homogenates by 4-pentenoic acid was partly prevented by the addition of CoA or carnitine, but was fully prevented by the simultaneous addition of both substances (Corredor *et al.*, 1969).

Based on these observations, they formulated the following hypothesis. MCPA and 4-pentenoic acid both form unmetabolizable or slowly metabolizable derivatives with carnitine and CoA, thereby lowering tissue levels of free carnitine and CoA. The unavailability of these cofactors results secondarily in the observed inhibition of long-chain-fatty-acid oxidation. The oxidation of short-chain fatty acids, which does not require carnitine, is less affected or entirely spared. Finally, gluconeogenesis is inhibited as a result of the insufficient production of acetyl-CoA and NADH from long-chain-fatty-acid oxidation (Bressler *et al.*, 1969). Williamson *et al.* (1970) supported this hypothesis.

Since the work of Corredor *et al.* (1967) discussed above, it was assumed that the mode of action of 4-pentenoic acid is identical to that of MCPA. Thus, for several years, all the experiments in this field were done with 4-pentenoic acid. The important structural difference between MCPA and 4-pentenoic acid, namely, the presence of a cyclopropyl structure, was completely neglected. Furthermore, no attention was paid to the fact that the hypoglycemic action of hypoglycin lasts much longer than that of 4-pentenoic acid.

7.4.1.2. Inhibition of Acyl-CoA Dehydrogenases by Methylenecyclopropylacetic Acid

Tanaka *et al.* (1971) initiated a series of studies on the mode of action of hypoglycin with a new approach. Several years prior, they described an inborn error of leucine metabolism, isovaleric acidemia (Tanaka, 1975a). Patients with this disease continuously excreted a large amount of isovalerylglycine and developed, episodically, accumulation of large quantities of isovaleric acid in serum (up to 30 mg/dl). The ability of patients' leukocytes to oxidize [1-^{14}C]isovaleric acid was diminished. Since no significant accumulation of the next intermediate in the leucine pathway, β-methylcrotonic acid (Fig. 5), or of other short-chain fatty acids including isobutyrate (from valine), butyrate, and α-methylbutyrate (from isoleucine) was observed, they proposed that isovaleryl CoA is dehydrogenated by a specific dehydrogenase, distinct from the green acyl-CoA dehydrogenase (G), and that patients with isovaleric acidemia have a deficiency of this isovaleryl CoA dehydrogenase. Tanaka *et al.* (1976b) later showed that the ability of their patients' fibroblasts to oxidize [2-^{14}C]leucine was less than 2% of that in controls. In these experiments, [^{14}C]isovalerate accumulated in the incubation medium with the patients' cells, but not

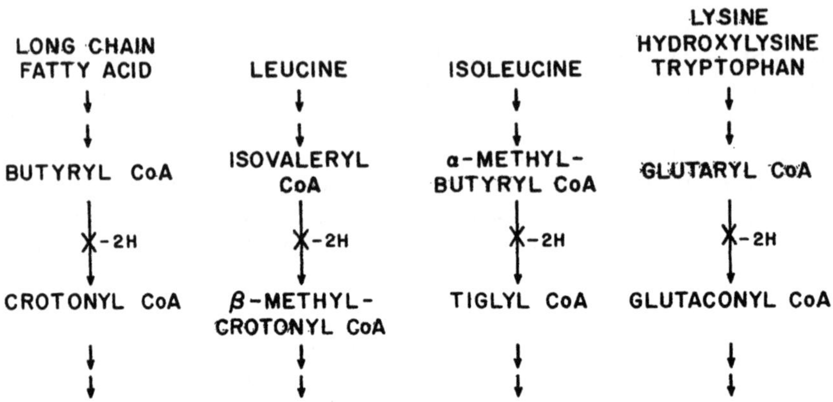

Fig. 5. Metabolic sequences for fatty acids and amino acids the catabolism of which proceeds via formation of acyl-CoA esters and their degradation by different acyl-CoA dehydrogenases. (X) Proposed metabolic blocks in Jamaican vomiting sickness and in glutaric aciduria type II.

with control cells. Direct assay of isovaleryl CoA dehydrogenase activity in crude cell homogenates was not possible, however, due to nonspecific reduction of artificial electron acceptors needed for the dehydrogenase assay.

To characterize isovaleryl CoA dehydrogenase activity further, Tanaka and colleagues sought an agent that might inhibit this enzyme specifically, and chose to examine hypoglycin. Overall oxidation of leucine by rat liver slices was inhibited by hypoglycin at some step beyond isovaleryl CoA formation, but precise localization of the inhibition was not accomplished. Oxidation of isoleucine and of valine, however, was not inhibited in these experiments (Tanaka, 1975a). Tanaka *et al.* (1971) speculated that leucine oxidation might be specifically inhibited by hypoglycin or its metabolites at the isovaleryl CoA dehydrogenase step, since the chemical structure of methylenecyclopropylacetyl CoA is very similar to that of isovaleryl CoA. They first tested this hypothesis *in vitro,* using DL-[2-^{14}C]leucine as a substrate and rat liver slices as an enzyme source. Inhibition of isovaleryl CoA dehydrogenase, coupled with activity of glycine-*N*-acylase, would theoretically yield isovalerylglycine as a product. They showed that this was in fact the case. Leucine oxidation to CO_2 was inhibited dramatically by 0.7 mM α-ketomethylenecyclopropylpropionic acid, the keto analogue of hypoglycin, and the labeled inhibitory product was recovered almost quantitatively as isovalerylglycine. Oxidation of isoleucine was also inhibited at its corresponding stage, α-methylbutyryl CoA dehydrogenation, but the extent of inhibition was less than that observed with leucine. Valine oxidation was not inhibited. The observed inhibition of isovaleryl CoA dehydrogenase activity was not the result of depletion of cofactors such as CoA or carnitine, for, if this had been the case, valine oxidation too would have been effected. Rather, it was the result of direct interaction between inhibitor and enzyme. These results from *in vitro* experiments were confirmed by *in vivo* loading with combinations of hypoglycin and branched-chain amino acids.

They also investigated in rats the time course of accumulation of branched-chain pentanoic acids (isovaleric and α-methylbutyric) in blood after a single dose (100 mg/kg) of hypoglycin A (Tanaka *et al.*, 1972). The concentration of branched pentanoic acids peaked at 45 mg/dl (800 times normal) 24 hr after administration. The ataxia and prostration observed in the rats during this period correlated well with the blood concentration of branched pentanoic acids. The results of analyses of serum short-chain fatty acids were similar to those in patients with isovaleric acidemia, but important differences existed. Small quantities of butyric, hexanoic, and methylenecyclopropylacetic acids were found in hypoglycin-treated rats, but not in the sera from patients with isovaleric acidemia. The other significant difference was that although the major peak of the branched pentanoic acids from the rat behaved as a single peak on gas chromatography, it actually consisted of two isomers, isovaleric and α-methylbutyric acids, with the former being 56% and the latter 44% as assessed by mass spectral analysis. In the sera of patients with isovaleric acidemia, isovaleric acid was the sole component (Tanaka and Yu, 1973).

Tanaka (1972) analyzed urines from hypoglycin-treated rats in search of isovalerylglycine, another clue to inhibition *in vivo* of isovaleryl CoA dehydrogenase activity. In fact, he detected a large amount of this compound, but also found several unusual organic acids in enormously large amounts. These compounds were not detected in significant amounts in urines from control or 4-pentenoic-acid-treated rats. These unusual metabolites were identified as aliphatic dicarboxylic acids with 5–10 carbons. Four were saturated compounds: glutarate (5 carbons), adipate (6 carbons), suberate (8 carbons), and sebacate (10 carbons). Three others were unsaturated dicarboxylic acids with 8 and 10 carbons. Hypoglycin was recovered almost quantitatively as MCPA-glycine, the end product. Butyrylglycine was also identified in large amounts (Tanaka, 1975b). Glutarate is produced from precursors distinctly different from those of other dicarboxylic acids. It has been shown by *in vivo* and *in vitro* studies using ^{14}C-labeled precursors that glutarate is produced by an inhibition of the metabolism of lysine (Tanaka, 1972) and tryptophan (Tanaka and Kerley, 1975) at the step of glutaryl CoA dehydrogenase (Fig. 5), not by the chain-shortening of adipate or the longer dicarboxylates. It should be mentioned that Tanaka and Kerley (1975) demonstrated that hypoglycin exhibits a strong synergistic hypoglycemic effect with tryptophan and lysine, the precursors of glutaryl CoA.

These workers also showed that glutaryl CoA inhibits the transmitochondrial malate shuttle, a key step in gluconeogenesis. Thus, they concluded that the accumulation of glutaryl CoA is one of the contributing factors to the hypoglycemic action of hypoglycin. This conclusion seems to be supported by the finding of severe hypoglycemia (12 mg/dl) seen in a patient with glutaric aciduria (Goodman *et al.*, 1977). The metabolic basis for the formation of the dicarboxylic acids with medium chain lengths, especially those with unsaturated bonds, is yet to be elucidated. They are probably produced from long-chain monocarboxylic acids such as palmitate and oleate. At present, however, it is not known whether these are first converted to dicarboxylic acids of the same chain length by ω-oxidation (due to depletion of carnitine) and then shortened by β-oxidation from both ends, or, alternatively, whether they are first oxidized to shorter-chain fatty acids and then ω-oxidized at these steps because of the inhibition of β-oxidation. Judging from the positions of double bonds in the unsaturated dicarboxylic acids, the former is more likely (Tanaka, 1972).

The studies by Tanaka and co-workers indicated that MCPA directly inhibits several acyl-CoA dehydrogenases, including those that oxidize isovaleryl CoA, butyryl CoA, and glutaryl CoA. These results were later confirmed by Billington *et al.* (1974) and Osmundsen and Sherratt (1975). Using partially purified rabbit liver enzymes, Kean (1976) showed that butyryl CoA dehydrogenase was strongly inhibited by MCPA-CoA, but palmityl CoA dehydrogenation was not. Both Sherratt and associates and Kean suggested that overall oxidation of palmitate was impaired due to the inhibition of oxidation it undergoes when shortened to 4–6 carbons (Fig. 5). It should be mentioned that the acyl-CoA dehydrogenase assays in these studies were done using artificial electron acceptors. In the natural state, electron-transferring flavoprotein (ETF), a flavoprotein with a molecular weight of 70,000, accepts hydrogen atoms from the substrates (Fig. 6). Therefore, MCPA-CoA inhibited the acyl-CoA dehydrogenases and not ETF.

7.4.1.3. Recent Studies on Jamaican Vomiting Sickness

Despite this substantial progress in understanding the mode of action of hypoglycin, detailed investigations of patients with Jamaican vomiting sickness have rarely been reported in the past 20 years. Evidence that

$$\mathrm{R{-}CH_2{-}CH_2{-}CO{-}CoA + ETF \xrightarrow[\text{DEHYDROGENASE}]{\text{ACYL CoA}} R{-}CH{=}CH{-}CO{-}CoA + H_2{-}ETF}$$

Fig. 6. General mechanism of acyl-CoA dehydrogenase reactions. (ETF) Electron-transferring flavoprotein.

directly links hypoglycin to this disease was therefore lacking. Neither hypoglycin and its metabolites nor the unusual dicarboxylic acids known to be produced by the action of hypoglycin had been identified in body fluids of patients. Tanaka *et al.* (1976a,c) recently extended their work to evaluation of urine from two patients with this disease. These patients had typical symptoms, and both of them died. In urines from these patients, dicarboxylic acids such as glutarate, adipate, suberate, sebacate, and unsaturated dicarboxylic acids with 8 and 10 carbons were detected in large quantities. Small but significant amounts of MCPA were also found in the urine. These two lines of evidence demonstrate convincingly that the intake of hypoglycin in unripe ackee is the cause of Jamaican vomiting sickness.

There were, however, a few significant differences in urinary metabolites in these patients compared with those in hypoglycin-treated rats. Although short-chain fatty acids such as isobutyric, *n*-butyric, isovaleric, and *n*-hexanoic acids accumulated up to 23 times the normal value in the blood of patients with vomiting sickness, the magnitude and specificity of increase in these short-chain fatty acids were not nearly as marked as the accumulation of isovaleric and α-methylbutyric acids in hypoglycin-treated rats. Furthermore, large amounts of ethylmalonic acid were found in the urine of patients, but no marked increase in this metabolite was found in urine from hypoglycin-treated rats. Ethylmalonic acid is known to be synthesized in mammals by two different pathways: carboxylation of butyryl CoA, and metabolism from isoleucine via 2-ethylhydracrylic acid. Since there was no appreciable increase of ethylhydracrylic acid in these two patients and the second route from isoleucine plays only a minor role in the formation of ethylmalonic acid, it can be assumed that the excessive ethylmalonic acid was produced by carboxylation of butyryl CoA.

They also analyzed urines from several patients with Reye's syndrome. Since the original description of Reye's syndrome in 1963, some pediatricians in Jamaica have suspected that Jamaican vomiting sickness may be identical to Reye's syndrome because clinical manifestations and histological findings are so similar in the two diseases. Urine samples from patients with Reye's syndrome, however, contained none of the dicarbosylic acids seen in Jamaican vomiting sickness. Thus, Reye's syndrome and Jamaican vomiting sickness are different conditions.

7.4.2. Glutaric Aciduria Type II

In 1976, a study on a newborn baby who died 44 hr after birth due to extreme hypoglycemia (5 mg/dl) and severe metabolic acidosis was reported by Przyrembel *et al.* (1976) from Germany. This infant's urine contained massive amounts of urinary organic acids, with a pattern almost identical to that found in patients with Jamaican vomiting sickness. Dicarboxylic acids including ethylmalonic, glutaric, adipic, suberic, and sebacic acids and unsaturated dicarboxylic acids with 8 or 10 carbons were found. Short-chain fatty acids such as isobutyric, isovaleric, and butyric acids were also found in abundance. The amount of glutarate, however, was by far the largest single component (11.8 mg/mg creatinine). Other dicarboxylic acids were present at about one-tenth the value of glutarate. These workers also showed that $^{14}CO_2$ production from [1,5-^{14}C]glutarate, [U-^{14}C]valine, [U-^{14}C]isoleucine, and α-[U-^{14}C]ketoisovalerate from intact, cultured fibroblasts was about 10–20% of control values, while that for [U-^{14}C]leucine approached 50% of normal. This disease was named *glutaric aciduria type II* to distinguish it from patients with glutaric aciduria who excreted mainly glutaric, glutaconic, and β-hydroxyglutaric acids (Goodman *et al.*, 1975; Stokke *et al.*, 1975). The abnormality in the latter patients is confined to the glutarate pathway and appears to be due to a deficiency of glutaconyl CoA decarboxylase. In contrast, the patient with glutaric aciduria type II seems to have defective activities of multiple medium-chain acyl-CoA dehydrogenases, judging from the similarity to Jamaican vomiting sickness.

Since the patient with glutaric aciduria type II had a sib who also died a few hours after birth, it is quite likely that this represents a hereditary metabolic disease. We must therefore seek a single mutation that might cause such inhibition of multiple enzyme reactions. The enzymatic reactions that are inhibited in this patient are all dehydrogenases for different acyl-CoAs. Clinical and enzymologic studies indicate that these acyl-CoA dehydrogenases are specific (Green and Allman, 1968; Besrat *et al.*, 1969). Thus, Przyrembel *et al.* (1976) speculated that these several dehydrogenases may have a common protein component essential for their function, and that this component is deficient in their patient. They also mentioned, as another general mechanism, lack of a common flavin coenzyme due to impaired vitamin transport or impaired coenzyme synthesis. It is important to note in this regard that other flavin enzymes such as pyruvate dehydrogenase seem to be intact in this patinet. It is also tempting to speculate that a single electron-transferring flavoprotein (ETF) functions for all these acyl-CoA dehydrogenases, and that ETF is deficient in this patient. Further studies with cultured cells from this patient may yield valuable information in this regard.

References

Albert, Z., Orlowski, M., and Szewczuk, A., 1961, Histochemical demonstration of gamma-glutamyltranspeptidase, *Nature (London)* **191**:767.

Bartholomé, K., Lutz, P., and Bickel, H., 1975, Determination of phenylalanine hydroxylase activity in patients with phenylketonuria and hyperphenylalaninemia, *Pediatr. Res.* **9**:899.

Besrat, A., Polan, C. E., and Henderson, L. M., 1969, Mammalian metabolism of glutaric acid, *J. Biol. Chem.* **244**:1461.

Beutler, E., 1976, Glutathione deficiency, pyroglutamic acidemia and amino acid transport, *N. Engl. J. Med.* **295**:441.

Billington, D., Kean, E. A., Osmundsen, H., and Sherratt, H. S. A., 1974, Inhibition of butyryl CoA dehydrogenase and isovaleryl CoA dehydrogenase in rat liver mitochondria by hypoglycin metabolites, *Int. Res. Commun. Syst. (Biochem. Pharmacol.)* **2**:1712.

Binkley, F., and Wiesemann, M. L., 1975, Glutathione and gamma glutamyl transferase in secretory process, *Life Sci.* **17**:1359.

Booth, A. G., and Kenney, A. J., 1974, A rapid method for the preparation of microvilli from rabbit kidney, *Biochem J.* **142**:575.

Bressler, R., Corredor, C., and Brendel, K., 1969, Hypoglycin and hypoglycin-like compounds, *Pharmacol. Rev.* **21**:105.

Cornell, J., and Meister, A., 1976, Glutathione and γ-glutamyl cycle enzymes in crypt and villus tip cells of rat jejunal mucosa, *Proc. Natl. Acad. Sci. U.S.A.* **73**:420.

Corredor, C., Brendel, K., and Bressler, R., 1967, Studies of the mechanism of the hypoglycemic action of 4-pentenoic acid, *Proc. Natl. Acad. Sci. U.S.A.* **58**:2299.

Corredor, C., Brendel, K., and Bressler, R., 1969, Effects of 4-pentenoic acid on carbohydrate metabolism in pigeon liver homogenate, *J. Biol. Chem.* **244**:1212.

DeLap, L. W., Tate, S. S., and Meister, A., 1975, Gamma-glutamyl transpeptidase of rat seminal vesicles: Effect of orchidectomy and hormone administration on the transpeptidase in relation to its possible role in secretory activity, *Life Sci.* **16**:691.

Dobson, J. C., Kushida, E., Williamson, M., and Friedman, E. G., 1976, Intellectual performance of 36 phenylketonuria patients and their nonaffected siblings, *Pediatrics* **58**:53.

Eldjarn, L., Jellum, E., and Stokke, O., 1972, Pyroglutamic aciduria: Studies on the enzymic block and on the metabolic origin of pyroglutamic acid, *Clin. Chim. Acta* **40**:461.

Eldjarn, L., Jellum, E., and Stokke, O., 1973, Pyroglutamic aciduria: Rate of formation and degradation of pyroglutamate, *Clin. Chim. Acta* **49**:311.

Enteman, M., and Bressler, R., 1967, The mechanism of action of hypoglycin on long chain fatty acid oxidation, *Mol. Pharmacol.* **3**:333.

Friedman, P. A., Fisher, D. B., Kang, E. S., and Kaufman, S., 1973, Detection of hepatic phenylalanine 4-hydroxylase in classical phenylketonuria, *Proc. Natl. Acad. Sci. U.S.A.* **70**:552.

Garvey, T. Q., Hyman, P. E., and Isselbacher, K. J., 1976, γ-Glutamyl transpeptidase of rat intestine: Localization and possible role in amino acid transport, *Gastroenterology* **71**:778.

Glenner, G. G., and Folk, J. E., 1961, Glutamyl peptidase in rat and guinea pig kidney slices, *Nature (London)* **192**:338.

Goodman, S. I., Mace, J. W., and Pollak, S., 1971, Serum gamma-glutamyl transpeptidase deficiency, *Lancet* **1**:234.

Goodman, S. I., Markey, S. P., Moe, P. G., Miles, B. S., and Teng, C. C., 1975, Glutaric aciduria: A "new" disorder of amino acid metabolism, *Biochem. Med.* **12**:12.

Goodman, S. I., Norenberg, M. D., Shikes, R. H., Breslin, D. J., and Moe, P. G., 1977, Glutaric aciduria: Biochemical and morphologic considerations, *J. Pediatr.* **90**:746.

Green, D. E., and Allman, D. W., 1968, Fatty acid oxidation, in: *Metabolic Pathways,* Vol. II, 3rd Ed. (D. M. Greenberg, ed.), pp. 1–36, Academic Press, New York.

Hagenfeldt, L., Larsson, A., and Zetterstrom, R., 1974, Pyroglutamic aciduria: Studies in an infant with chronic metabolic acidosis, *Acta Pediatr. Scand.* **63**:1.

Harris, H., 1975, Enzyme and protein diversity in human populations, in: *The Principles of Human Biochemical Genetics* (H. Harris, ed.), pp. 278–338, North-Holland/American Elsevier, Amsterdam.

Hassal, C. H., and Reyle, K., 1955, Hypoglycin A and B, two biological active polypeptides from *Blighia sapida, Biochem. J.* **60**:334.

Hill, K. R., 1952, The vomiting sickness of Jamaica: A review, *West Ind. Med. J.* **1**:243.

Hoffbauer, R. W., and Schrempf, G., 1976, Phenylketonuria hydroxylation in cultured fibroblasts from patients with PKU, *Lancet* **2**:194.

von Holt, C., and Benedict, I., 1959, Biochemie des Hypoglycins A. II. Der Einfluss des Hypoglycins auf die Oxydation von Glucose und Fettsäuren, *Biochem. Zschr.* **331**:430.

von Holt, C., von Holt, M., and Böhm, H., 1966, Metabolic effects of hypoglycin and methylenecyclopropaneacetic acid, *Biochim. Biophys. Acta* **125**:11.

Holtzman, N. A., Welcher, D. W., and Mellits, E. D., 1975, Termination of restricted diet in children with phenylketonuria: A randomized controlled study, *N. Engl. J. Med.* **293**:1121.

Jackson, R. C., 1969, Studies in the enzymology of glutathione metabolism in human erythrocytes, *Biochem. J.* **111**:309.

Jeliffe, D. B., and Stuart, K. L., 1954, Acute toxic hypoglycemia in the vomiting sickness of Jamaica, *Brit. Med. J.* **1**:75.

Jellum, E., Kluge, T., Borresen, H. C., Stokke, O., and Eldjarn, L., 1970, Pyroglutamic aciduria—a new inborn error of metabolism, *Scand. J. Clin. Lab. Invest.* **26**:327.

Kaufman, S., 1976, The phenylalanine hydroxylating system in phenylketonuria and its variants, *Biochem. Med.* **15**:42.

Kaufman, S., Holtzman, N. A., Milstien, S., Butler, I. J., and Krumholz, A., 1975a, Phenylketonuria due to a deficiency of dihydropteridine reductase, *N. Engl. J. Med.* **293**:785.

Kaufman, S., Max, E. E., and Kang, E. S., 1975b, Phenylalanine hydroxylase activity in liver biopsies from hyperphenylalaninemia heterozygotes: Deviation from proportionality with gene dosage, *Pediatr. Res.* **9**:632.

Kean, E. A., 1976, Selective inhibition of acyl-CoA dehydrogenases by a metabolite of hypoglycin, *Biochim. Biophys. Acta* **422**:8.

Knox, W. E., 1972, Phenylketonuria, in: *The Metabolic Basis of Inherited Disease* (J. B. Stanbury, J. P. Wyngaarden, and D. S. Fredrickson, eds.), pp. 266–295, McGraw-Hill, New York.

Koch, R., Blaskovics, M., Wenz, E., Fishler, K., and Schaeffler, G., 1974, Phenyl-

alaninemia and phenylketonuria, in: *Heritable Disorders of Amino Acid Metabolism: Patterns of Clinical Expression and Genetic Variation* (W. L. Nyhan, ed.), pp. 109–140, Wiley-Interscience, New York.
Larsson, A., and Mattson, B., 1976, On the mechanism of 5-oxoproline overproduction in 5-oxoprolinuria, *Clin Chim. Acta* **67**:245.
Larsson, A., Zetterstrom, R., Hagenfeldt, L., Anderson, R., Dreborg, S., and Hornell, H., 1974, Pyroglutamic aciduria (5-oxoprolinuria), an inborn error in glutathione metabolism *Pediatr. Res.* **8**:852.
Larsson, A., Zetterstrom, R., Hornell, H., and Porath, U., 1976, Erythrocytes glutathione synthetase in 5-oxoprolinuria: Kinetic studies of the mutant enzyme and detection of heterozygote, *Clin. Chim. Acta* **73**:19.
Louvard, D., Maroux, S., Vannier, C., and Desnuelle, P., 1975, Topological studies on the hydrolases bound to the intestinal brush border membrane, *Biochim. Biophys. Acta* **375**:236.
Marstein, S., Jellum, E., Halpern, B., Eldjarn, L., and Perry, T. L., 1976, Biochemical studies of erythrocytes in a patient with pyroglutamic acidemia (5-oxoprolinemia), *N. Engl. J. Med.* **295**:406.
McKerns, K. W., Bird, H. H., Kaleita, E., Coulomb, B. S., and DeRenzo, E. C., 1960, Effects of hypoglycin on certain aspects of glucose and fatty acid metabolism in the rat, *Biochem. Pharmacol.* **3**:305.
Meister, A., 1973, On the enzvmology of amino acid transport, *Science* **180**:33.
Meister, A., 1974, The γ-glutamyl cycle: Diseases associated with specific enzyme deficiencies, *Ann. Intern. Med.* **81**:247.
Meister, A., and Tate, S. S., 1976, Glutathione and related γ-glutamyl compounds: Biosynthesis and utilization, *Annu. Rev. Biochem.* **45**:557.
Milstien, S., and Kaufman, S., 1975, Production of antibodies to sheep liver dihydropteridine reductase: Characterization and use to study the enzyme defect in a variant form of phenylketonuria, *Biochem. Biophys. Res. Commun.* **66**:475.
Orlowski, M., and Meister, A., 1970, The γ-glutamyl cycle: A possible transport system for amino acids, *Proc. Natl. Acad. Sci. U.S.A.* **67**:1248.
Orlowski, M., and Wilk, S., 1975, Intermediate of the γ-glutamyl cycle in mouse tissues: Influence of administration of amino acids on pyrrolidone carboxylate and γ-glutamyl amino acids, *Eur. J. Biochem.* **53**:581.
Osmundsen, H., and Sherratt, H. S. A., 1975, A novel mechanism for inhibition of β-oxidation by methylenecyclopropylacetyl-CoA, a metabolite of hypoglycin, *FEBS Lett.* **55**:38.
Palekar, A. G., Tate, S. S., and Meister, A., 1974, Formation of 5-oxoproline from glutathione in erythrocytes by the γ-glutamyltranspeptidase–cyclotransferase cycle, *Proc. Natl. Acad. Sci. U.S.A.* **71**:293.
Pellefigue, F., Butler, J. D., Spielberg, P., Hollenberg, M. D., Goodman, S. I., and Schulman, J. D., 1976, Normal amino acid uptake by cultured human fibroblasts does not require gamma glutamyl cycle, *Biochem. Biophys. Res. Commun.* **73**:997.
Perry, T. L., Hansen, S., Tischler, B., Richards, F. M., and Sokol, M., 1973, Unrecognized adult phenylketonuria, *N. Engl. J. Med.* **289**:395.
Przyrembel, H., Wendel, U., Becker, K., Bremer, H. J., Bruinvis, L., Ketting, D., and Wadman, S. K., 1976, Glutaric aciduria Type II: Report on a previously undescribed metabolic disorder, *Clin. Chim. Acta* **66**:227.

Richman, P. G., and Meister, A., 1975, Regulation of gamma-glutamyl-cysteine synthetase by nonallosteric feedback inhibition by glutathione, *J. Biol. Chem.* **250**:1422.

Ross, L. L., Barber, L., Tate, S. S., and Meister, A., 1973, Enzymes of the gamma-glutamyl cycle in the ciliary body and lens, *Proc. Natl. Acad. Sci. U.S.A.* **70**:2211.

Schulman, J. D., Goodman, S. I., Mace, J. W., Patrick, A. D., Tietze, F., and Butler, E. J., 1975, Glutathionuria: Inborn error of metabolism due to tissue deficiency of gamma-glutamyl transpeptidase, *Biochem. Biophys. Res. Commun.* **65**:68.

Scriver, C. R., and Rosenberg, L. E. (eds.), 1973, Phenylalanine, in: *Amino Acid Metabolism and Its Disorders,* pp. 290–337, W. B. Saunders, Philadelphia.

Sekura, R., and Meister, A., 1974, Glutathione turnover in the kidney: Considerations relating to the γ-glutamyl cycle and the transport of amino acids, *Proc. Natl. Acad. Sci. U.S.A.* **71**:2969.

Smith, I., Clayton, B. E., and Wolff, O. H., 1975, New variant of phenylketonuria with progressive neurological illness unresponsive to phenylalanine restriction, *Lancet* **1**:1108.

Srivastava, S. K., Awasthi, Y. C., Miller, S. P., Yoshida, A., and Beutler, E., 1976, Studies on gamma-glutamyl transpeptidase in human and rabbit erythrocytes, *Blood* **47**:645.

Stokke, O., Goodman, S. I., Thompson, J. A., and Miles, B. S., 1975, Glutaric aciduria: Presence of glutaconic and beta-hydroxyglutaric acids in urine, *Biochem. Med.* **12**:386.

Strömme, J. H., and Eldjarn, L., 1972, The metabolism of L-pyroglutamic acid in fibroblasts from a patient with pyroglutamic aciduria: The demonstration of an L-pyroglutamate hydrolase system, *Scand. J. Clin. Lab. Invest.* **29**:335.

Tanaka, K., 1972, On the mode of action of hypoglycin A. III. Isolation and identification of *cis*-4-decene-1,10,-dioic, *cis,cis*-4,7-decadiene-1,10-dioic, *cis*-4-octene-1,8-dioic, glutaric and adipic acids, *N*-(methylenecyclopropyl) acetylglycine, and *N*-isovalerylglycine from urine of hypoglycin A treated rats, *J. Biol. Chem.* **247**:7465.

Tanaka, K., 1975a, Disorders of organic acid metabolism, in *Biology of Brain Dysfunction,* Vol. 3 (G. E. Gaull, ed.) pp. 145–214, Plenum Press, New York.

Tanaka, K., 1975b, Branched pentanoic acidemia and medium chain dicarboxylic aciduria induced by hypoglycin A: Inhibition of several short chain acyl CoA dehydrogenases, in: *Hypoglycin* (E. A. Kean, ed.), pp. 67–92, Academic Press, New York.

Tanaka, K., and Kerley, R., 1975, Synergistic hypoglycemic effects of lysine and tryptophan with hypoglycin A: Interrelationship between the inhibition of glutaryl CoA dehydrogenase and gluconeogenesis, in: *Hypoglycin* (E. A. Kean, ed.), pp. 163–173, Academic Press, New York.

Tanaka, K., and Yu, G., 1973, A method for the separate determination of isovalerate and α-methylbutyrate by use of GLC-mass spectrometer, *Clin. Chim. Acta* **43**:151.

Tanaka, K., Miller, E. M., and Isselbacher, K. J., 1971, Hypoglycin A: A specific inhibitor of isovaleryl CoA dehydrogenase, *Proc. Natl. Acad. Sci. U.S.A.* **68**:20.

Tanaka, K., Isselbacher, K. J., and Shih, V., 1972, Isovaleric acidemia and α-

methylbutyric acidemias induced by hypoglycin A: Mechanism of Jamaican vomiting sickness, *Science* **175**:69.

Tanaka, K., Kean, E. A., and Johnson, B., 1976a, Jamaican vomiting sickness: Biochemical investigation of two cases, *N. Engl. J. Med.* **295**:461.

Tanaka, K., Mandell, R., and Shih, V., 1976b, Metabolism of [1-^{14}C] and [2-^{14}C]leucine in cultured skin fibroblasts from patients with isovaleric acidemia, *J. Clin. Invest.* **58**:164.

Tanaka, K., Ramsdell, H. S., Baretz, B. H., Keefe, M. B., Johnson, B., and Kean, E. A., 1976c, Identification of ethylmalonic acid in urine of two patients with the vomiting sickness of Jamaica, *Clin. Chim. Acta* **69**:105.

Tate, S. S., Dunn, M. W., and Meister, A., 1975, Localization of γ-glutamyl transpeptidase in the retinal pigment epithelium and visual receptor cell, *Life Sci.* **18**:1145.

Van Der Werf, P., Orlowski, M., and Meister, A., 1971, Enzymic conversion of 5-oxoproline (L-pyrrolidone carboxylate) to L-glutamate coupled with cleavage of adenosine triphosphate to adenosine diphosphate, a reaction in the γ-glutamyl cycle, *Proc. Natl. Acad. Sci. U.S.A.* **68**:2982.

Van Der Werf, P., Stephani, R. A., and Meister, A., 1974, Accumulation of 5-oxoproline in mouse tissues after inhibition of 5-oxoprolinase and administration of amino acids: Evidence for function of the gamma-glutamyl cycle, *Proc. Natl. Acad. Sci. U.S.A.* **71**:1026.

Wellner, V. P., Sekura, R., Meister, R., and Larsson, A., 1974, Glutathione synthetase deficiency—an inborn error of metabolism involving the gamma-glutamyl cycle in patients with 5-oxoprolinuria (pyroglutamic aciduria), *Proc. Natl. Acad. Sci. U.S.A.* **71**:2505.

Williamson, J. R., Rostand, S. G., and Peterson, M. J., 1970, Control factors affecting gluconeogenesis in perfused rat liver. Effect of 4-pentenoic acid, *J. Biol. Chem.* **245**:3242.

Woolf, L. I., McBean, M. S., Woolf, F. M., and Cahalane, S. F., 1975, Phenylketonuria as a balanced polymorphism: The nature of the heterozygote advantage, *Ann. Hum. Genet.* **38**:461.

Young, J. D., Ellroy, J. C., and Tucker, E. M., 1975a, Amino acid transport defect in glutathione-deficient sheep erythrocytes, *Nature (London)* **254**:156.

Young, J. D., Ellroy, J. C., and Wright, P. C., 1975b, Evidence against the participation of the γ-glutamyltransferase–γ-glutamylcyclotransferase pathway in amino acid transport by rabbit erythrocytes, *Biochem. J.* **152**:713.

Young, J. D., Ellroy, J. C., and Tucker, E. M., 1976, Amino acid transport in normal and glutathione-deficient sheep erythrocytes, *Biochem. J.* **154**:43.

8

Disorders of Purine and Pyrimidine Metabolism

J. Edwin Seegmiller

8.1. Introduction

Substantial progress has been made in the past year in identifying new primary disorders associated with abnormalities of purine and pyrimidine metabolism, in defining more precisely the metabolic consequences of specific enzyme defects, and in deducing the mechanisms involved in producing their clinical expression. A new primary cause of purine overproduction has been identified in children with a type of genetically determined immunodeficiency disease involving a primary T-cell dysfunction (Cohen *et al.,* 1976; Wadman *et al.,* 1977; Stoop *et al.,* 1977). The condition, however, presents a curious metabolic paradox. Although the children overproduce purines, they produce virtually no uric acid and so can be conveniently identified by their marked hypouricemia and hypouricuria. The resolution of the paradox is found in the metabolic site of their enzyme deficiency—a gross deficiency of the enzyme purine nucleoside phosphorylase (PNP), which is responsible for processing purine

J. EDWIN SEEGMILLER • The University of California San Diego, La Jolla, California.

ribosides to their free purine bases. As a consequence, the ribosides inosine and guanosine and the corresponding deoxyribosides replace uric acid as the end products of purine metabolism and are produced in a remarkable abundance quite comparable to the record degree of purine overproduction excreted as uric acid by children with the Lesch–Nyhan syndrome. One such child excreted a new riboside of uric acid, *N*-9-ribosyl urate, not previously found in biological systems (Cohen *et al.*, 1976). Since the disorder was first described (Giblett *et al.*, 1975), four additional patients with this disorder have been identified, two of them, while they were still living.

Additional patients with severe combined immunodeficiency disease associated with gross deficiency of adenosine deaminase (ADA) were found (Polmar *et al.*, 1976; Mills *et al.*, 1976; Ackeret *et al.*, 1976; Keightley *et al.*, 1975; Trotta *et al.*, 1976; Cederbaum *et al.*, 1976), bringing the total number of cases to more than two dozen (Seegmiller *et al.*, 1977a,b).

The association of aberrations of purine metabolism with immunodeficiency disease has been further expanded to include a lowered activity of purine 5′-nucleotidase activity reported in lymphocytes of patients who have common variable agammaglobulinemia of adult onset (Johnson *et al.*, 1977). This enzyme is but the first in a metabolic pathway that includes in successive sequence ADA and PNP (see Fig. 1). The association of some degree of immunodeficiency with a diminished activity of any one of the three enzymes of this metabolic sequence remains at present merely a curious correlation that nevertheless suggests an important role for this pathway of purine nucleotide metabolism in the maintenance of competent cell function in the immune system. Whether the diminished activity of purine 5′-nucleotidase is a genetic or an acquired abnormality remains to be determined.

Two additional patients with adenine phosphoribosyltransferase (APRT) deficiency, one of whom presented with calculi of the urinary tract, were reported (Simmonds *et al.*, 1976; Van Acker *et al.*, 1977); there was also a more detailed report of the first such patient (Debray *et al.*, 1976). Four additional patients with xanthinuria were reported, two with the classic presentation of urinary tract obstruction from a ureteral calculus composed of xanthine (Kitamura *et al.*, 1976; Kenawi, 1976). One presented with only myalgias and arthralgias associated with crystalline deposits within the muscle cells (Isaacs *et al.*, 1975). All had hypouricemia with serum urate less than 1 mg/dl, hypouricuria, and excretions of xanthine with lesser amounts of hypoxanthine.

The medical history and clinical presentation of each of the patients mentioned above expanded substantially our concept of the possible clinical expression of these disorders to include not only immunodefi-

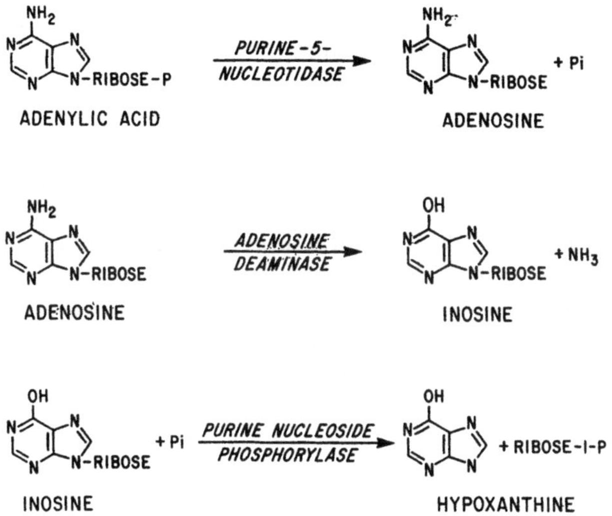

Fig. 1. Enzyme defects in purine metabolism associated with immunodeficiency.

ciency and purine overproduction in PNP deficiency, but also the possibility of some degree of neurological dysfunction with megaloblastic bone marrow and microcytic hypochromic erythrocytes and, in patients with APRT deficiency, a possible hypotonia. One patient with ADA deficiency also showed neurological symptoms consisting of a transient tremor (Polmar *et al.,* 1976). Whether or not these prove to be common or even frequent clinical accompaniments of these defects in purine metabolism must await the identification and detailed examination of a larger number of affected patients.

A new and simpler approach to treatment of immunodeficiency disease associated with ADA deficiency by enzyme replacement through transfusion of irradiated erythrocytes was also a significant development of the past year. This approach gives promise of supplanting transplantation of stem cells from marrow of a histocompatible donor or fetal liver as therapy for this condition (Polmer *et al.,* 1976). The remarkable therapeutic response achieved with the complete reversal of the immunodeficient state also has considerable implications for the pathogenic mechanism involved in the immunosuppression of this disease and points the direction for future pharmacological approaches to control of the immune response. Use of specific inhibitors of ADA or PNP could conceivably be used to produce a carefully controlled immunosuppression for therapeutic purposes. Preliminary reports of successful immunosuppression using inhibitors of ADA suggest the feasibility of this approach (Lum *et al.,*

1977; Chassin *et al.*, 1977). The etiological role of the primary deficiency of ADA in generation of severe combined immunodeficiency disease was further consolidated by the demonstration of elevated concentrations of adenosine in serum and erythrocytes (Mills *et al.*, 1976; Cohen *et al.*, 1977a) and by the presence of a similar clinical presentation of severe T-cell dysfunction with the degree of associated B-cell dysfunction varying from one family to another. The effect of ADA deficiency on development of cartilage and of the skeletal system was studied in greater detail by Cederbaum *et al.* (1976).

The converse of ADA deficiency, i.e., an excessive activity of the enzyme ADA, was also reported in the past year to be associated with a dominantly inherited hereditary disease. A total of 12 patients with non-spherocytic hemolytic anemia were described in a kindred of 23 individuals spanning three generations. All patients had a 40- to 75-fold increase above normal in ADA activity of their erthrocytes associated with lowered intracellular concentrations of ATP as a possible pathogenic mechanism (Valentine *et al.*, 1977). Less marked increases in ADA activity were also found in some patients with gout (Nishizawa *et al.*, 1975) and with gout and polycythemia vera (Snyder and Seegmiller, 1977).

The possibility of a more subtle form of immunodeficiency was suggested by Allison *et al.* (1975) in children with the Lesch–Nythan syndrome carrying a gross deficiency of hypoxanthine-guanine phosphoribosyltransferase (HPRT), the enzyme next in line in this metabolic sequence, but was not confirmed (Seegmiller *et al.*, 1977a,b). Some evidence was presented for an enhancing effect of added purine nucleosides on the immune response when tested both *in vitro* (Seegmiller *et al.*, 1977a,b) and *in vivo* (Hadden *et al.*, 1976a).

The aberrations of pyrimidine metabolism reported in the past year were additional patients with hemolytic anemia associated with deficiency of pyrimidine-5′-nucleotidase (Rochant *et al.*, 1975; Vives-Corrons *et al.*, 1976a,b) and depression of this enzyme activity in patients with hemolytic anemia of lead poisoning (Valentine *et al.*, 1976). Other reports centered on the effects on pyrimidine metabolism of drugs or of secondary effects of primary mutations in purine metabolism. An increased intracellular concentration of pyrimidine nucleotides was found in human azaguanine-resistant lymphoblast cell lines deficient in HPRT (Nuki *et al.*, 1977a,b), while treatment of lymphoblasts with adenosine, hypoxanthine, or adenine produced a lowered concentration of pyrimidine nucleotides (Snyder *et al.*, 1977a). A mild orotic aciduria was found in patients with PNP deficiency (Cohen *et al.*, 1977b).

During the past year, new and interesting aspects of purine metabolism were reviewed at two international symposia, both now published in book form. The first was held at Ciba House in London; it was published in *Ciba Foundation Symposium No. 48* (1977) and covers recent developments in both purine and pyrimidine metabolism. The second was held at Baden near Vienna, Austria, and appears in two volumes, one dealing with regulation of pathways and enzyme defects (Müller *et al.*, 1977a) and the second with physiology, pharmacology, and clinical aspects (Müller *et al.*, 1977b). In addition, a number of reviews on various topics were published, including the Lesch–Nyhan syndrome and its variants (Seegmiller, 1976c), the effects of drugs on uric acid in man (Kelley, 1975), regulation of purine biosynthesis and turnover (Wyngaarden, 1976), uric acid biosynthesis and its disorders (Watts, 1976), control of purine biosynthesis in normal and pathologic states (Holmes *et al.*, 1975–1976), uric acid metabolism in man (Balis, 1976), and a report of an earlier conference on purine metabolism and gout assembled as a supplement in *Arthritis and Rheumatism* (Klinenberg, 1975). In addition, books on gout and uric acid were published (Talbott and Yü, 1976; Wyngaarden and Kelley, 1976; Newcombe, 1975). Bloch (1973) and Robins (1975) reviewed the pharmocology of nucleosides. Conferences on immunodeficiency disease and purine metabolism were reported (Meuwissen *et al.*, 1975; Bergsma, 1975).

8.2. Purine Metabolism

Advances were made in our understanding of the physiological significance of purine metabolism, its role in maintaining the functional activity of various organs and tissues, and the control mechanism regulating the rate of synthesis of purine nucleotides. Through more detailed studies of specific human mutations, greater insight into the physiological and clinical importance of the normal operation of a number of enzyme systems was gained.

8.2.1. Role of Liver in Processing Purines of the Bloodstream

More definitive evidence was found that the liver not only degrades purines to uric acid irreversibly, but also plays an active role in generating adenosine as a nutritive supplement for other body cells. The presence of xanthine oxidase in highest activity in the liver makes it the primary site for the synthesis of uric acid in the human species. Studies of arteriovenous differences in the concentration of purine compounds in lightly anesthetized rabbits and rats by Pritchard *et al.* (1975) showed a removal of roughly 80% of hypoxanthine, xanthine, and urate in a single passage of blood through the liver. A substantial portion of the hypoxanthine, however, was converted to adenosine by the liver and excreted into the bloodstream to give a 10-fold increase in adenosine concentration during passage of portal or arterial blood through the liver (Fig. 2). When the liver was isolated and perfused with hypoxanthine, significant amounts of adenosine were formed from the hypoxanthine that disappeared, whether measured quantitatively by microbiological assay or qualitatively by analysis of the radioactive purines released from liver that had been prelabeled with [^{14}C]hypoxanthine.

This work now provides a clear delineation of the important role of the liver in this part of the purine reutilization cycle. Apparently, the liver takes up hypoxanthine generated by peripheral tissues and converts it in part to adenosine, which is liberated into the bloodstream, taken up by erythrocytes, and released to peripheral tissues such as kidney, brain, and possibly bone marrow, which have need of an augmented supply of purine compounds for optimal nutrition. Obviously, hepatic failure should greatly disrupt this purine cycle, but detailed examination of the possible role of such a disruption in the generation of clinical symptoms accompanying liver failure remains to be delineated.

8.2.2. Purines as a Source of Ammonia Production

Henderson *et al.* (1977) spoke a word of caution in extrapolating from the relative activity of enzymes in broken-cell preparations to the activity of the same enzymes in whole cells. Methods for assessment of the activity of various pathways being evaluated in whole cells must be developed. This perspective is especially pertinent to evidence presented in the past year supporting the view that the purine nucleotide cycle may be involved in the generation of ammonia by brain tissue (Schultz and Lowenstein, 1976) and kidney (Bogusky *et al.*, 1976).

Production of ammonia by the brain on incubation *in vitro* has been known for over half a century, but the precise origin of the ammonia has proved elusive. The observation has been confirmed both *in vivo* and *in vitro*. Furthermore, ammonia apparently disappears from brain during sleep and anesthesia. A common explanation of ammonia formation in the brain has been that it arises from transamination of amino acids with α-ketoglutarate to form glutamate and the subsequent deamination of glutamate by glutamate dehydrogenase. In studies by Schultz and Lowenstein (1976), the maximal activity of glutamate dehydrogenase found in cell-free extracts of rat brain was insufficient to account for the rates of ammonia production. On the other hand, activity of adenylic deaminase was sufficient to account for the maximum rate of ammonia production. Presumably, the ammonia originates from aspartic acid through its intermediate reaction with inosinic acid to form adenylosuccinate acid, followed by the formation of adenylic acid (Fig 3). The ammonia would then

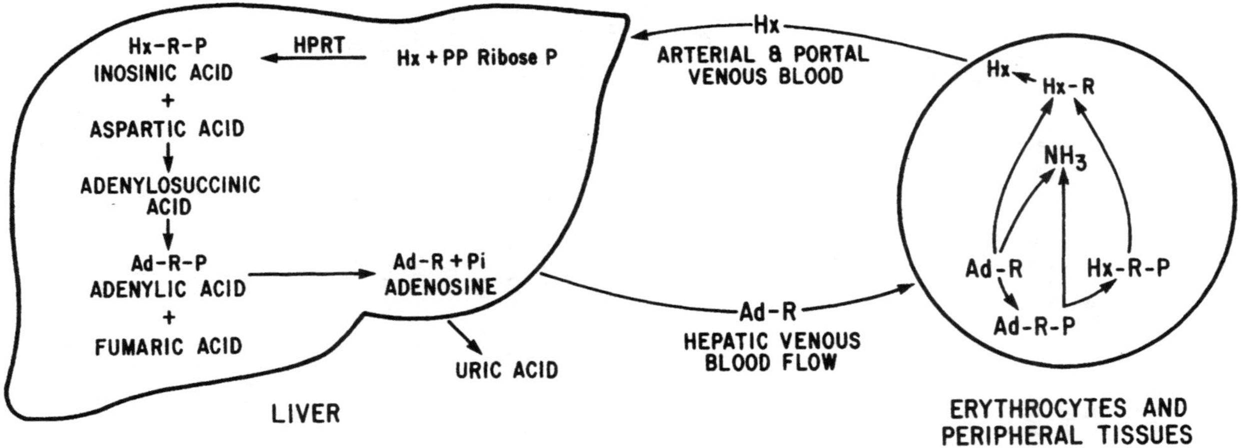

Fig. 2. Uptake of hypoxanthine (Hx) and excretion of adenosine (Ad-R) by the liver, and purine transport to peripheral tissues.

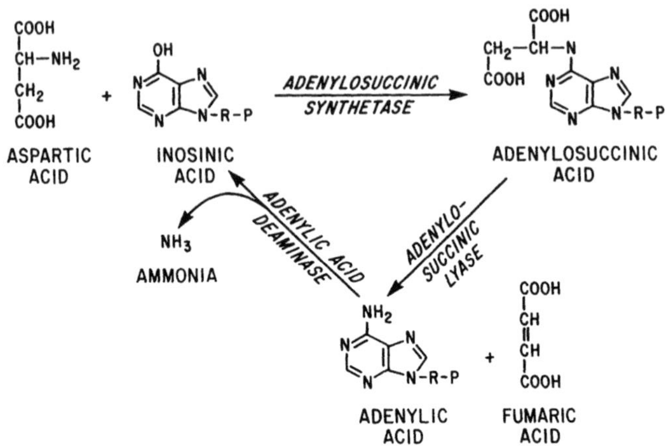

Fig. 3. Proposed origin of ammonia production via the adenylic acid cycle in brain and kidney from aspartic acid.

be released by the activity of the adenylic acid deaminase with regeneration of inosinic acid.

Although such a mechanism exists in brain, these experiments do not prove conclusively the operation of this cycle in intact mammalian brain cells. Similar particle-free extracts prepared from kidney cortex of rat catalyzed the formation of ammonia via the same nucleotide cycle (Bogusky *et al.*, 1976). The operational capacity of this cycle was accelerated by prior feeding of the rats with ammonium chloride for 2 days, and by potassium depletion with an accompanying increase in adenylosuccinate activity. Both these conditions are known to increase renal ammonia excretion in the intact rat. These observations introduce new considerations for evaluation of brain metabolism and the possible origin of ammonia in the kidney.

8.2.3. Regulation of Purine Synthesis

The addition of a variety of purine compounds to the media of cells cultured *in vitro* or administered to patients *in vivo* has long been known to suppress the rate of purine synthesis *de novo*. The relatively greater effect of adenine as compared with hypoxanthine or guanine in this regard can be related to the greater affinity of APRT for the rate-limiting substrate, phosphoribosylpyrophosphate (PP-ribose-P), as compared with the affinity of the enzyme HPRT for the same substrate (Seegmiller, 1974; Wyngaarden, 1976).

At the physiological concentrations of hypoxanthine normally present in plasma, a substantial amount of suppression of purine synthesis *de novo* is thereby operating in the normal individual. Children with the Lesch–Nyhan syndrome deficient in HPRT are in effect "blind" to the normal suppressive action of hypoxanthine in their plasma, even though it accumulates to much higher concentrations than are normally found. Preliminary studies of the incorporation of [^{14}C]formate into total purine compounds of lymphoblasts show that normal cells in the absence of exogenous hypoxanthine are capable of accelerating their rate of purine synthesis to values quite comparable to the rate observed in cells grossly deficient in HPRT. Successful demonstration of this enhanced rate of purine synthesis requires rigorous care, however, to exclude hypoxanthine from the incubation medium by thorough dialysis of fetal calf serum and prevention of cellular dissolution, which can also give rise to hypoxanthine (Hershfield *et al.*, 1977a; Hershfield and Seegmiller, 1977a). Normal lymphoblasts accumulate very little labeled hypoxanthine in the medium, but as would be expected, the HPRT-deficient cells show a 10-fold greater accumulation of label in hypoxanthine excreted into the medium than control cells. Studies by Holland *et al.* (1976b) also showed an enhanced excretion of labeled hypoxanthine by HPRT-deficient fibroblasts incubated with [^{14}C]formate.

A role for HPRT in transport of hypoxanthine was proposed by Quinlan and Hochstadt (1976) in microsomal vesicles isolated from mouse fibroblasts. Alford and Barnes (1976), however, concluded on the basis of their comparison of hypoxanthine transport by normal and HPRT-deficient cells that hypoxanthine is transported into Chinese hamster cells by means of carrier-mediated processes (facilitated diffusion) that operate independently of phosphoribosylation.

In the past few years, considerable evidence has accumulated to indicate a major role for the intracellular concentration of PP-ribose-P in the regulation of the rate of purine synthesis *de novo* (Seegmiller, 1974; Wyngaarden, 1976; Henderson *et al.*, 1977). A possible molecular mechanism for this regulation involving allosteric activation of PP-ribose-P-glutamine amidotransferase by PP-ribose-P was recently reviewed (Wyngaarden and Holmes, 1977).

Indirect evidence for the importance of PP-ribose-P in this regulation of the rate of purine synthesis also came from studies *in vivo* in rats (Zimmer and Gerlach, 1977) and in man (Zöllner and Gröbner, 1977). In the rat heart, stimulation of cardiac β-adrenergic receptors with isoproterenol resulted in a substantial ehhancement of the biosynthesis of adenine nucleotides from [^{14}C]glycine *in vivo* along with an elevation of the intracellular adenosine cyclic 3′,5′-monophosphate (cAMP). The pentoses D-ribose and D-xylose as well as the pentitols ribotol and xylitol all produced comparable degrees of enhanced synthesis of adenine nucleotides.

Presumably, this enhanced synthesis was mediated through an increased availability of PP-ribose-P. The ribose-5-P precursor xylitol greatly enhanced the effects of isoproterenol. Propranolol reduced the cAMP and also the rate of synthesis of adenine nucleotides *de novo*. Triiodo-L-thyronine also enhanced the rate of purine nucleotide synthesis and the β-receptor-blocking agent propranolol attenuated this response (Zimmer and Gerlach, 1977).

More recent studies of purine synthesis in human cells cultured *in vivo* suggested that PP-ribose-P concentrations are not always the sole determinants of the rate of purine synthesis. Becker (1976a, 1977b) showed a dissociation between the PP-ribose-P concentration and the rate of purine nucleotide synthesis in normal fibroblasts incubated with inosine. Presumably, the accompanying increase in intracellular concentrations of purine nucleotides exerts a feedback inhibition on *de novo* synthesis under these conditions in which he measured the incorporation of [^{14}C]formate into formylglycineamide ribonucleotide in the presence of the glutamine analogue azaserine to block the further metabolism.

In addition to suppressing *de novo* purine synthesis, the addition of the free purine base adenine or guanine produces a coordinate regulation of more distal steps at the stage of inosinic acid in the pathway of purine synthesis *de novo*. Hershfield and Seegmiller (1976, 1977b) showed not only a suppression of [^{14}C]formate incorporation into total purines by the addition of adenine, but also a coordinated inhibition of the conversion of inosinic acid to adenine nucleotides and an enhancement of total guanine nucleotide synthesis. Thus, concentrations of adenine that produce less than 40% inhibition of the overall rate of *de novo* purine synthesis do so by selectively inhibiting adenine nucleotide synthesis *de novo* by 50–70% while stimulating guanine nucleotide synthesis *de novo* by up to 20%. The reciprocal effect is produced by exogenous guanine. The adenosine analogue 6-methylmercaptopurine ribonucleoside selectively inhibits adenine nucleotide synthesis via the *de novo* pathway, but, most curiously, not adenine nucleotide synthesized from exogenous hypoxanthine.

An unusual purine compound with regulatory properties was first identified in bacterial systems and has now been found in mammalian cells in levels varying widely with the degree of proliferative activity of the tissue (Rapaport and Zamecnik, 1976b). This compound, diadenosine $5',5'''$-P_1,P_4-tetraphosphate (Ap_4A), was first described as a product of the reversal of the reaction of amino acid activation involved in protein synthesis in bacteria. It has now been identified in a variety of mammalian cells, and the concentration within the cells appears to be inversely related to their doubling time, varying from 0.1 to 20×10^{-4} of the cellular ATP levels. It shows a decrease of 30- to 50-fold on addition of the inhibitors of protein synthesis, pactamycin or puromycin. The possibility of Ap_4A

being a metabolic "signal nucleotide" that is formed at the onset of protein synthesis and is active in positive growth regulation (positive pleiotropic activation) was proposed by Rapaport and Zamecnik (1976b).

Inorganic orthophosphate has long been known to stimulate the activity of phosphoribosylpyrophosphate synthetase (PP-ribose-P synthetase). Studies by Planet and Fox (1976) provided evidence that the decreases in activity of this enzyme in human erythrocytes induced *in vitro* by exposure to purine nucleosides are mediated by a lowering of the intracellular concentrations of inorganic phosphate produced during phosphorolysis of the nucleoside.

Becker *et al.* (1975) purified PP-ribose-P synthetase from normal human erythrocytes and demonstrated a single repeating subunit of molecular weight 33,500 capable of reversible aggregation to polymeric states. The monomer and aggregates of up to 8 subunits are inactive or nearly inactive, while aggregates of 16 and 32 subunits have enzymatic activity. Both magnesium ATP and nucleotide inhibitors induce aggregation, and the latter exert their inhibitory effects on the aggregated enzyme. In contrast, 2,3-diphosphoglycerate suppresses PP-ribose-P synthetase activity by disaggregating the enzyme to the inactive forms. Neither inorganic phosphate nor ribose-5-phosphate alone causes enzyme aggregation, but these compounds do appear to exert a permissive effect on aggregation. These considerations suggest possible mechanisms by which an excessive enzyme activity with consequent overproduction of PP-ribose-P, purines, and uric acid could be achieved (see Section 8.9).

Rapaport and Zamecnik (1976a) obtained evidence compatible with an intracellular compartmentalization of ATP. They found that [^{3}H]adenosine was a much more effective precursor of ATP than was [^{3}H]adenine or [^{3}H]hypoxanthine, which gave higher labeling of AMP and ADP both in liver of the nude mouse and in a human hepatoma transplanted into the nude mouse. Siess and Wieland (1976) provided more direct evidence that the site of such a compartmentalization may be the cytosol of the hepatocyte. Addition of adenosine to isolated rat hepatocytes increased the ATP/ADP ratio in the cytosol and lowered the ratio in mitochondria.

8.2.4. Effects of Purine Compounds on the Immune System

Hadden *et al.* (1976a) reported a stimulation of mitogen-induced incorporation of [^{3}H]thymidine into human lymphocytes by the addition of the inosine-containing proprietary preparation Isoprinosine. Values as high as 1.6 times control values were obtained without concurrent change in the concentration of guanosine cyclic 3′,5′-monophosphate (GMP) within the cells. The authors failed to consider the possibility that the inosine in their preparation could have lowered the intracellular pyrimidine nucleotide concentrations in the same manner as hypoxanthine, adenine, or adenosine (Snyder *et al.*, 1977a; Carson and Seegmiller, 1976) and thereby enhanced the apparent incorporation of the [^{3}H]thymidine that was being used as an index of response to mitogens.

Adenosine, and to a lesser extent inosine, at concentrations of around 1 mM stimulated antibody production by cultured mouse spleen cells *in vitro* (Seegmiller *et al.*, 1977a,b), but at higher concentrations produced an inhibition.

Another possible role for purines in the biological processes was suggested by Gusella and Housman (1976). These investigators showed that hypoxanthine as well as 6-thioguanine and 6-mercaptopurine are extremely potent inducers of differentiation in cultured murine erythroleukemia cells, an effect that had been observed previously only with addition of dimethylsulfoxide. All three compounds were also potent inducers of erythrocyte differentiation in cell lines deficient in HPRT, suggesting that the inductive action is independent of formation of purine nucleotides.

Of significance for the possible role of purine compounds in the immune response is the report of the identification of hypoxanthine as a major UV-absorbing component of a chromatographic fraction of transfer factor by O'Dorisio *et al.* (1976). These workers used a Sephadex G-25 column to elute transfer factor capable of transferring delayed hypersentivity. The major component in this fraction proved to be hypoxanthine, identified by a variety of physical tests and by its conversion to uric acid by incubation with xanthine oxidase. It is worth noting that no concurrent measurements were made of transfer-factor activity in the same fractions they analyzed because of some recent difficulties they have encountered in obtaining active fractions; the analysis, however, was done on UV-absorbing peaks that in the past contained transfer-factor activity.

Evidence from three different sources has shown a differential sensitivity of various cells of the immune system to inhibition of ADA or adenosine toxicity. Seegmiller *et al.*, (1977a,b) showed a greater sensitivity of mouse T cells than B cells to growth inhibition by adenosine during mitogenic stimulation. Fischer *et al.* (1976) showed a 9-fold increase in specific activity of ADA accompanying the maturation of monocytes of peripheral blood into macrophages during 3 days of incubation *in vitro*. The increase in activity was associated with conversion of the high-molecular-weight (110,000) to the low-molecular-weight (30,000) form of ADA. The conversion of the monocyte to the macrophage was inhibited by a specific inhibitor of ADA, erythro-9-(2-hydroxy-3-nonyl) adenine (EHNA), suggesting a possible role of ADA in monocyte maturation. The structures of adenosine and of two inhibitors of ADA are shown in Fig. 4.

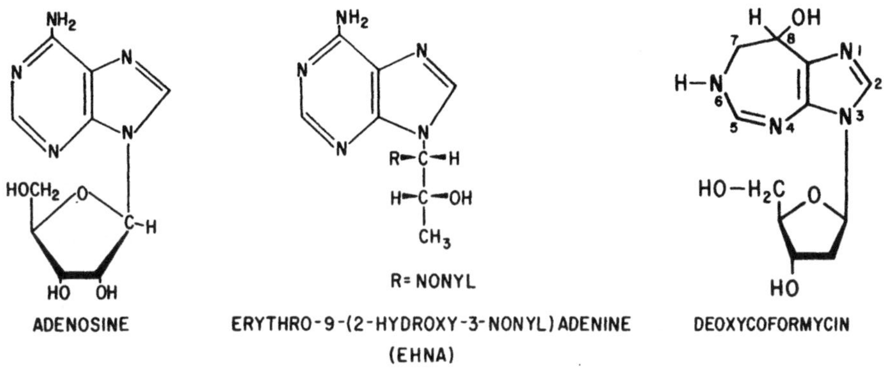

Fig. 4. Structure of adenosine compared with the structures of inhibitors of ADA.

In other studies, an impairment in maturation of precursors of lymphocytes was observed. Ballet *et al.* (1976) reported that coformycin, a potent inhibitor of ADA, at 1×10^{-6} M has no apparent effect on B-cell function *in vitro,* although a larger amount of this drug inhibits proliferative responses to mitogens. This concentration did, however, exert a profound inhibition on maturation of either T- or B-cell types when incubated under conditions that would otherwise result in substantial maturation of precursor cells into typical T and B lymphocytes. No actual measurements of degree of inhibition of ADA by the coformycin concentrations used were included in these studies.

Studies by Buckley *et al.* (1976) of peripheral blood lymphocytes from three infants with severe combined immunodeficiency disease provided evidence of a possible T-helper-cell defect or the inability of the T cells from immunodeficient children to produce soluble factors necessary for B-cell differentiation. The basis for their conclusion was the failure of lymphocytes from affected children to suppress the immune response when mixed with normal lymphocytes. Instead, the mixture produced an augmentation of immunoglobulin production from 310 to 560% over that expected on the basis of results obtained in the two individual cultures. Although not mentioned by the authors, the possibility that the addition of normal cells served to remove a soluble inhibitor should also be considered. This study has many points of similarity with that of Polmar *et al.* (1975), who found a 6-fold stimulation of mitogen response of ADA-deficient lymphocytes induced by addition of ADA to the medium.

The existence of immunodeficiency disease in association with both ADA and PNP deficiency provides strong evidence for an important role of purine metabolism in development of the immune system. The finding of an increase in intracellular adenine nucleotides in lymphocytes from a patient who had severe combined immunodeficiency disease from another cause (Goldblum *et al.*, 1976) suggests the possibility that alterations in intracellular nucleotide concentrations could be mediating the immunodeficiency disease of additional patients.

In contrast, leukocytes from patients with isolated defects in maturation of B lymphocytes when mixed with normal leukocytes inhibited the normal maturation of unaffected cells. In one such patient, removal of suppressor cells permitted the patient's remaining cells to differentiate into plasma cells *in vitro.* These finding support the view of a heterogeneous group of causes for the various clinical types of immunodeficiency disease (Siegal *et al.*, 1976; Waldmann *et al.*, 1974).

8.2.5. Changes in Adenosine Metabolism with Mitogenic Stimulation

Lymphocytes stimulated by plant lectins such as phytohemagglutinin (PHA) and concanavalin A (Con A) to undergo proliferation have provided an important model for studying *in vitro* the early events in the initiation of proliferation in resting (G_0) or restricted (G_1) cells. Binding of the lectin by lymphocytes is followed by aggregation of receptors and their removal from membrane surface (termed *patching* and *capping*); by increases in membrane transport of glucose, nucleosides, and potassium; and by increases in phospholipid synthesis, calcium influx, and intracellular concentrations of cGMP and cAMP. An increase in the rate of purine synthesis *de novo* form [^{14}C]glycine occurs within the first 2 hr, and may well be related to a 2- to 5-fold increase in intracellular PP-ribose-P concentrations observed within the first 30 min of addition of PHA to human lymphocytes (Hovi *et al.*, 1977). Proliferation in response to mitogenic stimulation requires purine synthesis *de novo,* but occurs at a normal rate in the absence of HPRT (Allison *et al.*, 1977; Seegmiller *et al.*, 1977a,b).

Several investigators have studied the changes in adenosine metabolism resulting from mitogenic stimulation of peripheral human lymphocytes and have observed the effects of adenosine and inhibitors of ADA on this process. Concentrations of the ADA inhibitor EHNA (see Fig. 4) as low as 0.3 μM inhibited ADA activity by over 90% and impaired the incorporation of tritiated leucine into protein, while it required 100 μM EHNA to produce inhibition of [^{3}H]thymidine uptake (Carson and Seegmiller, 1976). As little as 15 μM adenosine or 10 μM cAMP added to a Con-A-stimulated lymphocyte preparation inhibited [^{14}C]leucine uptake, while millimolar concentrations were required to inhibit [^{3}H]thymidine uptake. No evidence was found of any critical period early in mitogenic stimulation during which adenosine exerted its inhibitory effect to a greater extent. As might be expected, EHNA potentiated the effects of both adenosine and cAMP on leucine and thymidine uptake (Carson and Seegmiller, 1976).

Blastogenesis induced by PHA was not prevented by concentrations of coformycin that inhibited ADA activity more than 95% (Snyder *et al.*, 1976, 1977b); however, the combination of coformycin and adenosine substantially reduced both the viable cell count and the incorporation of thymidine into DNA (Snyder *et al.*, 1976, 1977b). Lymphocytes stimulated with PHA for 72 hr showed a 12-fold increase in the rate of deamination and a 6-fold increase in the rate of phosphorylation of adenosine. The specific activities of the enzymes carrying out these respective reactions remained essentially unchanged. At 72 hr, adenosine kinase activity was 92% of values obtained in unstimulated control cells, but ADA had decreased to 44% of control values. As much as 38% of initial lymphocyte ADA activity accumulated extracellularly. With concentrations of adenosine in the medium of less than 5 μM, phosphorylation was the principal route of metabolism, at greater concentrations, deamination constituted the major route in PHA-stimulated cells, but in unstimulated cells, deamination remained the principal route of adenosine metabolism. The metabolism of guanosine by PNP was also increased 6-fold by a 72 hr culture of lymphocytes with PHA stimulation without any significant change in the specific activity of this enzyme. Further evidence of the importance of adenosine in lymphocyte proliferation came from the work of Raivio and Hovi (1977) and Hovi *et al.* (1976), who reported a transient increase in ADA activity in human lymphocytes in response to PHA or pokeweed mitogen. The proliferative response was inhibited by adenosine at concentrations of 10^{-4} M or higher if use was made of horse serum, which lacks ADA. Coformycin was also an inhibitor of DNA synthesis and showed a synergistic action with adenosine.

8.2.6. Possible Role of Cyclic AMP in Immunosuppression

An inverse relationship between the cellular content of cAMP and cGMP has been observed with the intracellular concentration of cGMP increasing during PHA stimulation. At low to moderate concentrations, a succinylated derivative of Con A exerts a mitogenic action equivalent to that of native Con A, but differs from Con A in producing a progressive increase in mitogenic action at high concentration, while Con A at a similar concentration inhibits the mitogenic response. Hadden *et al.* (1976b) showed a progressive rise in cGMP with the proliferative response as measured by [^{3}H]thymidine incorporation, but no correlation with cAMP concentrations, which remained essentially unchanged. These results were presented as evidence that cGMP but not cAMP is involved in induction of the proliferative response of lymphocytes.

In earlier work, increases in cAMP levels in cultured human astrocytoma cell line, fetal rat brain, human lung fibroblast, bone cells, and lymphocytes were noted (Wolberg *et al.*, 1975) on the addition of adenosine. Clark and Seney (1976) demonstrated a 2- to 3-fold stimulation of adenylate cyclase isolated from human glioma cell lines by as little as 30 μM adenosine. Similar effects were also found in human fibroblast lines, particularly if phosphodiesterase inhibitors were added. A role for cGMP in induction of PP-ribose-P synthetase during lymphocyte activation was reported by Chambers *et al.* (1974).

One hypothesis of adenosine toxicity is that it acts by increasing the intracellular concentration of cAMP (Wolberg *et al.*, 1975). Evidence against this possibility was obtained from studies of three mutant cell lines that were resistant to killing by either isoproterenol or cholera toxin (Ullman *et al.*, 1976; see also the discussion by Martin in Seegmiller *et al.*, 1977a). Two of these lines were resistant to killing by dibutyryl cAMP as well, but all remained sensitive to killing by adenosine and EHNA. In the presence of EHNA or adenosine, the toxic effects of adenosine could be partially reversed by the addition of uridine. Thus, adenosine toxicity does not appear to be mediated by cAMP in the mouse T-cell lymphosarcoma cell line studied.

Effects similar to adenosine toxicity were observed on addition of cAMP to cultured cells, and a breakdown of cAMP to adenosine was demonstrated by enzyme activity in serum used in the culture medium (Snyder and Seegmiller, 1976).

Two binding proteins for cAMP were purified to homogeneity from rabbit erythrocytes. Each showed a molecular weight of 240,000 composed of 48,000-dalton subunits. Only adenosine significantly inhibited the binding of cAMP by these proteins, whereas cAMP had no effect on the binding of adenosine. These observations suggest the presence of two types of binding sites on receptor 1, one specific for adenosine and the other for cAMP (Yuh and Tao, 1974). Three major specific adenosine-binding proteins have been isolated from rat liver. The major adenosine-binding protein was associated with histone phosphokinase, which was stimulated 2-fold by binding cAMP. Adenosine inhibited this enzyme (Hsu, 1975).

8.2.7. Role of Adenosine Deaminase in Metabolism or Action of Drugs

The ADA activity of various tumors was correlated with their ability to inactivate the antitumor drugs 9-β-D-arabinofuranosyl-adenine (ara-A) and 9-β-D-xylofuranosyl-adenine (xyl-A) through deamination of these agents (Robins, 1975). Inhibitors of ADA activity or of the transport of these agents into blood cells were effective *in vivo* in prolonging the action of these agents.

The coronary vasodilator adenosine 5′-carboxylate and several of its esters do not inhibit ADA nor affect any aspect of purine ribonucleotide interconversions *in vitro* or *in vivo*; it does, however, increase the accumulation of [^{14}C]adenosine from [^{14}C]adenine in the presence of deoxyglucose and glucose, suggesting that it may inhibit ADA activity when relatively low concentrations of adenosine are generated (Henderson and Battell, 1976). Its potent physiological effects are thought to be mediated through a mechanism unrelated to an inhibition of specific aspects of intracellular purine metabolism.

8.3. Adenosine Deaminase (ADA) Deficiency Associated with Severe Combined Immunodeficiency Disease

The general clinical features of the syndrome associated with ADA deficiency were described in detail in *The Year in Metabolism 1975–1976* (Seegmiller, 1976a). Newly described patients continue to show a severe combined immunodeficiency disease (SCID) associated with severely depressed T-cell function and, in most families, evidence of B-cell impairment as well. The additional cases reported by Ackeret *et al.* (1976), Keightley *et al.* (1975), Mills *et al.* (1976), Polmar *et al.* (1976), Cederbaum *et al.* (1976), and Trotta *et al.* (1976) follow the same general features, with onset of infections during the first year of life with the presence of enlarged costochondral junctions, sparse lymphoid tissue, lymphopenia, marked reduction in immunoglobulin content of plasma, diminished response of lymphocytes to stimulation by mitogens, absence of delayed hypersensitivity response to common bacterial antigens, and less than 1% of normal ADA activity in erythrocytes. A new clinical feature consisting of a transient tremor not previously noted in ADA-deficient patients was described by Polmar *et al.* (1976).

Additional insight into the nature of the cartilage lesion was presented by Cederbaum *et al.* (1976). Three children, two of them siblings who died with SCID and ADA deficiency within the first 6 months of life, were examined at autopsy. The thymus showed evidence of early differentiation, and in one instance aborted Hassall's corpuscles. Radiographic abnormalities of a subtle nature summarized by Seegmiller (1976a) had been seen early in life at the costochondral junctions, at the apophysis of the iliac bones, and in the vertebral bodies. A histological study of the bone and cartilage showed a lack of normal columnar formation of cells in cartilage, large lacunae containing hypertrophied cells, and lack of trabecular formation with uninterrupted areas of calcified cartilage. These histological changes are distinctly different from those observed in metaphyseal chondrodysplasias or in chondrodystrophies. The one report of the presence of ADA deficiency in erythrocytes of a normal (!)Kung boy has been clarified with the demonstration of substantial amounts of ADA activity in his leukocytes (Jenkins *et al.*, 1976). Over two dozen patients are now known with an association of ADA deficiency and SCID (Meuwissen *et al.*, 1975; Seegmiller *et al.*, 1977a,b). This high association provides strong evidence that the enzyme defect may indeed be the primary cause of the disease.

8.3.1. Frequency

The frequency of ADA deficiency has been estimated at between one-third and one-half the small number of patients with the autosomal recessive type of SCID. In a retrospective study in Zurich, Switzerland, Ackeret *et al.* (1976) found the moderately reduced ADA activity characteristic of the heterozygous parents of 3 of 9 families who had produced an affected child and in 14 additional relatives. In a series of 10 immunodeficient children studied retrospectively in Boston, 5 had shown radiological evidence of the abnormalities of cartilage and bone associated with ADA deficiency (Rosen, 1977). In the majority of the family members, the heterozygous state is detectable by measurement of ADA activity in the erythrocytes of peripheral blood.

8.3.2. Metabolic Studies of ADA-Deficient Patients

Mills *et al.* (1976) used a fluorescent method for increasing the sensitivity of assay of adenine compounds sufficiently to allow their detection after separation with HCl on an ion-exchange chromatographic column. The reaction is based on the condensation of chloroacetaldehyde with adenine compounds to form a highly fluorescent derivative. Plasma of their ADA-deficient patient showed values for adenosine some 2- to 10-fold higher than that in plasma of control subjects along with increases in free adenine concentration 2- to 3-fold above normal. The free adenine of erythrocytes was increased 6- to 9-fold compared with that of controls, while the adenosine was unchanged. An increased excretion of free adenine was also found in the urine of the affected child. Erythrocytes of the affected patient show a nearly 2-fold increase in intracellular concentration of ATP. Pyrimidine nucleotide concentrations were normal, while orotic acid was not detected in the urine. The patient of Polmar and colleagues showed a 10-fold increase above normal in the ATP content of his erythrocytes, which was decreased to the normal range as he responded to the therapy decribed in Section 8.3.3 (Polmar *et al.*, 1976; Polmar, 1977).

Cohen *et al.* (1977a) were unable to confirm the presence of free adenine in erythrocytes, urine, or serum of an ADA-deficient child detected by screening tests and studied before onset of immunodeficiency. They reported adenosine concentrations in plasma of 1.5–2 μM compared with less than 0.5 μM in normal subjects. In erythrocytes, the adenosine content was substantially higher, 10–15 μM, compared with less than 0.5 μM in controls. No adenosine was detectable in the urine. The ATP content of erythrocytes of the ADA-deficient child was only around 10% greater than that of normal controls. These data raise the possibility of a partial or total hydrolysis of some of the adenine compounds by the hydrochloric acid used in preparation of the sample and for elution of the compounds from ion-exchange chromatographic column as performed by Mills *et al.* (1976).

The data cited above provide the first direct evidence of accumulation of adenosine in the cells or body fluids of ADA-deficient patients, and thus provide some objective support for the hypothesis of adenosine inhibiting the proliferation of lymphocytes in the ADA-deficient patient as a possible mechanism for the immunodeficiency. The concentrations of adenosine encountered in the ADA-deficient patients, however, were substantially lower than the concentrations of other purine nucleosides in patients with PNP deficiency (see Sections 8.5.2 and 8.5.3). The presence of an alternative pathway for adenosine by way of adenosine kinase could well contribute to this difference. The possibility of accumulation of another substrate for ADA such as deoxyadenosine should also be considered and attempts should be made to demonstrate its presence.

Trotta *et al.* (1976) reported a most curious increase in activity of ADA on storage at 4°C of lysates prepared from one of two affected children studied after successful bone marrow transplants. They noted a similar effect in heterozygous carriers of the family. The progressive increase in the apparent specific activity as the sample was progressively diluted before assay, and the inhibition observed on mixing with ADA partially purified from erythrocytes of normal individuals, were interpreted as indicating the presence of an inhibitor. Attempts by other investigators to verify the presence of such an inhibitor in other patients have been unsuccessful (Hirschhorn, 1977), suggesting that it may have been limited to one patient or to a peculiarity of the conditions used for the spectrophotometric assay.

8.3.3. New Approach to Treatment of ADA Deficiency

Hirschhorn *et al.* (1975) identified a male child with ADA deficiency prenatally, and the child was therefore studied from shortly after birth. During the first 6 weeks of life, both B and T lymphocytes were present and showed a proliferative response to mitogens as measured by [^{3}H]thymidine incorporation that was 25% of normal. Concurrent with his subsequent development of severe lymphopenia, the mitogen responsiveness was suppressed to less than 5% of control values. Addition of a partially purified preparation of calf intestinal ADA to the lymphocytes *in vitro* produced a 3- to 5-fold increase in [^{3}H]thymidine incorporation over values obtained in similarly stimulated cultures without ADA (Polmar *et al.*, 1975). The equivalent studies were then done *in vivo* using the ADA contained in frozen type O erythrocytes. The cells or plasma were first irradiated to kill any leukocytes and administered to this child with ADA deficiency associated with SCID (Polmar *et al.*, 1976). Administration of erythrocytes, but not plasma, restored the ability of this patient's lymphocytes to respond to mitogen *in vitro* and to synthesize immunoglobulins *in vivo*. The patient also responded to immunization with diptheria and tetanus toxoids, and his total lymphocyte count increased from less than 350 to over 1500/mm^3, with 44–48% T cells and 18–23% B cells. A thymus shadow appeared for the first time. Most telling was the ability of this child to remain free of infections for the next 17 months despite the discontinuation of all isolation procedures with retransfusion every 4–6 weeks.

As mentioned, one new clinical feature of this patient was the development of a very fine tremor of the hand, noted intermittently, beginning at the age of 3 months. In addition, the patient showed an intermittent dystonic posturing of extremely short duration when he reached for objects. When tremor was maximal, similar movements also occurred in the trunk and legs. These neurological symptoms gradually disappeared after the transfusion therapy was begun.

One additional child with ADA deficiency showed a beneficial response to the administration of frozen irradiated erythrocytes (Wolf *et al.*, 1976). In a third child, response was much less dramatic, although some doubling of the lymphocyte population of peripheral blood was observed (Goldblum, 1977).

Another approach to treatment using transplantation of allogenic fetal liver was successful in restoring the immune response in one child with SCID associated with ADA deficiency. Both T and B cells were immunocompetent, but the child died 1 year later from a fatal nephrotic syndrome associated with immune complex glomerulonephritis (Keightley *et al.*, 1975). In other children, transplantation of histocompatible bone marrow has restored immunocompetence with appearance of ADA in peripheral lymphocytes, but not in erythrocytes (Parkman *et al.*, 1975). Fetal liver and thymus have also been effective (Ackeret *et al.*, 1976).

8.3.4. Metabolic Consequences of ADA Deficiency

A variety of approaches have been taken to identify the mechanism by which ADA deficiency produces impairment of function of the cells and of the immune system. The effects of added adenosine on the growth or differentiation of various types of human cells in culture has been studied. In general, the toxic effects of adenosine were substantially greater in cells of lymphoid origin than in other cell types, and were accompanied by an excretion by the cells of orotic acid, a reduction in the intracellular concentration of pyrimidine nucleotides (Green, 1975), and a transient increase in the intracellular concentration of cAMP (Wolberg *et al.*, 1975). This reduction in intracellular pyrimidine nucleotides was traced to a profound depletion of intracellular PP-ribose-P (Snyder and Seegmiller, 1976).

The toxicity of adenosine appears to be independent of its phosphorylation to form adenine nucleotides, since the growth inhibition and the profound lowering of the intracellular concentration of PP-ribose-P in response to adenosine occurred in human lymphoblasts grossly deficient in adenosine kinase (Snyder *et al.*, 1977a; Hershfield *et al.*, 1977a). In like manner, the same investigators found adenine toxic to human lymphoblasts grossly deficient in APRT, indicating a mechanism of toxicity of adenine also independent of adenine nucleotide formation. Both adenine and adenosine produced marked depletion of PP-ribose-P, inhibition of growth, and a diminished concentration of intracellular pyrimidine nucleotides. Adenine toxicity differs from adenosine toxicity, however, in not producing an excretion of orotic acid and in the failure of uridine to reverse the growth inhibition produced by adenine as it does in part with adenosine toxicity (Snyder *et al.*, 1977a; Hershfield *et al.*, 1977a).

The effects of ADA deficiency on purine metabolism in erythrocytes and in fibroblasts cultured from affected patients has been studied. Agarwal *et al.* (1976) and Cohen *et al.* (1977a) showed that erythrocytes from heterozygous and normal individuals incorporated [^{14}C]adenosine primarily into inosinic acid, while erythrocytes from ADA-deficient patients incorporated [^{14}C]adenosine primarily into adenine nucleotides. The addition of coformycin as an inhibitor of ADA caused the normal and heterozygous cells to exhibit the same behavior as ADA-deficient cells. A similar effect was produced in normal erythrocytes by *p*-nitrobenzythioguanosine as a specific inhibitor of adenine transport.

The metabolism of adenine and adenosine was also studied in normal lymphocytes and in those obtained from patients deficient in ADA by Raivio and Hovi (1977) and Raivio *et al.* (1977). In the ADA-deficient lymphocytes, synthesis of [^{14}C]adenine into adenine nucleotides was approximately twice the rate found in normal lymphocytes, despite the presence of the same amount of APRT activity in both normal and ADA-deficient lymphocytes. Likewise, incorporation of [^{14}C]adenosine into adenine nucleotides in the ADA-deficient cells was almost twice that observed in the normal, and adenosine failed to disappear significantly on an hour's incubation of ADA-deficient cells, while it was rapidly converted to hypoxanthine and inosine by normal cells. The same difference in metabolism of [^{14}C]adenosine was also observed in fibroblasts cultured from affected patients by Cohen and Martin (1977) and by Benke and Dittmar (1976).

Another approach that has been used is to study the effect of inhibitors of ADA on the normal maturation of lymphocytes or on their response to stimulation by mitogens (Carson and Seegmiller, 1976; Snyder *et al.*, 1976, 1977b; Hovi *et al.*, 1976) (see Section 8.2.5).

8.3.5. Tissue Distribution of ADA

The distribution of ADA in various organs has been determined in the human. Adams and Harkness (1976a) found substantially higher specific activities in the thymus than in any other organ. In previous studies in animals, the highest specific activity had been reported in the spleen (Brady and O'Donovan, 1965). Adams and Harkness (1976a) found a 20-fold-higher specific activity in thymus obtained at postmortem examination. Another unusual observation was the finding that skin had twice the activity found in spleen, while liver and kidney showed activities on the order of 10 and 20%, respectively, of that of spleen. Substantially lower activities of human lymph node at autopsy, on the order of 20% of the values of spleen, were reported by Van der Weyden and Kelley (1976).

A severe immunodeficiency disease has been observed in foals of Arabian horses. Detailed studies of the activity of ADA, of xanthine oxidase, and of PNP in erythrocytes and various organs of affected foals failed to reveal any differences from the activities found in normal horses (McGuire *et al.*, 1976). The ADA activity of erythrocytes and of serum in normal horses is extremely low compared with that in other species.

8.3.6. Tissue Forms of ADA

Van der Weyden and Kelley (1976) and Daddona and Kelley (1977a,b) showed that ADA exists in three forms in human tissues: a small form of molecular weight 36,000, an intermediate form of molecular weight 114,000, and a large form of molecular weight 298,000. In addition, a particulate form accounts for approximately 3% of the total present in human lymphocytes. The large and intermediate forms of the enzyme dissociated spontaneously into the small form; the process was accelerated by incubation in succinate buffer at pH 3.4, but not at higher pH's. In contrast, the small form was converted to the large form by a tissue extract obtained from kidney or lung, both organs in which the large form predominates. The enzyme activity responsible for this conversion to the large form showed a molecular weight of 200,000. This conversion-factor activity is unusual in that the factor is consumed during the reaction. The large form of ADA predominates in tissue extracts exhibiting the lower specific activities of enzyme and abundant conversion activity. The molecular heterogeneity appears to be the result of posttranscriptional modification of the protein. The spleen of a patient who died with ADA deficiency showed only 1.5% of normal activity, with most of the residual activity residing in the intermediate-molecular-weight form of the enzyme (Van der Weyden *et al.*, 1974). ADA was purified 800,000-fold from erythrocyte using a highly specific antibody affinity column in the final step of the purification (Daddona and Kelley, 1977b). Adenosine was used as the ligand in an affinity column used for the final step in a 468,000-fold purification of ADA from human erythrocytes by Schrader *et al.* (1976) and in the purification by Carson *et al.* (1977a,b).

8.3.7. Genetic Heterogeneity of Residual ADA Activity

Hirschhorn *et al.* (1976) reported reduced but significant ADA activity in fibroblasts cultured from affected patients. It was present at around 20% of the activity found in normal fibroblasts and was of the same high-molecular-weight tissue isoenzyme found in normal fibroblasts, but showed an altered electrophoretic mobility and a greater than normal heat stability, and could be detected in fibroblasts cultured from obligate heterozygotes.

Carson *et al.* (1977a,b) reported substantially lower amounts of ADA activity in fibroblasts cultured from three affected patients. ADA activity in homozygous fibroblasts was 0.38% (range 0.28–0.55%) of that of normal fibroblasts, while heterozygous fibroblasts showed 38% of normal activity. Erythrocytes from one homozygote showed 2.7% of normal ADA activity, compared with 67% for erythrocytes from three heterozygotes. A lymphoblast line from one heterozygote showed 44.5% of the ADA activity found in normal lines.

Antibody prepared against ADA purified 45,000-fold from normal erthrocytes (Carson *et al.*, 1977a,b) showed the presence of 35% of the normal amount of cross-reactive material in extracts of fibroblasts cultured from one ADA-deficient patient, while fibroblast extracts from two other patients showed less than 5% of the normal values. These data present convincing evidence of the genetic heterogeneity in the primary mutations occurring at the ADA locus in the different patients. Similar evidence of genetic heterogeneity was found by Chen *et al.* (1975) from differences in electrophoretic migration.

8.3.8. Possible Pathogenetic Mechanism of ADA Deficiency

Consideration of the kinetic properties of the two enzymes that are involved in the metabolism of adenosine gives some insight into their relative roles within the cell. The enzyme adenosine kinase shows a very high affinity for adenosine but a relatively low capacity to process the substrate, while ADA has a substantially lower affinity for adenosine but a much higher capacity to process it. As a consequence, priority is given within the normal cell to the synthesis of adenylic acid when adenosine is present in relatively low concentrations, while at higher concentrations, the surplus quantities of adenosine are removed by deamination. Indeed, intact human lymphoblasts show such a response (Seegmiller *et al.*, 1977a; Synder *et al.*, 1977b; Raivio and Hovi, 1977; Raivio *et al.*, 1977).

In an *in vitro* antibody-synthesizing system, both inosine and, to a greater extent, adenosine produced a substantial stimulation of antibody production followed by an inhibition at increased concentrations of these agents in the growth media (Seegmiller *et al.*, 1977a,b). These studies were done in the presence of an abundant amount of ADA and PNP in the cells and in the fetal calf serum used in their culture medium. Addition of the ADA inhibitors EHNA (see Fig. 4) or coformycin resulted in both the stimulatory and the toxic effects occurring at a substantially lower concentration of the added nucleoside.

These findings suggest that the primary role of ADA is to remove excessive quantities of adenosine beyond those needed for maintenance of intracellular adenylic acid and ATP concentrations. The demonstrated ability of adenosine to inhibit proliferation of human lymphocytes induced by mitogens (Carson and Seegmiller, 1976; Snyder *et al.*, 1976, 1977b; Hovi *et al.*, 1976) coupled with the demonstrated accumulation of adenosine in cells and body fluid of affected children provides strong evidence for a primary role of adenosine as a mediator of the immunosuppression in this disease. The reversal of the pathology and the remarkable therapeutic response achieved by the infusion of normal erythrocytes containing ADA suggests that the inhibitor may be a small readily diffusible molecule and so provide additional evidence compatible with the view of the pathogenetic role of a substrate of ADA such as adenosine. The quantity of adenosine that accumulates in cells and plasma of ADA-deficient patients is not great, however, and detailed studies of the quantity of adenosine required to produce such an immunosuppression *in vivo* remain to be performed. The possibility of the accumulation of another substrate for ADA of greater lability and possibly of greater cytotoxicity, such as deoxyadenosine, must also be considered.

The diversion of adenosine into adenine nucleotide synthesis could readily account for the 10-fold increase in ATP found in lymphocytes (Polmar *et al.*, 1976; Polmar 1977; Schmalstieg *et al.*, 1976, 1977) and for the 65% increase in ATP in erythrocytes of ADA-deficient patients (Mills *et al.*, 1976). The process would be further amplified by the greater propensity of adenosine to be converted to ATP than to AMP and ADP as a result of the compartmentalization of ATP (Rapaport and Zamecnik, 1976b), presumably in the cytosol compartment of the cell (Siess and Wieland, 1976). The reversal of the immunodeficiency correlated with the decrease of erythrocyte ATP concentrations to normal with therapy suggests the possibility that the elevated ATP is involved in the biochemical mechanism of pathogenesis (Polmar *et al.*, 1976; Polmar, 1977). The finding of comparable elevations of adenine nucleotides in a 10-month-old male with deficiencies of T- and B-cell function but normal ADA and PNP provides further evidence in favor of this concept (Goldblum *et al.*, 1976) and points the direction for future biochemical investigations in other types of immunodeficiency disease. The identification of the nucleoside antibiotic 2′-deoxycoformycin (see Fig. 4) as a new and more potent inhibitor of ADA with a K_i of 2.5×10^{-12} (Johns and Adamson, 1976; Adamson *et al.*, 1977) and the preliminary report of its producing an immunosuppression, as shown by failure to reject a transpanted tumor in mice (Chassin *et al.*, 1977), are further evidence of the etiological role of impaired ADA function in generation of immunodeficiency. The report of similar results obtained by Lum *et al.* (1977) using EHNA, a less potent inhibitor, does not agree with the short biological half-life of this compound and the negative results obtained by others (Elion, 1977). Deoxycoformycin deserves further testing as a suppressor of the immune response.

8.4. Increased Activity of ADA in Red Cells Associated with Hereditary Hemolytic Anemia

Valentine *et al.* (1977) described a new enzyme abnormality consisting of an increased ADA activity associated with a dominantly inherited hereditary hemolytic anemia in 12 members of a family of 23 spanning three generations. In addition to the hemolytic anemia, which in some cases was mild and well compensated, affected patients showed splenomegaly, reticulocytosis up to 22%, a negative Coombs test for autoimmune hemolytic anemia, and no evidence of hemoglobinopathy.

The enzyme defect consisted of a 45- to 70-fold elevation of ADA of normal K_m activity in erythrocyte lysates and was found in all affected persons—5 of 10 males and 8 of 18 females in the pedigree. Red cells showed a shortened ^{51}Cr half-life of 5 days when tranfused, compared with 28 days' survival in normal persons. Reticulocytosis averaged 6%, the range being 3.3–11.7%. The adenine nucleotide concentration of erythrocytes of affected family members averaged about 60% of the normal control mean, and less than 50% of that of blood showing a comparable degree of reticulocytosis. The major decrease was in the ATP content of erythrocytes.

The possible mechanism for the decreased ATP concentration of erythrocytes is apparent when consideration is given to the metabolic fate of adenosine depending on the relative proportion deaminated as compared with that phosphorylated. As shown in Section 8.2.5, phosphorylation is favored at low substrate concentration by the 15- to 20-fold greater affinity of adenosine for the kinase than for ADA. In the presence of increased amounts of ADA, however, a relatively larger amount is presumably deaminated to account for the decreased conversion to AMP and the resultant decrease in concentration of adenine nucleotides, particularly ATP, in the erythrocytes of affected subjects.

This disorder becomes the second clinical disorder to be associated with a dominantly inherited increase in enzyme activity. An increased activity of PP-ribose-P synthetase is associated with gouty arthritis (see Section 8.9).

8.5. Purine Nucleoside Phosphorylase (PNP) Deficiency

Now that a total of five patients with PNP deficiency with deficient T-cell function have been reported, the occurrence of generalized vaccinia in three patients, which led to the death of two (Stoop *et al.*, 1976; Hamet *et al.*, 1977; Martin, 1977), emphasizes the marked vulnerability of these children to vaccinia infection. Obviously, vaccinia immunization is contraindicated in PNP-deficient children at our present state of knowledge.

8.5.1. Clinical Presentation

Since the original description of Giblett *et al.* (1975) of one child with a gross deficiency of PNP associated with a clinical presentation of immunodeficiency disease with isolated T-cell dysfunction, two additional patients with the same clinical picture and enzyme deficiency have been reported, both within the past year—one from France (Hamet *et al.*, 1977) and one from The Netherlands (Wadman *et al.*, 1976, 1977; Siegenbeek van Heukelom *et al.*, 1976, 1977) who had two older siblings who had died of a similar disorder (Wadman *et al.*, 1977; Stoop *et al.*, 1976, 1977). In addition to immunodeficiency, the surviving child in The Netherlands developed a neurological problem.

The patient reported from France was a boy whose only infection during the first year of life was a pharyngitis (Hamet *et al.*, 1977). He was successfully immunized with BCG vaccine at 2 months of age without abnormal reaction, and no complications occurred after administration of the killed vaccines for tetnus and diptheria immunization, or even the oral live-attenuated (Sabin) poliomyelitis vaccine; at 1½ years of age, however, he developed generalized spreading necrotic lesions 15 days following vaccinia immunization and required hospitalization.

His white cell count on admission was 12,300/mm^3, with 4% lymphocytes. Serum immunoglobulins were normal, with IgA 80 mg/dl, IgG 1100 mg/dl, and IgM 150 mg/dl. Investigations of blood group allohemagglutinins showed evidence of a severe T-cell deficiency. The patient was transfused twice with 250 ml irradiated (5000 rads) fresh blood, a fetal thymus was transplanted, and he was given hyperimmune antivaccinia serum and antibiotics. Lymphocytes from a donor recently immunized with vaccinia were transfused, but all to no avail, and his illness proved fatal at 20 months of age.

The patient reported from The Netherlands was a girl, the fourth child of healthy unrelated parents (Wadman *et al.*, 1976, 1977; Stoop *et al.*, 1977; Siegenbeek van Heukelom *et al.*, 1976, 1977). The first and second children of these parents were both girls, and both had suffered from a selective cellular immunodeficiency, but appeared to have normal humoral immune repsonse. The oldest developed a generalized vaccinia after vaccination at 9 months of age, and died of a lymphosarcoma at age 3 years. The second died from a graft-vs.-host reaction at age 1½ years following a blood transfusion given elsewhere (Stoop *et al.*, 1976). The third child, a boy, was entirely healthy.

At birth, the cord blood immunoglobulins of the fourth child were normal in amounts and lymphocytes were normal in number and function, with a normal response to PHA, pokeweed mitogen, and mixed lymphocyte culture. By 3 months of age, however, the patient had developed a lymphopenia with a diminished response of her lymphocytes to mitogens. By 1 year of life, the total number of lymphocytes had decreased to around 400/mm^3, with a marked decrease in the percentage of T lymphocytes. By 15 months of age, the responsiveness of her lymphocytes to stimulation by the mitogen PHA was only 10% of normal. Immunoglobulin concentrations were normal throughout. At 3 months of age, she showed no thymus shadow on X ray. No vaccinations were performed, however, and she remained healthy.

At 15 months of age, she was first admitted to the hospital because of a throat infection and otitis media, both of which responded to specific antibacterial therapy. No tonsilar tissue was present at that time, and no lymph nodes were palpable.

Neurological examination revealed a slight but definite spastic tetraparesis and a slight retardation of motor development. Bone-marrow examination revealed lymphopenia and megaloblastic changes in both the myloid and erythroid cells. Folic acid and B_{12} were present in normal amounts and, when examined by immunofluorescent staining procedures, lymphocytes showed a normal distribution of cells containing IgM, IgG, and IgA.

Her erythrocytes showed a microcytosis and a hypochromia with a hemoglobin of 13.3 g/dl, a hematocrit of 40%, erythrocyte sedimentation rate of 28 mm/hr, and erythrocyte count of 5.51 × 10^6/mm^3. Her erythrocyte indices showed a mean corpuscular volume of 72 fl, a mean corpuscular hemoglobin of 24.1 pg, and a mean corpuscular hemoglobulin concentration of 33.0 g/dl. Reticulocyte count was 1.2%, platelet count 337,000/mm^3, and leukocyte count 4300/mm^3, with a differential count of 76% neutrophils with a marked lymphopenia of 10% lymphocytes and 7% monocytes.

Of her peripheral lymphocytes, 38% formed rosettes with complement-bearing sheep erythrocyres, indicative of T cells, and 41% formed rosettes with bovine erythrocytes sensitized with IgG-type antibody (Fc receptor). The class distribution of Ig-bearing lymphocytes was IgM 12%, IgD 12%, IgG 0%, and IgA 0.2%; with anti-Ig conjugate, 13%. Because of the relatively high percentage of lymphocytes that could not be classified by these established markers, part of them must have represented the classic null lymphocyte.

Despite the low number of Ig-bearing B lymphocytes, the serum Ig concentrations had been normal at the age of 1 year. Futhermore, she showed the following antibody titers: anti-A isohemagglutinin (blood group B) was 1:16 at 12 months and 1:32 at 15 months, and anti-*Hemophilus influenza* was 1:250. Complement-fixing antibodies were found at the following titers: against parainfluenza virus at 1:16, *Herpes hominus* at 1:16, and Coxsackie at 1:32.

8.5.2. Metabolites in Urine

Detailed studies of the urinary metabolites, both of the original patient reported (Cohen *et al.*, 1976) and of the patient in The Netherlands (Stoop *et al.*, 1976; Wadman *et al.*, 1977; Siegenbeek van Heukelom *et al.*, 1977), showed an excretion of excessive amounts of total purines, primarily as inosine and guanosine, the amount of guanosine being about half that of the inosine, along with smaller amounts of deoxyinosine and deoxyguanosine. As would be expected, the uric acid content of both the urine and serum of both patients was very low. The inability of patients to form any appreciable amounts of uric acid points to a very simple diagnostic test for this disorder: demonstration of a very low serum urate concentration of less than 1 mg/dl of urinary uric acid/creatinine ratios, expressed in milligrams, on the order of less than 0.4:1.

The patient from The Netherlands excreted 0.16 mmol uric acid/g creatinine as the mean value of eight urine collections. Recalculated in terms of milligrams, this gave a uric acid/creatinine ratio of 0.27, which should be compared with a mean value of 1.4 found in normal children of similar age (Kaufman *et al.*, 1968). Xanthosine was low or absent, and no adenosine nor any appreciable amount of xanthine was detected. She excreted 16.1 mmol inosine/g creatinine. The total purine nucleoside excretion amounted to 28.46 mmol/g creatinine. This corresponds to a uric acid/creatinine ratio by weight of 4.78, a value 3–4 times greater than the mean, and is substantially above the normal range found for children of this age group. This amount of purine production is quite comparable in degree to the purine overproduction found in children with the Lesch–Nyhan syndrome.

The parents and the brother, all heterozygotes according to the enzyme determination, excreted inosine and a trace of guanosine in the urine, with normal amounts of uric acid. No elevation of the pseudouridine, uracil, or uridine in the urine was detected.

More detailed metabolic studies of the original patient with PNP deficiency, initially described by Giblett *et al.* (1975), were reported by Cohen and colleagues (Cohen *et al.*, 1976, 1977a,b; Cohen and Martin, 1977). The patient was 7 years of age, weighed 22 kg, and excreted 360 mg creatinine in her 24-hr urine. She showed a marked hypouricuria with excretion in the 24-hr urine of 38 mg uric acid on a regular diet, which decreased to 11mg/24 hr on a diet virtually free of purines. She also excreted 720 mg inosine, 440 mg guanosine, 439 mg deoxyinosine, 220 mg deoxyguanosine, and 100 mg *N*-9-ribosyl urate, a compound not previously identified in mammalian metabolism. The renal clearance of inosine was double that of creatinine, suggesting a tubular secretory process for its excretion. The large amount of inosine and guanosine produced constitutes very good evidence for the virtual absence of the kinase for these compounds in the human species.

For comparison with uric acid production in other defects of purine metabolism, the magnitude of the excretion of purine compounds was calculated in equivalent weight of uric acid. When compared with creatinine excretion by weight, the urate/creatinine ratio in the affected child was 4- to 6-fold greater than the mean value found in children of comparable age and nearly 3-fold above the upper limit of normal. This constitutes the third primary defect in purine metabolism that is associated with overproduction of purines (see Section 8.8 and 8.9). That the enzyme deficiency blocks the formation of hypoxanthine suggests that these children, like those whith the Lesch–Nyhan syndrome, may have their purine overproduction as a result of the lack of hypoxanthine, which, under physiological conditions, normally suppresses purine synthesis.

Cohen *et al.* (1977b) described the presence of small amounts of orotic acid in the urine of two children with PNP deficiency at concentrations of 74 and 52 μM, with an excretion of 27 and 34 μg/mg creatinine. After treatment of one patient with uridine, 100 μg/kg per day, the amount of orotic acid excreted in her urine was decreased to less than 5 μM, in a manner analogous to that seen in hereditary orotic aciduria; the amount of orotic acid excreted by these children was, however, only approximately 1/50 the amount excreted by untreated patients with orotic aciduria.

The presence of even mild orotic aciduria provides evidence of some degree of impairment of pyrimidine metabolism in PNP-deficient patients. Its correction by uridine suggests the possibility of clinical benefits from uridine therapy if the aberration of pyrimidine metabolism is of significance in the pathogenesis of the disease.

8.5.3. Metabolites in Blood and Serum

The mean uric acid concentration of eight different sera of the affected patient from The Netherlands was 0.5 mg/dl, the range being 0.2–1 mg/dl. Dietary restriction of purines had very little influence on either the serum urate concentration or the amount of purine excreted. Giblett's patient also exhibited marked hypouricemia, with serum urate values of 0.8–1.0 mg/dl (Cohen *et al.*, 1976).

Examination of the serum of the child from The Netherlands, as well as that of her two sisters, which ad been stored frozen, showed the presence of substantial amounts of purine nucleosides (Siegenbeek van Heukelom *et al.*, 1977). The concentration of inosine ranged from 13.9 to 37.4 μmol/liter serum, as compared with a highest value of 1.5 μmol/liter found in three control patients. The concentrations of inosine in the frozen cord blood of both the patient and her oldest sister were 3–4 times higher than the concentration found in either at 15 months of age. Guanosine concetration in the three patients ranged from 5.6 to 14.6 μm/liter, as compared with only a trace in the serum of controls. On the other hand, hypoxanthine concentration was, as might be expected, somewhat lower in the serum of the three affected patients (5.2–5.3 μmol/liter) than in the three centrol subjects (7–14 μmol/liter). Guanine concentrations tended to be only mildly elevated, again particularly so in the cord serum. The presence of even this amount of hypoxanthine or guanine in the serum of affected children is quite surprising, since virtually no hypoxanthine is generated from [^{14}C]inosine by their cells (see Section 8.5.4). Free guanine and hypoxanthine could have arisen in this assay by hydrolysis of the corresponding deoxyribonucleosides by the sulfosalicylic acid used in preparation of the sample for chromatographic analysis.

8.5.4. PNP Enzyme Activity and Metabolism of Erythrocytes and Fibroblasts

Erythrocytes from the patient previously reported by Giblett *et al.* (1975) showed no detectable activity of PNP, while her parents showed approximately half the normal level (Cohen *et al.,* 1976). Fibroblasts cultured from the patient in subconfluent culture showed less than 0.5% of the values found in normal fibroblasts. This value increased 10-fold when the patient's fibroblasts were confluent. The mother's fibroblasts showed essentially normal activity of PNP. Both the mother's erythrocytes and fibroblasts, however, contained a form of PNP with altered electrophoretic mobility, suggesting the presence of a hybrid PNP molecule that contained both altered and normal enzyme subunit molecules. No evidence of a diffusible enzyme inhibitor was found.

The patient from France (Hamet *et al.,* 1977) showed a PNP activity in her erythrocyte and lymphocyte lysates less than 0.1% of values found in normal lysates. Erythrocyte lysates of the mother and maternal grandfather showed values 45 and 55%, respectively, of normal. PNP activity in the child's cultured fibroblasts was 1.6% of normal. The father's erythrocytes showed an activity in the normal range despite the compatibility of his *HL-A* antgens and red cell group with his paternity (Hamet *et al.,* 1977).

Both parents, and a healthy brother, of the child in The Netherlands (Stoop *et al.,* 1977) showed PNP activities in hemolysates about one-half the activities found in control subjects, while there was no PNP activity detectable in lysates of either lymphocytes or erythrocytes of the affected child (Siegenbeek van Heukelom *et al.,* 1976). These findings are in agreement with the autosomal recessive inheritance noted in the original patient reported by Giblett *et al.* (1975). On mixing normal hemolysate with hemolysate from the patient, no evidence of inhibition of PNP was found. No PNP could be found in lysates of the lymphocytes of the patient isolated from her cord blood after storage in the frozen state.

Metabolic studies of PNP-deficient erythrocytes by Siegenbeek van Heukelom *et al.* (1977) showed a rapid conversion of [^{14}C]adenosine to inosine, with no detectable label appearing in hypoxanthine. Likewise, incubation of [^{14}C]inosine resulted in a rapid conversion to IMP in the normal erythrocyte, but not in erythrocytes of the PNP-deficient patient. The high intracellular PP-ribose-P of erythrocytes was thought to reflect an impaired consumption due to lack of substrate for the salvage enzyme,

HPRT. Normal activities of HPRT and APRT were demonstrated in the erythrocytes by incubation with [^{14}C]hypoxanthine and [^{14}C]adenine.

8.5.5. Purine Production in Cultured Fibroblasts

Despite the purine overproduction shown by affected patients, no evidence of an excessive rate of incorporation of [^{14}C]glycine into purines, as compared with proteins, was found in fibroblast cultures by Cohen *et al.* (1976). This is in contrast to the marked increase in this ratio observed in HPRT-deficient fibroblasts (Cohen *et al.*, 1976). Although erythrocytes of a PNP-deficient patient showed a 6-fold increase in PP-ribose-P concentration, the cultured fibroblasts showed normal concentration of PP-ribose-P quite in keeping with their lack of an excessive rate of purine synthesis. Conceivably, residual PNP activity in the fetal calf serum used in culturing the cells may have provided an enzyme replacement, or the serum could have provided hypoxanthine and thereby corrected the excessive rate of purine synthesis noted *in vivo.*

8.5.6. Possible Pathogenetic Mechanisms of PNP Deficiency

Since adenosine was not found in the serum and urine of PNP-deficient patients, it seems unlikely that a common mechanism is directly involved in the immunodeficiency of ADA and PNP deficiencies. An obvious explanation for the immunodeficiency disease associated with PNP deficiency would be an inhibitory action of one or more of the accumulated nucleosides on lymphocyte proliferation. Guanosine is such a compound. It inhibits substantially the growth of human lymphoblast cell lines in culture (Astrin, 1973; Brenton *et al.*, 1977). Lymphoblast lines are grossly deficient in the enzyme guanase, and are therefore unable to rapidly dispose of increased quantities of guanine. As a consequence, these cells show a substantial increase in the intracellular concentration of guanine nucleotides associated with the arrest of cellular growth when exposed to guanine or guanosine in the growth medium. Growth arrest is relieved after a lag period on removal of the guanine compounds from the media.

Recent studies of mitogen-stimulated human lymphocytes by Ito and Uchino (1976) showed an interference by guanosine with the induction of carbamyl phosphate synthetase and aspartate transcarbamylase, both enzymes carrying out the first two steps of *de novo* pyrimidine biosynthesis. The mild orotic aciduria of affected patients suggests an additional site for a defect in pyrimidine metabolism. Disturbance of nucleic acid biosynthesis in general could well account for the megaloblastic bone marrow associated with hypochromic microcytic erythrocytes of peripheral blood. Since somewhat similar but more pronounced hematological disturbances are present in congenital orotic aciduria, the possibility that an impaired pyrimidine metabolism could contribute to the hematological disturbance is an attractive and unifying hypothesis. The possibility of toxicity from deoxyinosine or deoxyguanosine has received very little attention in studies of mammalian cell systems in recent years.

The possibility that the lack of a product of the missing enzyme reactions could be responsible for the immunodeficiency seems unlikely. The product hypoxanthine cannot be used by patients with the Lesch–Nyhan syndrome, yet they appear to have no clinical problems with immunodeficiency. The product of ADA action, inosine, can also be formed by an alternative route by the reaction of ribose-1-phosphate with hypoxanthine catalyzed by PNP. Whatever the mechanism proves to be, it would need to account for the greater sensitivity of T cells than B cells to this metabolic effect.

The presence of mild orotic aciduria (Cohen *et al.*, 1977b) has led to the hypothesis that the PNP deficiency leads to a PP-ribose-P deficiency, which then leads to a secondary pyrimidine nucleotide deficiency. These data suggest the possibility of clinical treatment of this disorder with uridine in a manner analogous to that used in successful treatment of the clinical symptoms of orotic aciduria.

Against this view is the finding of overproduction of purines in the children in association with an increased erythrocyte concentration of PP-ribose-P, a presumed rate-limiting substrate in the control of purine synthesis.

Cohen *et al.* (1976, 1977a) discussed the possibility of similar mechanisms being involved in the overproduction of purines in PNP deficiency and in the Lesch–Nyhan syndrome. In both disorders, the ability to form inosinic acid is impaired. In the Lesch–Nyhan syndrome, the impairment results from the absence of an active HPRT enzyme, whereas in PNP deficiency, it results from the absence of the substrate, hypoxanthine, required for that reaction. That one patient with PNP deficiency has now been described with a mild spastic tetraplegia raises the possibility of some similarities in mechanism being responsible for the neurological problems in the two diseases. The hypothesis that an accumulation of inosine in PNP-deficient patients leads to secondary inhibition of ADA activity through an end-product inhibition of the enzyme, as a uniform explanation for the immunodeficient phenotypes of PNP deficiency and ADA deficiency in children, now seems very unlikely. The failure to find any accumulation of adenosine in PNP deficiency, while it definitely accumulates in the serum and cells in ADA deficiency (Mills *et al.*, 1976; Cohen *et al.*, 1977a), would argue against this hypothesis.

8.5.7. Properties of Purified PNP

A 4000-fold purification of PNP from rabbit liver was reported by Lewis and Glantz (1976) and by Treuman and Glantz (1977). The preparation gave a single band on both nondenaturing gel electrophoresis and sodium dodecyl sulfate gel electrophoresis. A molecular weight of 30,500 daltons was obtained for the presumed subunit and 62,000 daltons from material passed through a Sephadex G-100 gel filtration column. Two bands of 35,000 and 70,000 daltons were obtained in cross-linkage experiments using dimethyl suberimidate, indicating that the protein is a dimer.

PNP was purified 2800-fold from normal human erythrocyte lysate by a two-step procedure with a yield of 56% by Zannis *et al.* (1977a,b). The native enzyme has a molecular weight of 93,800, with a subunit molecular weight of 29,700. It thus appears to be a trimer. Gel electrophoresis of the purified human enzyme revealed four major separable subunits, all with the same molecular weight and presumably the result of posttranscriptional modifications.

Milman *et al.* (1976a) purified the PNP enzyme of Chinese hamsters to homogeneity from liver and kidney and from a cultured cell line, with formation of both dimers and trimers of a 30,000-molecular-weight subunit.

The mechanism of catalysis by PNP purified from rabbit liver was investigated by Lewis (1977). From his kinetic studies of initial velocities in product inhibition, he found evidence that strongly supports an ordered Theorell–Chance mechanism involving first the combination of nucleoside with the enzyme, followed by a transient attachment of inorganic orthophosphate during its formation and release of ribose-1-phosphate, followed by release of the free purine from the enzyme purine complex.

Siegenbeek van Heukelom *et al.* (1976) showed a normal pattern of six bands of PNP activity on electrophoretic migration of erythrocyte lysates from the heterozygote father, mother, and brother of a PNP-deficient patient. They showed a 2- to 3-fold-increased K_m for the substrate inosine, but with a normal pH optimum and a decreased heat stability.

8.6. Purine 5′-Nucleotidase Deficiency in Primary Hypogammaglobulinemia

An intrinsic defect in B lymphocytes is present in most patients with primary hypogammaglobulinemia, and is manifest clincially by a failure to produce significant antibody response *in vivo* and by failure to produce immunoglobulins *in vitro* (Broom *et al.*, 1976; Waldmann and Broder, 1977). In addition, a functional defect in the T lymphocytes is found in about one-third of the patients, particularly those whose disease began in adult life (Webster and Asherson, 1974).

8.6.1. Clinical Presentation

Substantially diminished activities of the membrane-bound enzyme purine 5′-nucleotidase were found in 9 of 11 patients with primary hypogammaglobulinemia (Johnson *et al.*, 1977). All these patients had "variable" types of the disease and none had affected relatives. Only one patient developed the disease in childhood; all the others began suffering from recurring infections as adults. All the patients showed a hypogammaglobulinemia affecting the IgG class, with a geometric mean concentration for IgG of 217 mg/dl serum. All had IgA deficiency, with a mean value of less than 5 mg/dl serum. One patient had a normal IgM concentration; the mean for the rest was 6 mg/dl serum. Normal values for comparison were: IgG 981 (643–1487), IgA 200 (72–552), and IgM 115 (50–261) mg/dl serum.

Six of the patients suffered from a chronic productive cough. All except one, who was admitted for treatment of a severe episode of bronchitis, were ambulant and in good health at the time of investigation. All but one were receiving regular injections of gammaglobulin.

Lymphocytes and monocytes were harvested from defibrinated blood after separation on a standard Ficoll–Triosil density gradient. Human erythrocytes have negligible purine 5′-nucleotidase activity (Shenoy and Clifford, 1975). The mean value of the 11 patients was only one-quarter of the value found in lymphocytes from 16 control patients (Johnson *et al.*, 1977).

Most patients with chronic lymphatic leukemia show low activities of purine 5′-nucleotidase in their lymphocytes. It is also significantly lowered during the acute phase of infectious mononucleosis, suggesting that virus infections may influence the activity of this enzyme. No differences from normal were found in a variety of common diseases including bacterial infections (Quagliata *et al.*, 1974).

In recent years, research on the etiology of primary hypogammaglobulinemia has centered on possible abnormalities in the action of suppressor T cells controlling B-lymphocyte response (Waldmann *et al.*, 1974; Waldmann and Broder, 1977). In other studies, a defect in the proliferative response of lymphocytes to PHA *in vitro* was found in at least a third of the patients with adult onset of primary hypogammaglobulinemia by Webster and Asherson (1974), and evidence of an abnormally high inhibiting action of suppressor T cells was found in three-fourths of the patients studied by Waldmann and Broder (1977).

Whether or not the lowered activity of purine 5′-nucleotidase in the patients discussed above is of primary importance in the etiology of the disease is not known. The possibility remains that the lowered activity could be explained by the active site of the enzyme being exposed on the cell surface and covered by "autoantibody" or by some other abnormality in metabolism that effects purine 5′-nucleotidase activity. With a lack of family history of agammaglobulinemia in these patients, a primary hereditary enzyme deficiency seems unlikely, but in future studies, this question will need to be resolved by appropriate family studies.

Of particular interest in future studies will be the intracellular concentration of purine and pyrimidine nucleotides in patients with hypogammaglobulinemia. If the concentration of purine nucleotidase of lymphocytes were rate-limiting, one might expect an elevated intracellular concentration of adenine nucleotides, particularly ATP, in this condition as well as in ADA deficiency (see Section 8.3).

The purine 5′-nucleotidase was purified from human placenta and its properties studied by Fox and Marchant (1976, 1977). The monomeric form of the enzyme had a molecular weight of 43,500, and a dimer and higher degrees of aggregation were identified, all with similar K_m, specific activity, and response to inhibitors. Since ADP and ATP were competitive inhibitors, a lowering of their intracellular concentration as occurs with fructose infusion should enhance the hydrolysis of mononucleotides by purine 5′-nucleotidase.

8.7. Hereditary Xanthinuria

Calculi of the urinary tract, composed of xanthine, provide the basis for the classic presentation of the metabolic disease, xanthinuria. They occurred in 6 of the 19 cases reported by Seegmiller, (1974). Of the 19 patients, however, 2 showed an entirely different type of presenting symptom consisting of arthralgias and myalgias associated with the crystalline deposits of xanthine and hypoxanthine inside the muscle cells. By far the majority of patients are asymptomatic and are now detected from the inadvertent discovery of profound hypouricemia during the routine determination of serum urate as part of a battery of tests routinely performed for other reasons. The discovery of a new cause of hypouricemia in PNP deficiency (see Section 8.5) makes the identification of the urinary metabolites xanthine and hypoxanthine with very little uric acid important in confirming the diagnosis of xanthinuria and distinguishing it from that produced by an increased renal clearance of uric acid resulting from an isolated defect in the renal tubule (Benjamin *et al.*, 1977).

Four additional patients presenting with these three types of presentation have recently been reported: (1) The patient of Holmes *et al.* (1974) was asymptomatic. (2) Kitamura *et al.* (1976) reported a case of xanthine calculus associated with a retrocaval ureter, and Kenawi (1976) reported a 5-year-old boy who presented with a 1-year history of dysuria and burning micturition, followed in 4 months by pain in the right iliac fossa with fever and chills. An introabdominal abscess was drained through an iliac incision. Although the origin of the infection was not identified, a non-functioning right kidney was found and was removed at surgery. The ureter below the pelvic brim was obstructed by a smooth, pale pinkish-yellow calculus that proved to be composed of almost pure xanthine. A postoperative jejunal biopsy was obtained by a Crosby capsule, and the homogenate of the biopsy showed no detectable xanthine oxidase activity by a radiochemical assay. The 24-hr urinary tract uric acid excretion was 29 mg (lower limit of normal was 80 mg/24 hr), urinary oxypurines were 172 mg/hr (highest limit of normal was 25 mg/24 hr). During the past 23 years, some type of surgical intervention has been required in 6 of the 8 patients who presented with xanthine calculi. (3) The fourth case was a report by Isaacs *et al.* (1975) of detailed studies of a woman in her early forties who presented with generalized aches and pains that were particularly troublesome in the knees and, to a lesser extent, in other joints. In addition, she complained of muscle pains, particularly in the shoulder region. Uric acid was almost absent from her serum. Muscle biopsy revealed high concentrations of xanthine and hypoxanthine with virtual absence of uric acid in the muscle extracts. Crystalline deposits of oxypurines in the skeletal muscle were found at biopsy. Chalmers (1975) commented on this type of clinical presentation and suggested the possibility of an alternative mechanism for the oxidation of the hypoxanthine to xanthine analogous to the oxidation of allopurinol to oxypurinol by xanthinuric patients *in vivo.* These reports confirm Chalmers's original observation and should alert the clinician to the possibility of this basis for clinical symptoms of arthralgia and myalgia.

The effect of allopurinol on oxypurine excretion in a patient with xanthinuria was reported by Salti *et al.* (1976). Allopurinol administration resulted in a 20% increase of oxypurine excretion and an elevation of the urinary xanthine/hypoxanthine ratio from 4.08 to 6.53. This rise was interpreted as evidence that residual xanthine oxidase activity was present. The authors also suggested that the excessive reutilization of hypoxanthine and xanthine in this disease prevents the allopurinol-induced inhibition of *de novo* purine synthesis seen in normal subjects.

8.8. Hypoxanthine-Guanine Phosphoribosyltransferase (HPRT) Deficiency

The clinical presentation, metabolic consequences, and enzyme characteristics of the varying degrees of deficiency of the HPRT enzyme were presented in comprehensive reviews by Seegmiller (1976c) and deBruyn (1976). Considerable evidence has accumulated of heterogeneity of this disease at many different levels. The disease shows a considerable range in the clinical presentation. At one extreme is the severe neurological involvement with choreoathetosis, spasticity, mental retardation, compulsive self-mutilation, and marked overproduction of uric acid that constitutes the classic Lesch–Nyhan syndrome associated with the virtually complete deficiency of the enzyme. At the other end of the spectrum are patients who present with gouty arthritis as a result of purine overproduction and, in general, less severe degrees of enzyme deficiency. An intermediate group shows, in addition, relatively mild neurological symptoms of considerable diversity.

Exceptions are being found in which the enzyme defect as measured in the assays *in vitro* under saturating conditions may not reflect the true enzyme activity of the enzyme in its natural state within the cell *in vivo*. Mutations affecting the affinity of the enzyme for one of its substrates are frequent causes of such disparity. Holland *et al.* (1976a) attempted to approximate the conditions *in vivo* by evaluating the activity of this enzyme in intact cultured fibroblasts obtained from patients with varying degrees of HPRT deficiency. The activity reported for the enzyme under these conditions was only a small fraction of the activity obtained in the lysates. The degree of lowering of enzyme activity required to produce hyperuricemia is the subject of continuing investigation among gouty patients.

Sweetman *et al.* (1977a) reported one patient who had as little as 40% of normal activity of HPRT in his erythrocytes, still in association with an increased content of PP-ribose-P in the erythrocytes. Whether or not the patient with an HPRT activity 80% of normal reported by Holland *et al.* (1976a) truly had a deficiency is a matter for controversy, since the normal range of enzyme activity could well extend to 80% of the mean in a normal population.

8.8.1. Clinical Correlations with HPRT Activity

A 25-yr-old patient, admitted for bilateral ureteral obstruction due to uric acid stone, gave a history of earlier episodic joint pain compatible with possible gouty arthritis. Henderson *et al.* (1976) found 44% of normal HPRT activity in lysates of his erythrocytes associated with a 15-fold increase in the K_m of the enzyme for the substrate PP-ribose-P. Five hemizygotes and nine heterozygotes for HPRT deficiency in five families all showed an excessive rate of turnover of [^{15}N]urate injected intravenously and an excessive incorporation of [^{14}C]glycine into urinary uric acid. Of the nine heterozygotes, only four showed excretion of an excessive amount of uric acid in the 24-hr urine, only two had hyperuricemia leading to gout, and one had a low urate clearance (Emmerson and Row, 1975).

Schneider *et al.* (1976) described absence of HPRT in a 20-yr-old man with spastic quadraplegia, choreoathetosis, oligophrenia, and hyperuricemia who had never shown any tendency toward self-mutilation. A similar absence of self-mutiliation with a normal intelligence and a gross deficiency of HPRT was described by Manzke (1976) in the patient originally described by Catel and Schmidt (1959), who is thus confirmed as the earliest reported case of this disease.

8.8.2. Biochemical Mechanism of the Neurological Defect

The mechanism by which the primary deficiency of HPRT in cells of the CNS leads to the neurological dysfunction characteristic of this disease has been one of the most puzzling aspects of this disorder (McKeran, 1977; Nyhan, 1976, 1977). Breakefield *et al.* (1976) reported a marked diminution in monoamine oxidase (MAO) activity in a murine neuroblastoma cell line lacking HPRT activity and in skin fibroblasts from four of six patients with the Lesch–Nyhan syndrome (Roth *et al.*, 1976). Skaper and Seegmiller (1976) reported a significant but far less marked decrease in MAO activity in rat glioma cell lines in cultures grossly deficient in HPRT. Whether of not a comparable decrease of MAO activity is present in basal ganglia and other cells of the CNS must await appropriate studies on the affected patient at autopsy. In the body, 5-hydroxytryptophan (5-HTP) is decarboxylated to 5-hydroxytryptamine (5-HT, serotonin), which is then deaminated and oxidized by MAO to 5-hydroxyindoleacetic acid (5-HIAA), which is excreted in the urine.The mean excretion of 5-HIAA in the 24 hr urine of ten children with the Lesch–Nyhan syndrome was nearly double that found in nine subjects of similar age range (Sweetman *et al.*, 1977b).

Earlier reports of a beneficial effect of 5-HTP in diminishing the self-mutilation in this disease (Mizuno and Yugari, 1974) were not confirmed in studies performed by Frith *et al.* (1976), Anderson *et al.* (1976), and discussion by Kelley in Nyhan (1977). Nyhan (1976, 1977) reported a transient improvement in some patients on treatment with 5-HTP, particularly when an inhibitor of peripheral decarboxylation, carbadopa, was used. In none of the patients, however, did this treatment provide sustained relief of symptoms. In each patient, the drug soon became ineffective. Anderson *et al.* (1977) reported the ineffectiveness of punishment reinforcement as a mode for diminishing the self-mutilation behavior, but positive reinforcement of non-self-mutilation behavior and "time-out" procedures were effective. These results emphasize the importance of environment in the management of behavioral aspects of this disease. Presumably, children with the Lesch–Nyhan syndrome are incapable of learning from aversive stimulation.

In recent years, some evidence has accumulated for a role for purine nucleotides as possible mediators of neurotransmission in the purinergic nerves of parts of the GI tract, cardiovascular system, and brain (Burnstock, 1977). If such a system proves to be of importance, than a more direct relationship between HPRT deficiency and abnormalities of function in the nervous systems could conceivably be established.

8.8.3. Nature of the Enzyme Abnormality

Considerable evidence has accrued for a variety of different types of mutations of the HPRT locus being responsible for HPRT deficiency (Nyhan, 1977; Bakay and Nyhan, 1975; Bakay *et al.*, 1976, 1977b). Hemolysates from 13 patients with the Lesch–Nyhan syndrome who have virtually total deficiency of HPRT activity and 2 patients with hyperuricemia with 2–5% of normal HPRT activity were unable to neutralize immunoglobulin produced against HPRT that had been highly purified from human erythrocytes. They showed no evidence whatever of cross-reacting material. Such material was found, however, in erythrocytes of 2 other patients with 4.5 and 50% of normal HPRT activity, and in a partially deficient heterozygous female with 34% of normal activity in her erythrocytes in a family with a less severe degree of impairment in HPRT activity (Bakay *et al.*, 1976, 1977b). A normal amount of cross-reacting material was found in only 1 of the 14 HPRT-deficient patients examined by Upchurch *et al.* (1975).

Three interconvertible variants of HPRT were detected by polyacrylamide gel electrophoresis by Arnold and Kelley (1975); all three were immunologically identical and had similar substrate utilization and end-product inhibition. All showed a molecular weight of 68,000 and a Stokes radius of 36 Å, and were composed of two noncovalently bound subunits of equal molecular weight of 34,000. Amino acid composition was nearly identical, and the electrophoretic differences were attributed to a post-transcriptional alteration of one or both subunits of HPRT.

The activity of HPRT in a wide variety of human and rat tissues was determined at various stages of development from fetal life onward by Adams and Harkness (1976b). After birth, activities were especially high in the testes and the CNS, with higher values found in adults in the gray matter of the cerebral cortex than in the basal nuclei or white matter.

8.8.4. Mechanism of Purine Overproduction

The marked overproduction of uric acid and the consistent elevation of PP-ribose-P of erythrocytes, cultured fibroblasts, or lymphoblasts continue to be consistent correlates of the Lesch–Nyhan syndrome.

An excessive rate of synthesis of purine nucleotides from [^{14}C]formate was reported by Brosh *et al.* (1976) in human peripheral blood leukocytes obtained from gouty patients affected with partial deficiency of HPRT. Some new considerations have been added, however, to the continuing discussion of the mechanism of purine overproduction in this disorder. Hershfield *et al.* (1977b) and Hershfield and Seegmiller (1977a) drew attention to the functional deprivation of hypoxanthine in HPRT deficiency as being a major cause of purine overproduction in this disease (see Section 8.2.3) and provided evidence that under these conditions, the concentration of PP-ribose-P inside the cell may not be the primary determinant of the rate of purine synthesis. The rise in intracellular PP-ribose-P that occurs in normal cells on stringent deprivation of hypoxanthine could conceivably create conditions in which the PP-ribose-P concentration is no longer rate-limiting.

Martin and Maler (1976) reported an increased activity of PP-ribose-P synthetase in fibroblasts from patients with complete or partial deficiency of HPRT or in HPRT-deficient hepatoma cells (Graf *et al.*, 1976), and proposed that this may well be the primary mechanism responsible for their excessive uric acid synthesis. Reem (1975) reported similar results in HPRT-deficient erythroleukemia cells. These results are at variance, however, with earlier studies by Rosenbloom *et al.* (1968) and by Becker *et al.* (1973) and Becker (1977b). One important consideration is the different assay systems used by the goups that obtained the divergent results. The procedure used by Martin and Maler and by Reem gives values for PP-ribose-P synthetase that are approximately one-fifth the values reported in the two-step reaction using partially purified APRT described by Rosenbloom *et al.* (1968) and by Becker and colleagues (Becker *et al.*, 1973; Becker, 1977b). A satisfactory resolution of these discordant results has not yet been made.

8.8.5. Genetics of HPRT Deficiency

HPRT deficiency continues to be a very useful genetic marker for manipulation of cells. Kahan and DeMars (1975) presented evidence for derepression of the gene for HPRT on the human inactive X chromosome obtained in hybrids of mouse and human cells. Milman *et al.* (1976b) presented a convenient system for detecting the various types of HPRT mutations in HeLa cells and evidence for activation of a silent gene in a revertant.

Genetic complementation of the HPRT deficiency was reported in hybrid cells derived from virus-induced hybrid mouse clones deficient in HPRT activity (Sekiguchi and Sekiguchi, 1973; Sekiguchi *et al.*, 1974, 1975a). Three complementation groups were identified, two of which correlated with the method used in selection, with one group obtained by using 6-thioguanine, and one by selection using 8-azaguanine. Transfer of the HPRT gene between two closely related cell lines was accomplished using metaphase chromosomes (Degnen *et al.*, 1976; Sekiguchi *et al.*, 1975b). The transferred HPRT gene is initially unstable, but in selective media is eventually stabilized. These data provide further evidence for the presence of genetic heterogeneity at the locus for HPRT (Nyhan, 1977). Emerson *et al.* (1977) presented autoradiographic evidence of two erythrocyte populations in a heterozygote family showing partial HPRT deficiency.

The frequency of new mutations of HPRT deficiency as revealed by the presence of two definable populations of cells in hair roots and in skin fibroblasts of mothers of affected children in 47 independent families was summarized by Francke *et al.* (1976) and Bakay *et al.* (1977a). Instead of the one-third predicted from theoretical considerations, only four probands were found to represent first mutations in a total of 47 families studied. The possibility of the new mutation arising in the germ cells of the maternal grandparents was suggested.

8.8.6. Other Conditions Associated with HPRT Deficiency

Allison *et al.* (1975, 1977) reported rather subtle abnormalities of the immune system in patients with the Lesch–Nyhan syndrome, including diminished plasma concentration of IgG, slight diminution in B cells in peripheral blood, and diminished isohemagglutinins. These observations seemed at variance with the clinical features of the disease. In none of these children has an unusual susceptibility to infections been reported. Other workers found the values for IgG of affected patients to be within the normal range for children (Seegmiller *et al.*, 1977b; see discussion by Scott in Allison *et al.*, 1977). The latter worker also found a normal concentration of B cells in peripheral blood.

8.9. Increased Activity of Phosphoribosylpyrophosphate Synthetase

The range of clinical presentation of patients with increased activity of PP-ribose-P synthetase has been extended substantially by identification of additional patients. Becker and Seegmiller (1975) and Becker (1976b, 1977a) identified two additional families with increased activity of this enzyme. Both propositi had gout and marked overproduction or uric acid, with a high incidence in one patient of renal calculi composed of uric acid. In one of the new families, the increased enzyme activity resulted from a K_m mutation of the enzyme resulting in a higher than normal affinity for ribose-5-phosphate, one of the substrates for PP-ribose-P synthetase. In still another family, the increased intracellular concentration of PP-ribose-P was related to an increase in intracellular concentration of ribose-5-phosphate, a substrate for PP-ribose-P synthetase. A resistance to feedback inhibitors is another cause of increased activity of PP-ribose-P synthetase (Sperling *et al.*, 1977a). The properties of the purified and normal enzyme have been described (Becker *et al.*, 1975, 1977).

8.9.1. Inheritance

The increased PP-ribose-P synthetase activity was inherited in a dominant manner compatible with either autosomal or X-linked transmission. Zoref *et al.* (1977b) presented evidence suggesting the presence of both normal and mutant cell populations in fibroblasts cultured from the mother of two affected patients, as would be expected for an X-linked gene from the random inactivation of one of the two X chromosomes that occurs in females. The evidence is based, however, on a greater resistance of the mutant cells to the lethal decrease in purine synthesis produced by methylmercaptopurine ribonucleoside. This resistance is also transferable to normal cells as a new form of metabolic cooperation (Zoref *et al.*, 1977a).

8.10. Adenine Phosphoribosyltransferase (APRT) Deficiency

8.10.1. Clinical Presentation

More detailed studies have now been reported of the case of urinary lithiasis in the original patient of Cartier and Hamet (1974), a child who showed gross deficiency of APRT. Clinical symptoms included abdominal colic from ureteral stones with elimination in the urine of crystals and small calculi (Debray *et al.*, 1976).

In addition, Simmonds *et al.* (1976, 1977) and Van Acker *et al.* (1977) identified gross deficiency of APRT in two young brothers. The father gave a history of surgery for right-sided calculus. The older brother was asymptomatic. The younger, aged 3 years, had passed gravel and small stones since birth. The stones varied in color from whitish-yellow to gray-blue, and ranged up to 3 mm in diameter. The crystals in the urine were first erroneously reported on routine laboratory examination to be uric acid, as was the chemical composition of the calculi.

At age 20 months, the patient showed no abnormal clinical findings on examination other than a marked muscular hypotonia and hyperlaxity of the joints. As a result of the hypotonia, subsequent motor developmental milestones were retarded, but intelligence was normal. No self-mutilation was ever observed. His kidneys showed a normal glomerular filtration rate. His serum urate was 6.3 mg/dl, and his uric acid excretion was 8.6 mg/kg per 24 hr by colorimetric procedure. No opacities were seen on X-ray films of the abdomen. One year later, the patient showed an appreciable diminution of the hypotonia and he was able to walk normally. EMGs and EEGs were normal.

Urine continued to show a sediment with a large number of crystals. More precise evaluation by the investigators showed the quantity of uric acid in the urine and plasma to be within the normal limits, when the enzymatic method was used, with a serum urate of 3 mg/dl and 24-hr uric acid excretion of 120–211 mg. More detailed examination of the urine by chromatography, however, revealed 17.6 mg adenine/24 hr, an amount more than 10-fold higher than the urinary adenine content of normal adults.

8.10.2. Chemical Composition of Calculi

Cartier and Hamet (1974) and Debray *et al.* (1976) presented evidence conclusively identifying the composition of their patient's calculi as 2,8-dihydroxyadenine by physical methods, including X-ray diffraction spectrum, chromatographic analysis on ion-exchange column, and IR and UV absorption spectra.

Direct analysis of an HCl extract of the stones of the patient reported by Simmonds *et al.* (1976, 1977) by UV spectrophotometry showed an absorption spectrum identical to that of a known sample of 2,8-dihydroxyadenine at pH 2. At pH 10, however, the spectrum was sufficiently close to that of uric acid to present a possible source of serious error in identification. Small fragments of various stones were further identified by introducing them into a mass spectrometer and determining their mass spectra at elevated temperatures. The spectrum of the major constituents was identical to that of a reference sample of 2,8-dihydroxyadenine. An HCl extract of the stones was resolved into six different compounds on high-voltage electrophoresis, followed by chromatography in the second dimension on thin-layer plates. The major component which constituted approximately 90% of the stone showed electrophoretic and chromatographic mobilities identical to those of authentic 2,8-dihydroxyadenine. Of the five minor components, only two were present in sufficent quantities to allow their identification as small amounts of uric acid with traces of xanthine. The identity of the same three components was also confirmed by IR absorption spectra.

8.10.3. Therapy

The patient of Cartier and Hamet (1974) and Debray *et al.* (1976) was lost to follow-up before definitive therapy could be started.

Treatment of the patient of Simmonds *et al.* (1976, 1977) with a low-purine diet and alloupurinol at a dose of 125 mg/day caused cessation of the gravel formation and of the renal colic over the full 3 months for which the patient was last observed (Simmonds *et al.,* 1977).

The muscular hypertonia was transient and can possibly be ascribed to a long-standing low-protein diet administered earlier as therapy for his calculus formation before admission. He did, however, retain hyperlaxity of the joints—which is also present to a lesser degree in his older brother—as the only clinical symptom. The precise difference in the two brothers responsible for the failure of the older to form renal stones (see Section 8.10.1) remains an enigma. The absence of a therapeutic effect during an earlier treatment of the child with allopurinol may have been related to the simultaneous treatment with alkali and to the lower dose administered.

8.10.4. APRT Activity in Erythrocytes

Erythrocyte hemolysates from this patient showed an HPRT activity in the normal range, but the APRT activity was less than 1% of normal, whereas the ARPT activity in the mother was 47% of normal; the father and other members of the family were not immediately available at the time of writing (Simmonds *et al.,* 1976; Van Acker *et al.,* 1977).

Of particular interest was the discovery of a comparable degree of APRT deficiency (with less than 0.8% of normal APRT) in the patient's older brother. This 7-year-old boy was of normal intelligence and entirely healthy without any complaint. He showed no abnormalities on clinical examination, except perhaps for a slight hyperlaxity of the joints. His urine also showed increased amounts of adenine and its oxidation product, 2,8-dioxyadenine, but no crystals were seen in the sediment and no stone formation was observed.

8.10.5. Adenine and Other Purine Metabolites in Urine

Although the quantities of uric acid, hypoxanthine, and xanthine excreted by the patient in the 24-hr urine were in the normal range, adenine and its two metabolites, 8-hydroxyadenine and 2,8-dihydroxyadenine, were present in increased amounts. His urinary excretion of 8-hydroxyadenine was 0.02 mmol/24 hr, while that of his brother was 0.01 mmol/24 hr. None was detectable in the urine of controls or of the heterozygote mother. The 2,8-dihydroxyadenine excreted by the patient was in a somewhat larger amount, 0.14 mmol/24hr, but his clinically unaffected brother excreted only 0.08 mmol/24 hr. The adenine excretion was 0.10 mmol/24 hr for the patient on a low-purine diet, while it was 0.20 mmol for the unaffected brother on a regular diet. The 24-hr uric acid production of the APRT-deficient patient with increased dietary purines was substantially greater than that of a normal control subject maintained on a similar diet (Simmonds *et al.*, 1977).

8.10.6. Genetics

The transmission and enzyme activity suggest an autosomal recessive pattern of inheritance. Five heterozygotes from the mother's side of the family were found with APRT activity in erythrocyte lysates ranging from 20 to 47% of normal. Another aspect of the immediate family history that may be of importance was the report of four spontaneous abortions. It is possible that these abortions represented a lethal form of APRT deficiency. Plasma uric acid in all the 14 relatives was in the normal range. The APRT activity of mixtures of the hemolysates of this patient, or that of his older brother, when mixed with hemolysates of a control subject showed no evidence of the presence of an inhibitor.

8.10.7. APRT Deficiency in Cell Culture

Fibroblasts were not obtained from the patient of Cartier and Hamet (1974), and no reports have yet appeared on metabolic studies on the cells from the child in Belgium. However, a cell line of human lymphoblasts grossly deficient in APRT activity was selected *in vitro* by their resistance to growth inhibition by 2,8-diaminopurine or 8-aza-adenine. These cells showed no increase in intracellular concentration of PP-ribose-P and no evidence of an enhanced rate of purine biosynthesis (Hershfield *et al.*, 1977b).

8.11. Nucleoside Triphosphate Pyrophosphohydrolase Deficiency

The accumulation of inosine triphosphate (ITP) in erythrocytes of certain persons was described and traced to a deficiency of the degradative enzyme, nucleoside triphosphate pyrophosphohydrolase (NTPH), by

Vanderheiden (1969). No specific pathology was noted initially. Recently, however, Vanderheiden (1976) found a somewhat increased frequency of elevated ITP in erythrocytes of inmates of a mental institution, especially among paranoid schizophrenics, as compared with the general population. The significance of this type of metabolic variation is not well delineated at present. The origin of ITP in the erythrocyte was studied by Henderson (1977), but its role in cellular metabolism remains obscure.

8.12. Gouty Arthritis

Further progress has been made in identifying and characterizing the primary enzyme defects leading to overproduction of uric acid and gout (Becker and Seegmiller, 1975; Becker, 1976b, 1977a). Nevertheless, such enzyme defects still account for the hyperuricemia of less than 5% of the gouty population and account for only a portion of patients who overproduce uric acid. In the majority of gouty patients, no basic enzyme disturbance has yet been identified, and a heterogeneous group of associations continues to be found with the hyperuricemia of gouty arthritis. These include obesity, hypertension, renal disease, lead poisoning as a late effect, ingestion of a wide range of drugs (Kelley, 1975), and associated disturbances of the endocrine or hematopoietic system (Seegmiller, 1974).

Significant progress has also been made in gaining new concepts of the possible sequence of events leading to deposition of monosodium urate crystals in and about the joints, their interaction with leukocytes, and the possible factors involved in the initiation and propagation of the acute gouty attack. Gout, uric acid, and related matters are the subjects of a number of recent reviews (Müller *et al.*, 1977a,b; Klinenberg, 1975; Kelley, 1975, 1976; Holmes *et al.*, 1975–1976; *Ciba Foundation Symposium No.* 48, 1977; Watts, 1976) and books (Newcombe, 1975; Talbott and Yü, 1976; Wyngaarden and Kelley, 1976). Relevant material also appears in reviews on urolithiasis research (Fleisch *et al.*, 1976; Van Reen, 1977).

8.12.1. Metabolic Abnormalities Associated with Gout

Additional types of mutations in the HPRT locus are being found as a cause of gout (see Section 8.8.3). Sweetman *et al.* (1977a) described a gouty patient with excessive production of uric acid and 60% of normal HPRT activity in lysates of his erythrocytes. His HPRT showed a decreased affinity of the enzyme for hypoxanthine and guanine with a 4-fold elevation in the K_m for these two substrates and a V_{max} 60% of normal, but a normal K_m for PP-ribose-P. Van Herwaarden *et al.* (1976) described partial HPRT deficiency in a gouty Celebesian family.

The high intracellular concentration of PP-ribose-P has provided a unifying concept in the mechanism of purine overproduction proposed for both severe and partial HPRT deficiency (see Section 8.8.4). The discovery of increased activity of PP-ribose-P synthetase in families correlated with an increased intracellular concentration of PP-ribose-P and excessive uric acid production in still other gouty families provided additional evidence in support of this concept (see Section 8.9).

A discordant factor in these considerations has been the lack of a consistent increase in the PP-ribose-P content of erythrocytes in all patients who showed a substantial overproduction of uric acid. The intracellular PP-ribose-P content was consistently increased, however, in fibroblasts cultured from 14 gouty patients who produce excessive amounts of uric acid. Furthermore, these cells also showed a consistent correlation between PP-ribose-P content and the rate of the early steps of purine biosynthesis as measured by the incorporation of [^{14}C]formate into formylglycineamide ribonucleotide in the presence of azaserine (Becker and Seegmiller, 1975; Becker, 1976b).

Consideration of these factors has resulted in a system for classification of purine overproduction (Becker and Seegmiller, 1975; Becker, 1976b). The increased intracellular concentration of ribose-5-phosphate found in cultured fibroblasts of one patient with an overproduction of uric acid (Becker, 1976b, 1977a) suggests the possibility of a primary abnormality at some step in the oxidative pathway of glucose to pentose. Sperling *et al.* (1977b), however, presented evidence that ribose-5-phosphate may not be rate-limiting, based on studies of the stimulation of the oxidative pathway of glucose produced by methylene blue or ascorbic acid.

Clifford *et al.* (1977) showed that serially cultured fibroblasts from gouty patients who overproduce uric acid displayed increased activities of various enzymes of purine metabolism with increasing cell passage, while fibroblasts from normal donors showed little change in such activity. The authors suggested that this might indicate an increase in the rate of purine turnover in aging gouty fibroblasts compared with normal fibroblasts.

The overproduction of uric acid observed in patients with glycogen storage disease Type 1 with glucose-6-phosphatase deficiency has been attributed to a more rapid breakdown of purine nucleotides, possibly related to an increase in the intracellular concentration of inorganic phosphate (Roe and Kogut, 1977). Continuous infusion of carbohydrates throughout the night, as treatment for this disease, decreased substantially the overproduction of uric acid, although it remained elevated about 2-fold compared with that of normal individuals (Greene *et al.*, 1976; Benke and Gold, 1977).

Nishizawa *et al.* (1976) reported a 14% lower activity of adenosine kinase in erythrocytes of 26 gouty patients. Moderate increases in activity of ADA in other gouty patients were also found (Nishizawa *et al.*, 1975; Snyder and Seegmiller, 1977). In a human lymphoblast line deficient in ADA, no evidence was found for an intrinsic overincorporation of formate into purine nucleotides, suggesting that this enzyme defect by itself does not lead to purine overproduction (Hershfield *et al.*, 1977a,b).

8.12.2. Clinical Features of Gouty Arthritis

The characteristics of gouty arthritis in females were reviewed by Yü (1977). Women showing onset of gout before the menopause usually have a strong family history of the disease, while those with onset of gout after the menopause often develop it in association with the use of diuretics. Renal calculi and tophi can precede the first acute attack of gout and may be the first indication of the presence of a blood dyscrasia; in this way, the presentation is no different from that in males.

A patient with leukemia in whom gouty arthritis and renal failure were the presenting symptoms was described by Morley *et al.* (1976). A patient with Downs syndrome who developed gout showed a normal range of incorporation of [^{15}N]glycine into urinary uric acid (Nishida *et al.*, 1976). The possibility that a recurrent superficial phlebitis in the lower extremity in a hyperuricemic patient was an isolated manifestation of an acute gouty inflammation was suggested on the basis of its response to colchicine and its prevention by lowering serum urate in a patient who had no prior history of gout (Pasero, 1977).

8.12.3. Local Conditions That Favor Urate Deposition

A tendency for acute gouty attacks and tophi to develop at the site of previous injury has long been known. Further evidence of the role of tissue damage in precipitation of crystals has come from several sources. Schumacher (1977) described two gouty patients who developed bullae containing massive numbers of monosodium urate crystals. In one patient, a burn had precipitated the bullae, demonstrating the role of local tissue injury in tophus localization.

Simkin (1977a,b) presented a thoughtful analysis of the possible role of local factors in urate deposition. The predilection for involvement of the first metatarsal phalangeal joint has previously been related to the unusually large amount of weight sustained over the relatively small area of the joint, which leads to an increased susceptibility of this joint to trauma during weight-bearing (Seegmiller, 1974). The presence of relatively minor structural abnormalities such as a halux valgus deformity may further accelerate the development of an early osteoarthritis. To account for acute attacks having their onset in early-morning hours, he proposes the accumulation of a minimal to moderate effusion in this joint during the sustained weight-bearing of walking, and its gradual resolution during the night when the feet are more elevated in the reclining position. He presented experimental evidence demonstrating a more than 2-fold greater rate of loss of water than of monosodium urate from a resolving effusion, thus providing a possible mechanism for the development of a substantial supersaturation of monosodium urate within the joint fluid. As a consequence, monosodium urate would accumulate within the resolving effusion at a substantially higher concentration than is present in the plasma, thus leading to more extreme degrees of supersaturation and thereby predisposing to urate crystal formation. Such a concentration mechanism could also account not only for the large deposits of crystals found within the gouty joint, but also for development of an acute gouty attack in particularly susceptible persons at concentration of serum urate within the upper range of normal and somewhat below the usually accepted saturating concentration. Additional predisposing effects include the lower temperature of peripheral joints and the tendency for seed crystal formation at the lower intraarticular pH. This, he proposes, is enhanced by trauma or injury of osteoarthritis as well as by the cavitation that occurs with normal use of the joint. Once the seed crystals are formed, crystal growth and additional crystal deposition could readily occur, leading to attacks of gouty arthritis. In keeping with this view of the role of even mild trauma of activity was the observation by Glynn and Clayton (1976) of marked tophaceous deposits in the active limb and their absence from the useless upper limb in the same hemiplegic patient.

Malawista (1977) reviewed the environmental factors involved in crystal formation and growth, with particular emphasis on the evidence suggesting that synovial tissue rather than the interarticular space can be the site of the gouty inflammation. He also concentrated on the interaction of leukocytes with crystals and the role of colchicine in suppressing this interaction. Spilberg *et al.* (1976) described the isolation of a chemotactic factor from leukocytes after their exposure to monosodium urate crystals. For phagocytosis to occur, the crystals must be coated with a γ-globulin or other protein (Kozin *et al.*, 1977; Skosey *et al.*, 1977). A hypothesis for a mechanism of urate crystal deposition involving proteoglycan destruction by lysosomal enzymes was proposed by Stuhlsatz *et al.* (1977).

8.12.4. Characteristics of the Monosodium Urate Crystal

The precise atomic and molecular features of the topography of monosodium urate crystals that lead them to disrupt lysosomal membranes during propagation of the gouty inflammation has been investigated. Mandel and Mandel (1976) and Mandel (1976) used X-ray diffraction analysis to derive the detailed arrangement of molecules on the surfaces of crystals. By comparison of models of the surface topography of crystals known to disrupt lysosomes and cause inflammation (monosodium urate monohydrate, calcium pyrophosphate dihydrate, and the silicon dioxide crystals: α-quartz, tridymite, and crystobalite) with that of crystals that fail to produce inflammation (cystine, titanium dioxide as anatase, and silicon dioxide in the form of stishovite), they deduced the molecular configurations at the surface shared by the two groups. The unifying feature allowing a crystal to disrupt a lysosomal membrane and thereby produce an inflammatory reaction is the presence of marked surface irregularities at the molecular level. In contrast, the noninflammatory crystals showed crystal faces that were smooth, regular, and boxlike.

8.12.5. Uric Acid and the Kidney

The mechanism of the bidirectional transport of uric acid by the human nephron was discussed in several publications and reviews (Rieselbach and Steele, 1975; Rieselbach, 1977; Klinenberg, 1975). Considerable evidence has accumulated supporting the view that urate is completely filtered at the glomerulus except for that bound to plasma proteins (Klinenberg *et al.*, 1977a) followed by a proximal and distal region of reabsorption with an interspersed region of tubular secretion. The role of uric acid in development of gouty nephropathy was reviewed by Emmerson and Row (1975). The pathogenesis of the early phase of acute urate nephropathy has been studied in the rat using sodium oxonate to inhibit uricase with infusion of large amounts of lithium urate intravenously. Not only was tubular obstruction noted in the collecting ducts but also obstruction of the distal renal vasculature was found. Whether or not this degree of obstruction is involved in the human disease, of course, remains unknown (Conger *et al.*, 1976).

Salicylate administration suppressed the urate nephropathy induced by sodium oxonate and urate (Klinenberg *et al.*, 1977b). The concepts of etiology and treatment of uric acid calculi were reviewed by Seegmiller (1976b) and de Vries and Sperling (1976, 1977).

8.12.6. Treatment of Gout

The treatment of gouty arthritis was reviewed by Kelley (1976). The effect of a wide variety of pharmacological agents on the serum urate was also reviewed by Kelley (1975). Studies by Sturge *et al.* (1977) showed that naproxen is equally effective as phenylbutazone in controlling the acute attacks of gouty arthritis. The risks of hyperuricemia and indications for treatment were presented at a panel discussion by an international group of specialists at the International Symposium on Purine Metabolism (Müller *et al.,* 1977b). The importance of the 24-hr excretion of uric acid as part of the evaluation of hyperuricemia and gouty patients was stressed. The upper limit of normal for the excretion of uric acid was generally taken as 800 mg/24 hr for persons on an unrestricted diet, and 600 mg/24 hr after a 3–5 day equilibration on a diet virtually free of purines. Obviously the latter test seems to be less subject to spurious values from consumption of high-purine foods such as fermented drinks, meat, or leguminous vegetables. Most participants agreed on the desirability of treating patients with asymptomatic hyperuricemia if the serum urate is consistently above 9 mg/dl. The correlation of hyperuricemia with obesity and other cardiac risk factors including subclinical diabetes and hyperlipidemia type IV was noted by Takkunen and Reunanen (1977) in a Finnish population, by Frank (1977) in an Austrian population, by Scott *et al.* (1977) in English and Scottish populations, and by Jacobs (1977) in a South African group. The value of weight reduction of obese patients was again stressed as a means of lowering the serum urate concentration (Scott *et al.,* 1977).

8.13. Abnormalities of Pyrimidine Metabolism

No new primary defects in pyrimidine metabolism were reported in the past year. Additional evidence was brought forth, however, for a very close interaction between purine and pyrimidine metabolism. Ito and Uchino (1976) reported an inhibition of the induction of the glutamine-utilizing carbamylphosphate synthetase (CPT) and aspartate transcarbamylase (AT) of PHA-stimulated periphral human lymphocytes by adenine guanine or guanosine. Surprisingly, adenosine showed relatively little effect. Guanine, and to a slightly lesser extent guanosine, inhibited the incorporation of $[^{14}C]NaHCO_3$ into uridine nucleotides in intact cells.

Nuki *et al.* (1977a,b) and Brenton *et al.* (1977) reported an increase in intracellular concentration of pyrimidine nucleotides in lymphoblast lines grossly deficient in HPRT. Presumably, the latter effect is related to their increased intracellular concentration of PP-ribose-P, which acts as an allosteric activator of CPT and AT. A similar accumulation of pyrimidine nucleotides was not found in fibroblasts cultured from Lesch–Nyhan patients. The marked increase in intracellular pyrimidine nucleotides produced by adenosine toxicity was discussed in Section 8.3.2 and 8.3.8.

8.13.1. Pyrimidine 5′-Nucleotidase Deficiency

Additional families with a gross deficiency of pyrimidine 5′-nucleotidase (PN) of erythrocytes were described (Ben-Bassat *et al.,* 1976; Rochant *et al.,* 1975). In all families, the defect was associated with congenital nonspherocytic hemolytic anemia. A recessive mode of inheritance is indicated by the diminished activity of PN in both parents, who were also first cousins, in a family in Spain with both a male and a female affected offspring (Vives-Corrons *et al.,* 1976a,b). Valentine *et al.* (1976) reported marked inhibition of PN in lead poisoning as a possible cause of the hemolytic anemia.

8.13.2. Hyperammonemia with Orotic Aciduria

A 3-year-old girl with mental and physical retardation was found by Beaudry *et al.* (1975) with chronic hyperammonemia and orotic aciduria. Plasma concentrations of glutamine, alanine, and proline were high. Increasing the protein intake induced symptoms of ammonia intoxication with convulsions. She excreted up to 693 mg orotic acid/day, and the amount excreted was directly correlated with blood ammonia levels. The ammonia rose with an ornithine load while citrulline was normally metabolized, thus providing evidence of a partial deficiency of ornithine carbamyltransferase. This enzyme was not present in normal leukocytes, rendering them useless for diagnosis.

8.13.3. Drug and Nutritional Factors That Affect Pyrimidine Metabolism

A consistent side effect of the administration of the uricase inhibitor sodium oxonate to the mouse is an increase in excretion of orotic acid in the urine (Mangoff and Milner, 1977). A potent inhibitor of pyrimidine biosynthesis was described by Kwong and Tsuboi (1977). This compound, *N*-(phosphonacetyl)-L-aspartate, acts as a competitive inhibitor with carbamylphosphate in the reaction catalyzed by aspartate transcarbamylase with a K_i of 1×10^{-8} M. Its inhibitory effect on cell growth continues for up to 15 days after removal of the inhibitor from the medium. Yet the inhibitory action on growth can be prevented or reversed by the addition of uridine to the culture medium. It shows antitumor activity against transplantable carcinoma of the colon in mice with prolongation of survival by 55%.

A dietary deficiency of arginine, like deficiencies of other amino acids involved in urea synthesis, produced a prompt increase in orotic acid excretion in rats, mice, hamsters, guinea pigs, and dogs of all ages. The excretion of ammonia, urea, and citric acid is not consistently correlated with arginine deficiency in all species and ages. Orotic acid excretion is thus the most reliable indicator of a dietary deficiency of arginine (Milner *et al.,* 1975).

The orotic aciduria associated with administration of allopurinol to gouty patients is corrected to a significant extent by the administration of RNA. UMP, CMP, GMP, and AMP each produced some degree of correction, while IMP, guanine, and adenine had little or no effect (Zöllner and Gröbner, 1977; Zöllner *et al.*, 1977).

Treatment of human cells in culture with adenine, but not adenosine, resulted in an excretion of orotic acid into the media (Snyder *et al.*, 1977a).

8.13.4. Orotic Aciduria Accompanying Other Errors of Metabolism

A mild orotic aciduria was found in patients with T-cell immunodeficiency disease associated with PNP deficiency (Cohen *et al.*, 1977b). This finding suggests the possibility that an impaired synthesis of pyrimidine nucleotides may underlie the metabolic derangement in this disease. If this were indeed true, uridine should provide a ready correction of this type of metabolic problem.

8.14. Chemotherapy of Malignancies and Viral Diseases

The wide range of analogues of purine and pyrimidine compounds used in the therapy of various malignancies or in the treatment of specific viral infections is a far greater subject than can be covered adequately in the space limitations of this chapter. Recent reviews were published by Robins, (1975), Bloch (1973), and Sartorelli and Johns (1975). The results being obtained in the clinical use of a number of antiviral drugs such as cytosine arabinoside (Ara-C) or adenine arabinoside (Ara-A), the latter used in the treatment of DNA virus infections including severe human infections with *Herpes hominis,* raise the prospect of extending our chemotherapy to include the treatment of other DNA viruses. Ribavirin is effective in therapy of a number of RNA virus infections in animals, and substantially prolonged the survival of NZB mice, an animal model of human lupus erythematosus (Klassen *et al.*, 1977). Viral bodies have been identified in the tissues of NZB mice. Ribavirin appears to be an inhibitor of RNA polymerase of viral but not of mammalian origin (Eriksson *et al.*, 1977).

The metabolism of purines and pyrimidines in malignant cells differs in many important ways from that of normal cells. The pattern of enzymes in the reutilization pathways of purine metabolism was assessed in normal and in leukemic leukocytes by Dietz and Czebotar (1977). In general, leukemic cells showed higher concentrations of adenine nucleotides, which were related to an increased activity of adenosine kinase and a diminished activity of ADA.

The prospect before us is one of greatly extending our ability to treat more rationally and effectively this large group of diseases through a reasoned use of specific inhibitors for treatments that are based on our knowledge of the metabolic differences in the various types of cells. It promises to be an area of continuing rapid development in the year ahead.

ACKNOWLEDGMENTS

This work was supported in part by grants AM-13622, AM-05646, and GM-17702 from the United States Public Health Service, and grants from the National Foundation and the Kroc Foundation.

References

Ackeret, C., Plüss, H. J., and Hitzig, W. H., 1976, Hereditary severe combined immunodeficiency and adenosine deaminase deficiency, *Pediatr. Res.* **10**:67–70.

Adams, A., and Harkness, R. A., 1976a, Adenosine deaminase activity in thymus and other human tissues, *Clin. Exp. Immonol.* **26**:647–649.

Adams, A., and Harkness, R. A., 1976b, Developmental changes in purine phosphoribosyltransferases in human and rat tissues, *Biochem. J.* **160**:565–576.

Adamson, R. H., Zaharevitz, D. W., and Johns, D. G., 1977, Enhancement of the biological activity of adenosine analogs by the adenosine deaminase inhibitor 2'-deoxycoformycin, *Pharmacology* **15**:84–89.

Agarwal, R. P., Crabtree, G. W., Parks, R. E., Jr., Nelson, J. A., Keightley, R., Parkman, R., Rosen, F. S., Stern, R. C., and Polmar, S. H., 1976, Purine nucleoside metabolism in the erythrocytes of patients with adenosine deaminase deficiency and severe combined immunodeficiency, *J. Clin. Invest.* **57**:1025–1035.

Alford, B. L., and Barnes, E. M., Jr., 1976, Hypoxanthine transport by cultured Chinese hamster lung fibroblasts, *J. Biol. Chem.* **251**:4823–4827.

Allison, A. C., Hovi, T., Watts, R. W. E., and Webster, A. D. B., 1975, Immunological observations on patients with Lesch–Nyhan syndrome, and on the role of *de novo* purine synthesis in lymphocyte transformation, *Lancet* **2**:1179–1183.

Allison, A. C., Hovi, T., Watts, R. W. E., and Webster, A. D. B., 1977, The role of *de novo* purine synthesis in lymphocyte transformation, in: *Ciba Found. Symp. No. 48: Purine and Pyrimidine Metabolism,* pp. 207–224, Elsevier/Excerpta Medica and North-Holland, Amsterdam and New York.

Anderson, L. T., Herrmann, L., and Dancis, J., 1976, The effect of L-5-hydroxytryptophan on self-mutilation in Lesch–Nyhan disease: A negative report, *Neuropaediatrie* **7**:439–442.

Anderson, L., Dancis, J., Alpert, M., and Herrmann, L., 1977, Punishment learning and self-mutilation in Lesch–Nyhan disease, *Nature (London) B* **265**:461–463.

Arnold, W. J., and Kelley, W. N., 1975, Studies on the electrophoretic variants of human hypoxanthine-guanine phosphoribosyltransferase, in: *Isozymes I: Physiological Function,* pp. 213–225, Academic Press, New York.

Astrin, K., 1973, Purine metabolism in cultured human lymphoid cells, Ph.D. thesis Department of Biology, University of California, San Diego, California.

Bakay, B., and Nyhan, W. L., 1975, Heterogeneity of hypoxanthine-guanine phosphoribosyl transferase from human erythrocytes, *Arch. Biochem. Biophys.* **168**:26–34.

Bakay, B., Becker, M. A., and Nyhan, W. L., 1976, Reaction of antibody to normal human hypoxanthine phosphoribosyltransferase with products of mutant genes, *Arch. Biochem. Biophys.* **177**:415–426.

Bakay, B., Francke, U., Nyhan, W. L., and Seegmiller, J. E., 1977a, Experience with detection of heterozygous carriers and prenatal diagnosis of Lesch–Nyhan disease, in: *Advances in Experimental Medicine and Biology,* Vol. 76A, *Purine Metabolism in Man II: Regulation of Pathways and Enzyme Defects* (M. M. Müller, E. Kaiser, and J. E. Seegmiller, eds.), pp. 351–358, Plenum Press, New York.

Bakay, B., Graf, M., Carey, S., and Nyhan, W. L., 1977b, Study of immunoreactive material in patients with deficient HPRT activity, in: *Advances in Experimental Medicine and Biology,* Vol. 76A, *Purine Metabolism in Man II: Regulation of Pathways and Enzyme Defects* (M. M. Müller, E. Kaiser, and J. E. Seegmiller, eds.), pp. 361–369, Plenum Press, New York.

Balis, M. E., 1976, Uric acid metabolism in man, *Adv. Clin. Chem.* **18**:213–246.

Ballet, J.-J., Insel, R., Merler, E., and Rosen, F. R., 1976, Inhibition of maturation of human precursor lymphocytes by coformycin, an inhibitor of the enzyme adenosine deaminase, *J. Exp. Med.* **143**:1271–1276.

Beaudry, M. A., Letarte, J., Collu, R., Leboeuf, G., Ducharme, J. R., Melancon, S. B., and Dallairf, L., 1975, Chronic hyperammonemia with orotic aciduria: Evidence of pyrimidine pathway stimulation (author's transl.), *Diabete Metab.* **1**:29–37.

Becker, M. A., 1976a, Regulation of purine nucleotide synthesis: Effects of inosine on normal and hypoxanthine-guanine phosphoribosyltransferase-deficient fibroblasts, *Biochim. Biophys. Acta* **435**:132–144.

Becker, M. A., 1976b, Patterns of phosphoribosylpyrophosphate and ribose-5-phosphate concentration and generation in fibroblasts from patients with gout and purine overproduction, *J. Clin. Invest.* **57**:308–318.

Becker, M. A., 1977a, Fibroblast phosphoribosylpyrophosphate and ribose-5-phosphate concentration and generation in gout with purine overproduction, in: *Advances in Experimental Medicine and Biology,* Vol. 76A, *Purine Metabolism in Man II: Regulation of Pathways and Enzyme Defects* (M. M. Müller, E. Kaiser, and J. E. Seegmiller, eds.), pp. 270–279, Plenum Press, New York.

Becker, M. A., 1977b, Effects of inosine on purine synthesis in normal and HGPRT-deficient fibroblasts, in: *Advances in Experimental Medicine and Biology,* Vol. 76A, *Purine Metabolism in Man II: Regulation of Pathways and Enzyme Defects*

(M. M. Müller, E. Kaiser, and J. E. Seegmiller, eds.), pp. 370–375, Plenum Press, New York.

Becker, M. A., and Seegmiller, J. E., 1975, Recent advances in the identificaiton of enzyme abnormalities underlying excessive purine synthesis in man, *Arthritis Rheum.* **18**(Suppl.):687–694.

Becker, M. A., Meyer, L. J., and Seegmiller, J. E., 1973, Gout with purine overproduction due to increased phosphoribosylpyrophosphate synthetase activity, *Am. J. Med.* **55**:232–242.

Becker, M. A., Kostel, P. J., and Meyer, L. J., 1975, Human phosphoribosylpyrophosphate synthetase: Comparison of purified normal and mutant enzymes, *J. Biol. Chem.* **250**:6822–6830.

Becker, M. A., Meyer, L. J., Huisman, W. H., Lazar, C. S., and Adams, W. B., 1977, Human phosphoribosylpyrophosphate synthetase: Relation of activity and quaternary structure, in: *Advances in Experimental Medicine and Biology,* Vol. 76A, *Purine Metabolism in Man II: Regulation of Pathways and Enzyme Defects* (M. M. Müller, E. Kaiser, and J. E. Seegmiller, eds.), pp. 71–79, Plenum Press, New York.

Ben-Bassat, I., Brok-Simoni, F., Kende, G., Holtzmann, F., and Ramot, B., 1976, A family with red cell pyrimidine 5′-nucleotidase deficiency, *Blood* **47**:919–922.

Benjamin, D., Sperling, O., Weinberger, A., Pinkas, J., and deVries, A., 1977, Familial renal hypouricemia due to isolated tubular defect, in: *Advances in Experimental Medicine and Biology,* Vol. 76B, *Purine Metabolism in Man II: Physiology, Pharmacology, and Clinical Aspects* (M. M. Müller, E. Kaiser, and J. E. Seegmiller, eds.), pp. 72–76, Plenum Press, New York.

Benke, P. J., and Dittmar, D., 1976, Purine dysfunction in cells from patients with adenosine deaminase activity, *Pediatr. Res.* **10**:642–646.

Benke, P. J., and Gold, S., 1977, Purine metabolism in therapy of von Gierke's disease, *Pediatr. Res.* **11**:511 (abstract).

Bergsma, D. (ed.), 1975, *Immunodeficiency in Man and Animals; Birth Defects, Vol. II, Sinauer Associates, Sunderland, Massachusetts.*

Bloch, A., 1973, The design of biologically active nucleosides, in: *Drug Design,* Vol. IV (E. J. Ariens, ed.), pp. 285–378, Academic Press, New York.

Bogusky, R. T., Lowenstein, L. M., and Lowenstein, J. M., 1976, The purine nucleotide cycle: A pathway for ammonia production in the rat kidney, *J. Clin. Invest.* **58**:326–335.

Brady, T. G., and O'Donovan, C. I., 1965, A study of the tissue distribution of adenosine deaminase in six mammal species, *Comp. Biochem. Physiol.* **14**:101–120.

Breakefield, X. O., Castiglione, C. M., and Edelstein, S. B., 1976, Monoamine oxidase activity decreased in cells lacking hypoxanthine phosphoribosyltransferase activity, *Science* **192**:1018–1020.

Brenton, D. P., Astrin, K. H., Cruikshank, M. K., and Seegmiller, J. E., 1977, Measurement of free nucleotides in cultured human lymphoid cells using high-pressure liquid chromatography, *Biochem. Med.* **17**:231–247.

Broom, B. C., De la Concha, E. G., Webster, A. D. B., Janossy, G. J., and Asherson,

G. L., 1976, Intracellular immunoglobulin production *in vitro* by lymphocytes from patients with hypogammaglobulinemia and their effect on normal lymphocytes, *Clin. Exp. Immunol.* **23**:73–77.

Brosh, S., Boer, P., Kupfer, B., deVries, A., and Sperling, O., 1976, *De novo* synthesis of purine nucleotides in human peripheral blood leukocytes: Excessive activity of the pathway in hypoxanthine-guanine phosphoribosyltransferase deficiency, *J. Clin. Invest.* **58**:289–297.

Buckley, R. H., Gilbertsen, R. B., Schiff, R. I., Ferreira, E., Sanal, S. O., and Waldmann, T. A., 1976, Heterogeneity of lymphocyte subpopulations in severe combined immunodeficiency: Evidence against a stem cell defect, *J. Clin. Invest.* **58**:130–136.

Burnstock, G., 1977, The purinergic nerve hypothesis, in: *Ciba Found. Symp. No. 48: Purine and Pyrimidine Metabolism,* pp. 295–314, Elsevier/Excerpta Medica and North-Holland, Amsterdam and New York.

Carson, D. A., and Seegmiller, J. E., 1976, Effect of adenosine deaminase inhibition upon human lymphocyte blastogenesis, *J. Clin. Invest.* **57**:274–282.

Carson, D. A., Goldblum, R., Keightley, R., and Seegmiller, J. E., 1977a, Immunoreactive adenosine deaminase (ADA) in cultured fibroblasts from patients with combined immunodeficiency disease, in: *Advances in Experimental Medicine and Biology,* Vol. 76A, *Purine Metabolism in Man II: Regulation of Pathways and Enzyme Defects* (M. M. Müller, E. Kaiser, and J. E. Seegmiller, eds.), pp. 463–470, Plenum Press, New York.

Carson, D. A., Goldblum, R., and Seegmiller, J. E., 1977b, Quantitative immunoassay of adenosine deaminase in combined immunodeficiency disease, *J. Immunol.* **118**:270–273.

Cartier, M. P., and Hamet, M., 1974, A new metabolic disease: The complete deficit of adenine phosphoribosyltransferase and lithiasis of 2,8-dihydroxyadenine, *C. R. Acad. Sci. (Paris)* **279**:883–886.

Catel, V. W., and Schmidt, J., 1959, Über familiare gichtische Diathese in Verbindung mit zerebralen und renalen Symptomen bei einem Kleinkind, *Deutsch. Med. Wochenschr.* **84**:2145–2147.

Cederbaum, S. D. Kaitila, I., Rimoin, D. L., and Stiehm, E. R., 1976, The chondroosseous dysplasia of adenosine deaminase deficiency with severe combined immunodeficiency , *J. Pediatr.* **89**:737–742.

Chalmers, R. A., 1975, Crystals in skeletal muscle in xanthinuria and in allopurinol-treated gout patients, *S. Afr. Med. J.* **49**:2072.

Chambers, D. A., Martin, D. W., and Weinstein, Y., 1974, The effect of cyclic nucleotides on purine biosynthesis and the induction of PRPP synthetase during lymphocyte activation, *Cell* **3**:375–380.

Chassin, M. M., Chirigos, M. A., Johns, D. G., and Adamson, R. H., 1977, Adenosine deaminase inhibition for immunosuppression, *N. Engl. J. Med.* **296**:1232.

Chen, S.-H., Scott, C. R., and Swedberg, K. R., 1975, Heterogeneity for adenosine deaminase deficiency: Expression of the enzyme in cultured skin fibroblasts and amniotic fluid cells, *Am. J. Hum. Genet.* **27**:46–52.

Ciba Foundation Symposium No. 48: Purine and Pyrimidine Metabolism, 1977, Elsevier/Excerpta Medica and North-Holland, Amsterdam and New York.

Clark, R. B., and Seney, M. N., 1976, Regulation of adenylate cyclase from cultured human cell lines by adenosine, *J. Biol. Chem.* **251**:4239–4246.
Clifford, A. J., Steine, L., and Castles, J. J., 1977, Activities of purine pathway enzymes in gouty human fibroblasts aged *in vitro, Clin. Chim. Acta* **74**:255–260.
Cohen, A., and Martin, D. W., Jr., 1977, Inosine uptake by cultured fibroblasts from normal and purine nucleoside phosphorylase deficient humans, *J. Biol. Chem.* **252**:4428–4430.
Cohen, A., Doyle, D., Martin, D. W. Jr., and Ammann, A. J., 1976, Abnormal purine metabolism and purine overproduction in a patient deficient in purine nucleoside phosphorylase, *N. Engl. J. Med.* **295**:1449–1454.
Cohen, A., Ammann, A. J., Staal, G. E. J., Borkowsky, W., Hirschhorn, R., and Martin, D. W., Jr., 1977a, Purine, pyrimidine and pyridine nucleotide levels in erythrocytes of purine nucleoside phosphorylase and adenosine deaminase deficient patients (personal communication).
Cohen, A., Staal, G. E. J., Stoop, J. W., Ammann, A. J., and Martin, D. W., Jr., 1977b, Orotic aciduria in two patients with inherited deficiencies of purine nucleoside phosphorylase, *J. Clin. Invest.* **60**:491–494.
Conger, J. D., Falk, S. A., Guggenheim, S. J., and Burke, T. J., 1976, A micropuncture study of the early phase of acute urate nephropathy, *J. Clin. Invest.* **58**:681–689.
Daddona, P. E., and Kelley, W. N., 1977a, Human adenosine deaminase: Purification and subunit structure, *J. Biol. Chem.* **252**:110–115.
Daddona, P. E., and Kelley, W. N., 1977b, Purification of human erythrocyte adenosine deaminase, in: *Advances in Experimental Medicine and Biology*, Vol. 76A, *Purine Metabolism in Man II: Regulation of Pathways and Enzyme Defects* (M. M. Müller, E. Kaiser, and J. E. Seegmiller, eds.), pp. 223–234, Plenum Press, New York.
Debray, H., Cartier, P., Temstet, A., and Cendron, J., 1976, Child's urinary lithiasis revealing a complete deficit in adenine phosphoribosyltransferase, *Pediatr. Res.* **10**:762–766.
deBruyn, C. H., 1976, Hypoxanthine-guanine phosphoribosyltransferase deficiency, *Hum. Genet.* **31**:127–150.
Degnen, G. E., Miller, I. L., Eisenstadt, J. M., and Adelberg, E. A., 1976, Chromosome-mediated gene transfer between closely related strains of cultured mouse cells, *Proc. Natl. Acad. Sci. U.S.A.* **73**:2838–2843.
deVries, A., and Sperling, O., 1976, Uric acid stone formation: Basic concepts of aetiology and treatment, in: *Scientific Foundations of Urology,* Vol. I (D. I. Williams and G. D. Chisholm, eds.), pp. 297–302, William Heinemann Medical Books, London.
deVries, A., and Sperling, O., 1977, Implications of disorders of purine metabolism for the kidney and the urinary tract, in: *Ciba Found. Symp. No. 48: Purine and Pyrimidine Metabolism,* pp. 179–206, Elsevier/Excerpta Medica and North-Holland, Amsterdam and New York.
Dietz, A. A., and Czebotar, V., 1977, Purine metabolic cycle in normal and leukemic leukocytes, *Cancer Res.* **37**:419–426.
Elion, G., 1977 (personal communication).

Emmerson, B. T., and Row, P. G., 1975, An evaluation of the pathogenesis of the gouty kidney (editorial), *Kidney Int.* **8**:65–71.

Emmerson, B. T., Gordon, R. B., and Johnson, L. A., 1976, Urate kinetics in hypoxanthine-guanine phosphoribosyltransferase deficiency: Their significance for the understanding of gout, *Q. J. Med.* **45**:49–61.

Emmerson, B. T., Johnson, L. A., and Gordon, R. B., 1977, HGPRT-positive and HGPRT-negative erythrocytes in heterozygotes for HGPRT deficiency, in: *Advances in Experimental Medicine and Biology,* Vol. 76A, *Purine Metabolism in Man II: Regulation of Pathways and Enzyme Defects* (M. M. Müller, E. Kaiser, and J. E. Seegmiller, eds.), pp. 359–360, Plenum Press, New York.

Eriksson, B., Helgstrand, E., Johannsson, N. G., Larsson, A., Misiorny, A., Noren, J. O., Philipson, L., Stenberg, K., Stening, G., Stridh, S., Oberg, B., 1977, Inhibition of influenza virus RNA polymerase by ribavirin triphosphate, *Antimicrob. Agents Chemother.* **11**:946–951.

Fischer, D., Van der Weyden, M. B., Snyderman, R., and Kelley, W. N., 1976, A role of adenosine deaminase in human monocyte maturation, *J. Clin. Invest.* **58**:399–407.

Fleisch, H., Robertson, W. G., Smith, L. H., and Vahlensieck, W. (eds.), 1976, *Urolithiasis Research,* Plenum Press, New York, 582 pp.

Fox, I. H., and Marchant, P. J., 1976, Purine catabolism in man: Characterization of placental microsomal 5′-nucleotidase, *Can. J. Biochem.* **54**:462–469.

Fox, I. H., and Marchant, P., 1977, Human 5′-nucleotidase: Multiple molecular forms and regulation, in: *Advances in Experimental Medicine and Biology,* Vol. 76A, *Purine Metabolism in Man II: Regulation of Pathways and Enzyme Defects* (M. M. Müller, E. Kaiser, and J. E. Seegmiller, eds.), pp. 249–253, Plenum Press, New York.

Francke, U., Felsenstein, J., Gartler, S. M. Migeon, B. R., Dancis, J., Seegmiller, J. E., Bakay, B., and Nyhan, W. L., 1976, The occurrence of new mutants in the X-linked recessive Lesch–Nyhan disease, *Am. J. Hum. Genet.* **28**:123–137.

Frank, O., 1977, Nutritional state and purine metabolism, in: *Advances in Experimental Medicine and Biology,* Vol. 76B, *Purine Metabolism in Man II: Physiology, Pharmacology, and Clinical Aspects* (M. M. Müller, E. Kaiser, and J. E. Seegmiller, eds.), pp. 266–268, Plenum Press, New York.

Frith, C. D., Johnstone, E. C., Joseph, M. H., Powell, R. J., and Watts, R. W. E., 1976, Double-blind clinical trial of 5-hydroxytryptophan in a case of Lesch–Nyhan syndrome, *J. Neurol. Neurosurg. Psychiatry* **39**:656–662.

Giblett, E. R., Ammann, A. J., Wara, D. W., Sandman, R., and Diamond, L. K., 1975, Nucleoside phosphorylase deficiency in a child with severely defective T-cell immunity and normal B-cell immunity, *Lancet* **1**:1010–1013.

Glynn, J. J., and Clayton, M. L., 1976, Sparing effect of hemiplegia on tophaceous gout, *Ann. Rheum. Dis.* **35**:534–535.

Goldblum, R. C., 1977 (personal communication).

Goldblum, R. C., Schmalstieg, F. C., Goldman, A. S., Nelson, J. A., and Monahan, T. M., 1976, Abnormal adenine metabolism in severe combined immunodeficiency (SCID) and normal adenosine deaminase (ADA) activity, *Pediatr. Res.* **10**:387.

Graf, L. H., Jr., McRoberts, J. A., Harrison, T. M., and Martin, D. W., Jr., 1976,

Increased PRPP synthetase activity in cultured rat hepatoma cells containing mutations in the hypoxanthine-guanine phosphoribosyltransferase gene, *J. Cell. Physiol.* **88**:331–342.

Green, H., 1975, Pyrimidine starvation induced by adenosine in cultured cells and its bearing on the lymphocyte deficiency disease associated with absence of adenosine deaminase, in: *Combined Immunodeficiency Disease and Adenosine Deaminase Deficiency: A Molecular Defect* (H. J. Meuwissen, R. J. Pickering, B. Pollara, and I. H. Porter, eds.), pp. 141–155, Academic Press, New York.

Greene, H. L., Slonim, A. E., O'Neill, J. A., Jr., and Burr, I. M., 1976, Continuous nocturnal intragastric feeding for management of Type I glycogen-storage disease, *N. Engl. J. Med.* **294**:423–425.

Gusella, J. F., and Housman, D., 1976, Induction of erythroid differentiation *in vitro* by purines and purine analogues, *Cell* **8**:263–269.

Hadden, J. W., Hadden, E. M., and Coffey, R. G., 1976a, Isoprinosine augmentation of phytohemagglutinin-induced lymphocyte proliferation, *Infect. Immun.* **13**:382–387.

Hadden, J. W., Hadden, E. M., Sadlik, J. R., and Coffey, R. G., 1976b, Effects of concanavalin A and succinylated derivatives on lymphocyte proliferation and cyclic nucleotide levels, *Proc. Natl. Acad. Sci. U.S.A.* **73**:1717–1721.

Hamet, M., Griscelli, C., Cartier, P., Ballay, J., deBruyn, C., and Hoslie, P., 1977, A second case of inosine phosphorylase deficiency with severe T-cell abnormalities, in: *Advances in Experimental Medicine and Biology*, Vol. 76A, *Purine Metabolism in Man II: Regulation of Pathways and Enzyme Defects* (M. M. Müller, E. Kaiser, and J. E. Seegmiller, eds.), pp. 477–480, Plenum Press, New York.

Henderson, J. F., 1977, Inosine triphosphate metabolism in human erythrocytes, in: *Advances in Experimental Medicine and Biology*, Vol. 76A, *Purine Metabolism in Man II: Regulation of Pathways and Enzyme Defects* (M. M. Müller, E. Kaiser, and J. E. Seegmiller, eds.), pp. 115–120, Plenum Press, New York.

Henderson, J. F., and Battell, M. L., 1976, Short communications: Metabolic effects of ethyl adenosine 5′-carboxylate in Ehrlich ascites tumor cells *in vitro*, *Biochem. Pharmacol.* **25**:1915–1916.

Henderson, J. F., Dossetor, J. B., Dasgupta, M. K., and Russel, A. S., 1976, Uric acid lithiasis associated with altered kinetics of hypoxanthine-guanine phosphoribosyltransferase, *Clin. Biochem.* **9**:4–8.

Henderson, J. F., Lowe, J. K., and Barankiewicz, J., 1977, Purine and pyrimidine metabolism: Pathways, pitfalls and perturbations, in: *Ciba Found. Symp. No. 48: Purine and Pyrimidine Metabolism*, pp. 3–22, Elsevier/Excerpta Medica and North-Holland, Amsterdam and New York.

Hershfield, M. S., and Seegmiller, J. E., 1976, Regulation of *de novo* purine biosynthesis in human lymphoblasts: Coordinate control of proximal (rate-determining) steps and the inosinic acid branch point, *J. Biol. Chem.* **251**:7348–7354.

Hershfield, M. S., and Seegmiller, J. E., 1977a, Regulation of *de novo* purine synthesis in human lymphoblasts: Similar rates of *de novo* synthesis during growth by normal cells and mutants deficient in hypoxanthine-guanine phosphoribosyltransferase activity, *J. Biol. Chem.* (in press).

Hershfield, M. S., and Seegmiller, J. E., 1977b, Coordinate regulation of the proximal and distal steps of the pathway of purine synthesis *de novo* in W1-L2 human lymphoblasts, in: *Advances in Experimental Medicine and Biology,* Vol. 76A, *Purine Metabolism in Man II: Regulation of Pathways and Enzyme Defects* (M. M. Müller, E. Kaiser, J. E. Seegmiller, eds.), pp. 19–29, Plenum Press, New York.

Hershfield, M. S., Snyder, F., and Seegmiller, J. E., 1977a, Adenine and adenosine are toxic to human lymphoblast mutants deficient in adenine phosphoribosyltransferase or adenosine kinase, *Science* **197**:1284–1286.

Hershfield, M. S., Spector, E. B., and Seegmiller, J. E., 1977b, Purine synthesis and excretion in mutants of the W1-L2 human lymphoblastoid line deficient in adenosine kinase (AK) and adenine phosphoribosyltransferase (APRT), in: *Advances in Experimental Medicine and Biology,* Vol. 76A, *Purine Metabolism in Man II: Regulation of Pathways and Enzyme Defects* (M. M. Müller, E. Kaiser, and J. E. Seegmiller, eds.), pp. 303–313, Plenum Press, New York.

Hirschhorn, R., 1977 (personal communication).

Hirschhorn, R., Beratis, N., Rosen, F. S., Parkman, R., Stern, R., and Polmar, S., 1975, Adenosine-deaminase deficiency in a child diagnosed prenatally, *Lancet* **1**:73–75.

Hirschhorn, R., Beratis, N., and Rosen, F. S., 1976, Characterization of residual enzyme activity in fibroblasts from patients with adenosine deaminase deficiency and combined immunodeficiency: Evidence for a mutant enzyme, *Proc. Natl. Acad. Sci. U.S.A.* **73**:213–217.

Holland, M. J. C., DiLorenzo, A. M., Dancis, J., Balis, M. E., Yü, T.-F., and Cox, R. P., 1976a, Hypoxanthine phosphoribosyltransferase activity in intact fibroblasts from patients with X-linked hyperuricemia, *J. Clin. Invest.* **57**:1600–1605.

Holland, M. J. C., Klein, N. C., Cox, R. P., Dancis, J., Yü, T.-F., Salser, J. S., and Balis, M. E., 1976b, Purine excretion by cultured skin fibroblasts from patients with abnormal purine metabolism, *Res. Commun. Chem. Pathol. Pharmacol.* **14**:331–342.

Holmes, E. W., Jr., Mason, D. H., Jr., Goldstein, L. I., Blount, R. E., Jr., and Kelley, W. N., 1974, Xanthine oxidase deficiency: Studies of a previously unreported case, *Clin. Chem.* **20**:1076–1079.

Holmes, E. W., Kelley, W. N., and Wyngaarden, J. B., 1975–1976, Control of purine biosynthesis in normal and pathologic states, *Bull. Rheum. Dis.* **26**:848–853.

Hovi, T., Smyth, J. F., Allison, A. C., and Williams, S. C., 1976, Role of adenosine deaminase in lymphocyte proliferation, *Clin. Exp. Immunol.* **23**:395–403.

Hovi, T., Allison, A. C., Raivio, K. O., and Vaheri, A., 1977, Purine metabolism and control of cell proliferation, in: *Ciba Found. Symp. No. 48: Purine and Pyrimidine Metabolism,* pp. 225–248, Elsevier/Excerpta Medica and North-Holland, Amsterdam and New York.

Hsu, H. H. T., 1975, Specific adenosine binding proteins from rat liver (38882), *Proc. Soc. Exp. Biol. Med.* **149**:698–701.

Isaacs, H., Heffron, J. J. A., Berman, L., Badenhorst, M., and Pickering, A., 1975, Xanthine, hypoxanthine and muscle pain: Histochemical and biochemical observations, *S. Afr. Med. J.* **49**:1035–1038.

Ito, K., and Uchino, H., 1976, Control of pyrimidine biosynthesis in human lymphocytes: Inhibitory effect of guanine and guanosine on induction of enzymes for pyrimidine biosynthesis *de novo* in phytohemagglutinin-stimulated lymphocytes, *J. Biol. Chem.* **251**:1427–1430.

Jacobs, D., 1977, Hyperuricemia as a risk factor in coronary heart disease, in: *Advances in Experimental Medicine and Biology;* Vol. 76B, *Purine Metabolism in Man II: Physiology, Pharmacology, and Clinical Aspects* (M. M. Müller, E. Kaiser, and J. E. Seegmiller, eds.), pp. 231–237, Plenum Press, New York.

Jenkins, R., Rabson, A. R., Nurse, G. T., Lane, A. B., and Hopkinson, D. A., 1976, Deficiency of adenosine deaminase not associated with severe combined immunodeficiency, *J. Pediatr.* **89**:732–736.

Johns, D. G., and Adamson, R. H., 1976, Enhancement of the biological activity of cordycepin (3′-deoxyadenosine) by the adenosine deaminase inhibitor 2′-deoxycoformycin, *Biochem. Pharmacol.* **25**:1441–1444.

Johnson, S. M., Asherson, G. L., Watts, R. W. E., North, M. E., Allsop, J., and Webster, A. D. B., 1977, Lymphocyte-purine 5′-nucleotidase deficiency in primary hypogammaglobulinaemia, *Lancet* **1**:168–170.

Kahan, B., and DeMars, R., 1975, Localized derepression on the human inactive X chromosome in mouse–human cell hybrids, *Proc. Natl. Acad. Sci. U.S.A.* **72**:1510–1514.

Kaufman, J. M., Greene, M. L., and Seegmiller, J. E., 1968, Urine uric acid to creatinine ratio: A screening test for inherited disorders of purine metabolism, *J. Pediatr.* **73**:583–592.

Keightley, R. G., Lawton, A. R., Cooper, M. D., and Yunis, E. J., 1975, Successful fetal liver transplantation in a child with severe combined immunodeficiency, *Lancet* **2**:850–883.

Kelley, W. N., 1975, Effect of drugs on uric acid in man, *Annu. Rev. Pharmacol.* **15**:327–350.

Kelley, W. N., 1976, Current therapy of gout and hyperuricemia, *Hosp. Pract.* **11**:69–76.

Kenawi, M. M., 1976, Xanthinuria and xanthine calculous pyonephrosis, *J. R. Coll. Surg. Edinburgh* **21**:95–99.

Kitamura, T., Kawamura, T. Kitagawa, R., and Ogawa, A., 1976, Xanthine stone and xanthinuria associated with retrocaval ureter: Report of a case and a review of the literature (author's transl.), *Jpn. J. Urol.* **67**:670–676.

Klassen, L. W., Budman, D. R., Williams, G. W., Steinberg, A. D., and Gerber, N. L., 1977, Ribavirin efficacy in the treatment of murine autoimmune disease, *Science* **195**:787–789.

Klinenberg, J. R. (ed.), 1975, Proceedings of the Second Conference on Gout and Purine Metabolism, *Arthritis Rheum.* (Suppl.):**18**:659–893.

Klinenberg, J. R., Campion, D. S., Olsen, R. W., Caughey, D., and Bluestone, R., 1977a, A relationship between free urate, protein-bound urate, hyperuricemia and gout in Caucasians and Maoris, in: *Advances in Experimental Medicine and Biology*, Vol. 76B, *Purine Metabolism in Man II: Physiology, Pharmacology, and Clinical Aspects* (M. M. Müller, E. Kaiser, and J. E. Seegmiller, eds.), pp. 159–162, Plenum Press, New York.

Klinenberg, J. R., Bluestone, R., and Waisman, J., 1977b, Suppression of experimental urate nephropathy by salicylate, in: *Advances in Experimental Medicine and Biology,* Vol. 76B, *Purine Metabolism in Man II: Physiology, Pharmacology, and Clinical Aspects* (M. M. Müller, E. Kaiser, and J. E. Seegmiller, eds.), pp. 176–178, Plenum Press, New York.

Kozin, F., Ginsberg, M., Karasek, V., Skosey, J., and McCarty, D., 1977, Protein binding to monosodium urate crystals and its effect on platelet degranulation, in: *Advances in Experimental Medicine and Biology,* Vol. 76B, *Purine Metabolism in Man II: Physiology, Pharmacology, and Clinical Aspects* (M. M. Müller, E. Kaiser, and J. E. Seegmiller, eds.), pp. 201–208, Plenum Press, New York.

Kwong, L. K., and Tsuboi, K. K., 1977, Selective inhibition of pyrimidine biosynthesis and effect on proliferative growth of colonic cancer cells, *Fed. Proc. Fed. Am. Soc. Exp. Biol.* **36**:774 (abstract).

Lewis, A. S., 1977, Purine nucleoside phosphorylase of rabbit liver: Mechanism of catalysis, *J. Biol. Chem.* **252**:732–738.

Lewis, A. S., and Glantz, M. D., 1976, Monomeric purine nucleoside phosphorylase from rabbit liver: Purification and characterization, *J. Biol. Chem.* **251**:407–413.

Lum, C. T., Sutherland, D. E. R., and Najarian, J. D., 1977, Inhibition for immunosuppression, *N. Engl. J. Med.* **296**:819.

Malawista, S. E., 1977, Gouty inflammation, *Arthritis Rheum.* (in press).

Mandel, N. S., 1976, The structural basis of crystal-induced membranolysis, *Arthritis Rheum.* **19**:439–445.

Mandel, N. S., and Mandel, G. S., 1976, Monosodium urate monohydrate, the gout culprit, *J. Am. Chem. Soc.* **98**:2319–2323.

Mangoff, S. C., and Milner, J. A., 1977, Oxonate induced uricosuria and orotic aciduria in mice, *Fed. Proc. Fed. Am. Soc. Exp. Biol.* **36**:1117 (abstract).

Manzke, H., 1976, Variable Expressivität der Genwirkung beim Lesch–Nyhan Syndrom, *Deutsch. Med. Wochenschr.* **101**:428–429.

Martin, D., 1977, (peronal communication).

Martin, D. W., Jr., and Maler, B. A., 1976, Phosphoribosylpyrophosphate synthetase is elevated in fibroblasts from patients with the Lesch–Nyhan syndrome, *Science* **193**:408–411.

McGuire, T. C., Pollara, B., Moore, J. J., and Poppie, M. J., 1976, Evaluation of adenosine deaminase and other purine salvage pathway enzymes in horses with combined immunodeficiency, *Infect. Immun.* **13**:995–997.

McKeran, R. O., 1977, Factors in the pathogenesis of the brain damage and anaemia in the Lesch–Nyhan syndrome, in: *Ciba Found. Symp. No. 48: Purine and Pyrimidine Metabolism,* pp. 83–96, Elsevier/Excerpta Medica and North-Holland, Amsterdam and New York.

Meuwissen, H. J., Pickering, R. J., Pollara, B., and Porter, I. H., (eds.), 1975, *Combined Immunodeficiency Disease and Adenosine Deaminase Deficiency: A Molecular Defect,* Academic Press, New York.

Mills, G. C., Schmalstieg, F. C., Trimmer, K. B., Goldman, A. S., and Goldblum, R. M., 1976, Purine metabolism in adenosine deaminase deficiency, *Proc. Natl. Acad. Sci. U.S.A.* **73**:2867–2871.

Milman, G., Anton, D. L., and Weber, J. L., 1976a, Chinese hamster purine-nucleoside phosphorylase: Purification, structural and catalytic properties, *Biochemistry* **15**:4967–4973.

Milman, G., Lee, E., Gurdev, S.-G., McLaughlin, J. R., and George, M., Jr., 1976b, Analysis of HeLa cell hypoxanthine phosphoribosyltransferase mutants and revertants by two-dimensional polyacrylamide gel electrophoresis: Evidence for silent gene activation, *Proc. Natl. Acad. Sci. U.S.A.* **73**:4589–4593.

Milner, J. A., Prior, R. L., and Visek, W. J., 1975, Arginine deficiency and orotic aciduria in mammals, *Proc. Soc. Exp. Biol. Med.* **150**:282–288.

Mizuno, T.-I., and Yugari, Y., 1974, Self mutilation in the Lesch–Nyhan syndrome, *Lancet* **1**:761.

Morely, C. J., Houston, I. B., and Morris-Jones, P., 1976, Acute renal failure and gout as presenting features of acute lymphoblastic leukaemia, *Arch. Dis. Child.* **51**:723–725.

Müller, M. M., Kaiser, E., and Seegmiller, J. E. (eds.), 1977a, *Advances in Experimental Medicine and Biology,* Vol. 76A, *Purine Metabolism in Man II: Regulation of Pathways and Enzyme Defects,* Plenum Press, New York, 641 pp.

Müller, M. M., Kaiser, E., and Seegmiller, J. E. (eds.), 1977b, *Advances in Experimental Medicine and Biology,* Vol. 76B, *Purine Metabolism in Man II: Physiology, Pharmacology, and Clinical Aspects,* Plenum Press, New York, 373 pp.

Newcombe, D. S., 1975, *Inherited Biochemical Disorders and Uric Acid Metabolism,* University Park Press, Baltimore, 282 pp.

Nishida, Y., Akaoka, I., Nishizawa, T., Maruki, M., Aikawa, T., Mitamura, T., Yokohari, R., and Horiuchi, Y., 1976, A case of gouty arthritis associated with Down's syndrome, *J. Ment. Defic. Res.* **20**:277–283.

Nishizawa, T., Nishida, Y., Akaoka, I., and Yoshimura, T., 1975, Erythrocyte adenosine deaminase and purine nucleoside phosphorylase activity in gout, *Clin. Chim. Acta* **58**:277–282.

Nishizawa, T., Nishida, Y., and Akaoka, I., 1976, Erythrocyte adenosine kinase activity in gout, *Clin. Chim. Acta* **67**:15–20.

Nuki, G., Astrin, K., Brenton, D., Cruikshank, M., Lever, J., and Seegmiller, J. E., 1977a, Purine and pyrimidine nucleotides in some mutant human lymphoblasts, in: *Ciba. Found. Symp. No. 48: Purine and Pyrimidine Metabolism,* pp. 127–142, Elsevier/Excerpta Medica and North-Holland, Amsterdam and New York.

Nuki, G., Astrin, K., Brenton, D., Cruikshank, M., Lever, J., and Seegmiller, J. E., 1977b, Purine and pyrimidine nucleotide concentrations in cells with decreased hypoxanthine-guanine phosphoribosyltransferase (HGPRT) activity, in: *Advances in Experimental Medicine and Biology,* Vol. 76A, *Purine Metabolism in Man II: Regulation of Pathways and Enzyme Defects* (M. M. Müller, E. Kaiser, and J. E. Seegmiller, eds.), pp. 326–340, Plenum Press, New York.

Nyhan, W. L., 1976, Behavior in the Lesch–Nyhan syndrome, *J. Autism Child. Schizophr.* **6**:235–252.

Nyhan, W. L., 1977, Genetic heterogeneity at the locus for hypoxanthine-guanine phosphoribosyltransferase, in: *Ciba Found. Symp. No. 48: Purine and Pyrimidine Metabolism,* pp. 65–82, Elsevier/Excerpta Medica and North-Holland, Amsterdam and New York.

O'Dorisio, M. S., Neidhart, J. A., Daniel, F. B., Balcerzak, S. P., and LoBuglio, A. F., 1976, Identification of hypoxanthine as the major component of a chromatographic fraction of transfer factor, *Cell. Immunol.* **23**:191–202.

Parkman, R., Gelfand, E. W., Rosen, F. S., Sanderson, A., and Hirschhorn, R.,

1975, Severe combined immunodeficiency and adenosine deaminase deficiency, *N. Engl. J. Med.* **292**:714–719.

Pasero, G., 1977, Recurrent gouty phlebitis without articular gout, in: *Advances in Experimental Medicine and Biology,* Vol. 76B, *Purine Metabolism in Man II: Physiology, Pharmacology, and Clinical Aspects* (M. M. Müller, E. Kaiser, and J. E. Seegmiller, eds.), pp. 245–248, Plenum Press, New York.

Planet, G., and Fox, I. H., 1976, Inhibition of phosphoribosylpyrophosphate synthesis by purine nucleosides in human erythrocytes, *J. Biol. Chem.* **251**:5839–5844.

Polmar, S. H., 1977, Enzyme replacement with red cells, *N. Engl. J. Med.* **296**:943.

Polmar, S. H., Wetzler, E. M., Stern, R. C., and Hirschhorn, R., 1975, Restoration of *in vitro* lymphocyte responses with exogenous adenosine deaminase in a patient with severe combined immunodeficiency, *Lancet* **2**:743–746.

Polmar, S. H., Stern, R. C., Schwartz, A. L., Wetzler, E. M., Chase, P. A., and Hirschhorn, R., 1976, Enzyme replacement therapy for adenosine deaminase deficiency and severe combined immunodeficiency, *N. Engl. J. Med.* **295**:1337–1343.

Pritchard, J. B., O'Connor, N., Oliver, J. M., and Berlin, R. D., 1975, Uptake and supply of purine compounds by the liver, *Am. J. Physiol.* **229**:967–972.

Quagliata, F., Faig, D., Conklyn, M., and Silber, R., 1974, Studies on the lymphocyte 5′-nucleotidase in chronic lymphocytic leukemia, infectious mononucleosis, normal subpopulations, and phytohemagglutinin-stimulated cells, *Cancer Res.* **34**:3197–3202.

Quinlan, D. C., and Hochstadt, J., 1976, Group translocation of the ribose moiety of inosine by vesicles of plasma membrane from 3T3 cells transformed by simian virus 40, *J. Biol. Chem.* **251**:344–354.

Raivio, K. O., and Hovi, T., 1977, Adenine and adenosine metabolism in phytochemagglutinin(PHA)-stimulated normal human lymphocytes, in: *Advances in Experimental Medicine and Biology,* Vol. 76A, *Purine Metabolism in Man II: Regulation of Pathways and Enzyme Defects* (M. M. Müller, E. Kaiser, and J. E. Seegmiller, eds), pp. 448–455, Plenum Press, New York.

Raivio, K. O., Schwartz, A. L., Stern, R. C., and Polmar, S. H., 1977, Adenine and adenosine metabolism in lymphocytes deficient in adenosine deaminase activity, in: *Advances in Experimental Medicine and Biology,* Vol. 76A, *Purine Metabolism in Man II: Regulation of Pathways and Enzyme Defects* (M. M. Müller, E. Kaiser, and J. E. Seegmiller, eds.), pp. 456–462, Plenum Press, New York.

Rapaport, E., and Zamecnik, P. C., 1976a, Incorporation of adenosine into ATP: Formation of compartmentalized ATP, *Proc. Natl. Acad. Sci. U.S.A.* **73**:3122–3125.

Rapaport, E., and Zamecnik, P. C., 1976b, Presence of diadenosine 5′,5‴-$P^1.P^4$-tetraphosphate (Ap_4A) in mammalian cells in levels varying widely with proliferative activity of the tissue: A possible positive "pleiotypic activator," *Proc. Natl. Acad. Sci. U.S.A.* **73**:3984–3988.

Reem, G. H., 1975, Phosphoribosylpyrophosphate overproduction, a new metabolic abnormality in the Lesch–Nyhan syndrome, *Science* **190**:1098–1099.

Rieselbach, R. E., 1977, Renal handling of uric acid, in: *Advances in Experimental Medicine and Biology,* Vol. 76B, *Purine Metabolism in Man II: Physiology, Pharma-*

cology, and Clinical Aspects (M. M. Müller, E. Kaiser, and J. E. Seegmiller, eds.), pp. 1–22, Plenum Press, New York.

Rieselbach, R. E., and Steele, T. H. (eds.), 1975, Symposium on influence of the kidney upon urate homeostasis in man, *Nephron* **14**:5–99.

Robins, R. K., 1975, Nucleosides and nucleotides: Past, present and future, *Ann. N. Y. Acad. Sci.* **255**:597–610.

Rochant, H., Dreyfus, B., Rosa, R., and Boiron, M., 1975, First case of pyrimidine 5′-nucleotidase deficiency in a male, International Society of Hematology, Europe and Africa, Third Meeting, London, August 24–28, p. 19 (abstract).

Roe, T. F., and Kogut, M. D., 1977, The pathogenesis of hyperuricemia in glycogen storage disease, Type 1, *Pediatr. Res.* **11**:664–669.

Rosen, F. S., 1977 (personal communication).

Rosenbloom, F. M., Henderson, J. F., Caldwell, I. C., Kelley, W. N., and Seegmiller, J. E., 1968, Biochemical bases of accelerated purine biosynthesis *de novo* in human fibroblasts lacking hypoxanthine-guanine phosphoribosyltransferase, *J. Biol. Chem.* **243**:1166–1173.

Roth, J. A., Breakefield, X. O., and Castiglione, C. M., 1976, Monoamine oxidase and catechol-O-methyltransferase activities in cultured human skin fibroblasts, *Life Sci.* **19**:1705–1710.

Salti, I. S., Kattuah, N., Alam, S., Wehby, V., and Frayha, R., 1976, The effect of allopurinol on oxypurine excretion in xanthinuria, *J. Rheum.* **3**:201–204.

Sartorelli, A. C., and Johns, D. G. (eds.), 1975, *Antineoplastic and Immunosuppressive Agents*, Vols. I and II, Springer-Verlag, New York–Heidelberg—Berlin.

Schmalstieg, F. C., Goldman, A. S., Mills, G. C., Monahan, T. M., Nelson, J. A., and Goldblum, R. M., 1976, Nucleotide metabolism in adenosine deaminase deficiency, *Pediatr. Res.* **10**:393 (abstract).

Schmalstieg, F. C., Nelson, J. A., Mills, G. C., Monahan, T. M., Goldman, A. S., and Goldblum, R. M., 1977, Purine nucleotides in ADA-deficient lymphocytes, *J. Pediatr.* **91**:48–51.

Schneider, W., Morgenstern, E., and Schindera, I., 1976, Lesch–Nyhan Syndrom ohne Selbstverstümmelungstendenz: Biochemische and morphologische Untersuchungen an Blutzellen eines Patienten, *Deutsch. Med. Wochenschr.* **101**:167–172.

Schrader, W. P., Stacy, A. R., and Pollara, B., 1976, Purification of human erythrocyte adenosine deaminase by affinity column chromatography, *J. Biol. Chem.* **251**:4026–4032.

Schultz, V., and Lowenstein, J. M., 1976, Purine nucleotide cycle, *J. Biol. Chem.* **251**:485–492.

Schumacher, H. R., 1977, Bullous tophi in gout, *Ann. Rheum. Dis.* **36**:91–93.

Scott, J. T., Sturge, R. A., Kennedy, A. C., Hart, D. P., and Buchanan, W. W., 1977, Serum uric acid levels in England and Scotland, in: *Advances in Experimental Medicine and Biology*, Vol. 76B, *Purine Metabolism in Man II: Physiology, Pharmacology, and Clinical Aspects* (M. M. Müller, E. Kaiser, and J. E. Seegmiller, eds.), pp. 214–222, Plenum Press, New York.

Seegmiller, J. E., 1974, Diseases of purine and pyrimidine metabolism, in: *Duncan's Diseases of Metabolism* (P. K. Bondy and L. E. Rosenberg, eds.), pp. 655–774, W. B. Saunders Co., Philadelphia.

Seegmiller, J. E., 1976a, Disorders of purine and pyrimidine metabolism, in: *The Year in Metabolism 1975–1976* (N. Freinkel, ed.), Chapt. 8, pp. 213–258, Plenum Press, New York.

Seegmiller, J. E., 1976b, Genetic defects in human purine metabolism leading to urolithiasis, International Symposium on Urolithiasis Research, Davos, Switzerland, in: *Urolithiasis Research* (H. Fleisch, W. G. Robertson, L. H. Smith, and W. Vahlensieck, eds.), pp. 147–154, Plenum Press, New York.

Seegmiller, J. E., 1976c, Inherited deficiency of hypoxanthine-guanine phosphoribosyltransferase in X-linked uric aciduria (the Lesch–Nyhan syndrome and its variants), in: *Advances in Human Genetics* (H. Harris and K. Hirschhorn, eds.), pp. 75–163, Plenum Press, New York.

Seegmiller, J. E., Watanabe, T., and Schreier, M. H., 1977a, The effect of adenosine on lymphoid cell proliferation and antibody formation, in: *Ciba Found. Symp. No. 48: Purine and Pyrimidine Metabolism,* pp. 249–266, Elsevier/Excerpta Medica and North-Holland, Amsterdam and New York.

Seegmiller, J. E., Watanabe, T., Schreier, M. H., and Waldmann, T. A., 1977b, Immunological aspects of purine metabolism, in: *Advances in Experimental Medicine and Biology,* Vol. 76A, *Purine Metabolism in Man II: Regulation of Pathways and Enzyme Defects* (M. M. Müller, E. Kaiser, and J. E. Seegmiller, eds.), pp. 412–433, Plenum Press, New York.

Sekiguchi, T., and Sekiguchi, F., 1973, Interallelic complementation in hybrid cells derived from Chinese hamster diploid clones deficient in hypoxanthine-guanine phosphoribosyl-transferase activity, *Exp. Cell Res.* **77**:391–403.

Sekiguchi, T., Sekiguchi, F., and Tomii, S., 1974, Complementation in hybrid cells derived from mutagen-induced mouse clones deficient in hypoxanthine-guanine phosphoribosyltransferase activity, *Exp. Cell Res.* **88**:410–414.

Sekiguchi, T., Sekiguchi, F., and Tomii, S., 1975a, Genetic complementation in hybrid cells derived from mutagen-induced mouse clones deficient in HGPRT activity, *Exp. Cell Res.* **93**:207–218.

Sekiguchi, T., Sekiguchi, F., Tachibana, T., Yamada, T., and Yoshida, M., 1975b, Gene expression of foreign metaphase chromosomes introduced into cultured mammalian cells, *Exp. Cell Res.* **94**:327–338.

Shenoy, T. S., and Clifford, A. J., 1975, Adenine nucleotide metabolism in relation to purine enzymes in liver, erythrocytes and cultured fibroblasts, *Biochim. Biophys. Acta* **411**:133–143.

Siegal, F. P., Siegal, M., and Good, R. A., 1976, Suppression of B-cell differentiation by leukocytes from hypogammaglobulinemic patients, *J. Clin. Invest.* **58**:109–122.

Siegenbeek van Heukelom, L. H., Staal, G. E. J., Stoop, J. W., and Zegers, B. J. M., 1976, An abnormal form of purine nucleoside phosphorylase in a family with a child with severe defective T-cell and normal B-cell immunity, *Clin. Chim. Acta* **72**:117–124.

Siegenbeek van Heukelom, L. H., Akkerman, J. W. N., Staal, G. E. J., deBruyn, C. H. M. M., Stoop, J. W., Zegers, B. J. M., deBree, P. K., and Wadman, S. K., 1977, A patient with purine nucleoside phosphorylase deficiency: Enzymological and metabolic aspects, *Clin. Chim. Acta* **74**:271–279.

Siess, E. A., and Wieland, O. H., 1976, Phosphorylation state of cytosolic and mitochondrial adenine nucleotides and of pyruvate dehydrogenase in isolated rat liver cells, *Biochem. J.* **156**:91–102.

Simkin, P. A., 1977a, Role of local factors in the precipitation of urate crystals, in: *Uric Acid: Handbook of Experimental Pharmacology* (B. Kelley and I. M. Weiner, eds.), : Springer-Verlag, Heidelberg (in press).

Simkin, P. A., 1977b, The pathogenesis of podagra, *Ann. Intern. Med.* **86**:230–233.

Simmonds, H. A., Van Acker, K. J., Cameron, J. S., and Snedden, W., 1976, The identification of 2,8-dihydroxyadenine, a new component of urinary stones, *Biochem. J.* **157**:485–487.

Simmonds, H. A., Van Acker, K. J., Cameron, J. S., and McBurney, A., 1977, Purine excretion in complete adenine phosphoribosyltransferase deficiency: Effect on diet and allopurional therapy, in: *Advance in Experimental Medicine and Biology*, Vol. 76B, *Purine Metabolism in Man II: Physiology, Pharmacology, and Clinical Aspects* (M. M. Müller, E. Kaiser, and J. E. Seegmiller, eds.), pp. 304–311, Plenum Press, New York.

Skaper, S. D., and Seegmiller, J. E., 1976, Hypoxanthine-guanine phosphoribosyltransferase mutant glioma cells: Diminished monoamine oxidase activity, *Science* **194**:1171–1173.

Skosey, J. L., Kozin, F., and Ginsberg, M., 1977, Protein adsorption to monosodium urate crystals: Differential responses of human peripheral blood neutrophils, in: *Advances in Experimental Medicine and Biology*, Vol. 76B, *Purine Metabolism in Man II: Physiology, Pharmacology, and Clinical Aspects* (M. M. Müller, E. Kaiser, and J. E. Seegmiller, eds.), pp. 209–213, Plenum Press, New York.

Snyder, F. F., and Seegmiller, J. E., 1976, The adenosine-like effect of exogenous cyclic AMP upon nucleotide and PP-ribose-P concentrations of cultured human lymphoblasts, *FEBS Lett.* **66**:102–106.

Snyder, F. F., and Seegmiller, J. E., 1977 (unpublished observation).

Snyder, F. F., Mendelsohn, J., and Seegmiller, J. E., 1976, Adenosine metabolism in phytohemagglutinin-stimulated human lymphocytes, *J. Clin. Invest.* **58**:654–666.

Snyder, F. F., Hershfield, M. S., and Seegmiller, J. E., 1977a, Purine toxicity in human lymphoblasts, in: *Advances in Experimental Medicine and Biology*, Vol. 76A, *Purine Metabolism in Man II: Regulation of Pathways and Enzyme Defects* (M. M. Müller, E. Kaiser, and J. E. Seegmiller, eds.), pp. 30–39, Plenum Press, New York.

Snyder, F. F., Mendelsohn, J., and Seegmiller, J. E., 1977b, Adenosine and guanosine metabolism during phytohemagglutinin-induced transfromation of human lymphocytes, in: *Advances in Experimental Medicine and Biology*, Vol. 76A, *Purine Metabolism in Man II: Regulation of Pathways and Enzyme Defects* (M. M. Müller, E. Kaiser, and J. E. Seegmiller, eds.), pp. 441–447, Plenum Press, New York.

Sperling, O., Boer, P., Brosh, S., Zoref, E., and deVries, A., 1977a, Superactivity of phosphoribosylpyrophosphate synthetase, due to feedback resistance, causing purine overproduction and gout, in: *Ciba Found. Symp. No. 48: Purine and Pyrimidine Metabolism*, pp. 143–164, Elsevier/Excerpta Medica and North-Holland, Amsterdam and New York.

Sperling, O., Boer, P., Lipstein, B., Kupfer, B., Brosh, S., Zoref, E., Bashkin, P., and deVries, A., 1977b, Regulation of *de novo* purine synthesis in human and rat tissue: Role of oxidative pentose phosphate pathway activity and of ribose-5-phosphate and phosphoribosylpyrophosphate availability, in: *Advances in Experimental Medicine and Biology,* Vol. 76A, *Purine Metabolism in Man II: Regulation of Pathways and Enzyme Defects* (M. M. Müller, E. Kaiser, and J. E. Seegmiller, eds.), pp. 481–487, Plenum Press, New York.

Spilberg, I., Gallacher, A., Mehta, J. M., and Mandell, B., 1976, Urate crystal-induced chemotactic factor: Isolation and partial characterization, *J. Clin. Invest.* **58**:815–819.

Stoop, J. W., Eijsvoogel, V. P., Zegers, B. J. M., Blok-Schut, B., van Bekkum, D. W., and Ballieux, R. E., 1976, Selective severe cellular immunodeficiency: Effect of thymus transplantation and transfer factor administration, *Clin. Immunol. Immunopathol.* **6**:289–298.

Stoop, J. W., Zegers, B. J. M., Hendricks, G. F. M., Siegenbeek van Heukelom, L. H., Staal, G. E. J., de Bree, P. K., Wadman, S. K., and Ballieux, R. E., 1977, Purine nucleoside phosphorylase deficiency associated with selective cellular immunodeficiency, *N. Engl. J. Med.* **296**:651–655.

Stuhlsatz, H. W., Enzensberger, W., and Greiling, H., 1977, Influence of urate on connective tissue metabolism, in: *Advances in Experimental Medicine and Biology,* Vol. 76B, *Purine Metabolism in Man II: Physiology, Pharmacology, and Clinical Aspects* (M. M. Müller, E. Kaiser, and J. E. Seegmiller, eds.), pp. 195–200, Plenum Press, New York.

Sturge, R. A., Scott, J. T., Hamilton, E. B. D., Liyanage, S. P., St. J. Dixon, A., and Engler, C., 1977, Multi-centre trial of naproxen and phenylbutazone in acute gout, in: *Advances in Experimental Medicine and Biology,* Vol. 76B, *Purine Metabolism in Man II: Physiology, Pharmacology, and Clinical Aspects* (M. M. Müller, E. Kaiser, and J. E. Seegmiller, eds.), pp. 290–296, Plenum Press, New York.

Sweetman, L., Borden, M., Lesch, P., Bakay, B., and Becker, M. A., 1977a, Diminished affinity for purine substrates as a basis for gout with mild deficiency of hypoxanthine-guanine phosphoribosyltransferase, in: *Advances in Experimental Medicine and Biology,* Vol. 76A, *Purine Metabolism in Man II: Regulation of Pathways and Enzyme Defects* (M. M. Müller, E. Kaiser, and J. E. Seegmiller, eds.), pp. 319–325, Plenum Press, New York.

Sweetman, L., Borden, M., Kulovich, S., Kaufman, I., and Nyhan, W. L., 1977b, Altered excretion of 5-hydroxyindoleacetic acid and glycine in patients with the Lesch–Nyhan disease, in: *Advances in Experimental Medicine and Biology,* Vol. 76A, *Purine Metabolism in Man II: Regulation of Pathways and Enzyme Defects* (M. M. Müller, E. Kaiser, and J. E. Seegmiller, eds.), pp. 398–404, Plenum Press, New York.

Takkunen, H., and Reunanen, A., 1977, Hyperuricemia and other cardiovascular risk factors, in: *Advances in Experimental Medicine and Biology,* Vol. 76B, *Purine Metabolism in Man II: Physiology, Pharmacology, and Clinical Aspects* (M. M. Müller, E. Kaiser, and J. E. Seegmiller, eds.), pp. 238–244, Plenum Press, New York.

Talbott, J. H., and Yü, T.-F., 1976, *Gout and Uric Acid Metabolism,* Stratton Intercontinental Medical Book Corp., New York, 303 pp.

Treuman, T. M., and Glantz, M. D., 1977, Isolation, purification and subunit structure of rabbit liver purine nucleoside phosphorylase, *Fed. Proc. Fed. Am. Soc. Exp. Biol.* **36**:873 (abstract).

Trotta, P. P., Smithwick, E. M., and Balis, M. E., 1976, A normal level of adenosine deaminase activity in the red cell lysates of carriers and patients with severe combined immunodeficiency disease, *Proc. Natl. Acad. Sci. U.S.A.* **73**:104–108.

Ullman, B., Cohen, A., and Martin, D. W., Jr., 1976, Characterization of a cell culture model for the study of adenosine deaminase and purine nucleoside phosphorylase-deficient immunologic disease, *Cell* **9**:205–211.

Upchurch, K. S., Leyva, A., Arnold, W. J., Holmes, E. W., and Kelley, W. N., 1975, Hypoxanthine phosphoribosyltransferase deficiency: Association of reduced catalytic activity with reduced levels of immunologically detectable enzyme protein, *Proc. Natl. Acad. Sci. U.S.A.* **72**:4142–4146.

Valentine, W. N., Paglia, D. E., Fink, K., and Madokoro, G., 1976, Lead poisoning: Association with hemolytic anemia, basophilic stippling, erythrocyte pyrimidine5′-nucleotidase deficiency, and intraerythrocyte accumulation of pyrimidine, *J. Clin. Invest.* **58**:926–932.

Valentine, W. N., Paglia, D. E., Tartaglia, A. P., and Gilsanz, F., 1977, Hereditary hemolytic anemia with increased red cell adenosine deaminase (45- to 70-fold) and decreased adenosine triphosphate, *Science* **195**:783–785.

Van Acker, K. J., Simmonds, H. A., and Cameron, J. S., 1977, Complete deficiency of adenine phosphoribosyltransferase: Report of a family, in: *Advances in Experimental Medicine and Biology*, Vol. 76A, *Purine Metabolism in Man II: Regulation of Pathways and Enzyme Defects* (M. M. Müller, E. Kaiser, and J. E. Seegmiller, eds.), pp. 295–302, Plenum Press, New York.

Vanderheiden, B. S., 1969, Genetic studies of human erythrocyte inosine triphosphatase, *Biochem. Genet.* **3**:289–297.

Vanderheiden, B. S., 1976, Erythrocyte ITP pyrophosphohydrolase deficiency in a psychiatric population, *Biol. Psychiatry* **11**:755–765.

Van der Weyden, M. B., and Kelley, W. N., 1976, Human adenosine deaminase: Distribution and properties, *J. Biol. Chem.* **251**:5448–5456.

Van der Weyden, M. B., Buckley , R. H., and Kelley, W. N., 1974, Molecular form of adenosine deaminase in severe combined immunodeficiency, *Biochem. Biophys. Res. Common.* **57**:590–595.

van Herwaarden, C. L., van der Korst, J. K., Boerbooms, A. M., de Bruyn, C. H., and Oei, T. L., 1976, Partial hypoxanthine-guanine phosphoribosyltransferase deficiency in a "Celebesian" family: A case of crippling gout associated with haematological disorders, *Neth. J. Med.* **19**:272–278.

Van Reen, R. (ed.), 1977, *Proceedings of the WHO Regional Symposium on Vesical Calculus Disease (1972)*, NIAMDD DHEW Publ. No. (NIH) 77-1191, 281 pp.

Vives-Corrons, J. L., Montserrat-Costa, E., Pujades, A., Woessner, S., and Rozman, C., 1976a, Congenital erythrocytic pyrimidine 5′-nucleotidase deficiency: A new type of haemolytic erythro-enzymopathy (author's transl.), *Sangre* **21**:827–835.

Vives-Corrons, J. L., Montserrat-Costa, E., and Rozman, C., 1976b, Hereditary hemolytic anemia with erythrocyte pyrimidine 5′-nucleotidase deficiency in Spain: Clinical, biological and familial studies, *Hum. Genet.* **34**:285–292.

Wadman, S. K., de Bree, P. K., van Gennip, A. H., Stoop, J. W., Zegers, B. J. M.,

Staal, G. E. J., and Siegenbeek van Heukelom, L. H., 1976, Urinary purines in a patient with a severely defective T cell immunity and a purine nucleoside phosphorylase deficiency, *Adv. Exp. Med. Biol.* **76A**:471.

Wadman, S. K., de Bree, P. K., van Gennip, A. H., Stoop, J. W., Zegers, B. J. M., Staal, G. E. J., and Siegenbeek van Heukelom, L. H., 1977, Urinary purines in a patient with a severely defective T cell immunity and a purine nucleoside phosphorylase deficiency, in: *Advances in Experimental Medicine and Biology,* Vol. 76A, *Purine Metabolism in Man II: Regulation of Pathways and Enzyme Defects* (M. M. Müller, E. Kaiser, and J. E. Seegmiller, eds.), pp. 471–476, Plenum Press, New York.

Waldmann, T. A., and Broder, S., 1977, Suppressor cells in the regulation of the immune response, in: *Progress in Clinical Immunology,* Vol. III (R. S. Schwartz, ed.), pp. 155–199, Grune & Stratton, New York.

Waldmann, T. A., Durm, M., Broder, S., Blackman, M., Blaese, R. M., and Strober, W., 1974, Role of suppressor T cells in pathogenesis of common variable hypogammaglobulinemia, *Lancet* **2**:609–613.

Watts, R. W. E., 1976, Uric acid biosynthesis and its disorders, *J. R. Coll. Physicians London* **11**:91–106.

Webster, A. D. B., and Asherson, G. L., 1974, Identification and function of T cells in the peripheral blood of patients with hypogammaglobulinemia, *Clin. Exp. Immunol.* **18**:499–504.

Wolberg, G. Zimmerman, T. P., Hiemstra, K., Winston, M., and Chu, L.-C., 1975, Adenosine inhibition of lymphocyte-mediated cytolysis: Possible rôle of cyclic adenosine monophosphate, *Science* **187**:957–959.

Wolf, J. W., Anderson, J. A., Reid, R. H., Weiss, L., and Lightbody, J. J., 1976, Syndrome of cellular immunodeficiency with immunoglobulins associated with adenosine deaminase deficiency, *Pediatr. Res.* **10**:394 (abstract).

Wyngaarden, J. B., 1976, Regulation of purine biosynthesis and turnover, *Adv. Enzyme Regul.* **14**:25–42.

Wyngaarden, J. B., and Holmes, E. W., Jr., 1977, Molecular nature of enzyme regulation in purine biosynthesis, in: *Ciba Found. Symp. No. 48: Purine and Pyrimidine Metabolism,* pp. 43–64, Elsevier/Excerpta Medica and North-Holland, Amsterdam and New York.

Wyngaarden, J. B., and Kelley, W. N., 1976, *Gout and Hyperuricemia,* Grune & Stratton, New York.

Yü, T. F., 1977, Some unusual features of gouty arthritis in females, *Semin. Arthritis Rheum.* **6**:247–255.

Yuh, K.-C. M., and Tao, M., 1974, Purification and characterization of adenosine-adenosine cyclic 3′,5′-monophosphate binding protein factors from rabbit erythrocytes, *Biochemistry* **13**:5220–5226.

Zannis, V., Doyle, D., and Martin, D. W., Jr., 1977a, Purification and characterization of human erythrocyte purine nucleoside phosphorylase and its subunits, *J. Biol. Chem.* (in press).

Zannis, V. I., Gudas, L. J., Doyle, D., and Martin, D. W., Jr., 1977b, Purification and characterization of hypoxanthine-guanine phosphoribosyl transferase from cultured HTC cells, in: *Advances in Experimental Medicine and Biology,* Vol. 76A, *Purine Metabolism in Man II: Regulation of Pathways and Enzyme Defects*

(M. M. Müller, E. Kaiser, and J. E. Seegmiller, eds.), pp. 162–171, Plenum Press, New York.

Zimmer, H.-G., and Gerlach, E., 1977, Studies on the regulation of the biosynthesis of myocardial adenine nucleotides, in: *Advances in Experimental Medicine and Biology,* Vol. 76A, *Purine Metabolism in Man II: Regulation of Pathways and Enzyme Defects* (M. M. Müller, E. Kaiser, and J. E. Seegmiller, eds.), pp. 40–49, Plenum Press, New York.

Zöllner, N., and Gröbner, W., 1977, Dietary feedback regulation of purine and pyrimidine biosynthesis in man, in: *Ciba Foundation Symp. No. 48: Purine and Pyrimidine Metabolism,* pp. 165–178, Elsevier/Excerpta Medica and North-Holland, Amsterdam and New York.

Zöllner, N., Gröbner, W., and Rauch-Janssen, A., 1977, The effect of different purines and pyrimidines on human pyrimidine biosynthesis, in: *Advances in Experimental Medicine and Biology,* Vol. 76B, *Purine Metabolism in Man II: Physiology, Pharmacology, and Clinical Aspects* (M. M. Müller, E. Kaiser, and J. E. Seegmiller, eds.), pp. 269–273, Plenum Press, New York.

Zoref, E., deVries, A., and Sperling, O., 1977a, Transfer of resistance to selective conditions from fiborblasts with mutant feedback-resistant phosphoribosylpyrophosphate snythetase to normal cells: A form of metabolic cooperation, in: *Advances in Experimental Medicine and Biology,* Vol. 76A, *Purine Metabolism in Man II: Regulation of Pathways and Enzyme Defects* (M. M. Müller, E. Kaiser, and J. E. Seegmiller, eds.), pp. 80–84, Plenum Press, New York.

Zoref, E., deVries, A., and Sperling, O., 1977b, X-linked pattern of inheritance of gout due to mutant feedback-resistant phosphoribosylpyrophosphate synthetase, in: *Advances in Experimental Medicine and Biology,* Vol. 76A, *Purine Metabolism in Man II: Regulation of Pathways and Enzyme Defects* (M. M. Müller, E. Kaiser, and J. E. Seegmiller, eds.), pp. 287–292, Plenum Press, New York.

9

Divalent Ion Metabolism

Jack W. Coburn, David L. Hartenbower, and, Charles R. Kleeman

9.1. Regulation of Calcium Homeostasis

The regulation of Ca homeostasis involves the precise control of Ca ion level in blood and extracellular fluid (ECF) and maintenance of the structural integrity of the skeleton. Under certain pathological conditions, the homeostatic mechanisms that regulate the Ca level in ECF may do so at the expense of skeletal integrity (e.g., renal osteodystrophy). The principal regulators of Ca include the serum level of inorganic phosphate and several hormones, including parathyroid hormone (PTH), calcitonin (CT), and vitamin D, or its active form, 1,25-dihydroxy-vitamin D_3 [$1,25(OH)_2D_3$]. The discussion of PTH will be limited to divalent ion control of its secretion, its actions on bone and kidney, and the immunoas-

---

JACK W. COBURN AND DAVID L. HARTENBOWER • Medical and Research Services, Veterans Administration Wadsworth Hospital Center and Department of Medicine, University of California Los Angeles School of Medicine, Los Angeles, California
CHARLES R. KLEEMAN • Department of Medicine, University of California Los Angeles School of Medicine, Los Angeles, California.

say of PTH. A more detailed description of recent developments in PTH research can be found in *The Year In Endocrinology 1977,* Chapter 4.

Bone contains enormous stores of Ca and PO_4, and it is generally held that the levels of Ca and PO_4 in blood are regulated by the exchange between the skeleton and the ECF. Large amounts of Ca and PO_4 are lost into glomerular filtrate and then reclaimed by renal tubular reabsorption. Variation in renal tubular reabsorption of Ca may be important in the control of serum Ca in some species, including man, particularly when skeletal turnover is low. A reciprocal interdependence exists between the levels of PO_4 and Ca in plasma, related, in part, to their solubility product. An increase in PO_4 causes a fall in Ca, with the movement of Ca and PO_4 into bone or nonosseous tissues or both. Generally, such an effect of changing serum PO_4 on the Ca level is largely offset by hormonal actions. Finally, variations in the efficiency of intestinal Ca absorption can influence Ca homeostasis.

9.1.1. Parathyroid Hormone

9.1.1.1. Divalent Ion Control of Parathyroid Hormone Secretion

It is generally accepted that a fall in the level of Ca^{2+} ion in the blood is the main factor that stimulates the secretion of PTH, although a fall in Mg concentration, β-adrenergic stimuli, and changes in the level of $1,25(OH)_2D_3$ may also affect PTH secretion. Studies by Habener *et al.* (1975) suggested that the glandular degradation of newly synthesized PTH may be affected by the Ca ion level and that PTH secretion may be influenced by the rate of degradation. They found that the PTH secretion rate was increased 5-fold in parathyroid slices as medium Ca was lowered from 2.0 to 1.0 mM. Some PTH secretion did occur even in the presence of 5 mM Ca. The biosynthesis of proparathyroid hormone (pro-PTH) was only slightly altered, and conversion of pro-PTH occurred invariably, independent of the extracellular Ca concentration. The parathyroid tissue content of PTH increased during an incubation in a high-Ca medium; however, the increase was far less than expected. Thus, a large fraction of newly synthesized PTH may be degraded within the tissues in the presence of a high extracellular Ca concentration, whereas little PTH may be degraded in the presence of a low Ca concentration. They suggested that parathyroid cells contain a Ca-sensitive mechanism for the degradation of PTH, and that such a pathway may be involved in regulation of PTH production and secretion.

To study the relative effects of Ca and Mg in stimulating PTH secretion, Habener and Potts (1976) measured the release of PTH from the synthesis of pro-PTH by bovine parathyroid slices that were incubated in media with varying concentrations of Ca and Mg. Hormone release varied in response to changes in concentrations of either Ca or Mg, but the two cations, although additive, were not equipotent. On a molar basis, Ca was 2.5 times more potent than Mg in producing a secretory response. Neither cation had much effect on biosynthesis of pro-PTH. These observations agree with previous interpretations of *in vivo* data that Ca is the predominant regulator of PTH secretion and synthesis within the range of normal physiological concentrations. Under certain unusual conditions, sufficient hypermagnesemia may develop to suppress PTH secretion. In a patient receiving magnesium sulfate therapy for toxemia of pregnancy, hypocalcemia developed in association with a low serum iPTH level. Following the return of serum Mg to normal, serum iPTH increased normally in response to hypocalcemia (Eisenbud and LoBue, 1976). Eisenbud and LoBue suggested that hypermagnesemia suppressed the parathyroid glands, with hypocalcemia occurring because of secondary hypoparathyroidism.

In a fascinating study, the response of normal parathyroid glands to hypercalcemia was measured *in vivo* in both awake and anesthetized calves (Mawer *et al.*, 1976). PTH levels were measured by radio-immunoassay in effluent venous samples draining the superior parathyroid gland and in peripheral blood. In each instance, the concentrations of iPTH in the venous effluent from the parathyroid glands of hypercalcemic calves exceeded the simultaneous levels found in the peripheral blood. The failure of hypercalcemia to suppress the secretion of normal parathyroid glands indicates that a fraction of PTH secretion occurs independent of the blood Ca concentration. Thus, continued PTH secretion, despite hypercalcemia, cannot be regarded as a unique feature of parathyroid hyperplasia or neoplasia, and may indicate the continued influence of other stimuli on parathyroid secretion.

It is generally assumed that changes in PTH secretion occur in response to long-term alterations in the body's need for Ca. The role of PTH in the adaptation of the organism to a low-Ca diet was reevaluated by Ramberg *et al.* (1976). Plasma iPTH levels were measured serially in nonlactating, nonpregnant cows, the diet of which was changed from a high to a very low Ca content. There was no change in plasma iPTH in response to the change in diet. Nonetheless, there was a decrease in the fraction of Ca absorbed in animals receiving the high-Ca diet, although the absolute net absorption of Ca was higher. Also, there was less bone resorption, but the net movement of Ca from gut and bone into the miscible Ca pool was unchanged with the high-Ca diet. These data suggest that the adaptive process may occur without a measurable change in parathyroid activity. Such observations are surprising, and it is possible that sampling of iPTH at more frequent intervals might have revealed differences in relation to changes in dietary Ca.

The effect of parathyroidectomy (PTX) on the ability of rats to adapt to a low-Ca diet was studied by Kemm (1976). When PTX was done before rats received the low-Ca diet, they exhibited a normal increase in fractional Ca absorption. When the PTX was carried out after the animals had "adapted" to the low-Ca diet, there was no alteration in the adaptation to the low Ca intake. When animals fed a high-Ca diet were given large doses of vitamin D, Ca absorption increased to equal that seen in rats fed the low-Ca diet. In accord with other data published by Kemm, these data suggest that PTH is not essential for the adaptation to a low-Ca diet. The observations that large doses of vitamin D increased Ca absorption in rats receiving a high-Ca diet provide some support for the view that vitamin D may be involved in the "adaptation" independent of PTH. Such data indicate that a role of the parathyroid glands in the long-term adaptation to changes in dietary Ca intake is certainly not firmly established.

9.1.1.2. Actions of Parathyroid Hormone on Bone

Although PTH is involved in stimulating the resorption and turnover of the skeleton and plasma homeostasis, there is increasing evidence that these are independent actions that can be separated (Kalu *et al.*, 1975) and that occur independently. An extensive review of the actions of PTH on bone turnover and on Ca homeostasis was recently published by Parfitt (1976a,b).

In bone as well as in other target tissues, PTH activates a membrane adenylate cyclase, which converts ATP to cyclic adenosine 3′,5′-monophosphate (cAMP). PTH, however, may also enhance the intracellular flux of Ca independent of its effect on adenylate cyclase. In a study evaluating the influence of PTH and cAMP on Ca uptake by isolated bone cells, Dziak and Stern (1975) found that PTH but not cAMP increased bone-cell permeability to Ca. These data support a hypothesis that Ca may be the intracellular mediator of PTH action on bone, which may be responsible for many of the characteristic effects of the hormone. Also the PTH action on Ca uptake is independent of increased levels of cAMP, suggesting that Ca and cAMP may be separate and independent mediators of PTH action on bone. Further evidence that all actions of PTH may not involve activation of adenylate cyclase is provided by Gebauer *et al.* (1976) through a study of the effect of diphosphonate on the skeletal responsiveness to PTH. The diphosphonate was capable of inhibiting bone reabsorption both *in vivo* and in tissue culture. Despite the development of resistance to PTH-induced bone resorption, bone cAMP was normal both under basal conditions and following PTH stimulation. Thus, an inhibition of adenylate cyclase is not necessary for the decrease in bone reasorption produced by the diphosphonates.

In a study of another aspect of PTH action on bone, Boelkins *et al.* (1976) found that PTH caused a reduction in blood flow to the bone coincident with the well-known early *hypocalcemic* phase of PTH action. Later, during the time of maximum hypercalcemic effect, blood flow was increased. These data raise the possibility that there may be a cause-and-effect relationship between Ca mobilization from bone and the rate of osseous blood flow. Compared with other tissues showing vascular reactivity to PTH, only bone showed a biphasic response that corresponds to the changes in serum Ca induced by PTH.

Because metabolic acidosis can induce a negative Ca balance and because bone resorption may increase during acidosis, Beck and Webster (1976) evaluated the effect of metabolic acidosis on Ca balance in PTX rats. Acute metabolic acidosis raised serum Ca directly and augmented the calcemic effect of PTH. These phenomena were seen in the absence of both the intestine and the kidneys, suggesting that acute metabolic acidosis augmented the skeletal response to PTH.

The mechanisms responsible for decreased sensitivity to PTH in vitamin D deficiency continue to be of interest. Kauta *et al.* (1975) confirmed previous observations that plasma Ca is not increased normally by PTH administration in the vitamin-D-deficient animal; however, the stimulation of adenylate cyclase by PTH was not different in bone-cell fractions from vitamin-D-deficient and vitamin-D-replete animals. These data suggest that the failure of PTH to elevate Ca is not due to impaired activation of adenylate cyclase in bone cells of vitamin-D-deficient animals. Forte *et al.* (1976) colleagues found that vitamin-D-deficient rats exhibited a smaller increase in renal excretion of both phosphate and cAMP in response to PTH administration than was observed in vitamin-D-replete animals. The adenylate cyclase in the plasma membrane fraction of the renal cortex of the vitamin-D-deficient animals was also less activated by PTH than that in samples obtained from vitamin-D-replete rats. These suggest that there is an association between the decreased phosphaturic response to PTH and a reduced activation of adenylate cyclase in vitamin D deficiency. Despite such observations in animals, humans with vitamin D deficiency exhibit low tubular reabsorption of P (TRP),and the TRP is rapidly increased as secondary hyperparathyroidism is reversed following initiation of vitamin D treatment. Thus, the renal resistance to PTH is only partial and of little clinical significance.

9.1.1.3. Actions of Parathyroid Hormone on the Kidney

The kidney is one of the primary target organs for PTH. An extensive review of the effects of PTH on glomeruler filtration rate; renal plasma flow; renal handling of PO_4, Ca, Mg, Na, K, and HCO_3; acid–base metabolism; and renal metabolism of $25(OH)D_3$ to $1,25(OH)_2D_3$ was recently published (Massry *et al.*, 1975).

The kidney may not be the major site of phosphorus regulation in the ruminant, where the salivary glands may be important in PO_4 regulation. Clark *et al.* (1975) evaluated the excretion of various electrolytes by both the kidney and the salivary glands of sheep given parathyroid extract. There was a mild increase in serum Ca, a fall in serum P, a modest decrease in urinary Ca and Mg, and an increase in urinary Na, HCO_3, K, and Cl, but there was no phosphaturia. Salivary phosphate concentration increased markedly and promptly after the administration of PTH. These data suggest that PTH regulates phosphate homeostasis in the ruminant primarily via its effect on the salivary glands, rather than via an action on the kidney.

9.1.1.4. Immunoassay for Parathyroid Hormone

There has been great interest in the use of the immunoassay for PTH as a clinical tool. Posen *et al.* (1976) suggested that the PTH immunoassay can provide a very useful adjunct for clinical decision-making. Among urinary stone-formers, the separation of hypercalcemic patients from those who are normocalcemic may be strengthened, because patients with primary hyperparathyroidism almost invariably had measurable plasma iPTH in conjuction with the hypercalcemia, while serum iPTH was normal or undetectable in normocalcemic stone-formers. Of 80 patients found to have abnormal parathyroid tissue at the time of neck surgery for hyperparathyroidism, 4 had no detectable iPTH in the peripheral blood, and serum iPTH was raised in 4 patients who lacked abnormal parathyroid tissue. Among patients with hypercalcemia due to malignancy, iPTH was detected in 25%. Patients with severe hypercalcemia due to primary hyperparathyroidism usually had iPTH levels 10–15 times the upper limit of normal, however, while iPTH was only twice the upper normal limit in patients with malignancy. Serum iPTH was undetectable in 4 of 6 patients with hypercalcemia due to hyperthyroidism. The assay of iPTH was considered useful in evaluating postsurgical hypoparathyroidism, in that the reappearance of measurable iPTH permitted them to discontinue treatment with vitamin D.

In a critical letter, Heath and Martin (1976) suggested that Posen and his colleagues overemphasized the usefulness of iPTH assay in the clinical evaluation of patients. They make an important point regarding the sensitivity of most PTH assays; thus, the values in many subjects are unmeasurable or very close to the limit of detection of the assay; hence, the measurement is subject to considerable error. There is reasonably good correlation between serum iPTH levels and serum Ca in patients with hyperparathyroidism, and the measurement of serum iPTH may be least helpful in patients with mild hypercalcemia, in whom one would expect the most equivocal increase in serum iPTH. Heath and Martin conclude that the measurement of serum iPTH levels is not necessary for the investigation of most patients with hypercalcemia or renal stones; they suggest that it is preferable for the patient to be evaluated by a clinician experienced with disorders affecting Ca metabolism, rather than to measure serum iPTH routinely. From our own clinical experience, we would agree with the latter viewpoint.

9.1.2. Vitamin D

Another hormone involved in Ca homeostasis is vitamin D. The sterol, cholecalciferol or vitamin D_3, produced naturally in the skin via sunlight or ingested in the diet, largely through fortified foods, is converted in the liver to 25-hydroxy-vitamin D_3 [25(OH)D_3]. The latter undergoes enterohepatic circulation, is reabsorbed from the gut, and is the major circulating form of vitamin D_3; its plasma "half-life" is approximately 20–25 days, and its metabolic turnover is believed to be 2–3 μg/day. It is converted to 1,25$(OH)_2D_3$ by a mitochondrial enzyme system localized in renal cortex. Three other naturally occurring forms of vitamin D are 24,25$(OH)_2$-vitamin D_3, 25,26$(OH)_2$-vitamin D_3, and 1,24,-25$(OH)_3$-vitamin D_3; the first is also produced in the kidney and has actions similar to those of 1,25$(OH)_2D_3$, probably after it is converted to 1,24,25$(OH)_3$. If we were to employ the terminology used for PTH, 1,25$(OH)_2D_3$ would probably be termed a hormone, 25(OH)D_3 a prohormone, and vitamin D_3 itself a pre-prohormone. Considerable evidence has accumulated to indicate that there is feedback regulation of the synthesis of 1,25$(OH)_2D_3$ related to the needs of the organism for Ca and perhaps PO_4 as well. There have been many developments in this field, and several reviews have recently appeared (DeLuca, 1976; Beale *et al.*, 1976; Boyle, 1976).

It is worthwhile to define the units of measurement currently being used and provide a comparison of the relative potencies of the naturally occurring forms of D_3. An International Unit (I.U.) of vitamin D has been defined as "equivalent to 0.025 μg crystalline vitamin D," while no definition of units for other sterols is provided. A comparison of the units of measure of other vitamin D compounds is summarized in Table I (Norman, 1972).

Although clinicians and nutritionsts have traditionally utilized units of vitamin D, it seems preferable to discuss the quantities used in terms of either micrograms or picomoles. Advances in the chemistry of these compounds have far outstripped the studies of relative biological potencies in various systems whereby the sterol was given *in vivo*. A summary of preliminary observations of potencies is given in Table II.

9.1.2.1. Chemistry and Metabolism of Vitamin D

9.1.2.1a. Conversion of D_3 to 25(OH)D_3. Previously reported data indicate that the conversion of vitamin D_3 to 25(OH)D_3 is not as rapid in animals or man provided with ample quantities of D as it is in the vitamin-D-deficient state. However, the factors that regulate the conversion of vitamin D_3 to 25(OH)D_3 have not been entirely clarified. *In vitro* studies of the hepatic microsomal enzyme, cholecalciferol-25-hydroxylase, suggest that product inhibition is induced by 25(OH)D_3, itself, but the significance of this mechanism in an intact animal is less certain.

The most recent data indicate that the liver plays the major role in conversion of vitamin D_3 to 25(OH)D_3 (Rojanasathit and Haddad, 1976; Olson *et al.*, 1976; Haddad and Rojanasathit, 1976). Arnaud *et al.* (1975) found that one-third of radioactivity, administered as [^{3}H]25(OH)D_3, was secreted into the lumen of the duodenum, probably via the bile, by 24 hr after its administration. Subsequently, over 85% of the secreted radioactivity was reabsorbed, suggesting that 25(OH)D_3 undergoes major enterohepatic circulation. The magnitude of the hepatic secretion and intestinal reabsorption is large enough to suggest that an alteration in the enterohepatic circulation of 25(OH)D_3 could be an important mechanism of acquired deficiency of vitamin D in certain gastrointestinal diseases. In man, Haddad and Rojanasathit (1976) observed prompt and predictable levels of serum 25(OH)D following oral administration of 25(OH)D_3. Such a predictable response may indicate some therapeutic advantage over vitamin D itself.

9.1.2.1b. 1α(OH)D_3. A synthetic sterol, 1α(OH)D_3, has been found to be biologically active without the necessity for renal 1α-hydroxylation. Certain interest has focused on this compound, because it may be useful clinically and because it was initially more readily synthesized than 1α,25$(OH)_2D_3$. This sterol is much more potent than either 25(OH)D_3 or vitamin D itself, and data, both *in vivo* (Holick, M. F., *et al.*, 1975, 1976; Holick, S. A., *et al.*, 1976; Fukushima *et al.*, 1976) and *in vitro* (Fukushima *et al.*, 1976), indicate that this analogue requires 25-hydroxylation by the liver to 1,25$(OH)_2D_3$ before it acts.

Table I. Quantitative Considerations of Vitamin D_3

Unit of measure	D_3	25(OH)D_3	1,25$(OH)_2D_3$
Molecular weight	385	400	416
μg/65 pmol	0.025	0.026	0.027
"units"/μg[a]	40.0	38.5	37.0
pmol/μg	2600	2499	2402

[a]Assume that 1 I.U. D_3 is 0.025 μg (65.0 pmol).

Table II. Relative Biological Effectiveness of D_3, 25(OH)D_3, and 1,25$(OH)_2D_3$[a]

Criteria of effectiveness	Species and condition	D_3	25(OH)D_3	1,25$(OH)_2D_3$
Intestinal Ca transport	−D chick	1.0	2.0	13–15
Line test	−D rat	1.0	1.4	2–3
Ca absorption	Normal man	–	1.0[b]	140
	Uremic man	–	1.0	400
Increase in serum Ca	Humans with hypoparathyroidism	–	1.0	80–100
	Vitamin-D-deficient infants	–	1.0	2.3–3.3

[a]Data summarized by Coburn *et al.* (1974), Kooh *et al.* (1975), or Colodro *et al.* (1976).
[b]Observations in normal man suggested that 25(OH)D_3, 20 μg/day, is more effective than vitamin D_3, 1.0 mg/day, in increasing Ca absorption.

In a comparison of the rapidity of onset and duration of action of 1α(OH)D_3 and 1,25$(OH)_3D_3$ in man, Brickman *et al.* (1976) found that 1α(OH)D_3 showed a slower onset of action and required a longer period for disipation of its effect, observations that were compatible with the need for hydroxylation of 1α(OH)D_3 to 1,25$(OH)_2D_3$ prior to exertion of its action in man. It is possible that 1α(OH)D_3 is somewhat more likely to produce hypercalcemia than 1,25$(OH)_2D_3$; moreover, there might be greater risk of a cumulative effect with 1α(OH)D_3.

9.1.2.1c. Conversion of 25(OH)D_3 to 1,25$(OH)_2D_3$. The conversion of 25(OH)D_3 to 1,25$(OH)_2D_3$ is the most closely regulated step in the feedback control of vitamin D metabolism. Although there is a lack of agreement about the relative importance of certain specific factors that stimulate or inhibit this step, it is generally agreed that there is increased production of 1,25$(OH)_2D_3$ under conditions of Ca deprivation, increased parathyroid activity, and phosphate deprivation. There is, however, a lack of consensus concerning the mechanisms whereby these stimuli exert their effect on the renal enzyme. It has been suggested that variations in dietary Ca intake exert an effect on 25(OH)D_3-1-hydroxylase solely through the action of PTH; other studies indicate, however, that Ca can have a direct effect, and this may explain how adaptation to a low-Ca diet can occur in the absence of the parathyroid glands (Kemm, 1976, Ramberg *et al.*, 1976).

Horiuchi *et al.* (1975) suggested that the metabolism of 25(OH)D_3 in the kidney is regulated by two independent mechanisms: (1) a long-term mechanism that may control the amount of the two enzymes, 25(OH)D_3-1-hydroxylase and 25(OH)D_3-24-hydroxylase, which is regulated by the amount of 1,25$(OH)_2D_3$ in the kidney; and (2) a second, short-term mechanism that may regulate enzyme activity and is sensitive to intracellular distribution of Ca. From a study of the interaction between the diphosphonate, EHPD, and a low-Ca diet on vitamin D metabolism, Taylor *et al.* (1975) suggested that the intracellular concentration of Ca may control the synthesis of 1,25$(OH)_2D_3$. Henry and Norman (1976) found that mitochondrial 25(OH)D_3-1-hydroxylase was inhibited as Ca ion concentration rose and suggested that the intramitochondrial concentration of Ca and PO_4 may play a role in enzyme regulation.

Previous studies indicated that 1,25$(OH)_2D_3$ itself can reduce the activity of the renal 25(OH)D_3-1-hydroxylase. Horiuchi *et al.* (1976) suggested, however, that 1,25$(OH)_2D_3$ inhibits the production of 1,25$(OH)_2D_3$, itself, through the direct inhibition of PTH secretion by this sterol.

Hughes *et al.* (1975) found that plasma 1,25$(OH)_2D_3$ levels measured by a radioreceptor assay were increased in rats fed a low-Ca or low-PO_4 diet. The increase in plasma 1,25$(OH)_2D_3$ in response to the low-Ca diet, but not to the low-P diet, was dependent on the presence of intact parathyroid or thyroid glands. Therefore, they propose that the effect of a low diet Ca on serum 1,25$(OH)_2D_3$ was mediated via PTH.

9.1.2.1d. 24,25(OH)₂D₃. The sterol 24,25$(OH)_2D_3$ is a major metabolite of vitamin D found in the chick, rat, or man following the administration of a radiolabeled precursor, vitamin D_3 or 25(OH)D_3. It is produced primarily by the kidneys; it may also be formed in other tissues. In general, 24,25$(OH)_2D_3$ is produced under conditions in which there is less need for 1,25$(OH)_2D_3$, and the true biological role of this sterol remains unknown at this time.

The biological actions of 24R,25$(OH)_2D_3$ in mobilizing bone calcium and stimulating intestinal Ca transport are eliminated by nephrectomy, suggesting that it must undergo renal 1-hydroxylation. The factors that stimulate the production of 24,25$(OH)_2D_3$ *in vivo* were evaluated by Tanaka *et al.* (1975). A single dose of 1,25$(OH)_2D_3$ given to chicks that were previously fed a vitamin-D-deficient, high-Ca diet suppressed the 1-hydroxylase and stimulated 24-hydroxylase within a period of hours. The administration of PTH also rapidly suppressed the 24(OH)D_3-24-hydroxylase. These changes occurred before there were changes in serum Ca or PO_4. On the basis of the rapid biological turnover of both 1- and 24-hydroxylase, these authors suggest that the regulation by 1,25$(OH)_2D_3$ and PTH involves changes in enzyme synthesis and degradation.

9.1.2.1e. 1,25$(OH)_2D_3$. The metabolic fate of ^{3}H-labeled 1,25$(OH)_2D_3$ given either intravenously or by repeated oral doses was studied in man by Mawer *et al.* (1976). The plasma decay curve showed two components, one with a rapid half-life of approximately 14 hr and a second slow component with a $t_{1/2}$ of 80 hr. Plasma radioactivity of the

$1,25(OH)_2D_3$ was much lower following oral than intravenous administration, but there were equivalent biological effects. They suggested that orally administered $1,25(OH)_2D_3$ may act directly on the intestine. These studies verify previous observations of rapid onset and disappearance of action of $1,25(OH)_2D_3$ in man.

9.1.2.1f. Plants with Vitamin D Activity. A number of plants contain a water-soluble material capable of producing hypercalcemia and even calcinosis. These plants were identified because animals eating them developed hypercalcemia or died with calcinosis. The effects observed were very similar to vitamin D toxicity. An aqueous extract from *Solanum glaucophyllum* (also known as *S. malacoxylon*), a plant common to Argentina, exerts effects very similar to those of $1,25(OH)_2D_3$ (Walling and Kimberg, 1975). Hydrolysis of the extract with a glycosidase resulted in a lipid-soluble material with an UV absorption spectrum identical to that of $1,25(OH)_2D_3$. Moreover, this compound displaced $1,25(OH)_2D_3$ from the intestinal chromatin-binding system and exhibited a mass-spectroscopy pattern identical to that of $1,25(OH)_2D_3$ (Haussler *et al.*, 1976a). *Cestrum diurnum,* a plant found in Florida, produces hypercalcemia and stimulates intestinal Ca transport in animals, including those lacking their kidneys. These and other characteristics in biological systems suggest that it acts in a manner identical to $1,25(OH)_2D_3$ (Wasserman *et al.*, 1976; Walling *et al.*, 1976), and it is currently believed that these plants produce a glycoside containing a secosterol that is presumably identical to $1,25(OH)_2D_3$. These plants are of importance because of accidental diseases in grazing animals and of interest to physiologists and biochemists because of their unique actions. It is also possible, however, that they might provide an inexpensive source of $1,25(OH)_2D_3$.

9.1.2.2. Actions of Vitamin D

The actions of vitamin D are summarized in Table III. Vitamin D, or more appropriately $1,25(OH)_2D_3$, stimulates intestinal absorption of Ca and PO_4 and augments bone resorption, actions that increase Ca and PO_4 in extracellular fluid. $1,25(OH)_2D_3$ is believed to act in the cell nucleus via messenger RNA (mRNA) to induce the synthesis of one or more new proteins, which facilitate Ca entry into cells. At least one protein, Ca-binding protein (CaBP), has been identified in response to vitamin D treatment. Despite its action in causing bone resorption, vitamin D also promotes mineralization of bone matrix in vitamin D deficiency. This may occur either because of favorable levels of Ca and PO_4 in fluid bathing the bone matrix or because vitamin D somehow promotes maturation of bone callagen to render it conducive to crystal deposition. Pharmacological quantities of $25(OH)D_3$ or $1,25(OH)_2D_3$ may enhance renal tubular reab-

Table III. Actions of Vitamin D [$1,25(OH)_2D_3$]

Intestine
Enhances Ca transport
Enhances PO_4 transport
Bone
Enhances bone resorption
Stimulates normal mineralization
Affects collagen maturation
Muscle
Restores normal function (?mechanism)
Parathyroid glands
?Inhibits PTH secretion
Kidney
?Stimulates PO_4 absorption
?Affects Ca and HCO_3 reabsorption
Other
Permits normal growth

sorption of PO_4, possibly by blocking PTH action. Whether vitamin D or its more active forms are involved in phosphate handling by the kidney under normal circumstances remains unknown.

9.1.2.2a. Intestinal Actions. The mechanism whereby $1,25(OH)_2D_3$ produces its actions has been the subject of continued investigation, and its stimulation of intestinal Ca transport has been studied to the greatest extent. When $1,25(OH)_2D_3$ enters the intestinal cells, it becomes bound to nuclear chromatin and leads to an increase in the chromatin template activity (Zerwekh *et al.,* 1976) measured with RNA polymerase by 2 hr after its administration, and preceding a biological response. Incubation of $1,25(OH)_2D_3$, with intestinal cytosol and the subsequent addition of this combination to intestinal mucosal nuclei is followed by a similar increase in template activity. These workers propose that stimulation of the chromatin template activity of the intestinal cell by $1,25(OH)_2D_3$ is required before initiation of the increased Ca transport.

For several years, there has been the suggestion that a CaBP, which is stimulated by vitamin D or $1,25(OH)_2D_3$, is an important mediator of intestinal Ca transport. CaBP is believed to be synthesized as a consequence of the stimulation of mRNA due to the interaction of $1,25(OH)_2D_3$ with the intestinal nucleus (Spencer *et al.,* 1976a). In experiments carried out *in vitro,* Freund and Bronner (1975) found that the addition of $1,25(OH)_2D_3$ to intestinal cells from vitamin-D-deficient rats doubled Ca uptake by the isolated cells within 90 min in association with the appearance of CaBP. It has been suggested that CaBP is important for Ca entry into the cell. A number of recent studies, however, cast some doubt on the primary role of CaBP in initiating vitamin-D-stimulated transcellular Ca transport. Spencer *et al.* (1976b) found that the vitamin-D stimulated intestinal Ca transport did not invariably correlate with an increase in CaBP, and they suggest that factors other than synthesis of CaBP are important for initiating Ca transport.

To date, no clinical disorder or pathophysiological state has been observed in which a primary excess or deficit of CaBP is the basic etiological cause.

It is well known that vitamin D can augment the intestinal absorption of phosphate. This effect can occur independent of any action on Ca transport; furthermore, Walling (unpublished) presented evidence that this is a saturable process that is sodium-dependent. Recently, Gennari *et al.* (1975) reported that vitamin D and $25(OH)D_3$ can enhance the intestinal absorption of radiophosphate in man. Studies in humans, with normal or altered vitamin D metabolism, indicate that $1,25(OH)_2D_3$ given in doses of 0.5–1.0 μg/day augments the net intestinal absorption of both Ca and P.

Many years ago, Nicholayson stated that increasing amounts of cholecalciferol were not needed to bring about the maximal adaptative responses of the intestine to a low-Ca diet, but only a minimal constant vitamin D intake was required. He proposed that an "endogenous factor," generated in the setting of a low-Ca diet, was responsible for the adaptation. It now appears that Nicholayson's endogenous factor is $1,25(OH)_2D_3$.

9.1.2.2b. Skeletal Actions. It is well known that vitamin D or $1,25(OH)_2D_3$ can elevate plasma Ca in a vitamin-D-deficient animal receiving a Ca-free diet; such observations provide evidence for vitamin-D-induced bone Ca mobilization. Also, $1,25(OH)_2D_3$ is potent in stimulating radiocalcium release from fetal bone, studied *in vitro*. The ingestion of minimal quantities of vitamin D is necessary for the prevention of rickets or osteomalacia, and the administration of vitamin D is known to produce normal mineralization of osteoid in vitamin D deficiency. It is our current concept based on our own observations and recently published data (Russell and Avioli, 1975; Edelstein *et al.*, 1976) that vitamin D, when present in physiological amounts, acts primarily to bring about bone mineralization, while bone resorption may predominate under conditions of vitamin D excess. It is likely that these actions, although modulated by other factors, such as PTH or mineral availability, occur as a result of vitamin D action on bone cells. Finally, the skeletal mechanisms whereby PTH maintains serum Ca in a normal range are dependent on the presence of normal vitamin D action on the skeleton. Alterations of one or more of these three fundamental actions of vitamin D on the skeleton can account for or encompass all the known clinical or pathophysiological states resulting from a deficiency of, resistance to, or excess action of vitamin D or one of its more metabolic forms.

The subcellular mechanism of vitamin D action on bone cells may be similar to that described earlier with respect to the intestinal mucosa. It does not appear to involve the activation of the adenylate cyclase–cAMP system as a second messenger. It is possible, however, that the well-known PTH stimulation of this system is modulated by vitamin D (Russell and Avioli, 1975; Forte *et al.*, 1976). Wezeman (1976) provided evidence from autoradiographic studies that radiolabeled $25(OH)D_3$ was selectively localized in hypertrophic epiphyseal cells, epiphyseal matrix, osteoid, osteoblasts, and the osteocytes of metaphyseal bone spicules. The radioactivity was localized only in areas of active mineralization of bone.

Vitamin D may also have a role in the development or maturation of collagen, and such an effect could permit the normal mineralization of the bone matrix. With the maturation of collagen, specific cross-linkages develop between the collagen molecules. Mechanic *et al.* (1975) studied the quantitative relationship between two of the major cross-linkages in diaphyseal collagen from chicks receiving either a vitamin-D-deficient diet, a normal vitamin D diet, or a diet with a high but nontoxic quantity of vitamin D for 1, 2, 3, and 4 weeks. The vitamin-D-deficient bone collagen showed an increase in the cross-link ratios before any observed change in growth rate. They suggest that such cross-link analysis may provide one of the earliest and most sensitive indications of a bone disturbance that is related to vitamin D deficiency. These data provide evidence that vitamin D may act to increase the normal maturation of bone collagen.

Another action of $1,25(OH)_2D_3$ that is particularly prominent in the vitamin-D-deficient rat, given a larger dose of the sterol, is a prompt increase in serum phosphorus level, which Castillo *et al.* (1975) suggest is derived, at least in part, from bone mineral. In human vitamin D deficiency, an increase in plasma P within the first 4 days of vitamin D treatment may be primarily the result of a fall in renal clearance of P and an augmentation of intestinal absorption of P.

9.1.2.2c. Actions on the Parathyroid Glands. Recently, it has been suggested that $1,25(OH)_2D_3$ may decrease PTH secretion via a direct action on the parathyroid glands. Thus, Chertow *et al.* (1975) found that $1,25(OH)_2D_3$ caused a significant decrease in serum iPTH in rats measured at 4 hr. Also, the $1,25(OH)_2D_3$ blocked the enhanced serum iPTH response to hypocalcemia. Studies with slices of bovine parathyroid tissue suggested that $1,25(OH)_2D_3$ inhibited the release of PTH. Following on the observation of Henry and Norman (1975) that radiolabeled $1,25(OH)_2D_3$ was preferentially localized in the parathyroid glands, Brumbaugh *et al.* (1975) found that $1,25(OH)_2D_3$ was specifically bound to macromolecular components in the cytoplasm and nucleus of the parathyroid glands of the vitamin-D-deficient chick. They considered these observations to be consistent with the action of a steroid-hormone on its target tissue and suggested that $1,25(OH)_2D_3$ may be involved in regulation of PTH synthesis or secretion or both.

Despite these "positive" experiments, we have found that exogenous $1,25(OH)_2D_3$ given either to normal man or to vitamin-D-deficient dogs failed to depress serum iPTH in the absence of an increase in serum Ca. Thus, it is too early to conclude that the homeostatic regulation of these two hormones involves the direct suppression of PTH secretion by $1,25(OH)_2D_3$.

9.1.2.2d. Actions on Muscle. Striking muscular weakness and a characteristic waddling gait are well-known features of vitamin D deficiency, and these abnormalities show a striking reversal following vitamin D treatment. The mechanism whereby vitamin D or its subsequent metabolically active forms produces this dramatic effect on muscle function is unknown.

9.1.2.2e. Neonatal–Maternal Interrelationships of Vitamin D. The mechanism whereby vitamin D metabolism is altered during pregnancy and the mechanisms for transfer of vitamin D from the maternal circulation to the fetus are subjects of considerable interest. Nicholson *et al.* (1976) found that estrogens enhanced the conversion of vitamin D_3 to $25(OH)D_3$ in homogenates of liver, while Kenny (1976) found greatly enhanced activity of the renal $25(OH)D_3$-1-hydroxylase during ovulation when estrogen secretion was high. It was recently reported that prolactin is potent in stimulating the renal production of $1,25(OH)_2D_3$ (Spanos *et al.*, 1976). The roles of estrogens and other factors associated with pregnancy and lactation that may affect Ca metabolism via an effect on vitamin D metabolism will be followed with great interest.

In pregnant humans (Hillman and Haddad, 1976), the plasma levels of $25(OH)D_3$, measured during the last trimester, revealed mean levels of 15 ± 6 ng/ml in February and 42 ± 14 ng/ml in August; no differences in serum Ca were noted. The plasma levels of 25(OH)D correlated weakly with vitamin D intake, but were considerably higher in the summer than in nonpregnant women studied in the same season (20.5 ± 1 ng/ml). Although the pregnant women were receiving larger amounts of vitamin D, the slightly higher intake may not have been totally responsible for the difference. The values of 25(OH)D in the winter were lower in pregnant women than those observed during winter in nonpregnant women (mean 23.6 ng/ml). Similar observations were reported from the United Kingdom by Turton *et al.* (1977). The last observations suggest that there may be an increased need for vitamin D during pregnancy. An increase in plasma binding of 25(OH)D might account for the higher values during the summer. No racial difference in 25(OH)D levels was seen in the patients, and serum 25(OH)D below 6.5 ng/ml, where significant deficiencies might be expected, were not observed.

9.1.2.3. Plasma Transport of Vitamin D

In studies designed to characterize the transport of vitamin D metabolites in plasma, Haddad and Walgate (1976) and Imawari *et al.* (1976) each reported isolation and characterization of a vitamin-D-binding protein in human plasma. The protein had an inter-α mobility and a molecular weight estimated at 59,000 and 52,000, respectively. There was binding of 1 mol vitamin D by 1 mol of the protein; also, the same protein is involved in transport of 25(OH)D_3. Under normal circumstances, only 2–3% of the vitamin D-binding protein was saturated. Haddad *et al.* (1976) also showed that 25(OH)-vitamin D_2 and 25(OH)-vitamin D_3 were equipotent in their ability to bind with serum binding sites in man. The binding capacities of sera from adults and sera from cord blood from newborn infants had similar binding capacities; however, maternal sera and sera from women receiving oral contraceptives exhibited an increase in binding capacity.

9.1.2.4. Assays for 25(OH)D, 1,25(OH)$_2$D, and other Vitamin D Sterols

With identification of specific binding proteins for vitamin D metabolites, assays to measure 25(OH)D_3 and other vitamin D sterols in plasma and other biological fluids have been developed. Most require preliminary chromatographic separation of plasma lipids followed by application of the binding protein. Bouillon *et al.* (1976) utilized Sephadex LH 20 chromatorgraphy of a lipid extract and the binding protein from normal rat serum. Plasma values of 25(OH)D in Belgium were 12.4 ± 4.1 μg/liter, while levels in patients with rickets were below 4 μg/l. During the treatment of renal osteodystrophy with vitamin D_3, 15 mg/week, values reached 220–500 μg/liter; after interruption of vitamin D_3 therapy, the values remained high for several months. Low 25(OH)D levels were found in the serum from epileptic patients receiving a combination of barbiturates and diphenylhydantoin. Bjorkhem and Holmberg (1976) reported a more specific method that utilizes ^{3}H-labeled 25(OH)D_3 as an internal standard and a mass fragmentographic techniques and that separates vitamin D_3 from vitamin D_2 derivatives. Garcia-Pascual *et al.* (1976) eliminated both the chromatography and the use of β-lipoproteins; their method may lack specificity but may have wider clinical applicability than others reported. The development of radioreceptor assays for

$1,25(OH)_2D$ is an important advancement. Haussler and colleagues (Haussler *et al.*, 1976b; Hughes *et al.*, 1976) developed a target-tissue assay system, consisting of a cytosol receptor protein, which binds the vitamin D metabolites, and nuclear chromatin, which has a limited number of acceptor sites. Several complex chromatographic purification steps are needed to remove interfering substances from plasma. There was slightly less efficient binding of the vitamin D_2 metabolite in a comparison of $1,25(OH)_2D_3$ and $1,25(OH)_2D_2$. Plasma levels were 25–40 ng/ml for 25(OH)D and 2.1–4.5 ng/100 ml for $1,25(OH)_2D$ in adults in Arizona. In a patient with hypervitaminosis D, the plasma 25(OH)D concentration was increased 15-fold, while the plasma level of $1,25(OH)_2D$ was not increased. Low levels of $1,25(OH)_2D_3$ were found in chronic renal failure, with a restoration to normal following renal transplantation. Patients with hypo- and pseudohypoparathyroidism had reduced plasma levels of $1,25(OH)_2D$, while levels of $1,25(OH)_2D$ were elevated in patients with parathyroid adenomas. Patients with idiopathic hypercalciuria and mild hypophosphatemia often demonstrated high levels of plasma $1,25(OH)_2D$. This experience in a variety of clinical syndromes represents one of the more convincing pieces of evidence for normal hormonal regulation of $1,25(OH)_2D_3$ production. Also, they provide evidence for disturbed vitamin D regulation in a number of conditions that alter Ca homeostasis.

The application of high-pressure liquid chromatography (Jones and DeLuca, 1975) in a chromatographic purification system and stabilization of the chick cytosolic binding protein was described by Eisman *et al.* (1976) in a binding assay for $1,25(OH)_2D$. Values of 29 ± 2 pg/ml in normal adults were similar to the values previously reported by Haussler. No detectable $1,25(OH)_2D$, could be found in the plasma of patients with end-stage renal failure.

Taylor *et al.* (1976) reported a competitive binding assay to measure $24,25(OH)_2$-vitamin D in biological samples. Sephadex LH 20 chromatography of the serum was necessary before the assay to avoid binding of $25(OH)D_3$ and $24,25(OH)_2D_3$. The level of $24,25(OH)_2D$ in normal individuals was 1.7 ± 0.82 ng/ml, while patients receiving therapeutic doses of vitamin D had higher levels. There appeared to be a close relationship between $24,25(OH)_2D$ and 25(OH)D levels.

9.1.2.5. Vitamin D Toxicity

With the passing of the fad of giving pharmacological large doses of vitamin D for disorders such as rheumatoid arthritis, clinical experience with marked vitamin D overdosage in humans is less common. Experimental data are not yet available concerning toxic actions of the new, highly active forms of vitamin D. New observations with the measurement of serum and tissue levels of various metabolites of vitamin D will be followed with interest. Surreptitious vitamin D ingestion, unknown to both the physician and the patient's relatives, can cause factitious hypercalcemia (Belchet *et al.,* 1976), and vitamin D intoxication occurs during treatment of patients with hypoparathyroidism (Shetty *et al.,* 1975). Under such conditions, there is considerable conversion of vitamin D to 25(OH)D, while the plasma levels of $1,25(OH)_2D$ may not be increased (Hughes *et al.,* 1976). Thus, the diagnostic dilemma presented by factitious hypercalcemia due to surreptitious ingestion of vitamin D or a related compound may be solved with the finding of low serum iPTH levels in conjunction with elevated levels of 25(OH)D (Jeremiah *et al.,* 1976; Belchetz *et al.,* 1976).

There is interest in a possible role of vitamin D, in quantities considered either physiological or preventive, in the pathogenesis of suprevalvular aortic stenosis and hypercalcemia of infancy. From *in vitro* studies utilizing skin fibroblasts, Becroft and Chambers (1976) noted increased sensitivity to vitamin D_2 in samples from children with the suprevalvular aortic stenosis–infantile hypercalcemia syndrome compared with controls. Such data strengthen their suggestion that this syndrome may represent a genetically predetermined hypersensitivity to vitamin D.

9.1.2.6. Absence of Vitamin D Action

The hypocalcemia and rickets or osteomalacia that occur due to lack of vitamin D can be conveniently classified according to the affected step in vitamin D metabolism, i.e., insufficient vitamin D, $25(OH)D_3$, or $1,25(OH)_2D_3$ (Coburn *et al.,* 1975). Several drugs, such as phenobarbital, diphenylhydantoin and glutethimide, are believed to hasten the conversion of vitamin D_3 to inactive forms by inducing hepatic microsomal steroid hydroxylases; the skeletal disorder can be corrected with small doses of $25(OH)D_3$. Vitamin-D-dependent rickets, characterized by rickets, hypocalcemia, and hypophosphatemia, responds to pharmacological doses of vitamin D_3; this condition is believed to be due to lack of the renal enzyme producing $1,25(OH)_2D_3$. Osteomalacia or impaired mineralization of bone can arise as a consequence of reduced vitamin D action or can also occur due to prolonged phosphate depletion and hypophosphatemia. Osteomalacia can occur with normal or only minimally reduced levels of serum Ca, and a bone biopsy may be needed for diagnosis.

9.1.2.6a. Deficiency of Vitamin D

Nutritional Rickets. With the present knowledge about the metabolism of vitamin D and newer methods to assess defects in bone mineralization, there has been a reassessment of the clinical features of rickets or osteomalacia due to vitamin D deficiency, so-called "nutritional rickets." Rickets is encountered more commonly in the United Kingdom than in the United States. Furthermore, in the United Kingdom, a much higher incidence of rickets has been reported among Asian immigrants, with evidence of either florid rickets or minimal active or healing rickets as high as 13% of Asian school children in one series (Goel *et al.,* 1976). A dietary survey revealed that 32% of all Asian children ingested less than 50 I.U. vitamin D/day. The Asians showed little or no tendency to adapt to Western foods, and all were chapati eaters. Only 8 of 54 Asian families used margarine (the food fortified with vitamin D_2 in the United Kindgom), and most used butter or ghee. Also, most Asian mothers discontinued vitamin supplements for their children after 1 year. The authors suggested that chapati, which is high in phytate, might reduce Ca absorption. Other investigators in the United Kingdom suggested that inositol polyphosphates and the high phosphate content of chapati contribute to the pathogenesis of rickets (Dunnigan *et al.,* 1976). Stamp (1975) noted that UV light was effective in curing the rickets present in Asian children, even while they continued to ingest a chapati diet.

Recent data indicate that nutritional rickets may occur in areas of the world exposed to a large quantity of sunlight, with reports of cases of nutritional rickets in children from Nigeria (Laditan and Adeniyi, 1975), New Dehli (Ahmed, S. H., *et al.*, 1975), and Jamaica (Miller and Chutkan, 1976). In each series, malnutrition and reduced exposure to sunlight were believed to be major etiological factors. In the report from New Dehli, the authors concluded that the retention fraction of an intravenous Ca load provided the most consistently abnormal and best diagnostic test for identification of rickets.

Plasma measurement of 25(OH)D have now been reported in several series of patients with nutritional rickets. Preece *et al.* (1975) found little overlap of the values in patients with rickets or osteomalacia and those in normal subjects. Stanbury *et al.* (1975) also reported good separation of values in osteomalacic compared with normal subjects; however, Goel *et al.* (1976) and Arnaud *et al.* (1976) noted overlap between the values of 25(OH)D, found in patients with all degrees of rickets and controls except in those with florid rickets. It is well known that there is seasonal variation in plasma 25(OH)D levels, and it is possible that a greater attention to values in "season-matched" normals may make measurements of plasma 25(OH)D levels more useful for the identification of vitamin D_3 deficiency. Preece *et al.* (1975) demonstrated a substantial fall in plasma 25(OH)D levels in submariners after 2 months on patrol without exposure to sunlight, indicating the important role of UV light and the rapidity of fall in plasma 25(OH)D when one source was removed.

Attempts to define the vitamin D requirements in both children and adults have been difficult. Vitamin D deficiency may develop in adults consuming less than 70–80 I.U. vitamin D/day, and it is believed that the requirements are somewhat greater in children. This matter is the subject of a brief but thoughtful review by Bergstrom (1975), who reviews the evidence that 200 I.U. vitamin D is adequate to prevent rickets in children. With a Recommended Daily Allowance of 400 I.U., it is assumed that most children will readily ingest the lower quantity. With consumption of a self-selected diet, the amount could readily be twice the RDA, and the Committee on Nutrition of the American Academy of Pediatrics recommended several years ago that milk be the only food that is supplemented. Bread and certain other foods are regularly supplemented in the United States, however, so that intakes greater than 400 I.U./day may be common. It is possible that measurements of plasma 25(OH)D may help in identification of the optimal quantity of vitamin D that should be added to foods to assure the prevention of rickets and yet avoid overdosages.

The response of endogenous PTH to vitamin D deficiency has been a subject of some interest. Arnaud *et al.* (1976) found that the serum iPTH levels were appropriately elevated for the degree of hypocalcemia, while Stanbury *et al.* (1975) found a normal rapid decrease in the elevated levels of serum iPTH during a Ca infusion as the serum Ca was increased in the majority of patients with vitamin D deficiency. To point out an interaction between vitamin D and PTH at the clinical level, Arnaud *et al.* (1976) suggested that PTH itself may hasten the metabolism of 25(OH)D_3 to 1,25$(OH)_2D_3$ and thus accelerate the development of vitamin D_3 deficiency when D_3 intake is low or sunlight exposure is minimal. Some support for this view is provided by the finding (Sann *et al.*, 1976) of low levels of plasma 25(OH)D despite treatment with large doses of vitamin D in an infant with secondary hyperparathyroidism due to maternal hypoparathyroidism.

Malabsorption of Vitamin D. The most common causes of vitamin D deficiency in the United States are intestinal disorders that produce malabsorption of vitamin D, and the intestinal absorption of vitamin D may be reduced in all conditions causing steatorrhea. The nature and cause of an increased incidence of osteomalacia in patients following partial gastrectomy are less well defined, but demineralization of the skeleton after subtotal gastrectomy has been documented by a number of investigators. Alhava *et al.* (1975) prospectively evaluated the influence of supplemental Ca, with or without 1000 I.U. vitamin D_2, in patients who had undergone partial gastric resection. The patients were randomly assigned to treatment with oral Ca (2.0 g/day), oral Ca plus vitamin D_2, or their usual diet (controls). They found that either Ca or Ca plus vitamin D_2 increased bone density, measured by photon absorption, in male patients compared with the controls, while no differences were seen in a smaller group of female patients. Urinary Ca increased in all Ca-supplemented groups, and there was a small decrease in plasma alkaline phosphatase in the males receiving Ca and vitamin D_2. They concluded that prophylactic treatment is required after partial gastrectomy, but further data are needed to establish suitable management for female patients.

9.1.2.6b. Defective Production of 25(OH)D_3. Several clinical conditions, which are associated with an increased incidence of skeletal disease, probably involve abnormal 25-hydroxylation of vitamin D.

Liver Disease. Parenchymal liver disease and abnormalities of the biliary tract can affect homeostasis of Ca and vitamin D, although there is disagreement about the mechanism of this effect. In a survey of patients with both parenchymal and cholestatic liver disease, Long *et al.* (1976) found low mean plasma levels of 25(OH)D in groups of patients with chronic active hepatitis, alcoholic hepatitis and cirrhosis, lupoid and cryptogenic cirrhosis, symptomatic primary biliary cirrhosis, and acute and chronic biliary disease. Plasma levels of 25(OH)D were normal in asymptomatic patients with biliary cirrhosis, and they concluded that 25(OH)D levels may be reduced in patients with significant parenchymal or cholestatic hepatic disease. Hepner *et al.* (1976) measured plasma 25(OH)D levels in alcoholic cirrhotics, alcoholic patients without abnormal liver function tests, and "inactive" cirrhotics whose alcoholism was in remission. Cirrhosis but not alcoholism was associated with lower serum levels of 25(OH)D. Results from this aminopyrine breath test, which measures the metabolism of aminopyrine by hepatic microsomes, correlated closely with plasma levels of 25(OH)D in the patients with "inactive" cirrhosis. The intravenous administration of vitamin D_3 was followed by an increase in serum 25(OH)D levels in patients with celiac disease, but not in those with cirrhosis. They suggested that impaired 25-hydroxylation of vitamin D to 25(OH)D is related to the degree of hepatic malfunction in cirrhosis.

In patients with primary biliary cirrhosis, Wagonfeld *et al.* (1976) reported that neither oral nor intravenous vitamin D affected plasma 25(OH)D levels or prevented the progression of skeletal demineralization. In contrast, the oral administration of 25(OH)D_3, 100–200 μg, enhanced plasma levels of 25(OH)D, while bone mineral content either stabilized or improved. They concluded that 25(OH)D_3 may be the preferred therapeutic form of vitamin D in patients with biliary cirrhosis. In another report, Daum *et al.* (1976) noted low plasma levels of 25(OH)D in children with extrahepatic biliary atresia; oral treatment with 25(OH)D_3, 50 μg/day, augmented plasma 25(OH)D levels and was associated with clinical improvement. It should be noted that the quantities of 25(OH)D_3 given to these patients with biliary tract disease considerably exceeds the amount believed to turn over normally; further data are needed to demonstrate whether these patients can respond to quantities of $25(OH)D_3$ that are truly physiological, since it is possible that the intestinal absorption of $25(OH)D_3$ may be abnormal. Nonetheless, these studies provide evidence for considerable advantage in using $25(OH)D_3$ to bypass the need for hepatic 25-hydroxylation.

Alcoholism. Although alcoholism, *per se,* may not affect the plasma levels of 25(OH)D, it is known that skeletal demineralization is common in alcoholic patients. In a prospective study of bone mineral content using X-ray spectrophotometry, Dalen and Lamke (1976) found that mean bone loss in the alcoholic patients was 2% greater than in controls. Also, Krawitt *et al.* (1975) found a significant reduction in intestinal Ca transport in rats given alcohol for 12 days. The administration of $1,25(OH)_2D_3$ failed to restore the ethanol-induced Ca transport to normal, and they suggested that alcohol affects Ca metabolism in a step that is independent of vitamin D metabolism.

Anticonvulsants. The prolonged use of anticonvulsant drugs, phenobarbital or diphenylhydantoin, may lead to hypocalcemia and even florid ostemalacia. Hahn and Avioli (1975) reviewed evidence for the induction of hepatic microsomal mixed oxidase enzyme activity following the long-term administration of phenobarbital to rats. They discuss clinical observations of a mild decrease in serum Ca, a moderate reduction in plasma 25(OH)D levels, and in increase in serum alkaline phosphatase activity (both hepatic and bone isoenzymes) in patients receiving phenobarbital and diphenylhydantoin. The precise epidemiological factors associated with such osteomalacia are disputed, and it has been suggested that clinically significant disease may be present only in institutionalized patients receiving large quantities of anticonvulsants. Mosekilde and Melsen (1976), however, reported results of bone biopsies in 60 ambulatory patients treated with anticonvulsants. Biochemical evaluation revealed hypocalcemia in 7% and elevated alkaline phosphatase in 42%; bone biopsies showed an increase in unmineralized bone in 53%; the osteoclastic resorption surfaces and the mean volume of periosteocytic lacunae were elevated in 69 and 75%, respectively. These data suggest a defect in mineralization analagous to osteomalacia in conjunction with secondary hyperparathyroidism. In institutionalized patients, those receiving anticonvulsants had a 25% reduction in plasma 25(OH)D and a 52% increase in serum iPTH in conjunction with a very slight decrease in serum Ca, i.e., 9.2 ± 0.4 vs. 9.6 ± 0.3 mg/dl in controls (Bouillon *et al.*, 1975). The administration of vitamin D_3, 2000 I.U./day, increased serum 25(OH)D slightly, but serum Ca and iPTH remained abnormal. These data provide additional support for the view that anticonvulsant therapy can lead to mild "vitamin D deficiency" with secondary hyperparathyroidism.

The methods used to identify patients with a significant abnormality remain uncertain. Fraser *et al.* (1976) suggested that the antipyrine half-life, in saliva, is useful to detect the existence of enzyme induction. The use of salivary samples obviated the need for frequent venipunctures.

Several recent studies have reexplored the pathophysiology of the osteomalacia of anticonvulsant therapy. In rats treated with PB and given radiolabeled 25(OH)D_3, Burt *et al.* (1976) found rates of disappearance of 25(OH)D_3 and appearance of 1,25$(OH)_2D_3$ to be normal. They concluded that the biotransformation of 25(OH)D_3 is not abnormal during PB treatment. Norman *et al.* (1976) found that phenobarbital treatment of rachitic chicks reduced the ability of D_3 and 25(OH)D_3 but not of 1,25$(OH)_2D_3$ to stimulate intestinal Ca absorption. Also, phenobarbital treatment was associated with reduced quantities of 1,25$(OH)_2D_3$ in bone, but not in the intestine. Corradino (1976) noted that diphenylhydantoin directly inhibited the vitamin-D_3-stimulated Ca absorption in a model whereby Ca transport is measured in organ culture. Since the intestine is not known to convert vitamin D into a more active metabolite, these data suggest that diphenylhydantoin may directly affect the Ca-absorptive mechanism. Such data suggest that anticonvulsant treatment may have as yet undefined actions on both vitamin D metabolism and action.

In a study of the metabolism of vitamin D during anticonvulsant therapy in man, Matheson *et al.* (1976) measured the intestinal absorption of vitamin D_3 and its subsequent metabolic transformation to 25(OH)D_3. The intestinal absorption of D_3 was identical to that observed in controls; however, the biotransformation of D_3 to 25(OH)D_3 was significantly accelerated in the anticonvulsant-treated patients. These observations, in conjunction with low plasma levels of 25(OH)D, are consistent with the rapid conversion of D_3 into inactive forms with anticonvulsant treatment. There may also be abnormalities of end-organ response to the active vitamin D sterols, although the latter theory is not proved in man.

In a clinical study concerned with the prevention or management of anticonvulsant-associated osteomalacia, Peterson *et al.* (1976) found that the metabolic balance for Ca became positive in anticonvulsant-treated patients receiving a daily vitamin D_3 dose of 975 I.U./day, compared with 380 I.U. D_3/day in patients not receiving anticonvulsants. On the basis of the quantity of vitamin D_3 needed to correct vitamin D deficiency in anticonvulsant-treated patients, Silver (1975) suggested that anticonvulsants increased the vitamin D requirement by 10 μg (400 I.U.)/day.

Two reports point out an interesting drug interaction that might produce severe skeletal disease in patients with seizure disorders. Thus, Matsuda *et al.* (1975) and Mallette (1975) reported the development of osteomalacia during the simultaneous treatment with anticonvulsant and acetazolamide. Acetazolamide treatment was associated with hypercalciuria and marked metabolic acidosis, which probably accelerated the development of bone disease and secondary hyperparathyroidism. With vitamin D treatment, supplemental phosphate, and deletion of treatment with acetazolamide, there was recovery from the osteomalacia.

9.1.2.6c. Defective Production of 1,25(OH)$_2$D$_3$. With knowledge that the conversion of 25(OH)D$_3$ to 1,25(OH)$_2$D$_3$ is the most carefully controlled step in vitamin D metabolism, there has been considerable interest in disorders involving altered synthesis of 1,25(OH)$_2$D$_3$.

Vitamin-D-Dependent Rickets. One hereditary disorder, vitamin-D-dependent rickets, may arise because of impaired synthesis of 1,25(OH)$_2$D$_3$. This disorder differs from the more common syndrome of sex-linked hypophosphatemic rickets in that there is marked hypocalcemia, and it differs from nutritional rickets in that pharmacological amounts of vitamin D are required to correct the abnormality. Vitamin D$_2$ in doses of 0.25–1.25 mg/day (10,000–50,000 I.U./day) can correct the abnormality; however, these patients respond to only 1.0 μg 1,25(OH)$_2$D$_3$/day while substantially larger amounts of 25(OH)D$_3$ are necessary. Such observations led to the theory that this disorder represents a deficiency of the renal enzyme, 25(OH)D$_3$-1-hydroxylase. To date, there has been no direct measurement of enzyme activity, and this is merely a hypothesis. Balsan *et al.* (1975) compared the efficacy of 1,25(OH)$_2$D$_3$ or 1α(OH)D$_3$ in children with nutritional rickets compared to those with vitamin D dependent rickets. They found that children with nutritional rickets uniformly responded to 0.5 μg/day of either drug, while this quantity was only partially active in those with vitamin-D-dependent rickets. On the basis of such data, they suggest that the hypothesis that vitamin-D-dependent rickets occurs because of reduced or absent generation of 1,25(OH)$_2$D$_3$ must be regarded as tentative.

Chronic Renal Failure. Chronic renal insufficiency is one of the most common conditions believed to adversely affect the conversion of 25(OH)D$_3$ to 1,25(OH)$_2$D$_3$. Moreover, this abnormality is believed to be one of the major factors contributing to secondary hyperparathyroidism in uremia. A discussion of the recent advances in vitamin D metabolism as they pertain to chronic renal failure was recently published (Coburn *et al.*, 1976).

The severity of defective calcium transport in patients with chronic renal disease was studied by Vergne-Marini *et al.* (1976), who studied Ca absorption in segments of the jejunum or ileum during the constant perfusion of test solutions. Ca absorption was markedly depressed in patients with chronic renal disease due to an abnormality of net flux out of the lumen; the flux from blood into the lumen was normal. In normal individuals, there is evidence for active Ca absorption by both jejunum and ileum, while patients with chronic renal failure displayed no evidence for active Ca transport. Treatment with 1α(OH)D$_3$, 2 μg/day for 1 week, restored Ca absorption and the unidirectional Ca flux out of the lumen to normal in the jejunum. Ca absorption by the ileum was increased to 60–83% of normal. The $1\alpha(OH)D_3$ had no effect on xylose or electrolyte absorption or on Ca flux into the lumen. Such data indicate the marked abnormality of intestinal Ca transport in renal failure; they document that the major abnormality exists in the proximal small intestine. A possible role of altered vitamin D metabolism in the pathogenesis of skeletal resistance to the calcemic action of PTH was suggested by Massry *et al.* (1976). Acute renal failure produced in dogs by bilateral nephrectomy reduced the calcemic response to PTH, and the administration of $1{,}25(OH)_2D_3$ partially restored this response toward normal. In an organ-culture system for' bone, Wills and Jenkins (1976) found that serum obtained from uremic patients prior to hemodialysis inhibited the PTH-stimulated release of Ca from bone. With the addition of several individual uremic metabolites, a similar inhibition was produced, but only in higher concentrations than those observed *in vivo.* They concluded that if uremic metabolites play a role causing the resistance to PTH, *in vivo,* it is due to a cumulative phenomenon. The possible effects of alterations of collagen metabolism on uremic skeletal disease were recently reviewed by Heidbreder *et al.* (1976). Abnormalities of collagen metabolism in uremia may contribute to the changes in turnover and maturation of normal bone crystals, which may in turn impair the mechanical strength of the skeleton. The effects of $25(OH)D_3$ and a diphosphonate, dichlormethylenediphosphate (Cl_2MDP), on experimental renal osteodystrophy were reported by Russell *et al.* (1975). There was an excess of less dense, more immature collagen and a preponderance of abnormal hydroxyapatite crystals in untreated uremic animals. These abnormalities were largely reversed in uremic animals with both $25(OH)D_3$ and Cl_2MDP. Also, the degree of soft-tissue calcification was reduced. These observations underscore the occurrence of abnormal collagen formation and crystal maturation in the skeleton of uremic animals; however, the relationship between such findings and the abnormalities in vitamin D metabolism remains to be established.

Pierides *et al.* (1976a) considered that barbiturate and anticonvulsant treatment may contribute to osteomalacia in patients undergoing hemodialysis and following renal transplantation. Pathological fractures and evidence of osteomalacia were more common in hemodialysis patients who received barbiturates than in those who did not. Moreover, osteomalacia was also more common in transplant recipients receiving barbiturates. They suggested that barbiturates and diphenolhydantoin should be avoided if possible in uremic patients undergoing hemodialysis and in transplant recipients. In another report from the same laboratory (Pierides *et al.,* 1976b), the failure of response of renal osteodystrophy to

$1\alpha(OH)D_3$ in a patient receiving anticonvulsant therapy was compared with a favorable response in another patient who was not receiving barbiturates and treated with a smaller quantity of $1\alpha(OH)D_3$. Eastwood *et al.* (1976) evaluated plasma levels of 25(OH)D and bone biopsis in patients with chronic renal failure and found that osteomalacia was present only in the patients with relatively low levels of 25(OH)D; they suggest that osteomalacia can occur in chronic renal failure due to lack of $25(OH)D_3$ or an abnormal ability to convert $25(OH)D_3$ to $1,25(OH)_2D_3$.

Certain uremic patients may have considerable impairment of phosphate absorption. Thus, K. Y. Ahmed *et al.* (1976) described 4 patients undergoing regular hemodialysis for 3–7 years who became hypophosphatemic even when they were not taking phosphate-binding antacids. Bone histology revealed excess osteoid, and there was a subnormal increase in plasma phosphate following an oral phosphate load. On treatment with dihydrotachysterol, there was improved absorption of phosphate. We have observed increased phosphate absorption with $1,25(OH)_2D_3$ treatment in uremia. In contrast, Pierides *et al.* (1976c) reported that uremic patients who were phosphate-depleted do not respond to $1\alpha(OH)D_3$; they suggest that phosphate depletion can contribute in a major way to the pathogenesis of the skeletal disease in certain patients with chronic renal failure. If this problem occurs in the United States, it is probably far less common than has been reported by the group at Newcastle upon Tyne.

A number of studies described therapeutic results following treatment with various vitamin D compounds. Pogglitsch *et al.* (1976) evaluated the use of dihydrotachysterol (DHT), 0.2 mg/day for 2 months followed by 0.45 mg/day for 2 months, in patients undergoing long-term dialysis. The DHT-treated patients showed a significant progression of skeletal demineralization, while there was no change in bone mineralization in the patients receiving no vitamin D. The doses of DHT employed may be large enough to enhance bone resorption in these patients, and further studies in larger numbers of patients are needed.

There has been interest in $1,25(OH)_2D_3$ or $1\alpha(OH)D_3$ in the management of uremia because these sterols do not require 1-hydroxylation by the kidney; however, Rutherford *et al.* (1975) showed that Ca absorption can be increased substantially following oral treatment with $25(OH)D_3$, 100 or 500 μg/day. Augmented Ca absorption occurred even in anephric patients, indicating that $25(OH)D_3$ may enhance Ca absorption even without the presence of renal tissue. It should be noted that the quantities of $25(OH)D_3$ employed are greater than the physiological amounts normally produced, and the effects observed probably represent pharmacological actions. Nonetheless, the quantities of $25(OH)D_3$ necessary to produce an effect are considerably smaller than the amounts of vitamin

D_2 or D_3 needed to increase Ca absorption in uremia. Teitelbaum *et al.* (1976) reported the results of long-term treatment of 5 uremic patients with $25(OH)D_3$, 40–100 μg/day. Skeletal biopsies showed a decrease in the number of osteoclasts and a fall in the percentage of osteoid surface covered with active osteoclasts. Osteitis fibrosa improved and serum iPTH activity decreased. Serum Ca rose above 12 mg/dl in 3 of 5 patients, indicating that treatment with $25(OH)D_3$, as well as $1,25(OH)_2D_3$, carries a significant risk of hypercalcemia.

The effects of $1\alpha(OH)D_3$ in patients with chronic renal failure were described in several reports. Davie *et al.* (1976) treated 4 patients with $1\alpha(OH)D_3$, 1.5–2 μg/day for periods up to 1 year; they noted increased Ca absorption, positive Ca and P balances, a modest increase in serum Ca, a reduction in serum alkaline phosphatase and iPTH, and improved skeletal X-rays and histological findings. Proximal myopathy improved strikingly in one patient. They concluded that $1\alpha(OH)D_3$ is an effective means for treating renal osteodystrophy. Neilsen *et al.* (1976) reported favorable results in 3 adolescents with azotemic osteodystrophy treated with $1\alpha(OH)D_3$ for 7 months; hypercalcemia was reversed quickly following withdrawal of treatment. Naik *et al.* (1976) utilized body Ca measurements by neutron activation to follow the course of patients receiving $1\alpha(OH)D_3$. Total body Ca increased in association with radiological and histological improvement. There was no change in whole-body Ca in patients who showed no histological improvement of skeletal lesions. Thus, $1\alpha(OH)D_3$ may be of value in certain patients, while no response may occur in others; the authors suggest that measurement of total-body Ca may provide a sensitive and noninvasive index of the response to treatment. The facilities for such measurements, however, are not readily available. In a double-blind study, Tougaard *et al.* (1976) administered $1\alpha(OH)D_3$ (1.0 μg/day) or a placebo to patients with chronic renal failure for 11 weeks. Treatment with $1\alpha(OH)D_3$ increased intestinal absorption of Ca associated with a fall in serum iPTH. Plasma phosphorus, alkaline phosphatase, and bone mineralization, measured by the phosphorus/hydroxyproline ratio, were not changed. Bone mineral content, however, measured by photoabsorption, decreased to the same extent in both groups. They concluded that treatment with $1\alpha(OH)D_3$ may not affect a progressive loss of Ca from bone despite normalization of plasma Ca and iPTH. These studies are of interest, but a longer period of study and the use of a larger number of patients are needed before firm conclusions can be drawn.

Several reports corroborated early observations indicating that treatment with $1,25(OH)_2D_3$ is associated with prompt improvement in certain patients with renal osteodystrophy (Smith *et al.*, 1975). Pierides *et al.* (1976d) found improved Ca absorption, a reversal of secondary hypoparathyroidism, histologically and radiologically, and a fall in serum iPTH and alkaline phosphatase in patients given $1,25(OH)_2D_3$. Muscle function improved, both clinically and electromyographically, and there was improved skeletal mineralization, but this change was slow and less marked. Our present experience indicates that many patients with symptomatic overt renal osteodystrophy respond favorably to treatment with these highly active forms of vitamin D; however, certain patients do not improve. A failure to improve may be due to other superimposed factors, such as phosphate depletion (Pierides *et al.*, 1976c) and other poorly defined abnormalities that alter bone metabolism.

Diabetes Mellitus. Recently, the possibility that an alteration in vitamin D metabolism or sensitivity may occur in diabetes mellitus has been suggested as a result of a series of experiments carried out in animals with experimental diabetes. Previously reported data indicate that uncontrolled alloxan or streptozotocin diabetes in the rat is associated with reduced intestinal transport of Ca. This abnormality is associated with a decrease in intestinal CaBP, and it occurs despite the animals being fed a diet adequate in vitamin D. Treatment of the diabetes with insulin results in a restoration of Ca transport toward normal. Schneider *et al.* (1975) reported that the administration of an extract of *Solanum malacoxylon,* given as a presumed source of $1,25(OH)_2D_3$, restores the intestinal Ca transport of diabetic rats to normal. In another study, Schneider *et al.* (1976) found that the impaired intestinal Ca absorption in diabetes could be restored by $1,25(OH)_2D_3$ or $1\alpha(OH)D_3$, but not by D_3 or $25(OH)D_3$. Such observations provide strong support for the view that the production of $1,25(OH)_2D_3$ may be impaired in this model of diabetes. In light of the recognized nephrotoxic actions of streptozocin and alloran, the clinical significance of these recent observations is uncertain at present. There are, however, data indicating that osteopenia, osteoporosis, and certain types of fractures are more common in diabetic patients than in age-matched nondiabetic controls.

Pseudohypoparathyroidism. The possibility that vitamin D metabolism or action may be altered in pseudohypoparathyroidism was recently suggested. Drezner *et al.* (1976) found plasma levels of $1,25(OH)_2D_3$ to be low in patients with type I pseudohypoparathyroidism. Treatment with pharmacological doses of vitamin D_2 restored both the serum Ca and the calcemic response to PTE to normal; however, the renal response remained abnormal. Skeletal biopsies revealed both increased osteoclastic resorption and osteomalacia. They suggested that abnormal renal production of $1,25(OH)_2D_3$ may be responsible for the pathogenesis of this syndrome. Sinha and Bell (1976) provided indirect support for this view with observations that treatment of patients with pseudohypoparathyroidism with $1,25(OH)_2D_3$, 1 μg/day, restored the intestinal absorption of Ca, serum Ca and P, and serum iPTH to normal. It was recently shown that the serum prolactin (Carlson *et al.*, 1977) levels are reduced in these patients, and it was recently reported that prolactin is a potent factor stimulating the renal production of $1,25(OH)_2D_3$ (Spanos *et al.*, 1976). Thus, it seems possible that reduced serum levels of $1,25(OH)_2D_3$ could occur as a result of deficient prolactin.

9.1.3. Other Factors that Affect Calcium Homeostasis

Immobilization is known to be associated with a negative Ca balance and increased urinary Ca, and the effect of weightlessness on mineral balance during the prolonged space flight of the Second Manned Skylab Mission was studied by Whedon *et al.* (1976). There was a substantial increase in urinary Ca in all 3 crewmen during the 60 day flight period with no reduction in the loss during the course of the flight; moreover, the losses occurred despite regular strenuous exercise. These observations emphasize the importance of physical stress or weight-bearing on the integrity of bone.

9.1.3.1. Calcium-Handling by the Kidney

The renal tubular reabsorption of Ca lost into the tubule by glomerular filtration is a factor that affects the level of blood Ca. In man, only 0.5–1.0% filtered Ca is lost in the urine because of remarkably effective mechanisms for tubular reabsorption. Several hormonal and nonhormonal factors alter the renal handling of Ca and change its excretory rate. There is a close association between the renal tubular reabsorption of Ca and that of Na, and many maneuvers that alter tubular reabsorption of Na have a similar effect on that of Ca; such factors include saline infusion, renal vasodilatation, and the administration of certain diuretics, such as furosemide or ethacrynic acid.

PTH lowers urinary Ca by means of an increase in net Ca reabsorption. The relative contribution of the kidney toward the regulation of plasma Ca is controversial. It is generally believed that the rate of movement of Ca from the skeleton is the primary determinant of serum Ca, while others maintain that the kidney is an important regulator of serum Ca concentration (Nordin, 1976).

The thiazide diuretics as well as PTH are among the few substances that reduce the renal clearance of Ca relative to that of Na. Observations in man suggest that the thiazide diuretics do not reduce urinary Ca in patients with hypoparathyroidism, suggesting that the hypocalciuric action of thiazides may not occur in the absence of PTH. Costanzo *et al.* (1975) evaluated the acute effects of thiazide diuretics on the clearances of

Ca and Na in patients with hypoparathyroidism; there was a 65% decrease in the Ca/Na clearance ratios in normal subjects and in patients with hypoparathyroidism, indicating that the acute action of thiazides is not impaired in hypoparathyroidism. Other observations by Quamme *et al.* (1975) provide further evidence that the dissociative actions of thiazides on transport of Na and Ca in the distal nephron do not involve PTH. It is possible that the administration of pharmacological doses of vitamin D to patients with hypoparathyroidism prevented the appearance of hypocalciuria during long-term administration of thiazide diuretics.

The possible actions of vitamin D and its metabolites on the renal handling of Ca are variable; these data were reviewed elsewhere (Coburn *et al.*, 1976). Bonjour *et al.* (1975) reported that $1,25(OH)_2D_3$, caused a quantitatively similar increase in both urinary Ca excretion and intestinal Ca absorption. These observations resemble results found in normal humans given $1,25(OH)_2D_3$, although they are opposite to the effects of renal Ca reabsorption observed in micropuncture studies.

9.2. Phosphate Metabolism

9.2.1. Regulation by the Kidney

In many mammals, the kidney plays a major role in phosphate homeostasis, and urinary phosphorus is believed to represent the difference between the quantity filtered and the amount reabsorbed by the tubule. The regulation of tubular reabsorption is influenced by a number of factors and is a primary determinant of body phosphate stores. The factors that are known to affect the renal tubular reabsorption of phosphate include: (1) the filtered load of PO_4; (2) PTH; (3) the state of extracellular volume; (4) the level of serum calcium; (5) tissue stores of PO_4 and previous dietary intake; and (6) acid–base status.

9.2.1.1. Effects of Dietary Intake of Phosphorus

The influence of previous dietary phosphate intake on its renal handling was assessed by Steele and DeLuca (1976) and by Trohler *et al.* (1976), who independently carried out studies in thyroparathyroidectomized (TPTX) rats fed either a high- or a low-PO_4 diet and then given phosphate infusions. At any given level of serum PO_4, there was as much as a 100-fold change in PO_4 excretion, depending on the previous dietary intake of phosphate and even independent of presence or absence of PTH. In contrast, the addition of PTH increased the fractional excretion of PO_4 only 2- to 5-fold, at similar filtered loads of phosphate. These data indicate that changes in dietary phosphate intake can significantly alter tubular PO_4 reabsorption under a number of circumstances; thus, the previous dietary intake of PO_4 needs to be taken into consideration when one evaluates any given factor affecting renal phosphate transport.

9.2.1.2. Effects of Parathyroid Hormone

Disagreement persists about the sites of the nephron where phosphate transport takes place, and there is uncertainty about the nephron sites that are sensitive to the action of PTH. It has been assumed that all phosphate transport takes place in the proximal tubule, although certain observations suggest that significant distal PO_4 transport exists. To evaluate this, Knox and Lechene (1975) carried out micropuncture studies in TPTX dogs given bovine PTH. The latter decreased the proximal-tubular-fluid/plasma-inulin ratio, indicating a decrease in proximal fluid reabsorption; the delivery of phosphate from the accessible part of proximal tubule was increased from 26 to 37% of the filtered load, and the fraction of filtered PO_4 appearing in the urine increased from 2.5 to 21.5%.

Saline infusion produced the same fall in tubular-fluid/plasma-inulin ratio in the proximal tubule, but there was an insignificant augmentation of the fraction of filtered PO_4 appearing in the final urine. These observations indicate that there is a substantial action of PTH distal to the accessible portion of the proximal tubule. However, such changes in PO_4 transport might well occur in the proximal tubule beyond the point of micropuncture. The possibility that PTH and acetazolamide have a common mechanism of action on PO_4 reabsorption was studied by Knox *et al.* (1976); they measured the effect of PTH, given with or without acetazolamide, in TPTX dogs. In the absence of acetazolamide, PTH increased the fractional delivery of PO_4 from the proximal tubule from 28 to 38%, while the fractional excretion of P increased from 4 to 20%. With concomitant acetazolamide treatment, PTH increased the fractional delivery of P out of the proximal tubule from 50 to 58% and augmented the fractional excretion of P in the urine from 9 to 31%. Thus, the action of PTH was additive to the effect of maximal inhibition of carbonic anhydrase, suggesting that PTH and acetazolamide have different mechanisms of action on PO_4 reabsorption. Also, phosphate reabsorption was inhibited to a greater degree by PTH than by acetazolamide beyond the point of micropuncture. Such observations do not support the previous contention that PTH may act as a carbonic anhydrase inhibitor in the proximal tubule.

Slatopolsky *et al.* (1976) studied the renal responsiveness to PTH in intact and TPTX dogs before and after inducing acute hypermagnesemia. Hypermagnesemia blunted both the phosphaturia and increased urinary cAMP seen in response to a submaximal infusion of PTH. When dibutyryl cAMP was infused, the phosphaturic response was not altered by hypermagnesemia. Also, an elevation of the Mg concentration in kidney slices reduced the production of cAMP in response to PTH. These observations suggest that an increase in plasma Mg can alter the end-organ responsiveness to PTH, presumably due to changes in PTH activation of adenylate cyclase.

9.2.1.3. Effects of Serum Calcium Level

Variations in the level of plasma Ca can affect renal phosphate-handling, independent of changes in PTH. Cuche *et al.* (1976) evaluated the effect of altering intrarenal Ca on renal phosphate-handling. When acutely TPTX dogs were given a constant infusion of bovine PTH and a calcium chloride infusion was superimposed, there was an increase in the fractional excretion of phosphate as serum Ca increased by 20%. Such changes occurred when Ca was given intravenously or into one renal artery. There was no change or there was even a fall in the fractional excretion of phosphate, however, when serum Ca was increased by 75%. In the dog, as in man, an acute elevation of serum Ca is associated with an increase in the serum P. Even when this change in serum P is considered, these data suggest that a small increase in serum Ca can decrease the tubular reabsorption of phosphate. These results are consistent with the previous demonstration of phosphaturia despite a fall in serum P in hypoparathyroid patients during a prolonged Ca infusion. Amiel *et al.* (1976) evaluated renal PO_4 handling in PTX rats as they increased plasma Ca from a very low level to subnormal levels. They found an increase in reabsorptive capacity for phosphate in both the proximal tubule and more distal portion of the nephron when Ca was infused. They concluded that there is a PTH-independent mechanism for phosphate transport that is augmented by raising serum Ca independent of PTH. The results from these two laboratories show opposite effects of raising serum Ca. At present, it is not known whether differences in techniques (i.e., rate of increase in serum Ca) or the use of different species could account for the divergent results reported.

9.2.1.4. Actions of Vitamin D

The knowledge that $25(OH)D_3$ is localized in the kidney, where it is further converted to either $1,25(OH)_2D_3$ or $24,25(OH)_2D_3$, indicates the existence of an intimate relationship between vitamin D and the kidney. Moreover, such information has intensified the search for possible direct action of vitamin D or one of its more active metabolic forms on electrolyte transport by the kidney. The evidence that vitamin D_3, $25(OH)D_3$, or $1,25(OH)_2D_3$ may affect phosphate reabsorption was considered in a recent review (Coburn *et al.,* 1976). Data suggest that pharmacological, but nontoxic, quantities of vitamin D, $25(OH)D_3$, or $1,25(OH)_2D_3$ enhance the renal tubular reabsorption of phosphate. Thus, the effect of vitamin D on phosphate transport may be opposite to that of PTH, and other observations suggest that vitamin D or an analogue may block the action of PTH on phosphate transport in the renal tubule. Whether such an effect of vitamin D on renal phosphate transport is of any physiological importance remains unknown. Observations that a low dietary phosphate stimulates the renal production of $1,25(OH)_2D_3$ raise the possibility that an action of $1,25(OH)_2D_3$ to enhance renal tubular phosphate reabsorption could be a defense mechanism that prevents more severe phosphate depletion. Vitamin D is known to stimulate the transepithelial transport of both Ca and PO_4 in the intestine, and it is possible that the sterol acts in an analogous manner on the kidney. Further studies are necessary to clarify whether vitamin D plays a physiological role in phosphate homeostasis by the kidney.

Studies from Garabedian *et al.* (1976) and Steele *et al.* (1975) emphasize that $1,25(OH)_2D_3$ can exert an early and potent phosphatemic action in rats. Such an effect might be related in part to a renal action, but it probably arises from an action on bone. Such an immediate effect on serum phosphorus level has not been apparent in dog or in man.

9.2.1.5. Other Factors that Affect Renal Phosphate-Handling

Observations that lithium-induced nephrogenic diabetes insipidus is associated with impaired activation of vasopressin-sensitive renal medullary adenylate cyclase led Steele (1976) to study the effect of lithium on the phosphaturic response to both PTH and large doses of pitressin. Lithium treatment inhibited the phosphaturic response to certain doses of both PTH and vasopressin. He suggested that lithium may affect the adenylate cyclase systems that are stimulated by PTH and vasopressin, but these effects are modified by the renal reabsorption and tissue uptake of lithium itself.

It is known that extracellular volume expansion (ECVE) can cause phosphaturia and that PTH secretion is stimulated during certain maneuvers that produce ECVE. To evaluate the role of expansion of blood volume on PTH secretion and on renal phosphate-handling, Epstein *et al.* (1976) studied the effects of expansion of central blood volume, using a method whereby ionized blood Ca remains unchanged. The model used was water immersion to the neck, a procedure shown to cause natriuresis, bicarbonaturia, and, presumably, an increase in delivery of sodium to the distal tubule. During water immersion, there was no change in serum iPTH or in urinary PO_4 excretion despite substantial natriuresis. These data suggest that PTH is not involved in volume homeostasis in man; the absence of phosphaturia, despite the probability that distal phosphate delivery was enchanced, suggests the possibility that distal sites for phosphate reabsorption exist in the human kidney.

9.2.2. Phosphate Depletion

The reader interested in the pathophysiology and metabolic aspects of phosphate (P) depletion and hypophosphatemia should read a series of classic articles dating back to the early 1920's (Sherman and Pappenheimer, 1921; Theiler *et al.,* 1927; Theiler, 1931; Theiler and Green, 1932; Riddell *et al.,* 1934; Aubel, 1936; Day and McCollum, 1939; Bloom and Flinchum, 1960; Lotz *et al.,* 1966). These laboratory and clinical studies did not excite great attention until the relationship of P depletion to clinical symptomatology was "rediscovered" in chronic hemodialysis patients dialyzed with P-free solutions and ingesting large amounts of P-binding antacids (Knochel *et al.,* 1975; Jacob, 1975); stable chronic renal failure patients and post-renal-transplantation patients ingesting comparable or even larger amounts of these antacids, patients during and after severe debilitating medical and surgical illnesses receiving gastric or parenteral "total" nutrition with inadequate P supplementation (Craddock *et al.,* 1974; Yawata *et al.,* 1973); and acute and chronic alcoholic patients subsisting on almost P-free rations and receiving more of the same with parenteral solutions utilized early after their hospitalization (Knochel *et al.,* 1975).

Recent reviews by Knochel (1977), Lee and Kleeman (1976), and Jacob (1975) have brought up to date our understanding of the syndromes associated with P depletion and hypophosphatemia. Many hypophosphatemic disorders such as primary hyperparathyroidism, Fanconi's syndrome, congenital and acquired renal tubular acidosis with phosphate wasting, vitamin-D-deficient and vitamin-D-resistant rickets, and osteomalacia cause an *increased* renal clearance of P. These disorders do not appear to show the marked soft-tissue abnormalities of the classic P-depletion syndrome associated with a true deficiency of P, while the latter and the former may both display classic osteomalacia. The P-depletion syndrome is seen on an acute or chronic basis when the diet ingested or infused is truly deficient in P or P is inadequately absorbed from the G.I. tract, as with the excessive administration of P-binding antacids.

In the experimental animal with dietary P depletion, we observe a constantly reproducible set of biochemical changes: severe hypophosphatemia; hypophosphaturia, or a urine free of P; marked hypercalciuria;

and often frank hypercalcemia. This hypercalcemia is primarily the result of markedly increased bone reabsorption (Baylink *et al.*, 1971), although at times it is accompanied by enhanced absorption of Ca from the G.I. tract (Hughes *et al.*, 1975; Dominguez *et al.*, 1976). Hypercalcemia is not usually observed in P-depleted humans (Lee and Kleeman, 1976; Dominguez *et al.*, 1976). Despite the normo- or hypercalcemic state, the evidence indicates that circulating PTH is low, or not measurable, and associated with marked hyposecretion of the parathyroid glands. Therefore, P depletion is a state of physiological hypoparathyroidism.

As was stated earlier, one of the most potent stimuli to the 1α-hydroxylase enzyme in the renal cortex responsible for the synthesis of $1\alpha,25(OH)_2D_3$ is P depletion. It has now been demonstrated that the blood level of $1\alpha,25(OH)_2D_3$ is significantly increased in the P-depleted rat (Hughes *et al.*, 1975). Therefore, P depletion may also be a state of physiological "hypervitaminosis D." The role of excess circulating $1,25(OH)_2D_3$ in the biochemical manifestations of P depletion has not been delineated; it is now clear, however, that these manifestations may all be seen when P depletion is superimposed on vitamin D deficiency in the rat (Brautbar *et al.*, 1977a). That is, D deficiency does not prevent these biochemical changes. These authors found that large and probably pharmacological doses of $1,25(OH_2D_3$ given to P-depleted animals can cause a return of the serum P toward normal, but this appears to be due to vitamin-D-induced further bone resorption in a setting in which the released P stays in the circulation because of the remarkably reduced P excretion. It should be noted that the elevated $1,25(OH)_2D_3$ observed in P-depleted rats does not prevent the hypophosphatemia in these animals. Early in P depletion, the urine becomes P-free, and this avid tubular reabsorption of P is markedly resistent to PTH (Steele and DeLuca, 1976) and even to acute increases in the filtered load of P produced by P infusion. The exact cause of the extreme reduction and elevation in the renal clearance of P and Ca, respectively, in the P-depleted state is unknown. It is not due simply to the physiological hypoparathyroidism, and it cannot be corrected by administration of PTH. Studies utilizing the isolated perfused rabbit kidney obtained from normal and P-depleted rabbits strongly suggest that two factors are responsible for the decreased tubular reabsorption of Ca: (1) a humoral factor circulating in the blood of the P-depleted rabbit inhibited the reabsorption of Ca when perfused into the normal kidney; and (2) the kidney from the P-depleted rabbit, when perfused with normal rabbit blood, also demonstrated impaired reabsorption of Ca (Ben-Issac *et al.*, 1975). There is little question that for any given metabolic setting or filtered load of P, the dietary intake of P greatly influences the net tubular reabsorption of P (Trohler *et al.*, 1976).

The hypercalciuria and hypophosphatemia plus the renal resistance to PTH resemble the effects of growth hormone on the renal excretion of Ca and P. Considering the possibility that P depletion caused an increased secretion of growth hormone, Brautbar *et al.* (1977b) studied the effect of hypophysectomy in young, rapidly growing rats on the biochemical picture of P depletion. The rats were maintained on ACTH and thyroxine. Hypophysectomy significantly ameliorated the major biochemical changes associated with P depletion (hypercalcemia, hypophosphatemia, hypercalciuria, and hypophosphaturia); however, it is not certain whether this amelioration is a *direct* consequence of the absence of growth hormone or is due to the inhibition of growth in the hypophysectomized animals. Studies are in progress to determine whether paired feeding of the normal animals can inhibit their growth to the level of hypophysectomized animals and thereby greatly ameliorate the biochemical changes of P depletion. Dominguez *et al.* (1976) reviewed the effects of sex on the biochemical pattern of P depletion carried out for short periods (16–19 days) in 6 healthy women aged 18–22 and 5 healthy men aged 19–25. In both groups, they observed almost complete disappearance of P from the urine; however, the serum P of the men did not significantly decrease, while that of the women fell from a mean of 1.45 mM to a mean of 0.76 mM, emphasizing the dissociation of the P-free urine from the filtered load of P. Hypercalciuria appeared by the second day of P restriction and reached a plateau in the males by the 8th day, approximately 3-fold greater than control rates of Ca excretion. The latter continued to rise in the women to reach a level 4–5 times greater than control. In both males and females, enhanced intestinal absorption of Ca was observed, but the magnitude of the hypercalciuria in the women resulted in a frankly negative balance of Ca during the latter part of the study. Both groups demonstrated a significantly faster disappearance of $[^3H]$- or $[^{14}C]25(OH)D_3$ from the circulation. The authors concluded that this represented an enhanced production of $1,25(OH)_2D_3$ in the kidney from the circulating $25(OH)D_3$. At the same time, a significant fall in serum iPTH (*COOH*-terminal) was found. The positive correlation in both groups between the net intestinal absorption of Ca and plasma $25(OH)D_3$ turnover was very close ($r = 0.80$). The decrease in iPTH in these studies probably cannot be explained by a rise in serum Ca, because if any changes in the latter occurred, it was actually a slight mean decrease (-0.06 ± 0.02 mM/liter). Unfortunately, the concentration of free Ca^{2+} in the blood was not measured in these experiments. In the rat, hypercalcemia occurs in P depletion despite the hypoparathyroid state and may even contribute to this state. It is possible that the physiological hypoparathyroidism that is clearly present in P-depleted animals and humans is due to a direct "feedback" inhibition of PTH secretion by the increased $1,25(OH)_2D_3$ (see earlier discussion), or it may well be that the "P-depleted" parathyroid gland actually "sees" a normal Ca^{2+} ion concentration in the perfusing blood as an increased one. An important unsettled question in the P-depleted animal is what the true values are for free intracellular Ca^{2+} and inorganic P. Major methodological problems must be overcome before exact intracellular (cytoplasmic and mitochondrial) measurements of these ions can be achieved.

Dominguez *et al.* (1976) suggested that sex difference in response to dietary P restriction may have been due to the greater muscle mass in the males as a source for P, rather than the skeleton as the primary suggested source in women. Additional studies in rapidly growing and adult male and female dogs and rats and male animals receiving exogenous estrogens must be carried out to arrive at a more definite conclusion.

Dominguez *et al.* (1976) stated, "Overall, the low P diet was well tolerated by each subject and none developed any symptoms of muscle weakness or bone pain." This, of course, is the direct consequence of the brief duration of the study and the minimal degree of P depletion. As reviewed in detail by Knochel (1977), Lee and Kleeman (1976), and Jacob (1975), it is clear that chronic P depletion in humans can cause severe demineralization of the skeleton and classic osteomalacia despite adequate vitamin D intake. Furthermore, chronic P depletion and severe actue (days to weeks) depletion as is observed in total parenteral nutrition without supplemental P, chronic and actue alcoholism, or large antacid ingestion together with P-free hemo- or peritoneal dialysis can result in the following severe clinically evident organ system dysfunctions:

- *Nervous system:* irritability, confusion, obtundation-coma, dysarthria, anisocoria, ballismus, parasthesias, impaired peripheral nerve conduction
- *Muscular system:* profound muscle weakness, true myopathy with low transmembrane resting potential, filbrillation pattern by EMG and increased serum CPK and aldolase
- *Hematological system:* abnormal rigidity of the red cell with shortened red-cell life span and overt hemolytic anemia, impaired O_2 release from the red cell due to an intracellular deficiency of 2,3-diphosphoglycerate, phatelet dysfunction, impaired leukocyte phagocytosis
- *Liver:* abnormal liver function tests
- *GI tract:* profound loss of appetite, nausea and vomiting
- *Kidney:* renal tubular dysfunction with impaired reabsorption of glucose and bicarbonate

With respect to the latter, Emmett *et al.* (1977) documented a severe bicarbonaturia in the P-depleted rat, but despite this finding the animals do not demonstrate systemic acidosis. These authors showed indirectly, but quite conclusively, that the bone breakdown and bicarbonate mobilization from the skeleton of these animals protect them from the development of metabolic acidosis despite the marked renal "wasting" of bicarbonate.

P depletion appears to produce these abnormal effects in the soft tissue and possibly even in the bone cells by interfering with the normal production of essential intracellular organic phosphates, especially ATP. The exact role of low intracellular inorganic P and possibly a raised intracellular free Ca^{2+} ion concentration in the pathophysiology of the P-depletion "syndrome" may be clearer at the time of our next edition.

9.3. Magnesium Metabolism

Of body Mg, 60% is found in bone, with 30% within the cells, and Mg is quantitatively second to K as a major intracellular cation. In cells, Mg is largely bound to intracellular organelles or complexed to enzymes. A readily exchangeable pool consists of Mg in ECF and a labile component in bone. Of dietary Mg, 30–60% is absorbed regardless of the needs of the body, the excess Mg being excreted in the urine as a renal tubular reabsorptive maximum (T_m) is exceeded. With reduced magnesium intake, filtered Mg is avidly reabsorbed. Brannan *et al.* (1976) studies Mg transport in man utilizing the technique of intestinal perfusion with a triple-lumen catheter; Mg absorption by the jejunum increased with its luminal concentration, with a tendency for saturation to occur at high concentrations. The absorption of Mg was reduced in patients with chronic renal failure, while patients with hypercalciuria and hyperabsorption of Ca exhibited normal absorption of Mg. The authors suggested that the processes responsible for Mg absorption differ from those necessary for Ca transport; on the basis of the observations in renal failure, however, they suggested that Mg absorption may depend on vitamin D.

9.3.1. The Kidney in Magnesium Homeostasis

Because of the major role of the kidney in regulation of body Mg homeostasis, there is continued interest in the physiology of renal Mg-handling. Results of micropuncture studies of Mg reabsorption in the proximal tubule, loop of Henle, and distal tubule of Mg-loaded rats were compared with data obtained without Mg loading (Brunette *et al.*, 1975). In nonloaded animals the fractions of filtered Mg remaining in the early and late proximal tubule were 0.78 and 0.70, respectively; comparable fractions in the deep loop of Henle, the early and late distal tubules, and the final urine were 0.72, 0.15, 0.10, and 0.10, respectively. In Mg-loaded rats, there was no change in proximal tubular fluid reabsorption, but the fractions of Mg remaining in the early and late proximal tubules increased to 1.00 and 0.90, respectively. The fractions of filtered Mg remaining in the deep loops of Henle, the early and late distal tubules, and the final urine average 1.30, 0.58, 0.54 and 0.56, respectively. Thus, a smaller fraction of filtered Mg was reabsorbed in the proximal tubule in nonloaded animals than had been identified in the past. A large fraction of Mg was absorbed between the tip of Henle's loop and the early distal tubule, with very little Mg reabsorption occurring at more distal sites. During Mg loading, there was little or no proximal reabsorption, and there was net flux of Mg *into* the tubular lumen between the accessible portion of the proximal tubule and the tip of Henle's loop, with a considerable fraction reabsorbed in the ascending limb. These studies suggest an apparent site of Mg secretion, which can be identified during Mg loading. Moreover, the ascending limb is a major site of Mg reabsorption; such transport occurred independent of whether there had been loading with Mg or not. It is possible that such absorption is dependent on chloride transport and could explain why net Mg secretion can be seen when this component is inhibited during the administration of "loop" diuretics such as furosemide.

9.3.2. Magnesium Depletion

Mg depletion can arise (1) due to a low dietary intake or impaired of Mg, (2) due to defective renal tubular reabsorption of Mg, or (3) as a consequence of Mg incorporation into cells or into the skeleton during a period of rapid metabolic repair. Hypocalcemia and hypokalemia are common in Mg depletion. Since serum levels of Ca and K are measured routinely, many features of Mg depletion are often attributed incorrectly to hypocalcemia or hypokalemia. The hypocalcemia that develops with Mg depletion is multifactorial and arises due to failure of PTH secretion and because of reduced end-organ response of the bone and kidney to the PTH that is secreted. Also, Mg depletion may favor the precipitation of $CaPO_4$ in the skeleton. Rude *et al.* (1976) studied 20 patients with hypomagnesemia and hypocalcemia, with malabsorption, alcoholism, and prolonged therapy with parenteral fluids accounting for most cases. Serum iPTH was either undetectable or normal in all but 2 of 26 hypocalcemic patients. When 150–300 mg Mg was given intravenously, serum iPTH increased markedly within 1 min, although there was no change in serum Ca. With more prolonged replacement of Mg salts over several days, the authors noted a sustained increase in serum iPTH and a slow rise in serum Ca. There was a sluggish or negligible increment in urinary excretion of cAMP in response to exogenous PTE in 2 patients studied. They suggested that there is a major defect in the secretion of PTH in hypomagnesemia, and, in addition, there may be defective renal generation of cAMP in response to PTH. In the study of a patient with intestinal malabsorption of Mg, Anast *et al.* (1976) also reported that the administration of Mg to a hypomagnesemic patient was followed by a prominent and very rapid increase in serum iPTH. These observations point to the existence of a defect in the secretion of PTH in Mg depletion, although the observations of Rude *et al.* (1976) indicate that end-organ resistance may exist, as well. From results of the measurement of adenylate cyclase activity in rats with Mg depletion, Ashby and Heaton (1975) concluded that the metabolism of cAMP may be abnormal as a secondary result of other events that occur as a consequence of a Mg deficiency.

The effect of Mg depletion on vitamin D metabolism and action has been the subject of recent studies. Most data indicate that the intestinal absorption of Ca is increased during Mg depletion, and there is no evidence for altered metabolism of vitamin D. Two recent studies suggest that there may be skeletal resistance to the pharmacological actions of vitamin D on bone resorption during Mg depletion (Rayssiguier *et al.*, 1975; Medalle *et al.*, 1976).

Interesting clinical and laboratory observations noted in association with hypomagnesemia were described by Passer (1976). Two patients with hypocalcemia and hypomagnesemia were found to have mild distal renal tubular acidosis and increased serum iPTH levels. Following the administration of Mg, the hypocalcemia and the renal acidifying defect disappeared. The explanation for the reversible renal acidifying defect is obscure.

The factors responsible for the hypocalcemia that commonly accompanies hypomagnesemia are under continued investigation. Recent data suggest that there may be decreased synthesis or secretion of PTH, that there is resistance to the action of PTH on target tissues, and that alterations in the skeleton may favor the deposition of Ca into osteoid.

Acknowledgments

We are greatly indebted to Carolyn Schaefer and Judith Bernstein for their secretarial assistance; to Frieda Oxman, Research Librarian, for her assistance with the bibliographic searches; and to Mary Scott for her editorial assistance. Without their assistance, this review could not have been completed.

References

Ahmed, K. Y., Varghese, Z., Wills, M. R., Meinhard, E., Skinner, R. K., Baillod, R. A., and Moorhead, J. F., 1976, Persistent hypophosphataemia and osteomalacia in dialysis patients not on oral phosphate-binders: Response to dihydrotachysterol therapy, *Lancet* **2**:439.

Ahmed, S. H., Rizvi, S. N., and Vaishnava, S., 1975, A diagnostic study of 120 cases of nutritional rickets, *Indian Pediatr.* **12**:1141.

Alhava, E. M., Aukee, S., Karjalainen, P., Kettunen, P., and Juuti, M., 1975, The influence of calcium and calcium + vitamin D_2 treatment on bone mineral after partial gastrectomy, *Scand. J. Gastroenterol.* **10**:689.

Amiel, C., Kuntziger, H., Couette, S., Coureau C., and Bergounioux, N., 1976, Evidence for a parathyroid hormone-independent calcium modulation of phosphate transport along the nephron, *J. Clin. Invest.* **57**:256.

Anast, C. S., Winnacker, J. L., Forte, L. R., and Burns, T. W., 1976, Impaired release of parathyroid hormone in magnesium deficiency, *J. Clin. Endocrinol. Metab.* **42**:707.

Arnaud, S. B., Goldsmith, R. S., Lambert, P. W., and Go, V. L., 1975, 25-Hydroxyvitamin D_3: Evidence of an enterohepatic circulation in man, *Proc. Soc. Exp. Biol. Med.* **149**:570.

Arnaud, S. B., Stickler, G. B., and Haworth, J. C., 1976, Serum 25-hydroxyvitamin D in infantile rickets, *Pediatrics* **57**:221.

Ashby, J. P., and Heaton F. W., 1975, Effect of magnesium deficiency and parathyroid hormone on cyclic AMP metabolism in rat renal cortex, *J. Endocrinol.* **67**:105.

Aubel, C. E., 1936, The effects of low phosphorus rations on growing pigs, *J. Agric. Res. (Washington)* **52**:149.

Balsan, S., Garabedian, M., Sorgniard, R., Holick, M. F., and DeLuca, H. F., 1975, 1,25-Dihydroxyvitamin D_3 and 1,alpha-hydroxyvitamin D_3 in children: Biologic and therapeutic effects in nutritional rickets and different types of vitamin D resistance, *Pediatr. Res.* **9**:586.

Baylink, D., Wergedal, J., and Stauffer, M., 1971, Formation, mineralization and resorption of bone in hypophosphatemic rats, *J. Clin. Invest.* **50**:2519.

Beale, M. G., Chan, J. C. M., Oldham, S. B., and DeLuca, H. F., 1976, Vitamin D: The discovery of its metabolites and their therapeutic applications, *Pediatrics* **57**:729.

Beck, N., and Webster, S. K., 1976, Effects of acute metabolic acidosis on parathyroid hormone action and calcium mobilization, *Am. J. Physiol.* **230**:127.

Becroft, D. M. O., and Chambers, D., 1976, Supravalvular aortic stenosis–infantile hypercalcaemia syndrome: *In vitro* hypersensitivity to vitamin D_2 and calcium, *J. Med. Genet.* **13**:223.

Belchetz, P. E., Cohen, R. D., O'Riordan, J. L., and Tomlinson, S., 1976, Factitious hypercalcaemia, *Br. Med. J.* **1**:690.

Ben-Isaac, C., Massry, S. G., Rosenfeld, S., Kleeman, C. R., and Bick, M., 1975,

Evidence for humoral factor responsible for the hypercalciuria of phosphate depletion, *Clin. Res.* **23**:134A.

Bergstrom, W. H., 1975, Calciferol deficiency here and now, *Am. J. Dis. Child.* **129**:1137.

Bjorkhem, I., and Holmberg, I., 1976, A novel specific assay of 25-hydroxyvitamin D, *Clin. Chim. Acta* **68**:215.

Bloom, W. L., and Flinchum, D., 1960, Osteomalacia with pseudofractures caused by the ingestion of aluminum hydroxide, *J. Am. Med. Assoc.* **174**:1327.

Boelkins, J. N., Mazurkiewicz, M., Mazur, P. E., and Mueller, W. J., 1976, Changes in blood flow to bones during the hypocalcemic and hypercalcemic phases of the response to parathyroid hormone, *Endocrinology* **98**:403.

Bonjour, J. P., Trechsel, U., Fleisch, H., Schenk, R., DeLuca, H. F., and Baxter, L. A., 1975, Action of 1,25-dihydroxyvitamin D_3 and a diphosphonate on calcium metabolism in rats, *Am. J. Physiol.* **229**:402.

Bouillon, R., Reynaert, J., Claes, J. H., Lissens, W., and De Moor, P., 1975, The effect of anticonvulsant therapy of serum levels of 25-hydroxy-vitamin D, calcium and parathyroid hormone, *J. Clin. Endocrinol. Metab.* **41**:1130.

Bouillon, R., Kerkhove, P. V., and De Moor, P., 1976, Measurement of 25-hydroxyvitamin D_3 in serum, *Clin. Chem.* **22**:364.

Boyle, I. T., 1976, Vitamin D and the kidney, *Proc. Eur. Dial. Transplant Assoc.* **12**:113.

Brannan, P. G., Vergne-Marini, P., Pak, C. Y., Hull, A. R., and Fordtran, J. S., 1976, Magnesium absorption in the human small intestine: Results in normal subjects, patients with chronic renal disease, and patients with absorptive hypercalciuria, *J. Clin. Invest.* **57**:1412.

Brautbar, N., Walling, M. W., and Coburn, J. W., 1977a, Effects of $1,25(OH)_2D_3$ on tissue P in phosphate depletion, *Clin. Res.* **25**:158A.

Brautbar, N., Lee, D. B. N., Carlson, H. E., Coburn, J. W., and Kleeman, C. R., 1977b, Experimental phosphorus depletion: Attenuation of biochemical changes in hypophysectomized rats, *Clin. Res.* **25**:165A.

Brickman, A. S., Coburn, J. W., Friedman, G. R., Okamura, W. H., Massry, S. G., and Norman, A. W., 1976, Comparison of effects of 1-alpha-hydroxy-vitamin D_3 and 1,25-dihydroxy-vitamin D_3 in man, *J. Clin. Invest.* **57**:1540.

Brumbaugh, P. F., Hughes, M. R., and Haussler, M. R., 1975, Cytoplasmic and nuclear binding components for 1-alpha-25-dihydroxyvitamin D_3 in chick parathyroid glands, *Proc. Natl. Acad. Sci. U.S.A.* **72**:4871.

Brunette, M. G., Vigneault, N., and Cariere, S., 1975, Micropunture study of renal magnesium transport in magnesium-loaded rats, *Am. J. Physiol.* **229**:1695.

Burt, R., Freston, J. W., and Tolman, K. G., 1976, The influence of phenobarbital on biotransformation of 25-hydroxycholecalciferol, *J. Clin. Pharmacol.* **16**:393.

Carlson, H. E., Brickman, A. S., and Bottazzo, G. F., 1977, Prolactin deficiency in pseudohypoparathyroidism, *N. Engl. J. Med.* **296**:140.

Castillo, L., Tanaka, Y., and DeLuca, H. F., 1975, The mobilization of bone mineral by 1,25-dihydroxyvitamin D_3 in hypophosphatemic rats, *Endocrinology* **97**:995.

Chertow, B. S., Baylink, D. J., Wergedal, J. E., Su, M. H., and Norman, A. W., 1975, Decrease in serum immunoreactive parathyroid hormone in rats and in parathyroid hormone secretion *in vitro* by 1,25-dihydroxycholecalciferol, *J. Clin. Invest.* **56**:668.

Clark, R. C., French, T. J., Beal, A. M., Cross, R. B., and Budtz-Olsen, D. E., 1975, The actue effects of intravenous infusion of parathyroid hormone on urine, plasma and saliva in the sheep, *J. Exp. Physiol.* **60**:95.

Coburn, J. W., Hartenbower, D. L., and Norman, A. W., 1974, Metabolism and action of the hormone vitamin D: Its relation to diseases of calcium homeostasis, *West. J. Med.* **121**:22–24.

Coburn, J. W., Brickman, A. S., and Hartenbower, D. L., 1975, Clinical disorders of calcium metabolism in relation to vitamin D, in: *Vitamin D and Problems Related to Uremic Bone Disease* (A. W. Norman, K. Schaefer, H. G. Griyoleit, D. Von Merrath, and E. Ritz, eds.), pp. 219–240, Walter de Gruyter, Berlin and New York.

Coburn, J. W., Saltzman, R. L., and Massry, S. G., 1976, Interactions between vitamin D and the kidney, in: *Methods in Pharmacology,* Vol. 4A (M. Martinez-Maldanado, ed.) pp. 227–267, Plenum Press, New York.

Colodro, I. H., Brickman, A. S., Coburn, J. W., Osborn, T. W., and Norman, A. W., 1976, Comparison of effects of 25(OH)D_3 vitamin on intestinal Ca absorption in normal and uremic man, *Clin. Res.* **24**:125A.

Corradino, R. A., 1976, Diphenylhydantoin: Direct inhibition of the vitamin D_3-mediated calcium absorptive mechanism in organ-cultured duodenum, *Biochem. Pharmacol.* **25**:863.

Costanzo, L. S., Moses, A. M., Rao, K. J., and Weiner, I. M., 1975, Dissociation of calcium and sodium clearances in patients with hypoparathyroidism by infusion of chlorothiazide, *Metabolism* **24**:1367.

Craddock, P. R., Yawata, Y., and Van Santen, L., 1974, Acquired phagocyte dysfunction a complication of the hypophosphatemia of parenteral hyperalimentation, *N. Engl. J. Med.* **290**:1403.

Cuche, J. L., Ott, E. C., Marchand, G. R., Diaz-Buxo, J. A., and Knox, F. G., 1976, Intrarenal calcium in phosphate handling, *Am. J. Physiol.* **230**:790.

Dalen, N., and Lamke, B., 1976, Bone mineral losses in alcoholics, *Acta Orthop. Scand.* **47**:469.

Daum, F., Rosen, J. F., Roginsky, M., Cohen, M. I., and Finberg, L., 1976, 25-Hydroxycholecalciferol in the management of rickets associated with extrahepatic biliary atresia, *J. Pediatr.* **88**:1041.

Davie, M. W., Chalmers, T. M., Hunter, J. D., Pelo, B., and Kodicek, E., 1976, 1-α-hydroxycholecalciferol in chronic renal failure: Studies of the effect of oral doses, *Ann. Intern. Med.* **84**:281.

Day, H. G., and McCollum, E. V., 1939, Mineral metabolism, growth, and symptomatology of rats on diet extremely deficient in phosphorus, *J. Biol. Chem.* **130**:269.

DeLuca, H. F., 1975, Regulation of vitamin D metabolism, *Life Sci.* **17**:1351.

Dominiguez, J. H., Gray, R. W., and Lemann, J., Jr., 1976, Dietary phosphate deprivation in women and men: Effects on mineral and acid balances, parathyroid hormone, and the metabolism of 25-OH-vitamin D, *J. Clin. Endocrinol. Metab.* **43**:1056.

Drezner, M. K., Neelon, F. A., Haussler, M., McPherson, H. T., and Lebovitz, H. E., 1976, 1,25-Dihydroxycholecalciferol deficiency: The probable cause of hypocalcemia and metabolic bone disease in pseudohypoparathyroidism, *J. Clin. Endocrinol. Metab.* **42**:621.

Dunnigan, M. G., McIntosh, W. B., and Ford, J. A., 1976, Rickets in Asian immigrants, *Lancet* **1**:1346.

Dziak, R., and Stern, P. H., 1975, Calcium transport in isolated bone cells. III. Effects of parathryoid hormone and cyclic 3',5'-AMP, *Endocrinology* **97**:1281.

Eastwood, J. B., Harris, E., Stamp, T. C. B., and De Wardener, H. E., 1976, Vitamin D deficiency in the osteomalacia of chronic renal failure, *Lancet* **2**:1209.

Edelstein, S., Sapir, R., and Harell, A., 1976, The action of vitamin D on bone, *Clin. Endocrinol.* **5**:145S.

Eisenbud, E., and Lobue, C. C., 1976, Hypocalcemia after therapeutic use of magnesium sulfate, *Arch. Intern. Med.* **136**:688.

Eisman, J. A., Hamstra, A. J., Kream, B. E., and DeLuca, H. F., 1976, 1,25-Dihydroxy-vitamin D in biological fluids: A simplified and sensitive assay, *Science* **193**:1021.

Emmett, M., Goldfarb, S., Agus, F. S., and Narins, R. G., 1977, The pathophysiology of acid–base changes in chronically phosphate-depleted rats: Bone–kidney interactions, *J. Clin. Invest.* **59**:291.

Epstein, M., Pins, D. S., Silvers, W., Loutzenhiser, R., Canterbury, J. M., and Reiss, E., 1976, Failure of water immersion to influence parathyroid hormone secretion and renal phosphate handling in normal man, *J. Lab. Clin. Med.* **87**:218.

Forte, L. R., Nickols, G. A., and Anast, C. S., 1976, Renal adenylate cyclase and the interrelationship between parathyroid hormone and vitamin D in the regulation of urinary phosphate and adenosine cylcic 3',5'-monophosphate excretion, *J. Clin. Invest.* **57**:559.

Fraser, H. S., Thompson, D., and Khan, C, 1976, Clinical application of antipyrine half life in saliva in a patient with osteomalacia, *Br. Med. J.* **1**:1507.

Freund, T., and Bronner, F., 1975, Stimulation *in vitro* by 1,25-dihydroxy-vitamin D_3 of intestinal cell calcium uptake and calcium-binding protein, *Science* **190**:1300.

Fukushima, M., Suzuki, Y., Tohira, Y., Nishii, Y., and Suzuki, M., 1976, 25-Hydroxylation of 1-α-hydroxyvitamin D_3 *in vivo* and in perfused rat liver, *FEBS. Lett.* **65**:211.

Garabedian, M., Pezant, E., Maravet, L., Fellot, C., and Balsan, S., 1976, 1,25-Dihydroxycholecalciferol effect on serum phosphorus homeostasis in rats, *Endocrinology* **98**:794.

Garcia-Pascual, B., Peytremann, A., Courvoisier, B., and Lawson D. E., 1976, A simplified competitive protein-binding assay for 25-hydroxycalciferol, *Clin. Chim. Acta* **68**:99.

Gebauer, U., Russell, R. G., Touabi, M., and Fleisch, H., 1976, Effect of diphosphonates on adenosine 3'5'-cyclic monophosphate in mouse calvaria after stimulation by parathyroid hormone *in vitro, Clin. Sci. Mol. Med.* **50**:473.

Gennari, C., Vattimo, A., and Nardi, P., 1975, Effect of vitamin D_2 and 25-hydroxycholecalciferol on intestinal absorption of radiophosphate in man, *Boll. Soc. Ital. Biol. Sper.* **51**:86.

Goel, K. M., Sweet, E. M., Logan, R. W., Warren, J. M., Arneil, G. C., and Shanks, R. A., 1976, Florid and subclinical rickets among immigrant children in Glasgow, *Lancet* **1**:1141.

Habener, J. F., and Potts, J. T., Jr., 1976, Relative effectiveness of magnesium and calcium on the secretion and biosynthesis of parathyroid hormone *in vitro, Endocrinology* **98**:197.

Habener, J. F., Kemper, B., and Potts, J. T., Jr., 1975, Calcium-dependent intracellular degradation of parathyroid hormone: A possible mechanism for the regulation of hormone stores, *Endocrinology* **97**:431.

Haddad, J. G., Jr. and Rojanasathit, S., 1976, Acute administration of 25-hydroxycholecalciferol in man, *J. Clin. Endocrinol. Metab.* **42**:284.

Haddad, J. G., Jr., and Walgate, J., 1976, 25-Hydroxyvitamin D transport in human plasma: Isolation and partial characterization of calcifidiol-binding protein, *J. Biol. Chem.* **251**:4803.

Haddad, J. G., Hillman, L., and Rojanasathit, S., 1976, Human serum binding capacity and affinity for 25-hydroxyergocalciferol and 25-hydroxycholecalciferol, *J. Clin. Endrocrinol. Metab.* **43**:86.

Hahn, T. S., and Avioli, L. V., 1975, Anticonvulsant ostemalacia, *Arch. Intern. Med.* **135**:997.

Haussler, M. R., Wasserman, R. H., McCain, T. A., Peterlik, M., Bursac, K. M., and Hughes, M. R., 1976a, 1,25-Dihydroxyvitamin D_3-glycoside: Identification of a calcinogenic principle of *Solanium malacoxylon, Life Sci.* **18**:1049.

Haussler, M. R., Baylink, D. J., Hughes, M. R., Brumbaugh, P. F., Wergedal, J. E., Shen, F. H., Nielsen, R. L., Counts, S. I., Bursac, K. M., and McCain, T. A., 1976b, The assay of 1-alpha-dihydroxyvitamin D_3: Physiologic and pathologic modulation of circulating hormone levels, *Clin. Endocrinol.* **5**:151s.

Heath, D. A., and Martin, T. J., 1976, Parathyroid hormone assay, *Br. Med. J.* **1**:277.

Heidbreder, E., Luke, F., and Heidland, A., 1976, Collagen metabolism and mineralization of uremic bone—aspects of the molecular pathology of renal osteodystrophy, *Klin. Wochenschr.* **54**:341.

Henry, H. C., and Norman, A. W., 1975, Studies on the mechanism of action of calciferol. VII. Localization of 1,25-dihydroxy-vitamin D_3 in chick parathyroid glands, *Biochem. Biophys. Res. Commun.* **62**:781.

Henry, H. C., and Norman, A. W., 1976, Studies on calciferol metabolism: Regulation of 25-hydroxyvitamin D_3-1-hydroxylase in isolated renal mitochondria, *Arch. Biochem. Biphys.* **172**:582.

Hepner, G. W., Roginsky, M., and Moo, H. F., Abnormal vitamin D metabolism in patients with cirrhosis, *Am. J. Dig. Dis.* **21**:527.

Hillman, L. S., and Haddad, J. G., 1976, Perinatal vitamin D metabolism. III.

Factors influencing late gestational human serum 25-hydroxyvitamin D, *Am. J. Obstet. Gynecol.* **125**:196.

Holick, M. F., Holick, S. A., Tavela, T., Gallagher, B., Schnoes, H. K., and Deluca, H. F., 1975, Synthesis of (6-^{3}H)-1alpha-hydroxyvitamin D_3 and its metabolism *in vivo* to (^{3}H)-1alpha,25-dihydroxyvitamin D_3, *Science* **190**:576.

Holick, M. F., Tavela, T. E., Holick, S. A., Schnoes, H. K., DeLuca, H. F., and Gallagher, B. M., 1976, Synthesis of 1alpha-hydroxy[6-3H]vitamin D_3 and its metabolism to 1alpha,25-dihydroxyvitamin[6-3H]vitamin D_3 in the rat, *J. Biol. Chem.* **251**:1020.

Holick, S. A., Holick. M. F., Tavela, T. E., Schnoes, H. K., and DeLuca, H. F., 1976, Metabolism of 1alpha-hydroxyvitamin D_3 in the chick, *J. Biol. Chem.* **251**:1025.

Horiuchi, N., Suda, T., Sasaki, S., Ogata, E., and Ezawa, I., 1975, The regulatory role of calcium in 25-hydroxycholecalciferol metabolism in chick kidney *in vitro, Arch. Biochem. Biphys.* **171**:540.

Horiuchi, N., Suda, T., Sasaki, S., Takahashi, H., Shimazawa, E., and Ogata, E., 1976, Absence of regulatory effects of 1-α,25-dihydryxyvitamin D_3 on 25-hydroxy-vitamin D_3 metabolism in rats constantly infused with parathyroid hormone, *Biochem. Biophys. Res. Commun.* **73**:869.

Hughes, M. R., Brumbaugh, P. F., Haussler, M. R. Wergedal, J. E., and Baylink, D. J., 1975, Regulation of serum 1-α,25-dihydroxyvitamin D_3 by calcium and phosphate in the rat, *Science* **190**:578.

Hughes, M. R., Baylink, D. J., Jones, P. G., and Haussler, M. R., 1976, Radioligand receptor assay for 25-hydroxyvitamin D2/D2 and 1-α,25-dihydroxyvitamin D_2/D_3, *J. Clin. Invest.* **58**:61.

Imawari, M., Kida, K., and Goodman, D. S., 1976, The transport of vitamin D and its 25-hydroxy metabolite in human plasma, *J. Clin. Invest.* **58**:514.

Jacob, H. S., 1975, Severe hypophosphatemia: A previously ignored cause of cellular dysfunction, *West J. Med.* **122**:501.

Jeremiah, G. M., Compston, J. E., and Bacchus, R. A., 1976, Hypercalcaemia, *Lancet* **1**:547.

Jones, G., and DeLuca, H. F., 1975, High-pressure liquid chromatography: Separation of the metabolites of vitamin D_2 and D_3 on small-particle silica columns, *J. Lipid. Res.* **16**:448.

Kakuta, S., Suda, T., Sasaki, S., Kimura, N., and Nagata, N., 1975, Effects of parathyroid hormone on the accumulation of cyclic AMP in bone of vitamin-D deficient rats, *Endocrinology* **97**:1288.

Kalu, D. N., Hadji-Georgopoulos, A., and Foster, G. V., 1975, A dissociation of the effects of PTH on bone matrix and calcium in rats, *Horm. Metab. Res.* **7**:443.

Kemm, J. R., 1976, The effect of parathyroidectomy and large doses of cholecalciferol on the ability of rats to adapt to changes in dietary intake of calcium, *J. Physiol. (London)* **256**:103.

Kenny, A. D., 1976, Vitamin D metabolism: Physiological regulation in egg-laying Japanese quail, *Am. J. Physiol.* **230**:1609.

Knochel, J. P., 1977, The pathophysiology and clinical characteristics of severe hypophosphatemia, *Arch. Intern. Med.* **137**:203.

Knochel, J. P., Bilbrey, G. L., and Fuller, T. J., 1975, The muscle cell in chronic alcoholism: The possible role of phosphate depletion in alcoholic myopathy, *Ann. N.Y. Acad. Sci.* **252**:274.

Knox ,F. G., and Lechene, C., 1975, Distal site of action of parathyroid hormone on phosphate reabsorption, *Am. J. Physiol.* **229**:1556.

Knox, F. G., Haas, J. A., and Lechene, C. P., 1976, Effect of parathyroid hormone on phosphate reabsorption in the presence of acetazolamide, *Kidney Int.* **10**:216.

Kooh, S. W., Fraser, D., DeLuca, H. F., Holick, M. F., Belsey, R. E., Clark, M. B., and Murray, T. M., 1975, Treatment of hypoparathyroidism and pseudohypoparathyroidism with metabolities of vitamin D: Evidence for impaired conversion of 25-hydroxyvitamin D to 1α,25-dihydroxyvitamin D., *New Engl. J. Med.* **293**:840.

Krawitt, E. L., Sampson, H. W., and Katagiri, C. A., 1975, Effect of 1,25-dihydroxycholecalciferol on ethanol mediated suppression of calcium absorption, *Calcif. Tissue Res.* **18**:119.

Laditan, A. A., and Adeniyi, A., 1975, Rickets in Nigerian children—response to vitamin D, *J. Trop. Med. Hyg.* **78**:206.

Lee, D. B. N., and Kleeman, C. R., 1976, *Phosphorus Depletion in Man* McGaw Medical Monographs (G, Banks, ed), Irvine, California.

Long, R. G., Skinner, R. K., Wills, M. R., and Sherlock, S., 1976, Serum-25-hydroxy-vitamin-D in untreated parenchymal and cholestatic liver disease, *Lancet* **2**:650.

Lotz, M., Zigman, E., and Bartta, F. C., 1966, Evidence for a phosphorus-depletion syndrome in man, *N. Engl. J. Med.* **278**:409.

Mallette, L. E., 1975, Anticonvulsants, acetazolamide and osteomalacia, *N. Engl. J. Med.* **293**:668.

Massry, S. G., Coburn, J. W., Friedler, R. M., Kurokawa, K., and Singer, F. R., 1975, Relationship between the kidney and parathyroid hormone, *Nephron* **15**:197.

Massry, S. G., Stein, R., Garty, J., Arieff, A. I., Coburn, J. W., Norman, A. W., and Friedler, R. M., 1976, Skeletal resistance to the calcemic action of parathyroid hormone in uremia: Role of 1,25$(OH)_2D_3$ *Kidney Int.* **9**:467.

Matheson, R. T., Herbst, J. J., Jubiz, W., Freston, J. W., and Tolman, K. G., 1976, Absorption and biotransformation of cholecalciferol in drug-induced osteomalacia, *J. Clin. Pharmacol.* **16**:426.

Matsuda, I., Takekoshi, Y., Shida, N., Fujieda, K., Nagai, B., Arishima, S., Anakura, M., and Oka, Y., 1975, Renal tubular acidosis and skeletal demineralization in patients on long-term anticonvulsant therapy, *J. Pediatr.* **87**:202.

Mawer, E. B., Backhous, J., Davies, M., Hill, L. F., and Taylor, C. M., 1976, Metabolic fate of administered 1,25-dihydroxycholecalciferol in controls and in patients with hypoparathyroidism, *Lancet* **1**:1203.

Mechanic, G. L., Toverud, S. U., Ramp, W. K., and Gonnerman, W. A., 1975, The effect of vitamin D on the structural crosslinks and maturation of chick bone collagen, *Biochim. Biophys. Acta* **393**:419.

Medalle, R., Waterhouse, C., and Hahn, T. J., 1976, Vitamin D resistance in magnesium deficiency, *Am. J. Clin. Nutr.* **29**:854.

Miller, C. G., and Chutkan, W., 1976, Vitamin-D deficiency rickets in Jamaican children *Arch. Dis. Child.* **51**:214.

Mosekilde, L., and Melsen, F., 1976, Anticonvulsant ostemalacia determined by quantitative analysis of bone changes: Population study and possible risk factors, *Acta Med. Scand.* **199**:349.

Naik, R. B., Gosling, P., Price, C. P., Robinson, B. H., Dabek, J. T., Heath, D. A., James, H. M., Kanis, J. A., and Smith, R., 1976, Whole-body *in-vivo* neutron activation analysis in assessing treatment of renal osteodystrophy with 1-alpha-hydroxycholecalciferol, *Br. Med. Jr.* **2**:79.

Nicholaysen, R., 1943, The absorption of calcium, *Acta Physiol. Scand.* **6**:201.

Nicholson, R., Akhtar, M., and Taylor, T. G., 1976, Proceedings: Oestradiol as a regulator of the metabolism of vitamin D_3 in the liver of Japanese quail, *J. Endocrinol.* **68**:16P.

Nielsen, S. P., Binderup, E., Godtfredsen, W. O., Jensen, H., and Ladefoged, J., 1976, 1-Alpha-hydroxycholecalciferol: Long-term treatment of patients with uraemic osteodystrophy, *Nephron* **16**:359.

Nordin, B. E. C., 1976, *Calcium, Phosphate and Magnesium Metabolism: Clinical Physiology and Diagnostic Procedures,* Longman Group, Essex, England.

Norman, A. W., 1972, Problems relating to the definitions of International Unit for vitamin D and its metabolites, *J. Nutr.* **102**:1243.

Norman, A. W., Bayless, J. D., and Tsai, H. C., 1976, Biologic effects of short-term phenobarbital treatment on the response to vitamin D and its metabolites in the chick, *Biochem. Pharmacol.* **25**:163.

Olson, E. B., Jr., Knutson, J. C., Bhattacharyya, M. H., and Deluca, H. F., 1976, The effect of hepatectomy on the synthesis of 25-hydroxyvitamin D_3, *J. Clin. Invest.* **57**:1213.

Parfitt, A. M., 1976a, The actions of parathyroid hormone on bone: Relation to bone remodeling and turnover, calcium homeostasis, and metabolic bone disease. I. Mechanism of calcium transfer between blood and bone and their cellular basis: Morphological and kinetic approaches to bone turnover, *Metabolism* **25**:809.

Parfitt, A. M., 1976b, The action of parathyroid hormone on bone: Relation to bone remodeling and turnover, calcium homeostasis, and metabolic bone disease. II. PTH and bone cells: Bone turnover and plasma calcium regulation, *Metabolism* **25**:909.

Passer, J., 1976, Incomplete distal renal tubular acidosis in hypomagnesemia-dependent hypocalcemia, *Arch. Intern. Med.* **136**:462.

Peterson, P., Gray, P., and Tolman, K. G., 1976, Calcium balance in drug-induced osteomalacia: Response to vitamin D, *Clin. Pharmacol. Ther.* **19**:63.

Pierides, A. M., Ellis, H. A., Ward, M., Simpson, W., Peart, K. M., Alvarez-Ude, F., Uldall, P. R., and Kerr, D. N., 1976a, Barbiturate and anticonvulsant treatment in relation to osteomalacia with hoemodialysis and renal transplantation, *Br. Med. Jr.* **1**:190.

Pierides, A. M., Kerr, D. N., Ellis, H. A., Peart, K. M., O'Riordan, J. L., and DeLuca, H. F., 1976b, 1-Alpha-hydroxycholecalciferol in hemodialysis renal osteodystrophy: Adverse effects of anticonvulsant therapy, *Clin. Nephrol.* **514**:189.

Pierides, A. M., Ellis, H. A., Simpson, W., Dewar, J. H., Ward, M. K., and Kerr, D. N., 1976c, Variable response to long-term 1-alpha-hydroxycholecalciferol in haemodialysis osteodystrophy, *Lancet* **1**:1092.

Pierides, A. M., Ward, M. K., Alvarez-Ude, F., Ellis, H. A., Peart, K. M., Simpson, W., Kerr, D. N., and Norman, A., 1976d, Long term therapy with $1,25(OH)_2D_3$ in dialysis bone disease, *Proc. Eur. Dial. Tranplant Assoc.* **12**:237.

Pogglitsch, H., Schmidberger, H., and Gell, G., 1976, Renal osteopathy and bone mineralisation in patients treated with dihydrotachysterol during long term dialysis (author's transl.), *Muench. Med. Wochenschr.* **188**:131.

Posen, S., Kleerekoper, M., Ingham, J. P., and Hirshorn, J. E., 1976, Parathyroid hormone assay in clinical decision making, *Br. Med. J.* **1**:16.

Preece, M. A., Tomlinson, S., Ribot, C. A., Pietrek, J., Korn, H. T., Davies, D. M., Ford, J. A., Dunnigan, M. G., and O'Riordan, J. L., 1975, Studies of vitamin D deficiency in man, *Q. J. Med.* **44**:575.

Quamme, G. A., Wong, N. L. M., Sutton, R. A. L., and Dirks, J. H., 1975, Interrelationship of chlorothiazide and parathyroid hormone: A micropuncture study, *Am. J. Physiol.* **229**:200.

Ramberg, C. F., Jr., Mayer, G. P., Kronfeld, D. S., and Potts, J. T., Jr., 1976, Dietary calcium, calcium kinetics and plasma parathyroid hormone concentration in cows, *J. Nutr.* **106**:671.

Rayssiguier, Y., Carré, M., Ayigbédé, O., and Miravet, L., 1975, The effect of 1-25 dihydroxycholecalciferol in magnesium-deficient rats, *C. R. Acad. Sci. Ser.* D **281**:731.

Riddell, W. H., Hughes, J. S., and Fitch, J. B., 1934, The relation of phosphorus deficiency to the utilization of feed of diary cattle, *Kans. Agric. Exp. Stn. Tech. Bull.* **36**:54.

Rojanasathit, S., and Haddad, J. G., 1976, Hepatic accumulation of vitamin D_3 and 25-hydroxyvitamin D_3, *Biochim. Biophys. Acta* **421**:12.

Rude, R. K., Oldham, S. B., and Singer, F. R., 1976, Functional hypoparathyroidism and parathyroid hormone end-organ resistance in human magnesium deficiency, *Clin. Endocrinol.* **5**:209.

Russell, J. E., and Avioli, L. V., 1975, 25-Hydroxycholecalciferol-enhanced bone maturation in the parathyroprivic state, *J. Clin. Invest.* **56**:792.

Russell, J. E., Termine, J. D., and Avioli, L. V., 1975, Experimental renal osteodystrophy: The response to 25-dyhroxycholecalciferol and dicholomethylene diphosphate therapy, *J. Clin. Invest.* **56**:548.

Rutherford, W. E., Blondin, J., Hruska, K., Kopelman, R., Klahr, S., and Slatopolsky, E., 1975, Effect of 25-hydroxycholecalciferol on calcium absorption in chronic renal disease, *Kidney Int.* **8**:320.

Sann, L., David, L., Thomas, A., Frederick, A., Chapuy, M. C., and Francois, R., 1976, Congenital hyperparathyroidism and vitamin D deficiency secondary to maternal hypoparathyroidism, *Acta Pediatr. Scand.* **65**:381.

Schneider, L. E., Wasserman, R. H., and Schedl, H. P., 1975, Depressed duodenal calcium absorption in the diabetic rat: Restoration by *Solanum malacoxylon, Endocrinology* **97**:649.

Schneider, L. E., Omdahl, J., and Schedl, H. P., 1976, Effects of vitamin D and its metabolites on calcium transport in the diabetic rat, *Endocrinology* **99**:793.

Sherman, H. C., and Pappenheimer, A. M., 1921, A dietetic production of rickets in rats and its prevention by an inorganic salt, *Proc. Soc. Exp. Biol. Med.* **18**:193.

Sheety, K. R., Ajlouni, K., Rosenfeld, P. S., and Hagen, T. C., 1975, Protracted vitamin D intoxication, *Arch. Intern. Med.* **135**:986.

Silver, J., 1975, Vitamin D therapy for children on anticonvulsants, *N. Engl. J. Med.* **293**:1106.

Sinha, T. K., and Bell, N. H., 1976, 1,25-Dihydroxyvitamin D_3 and pseudohypoparathyroidism, *N. Engl. J. Med.* **294**:612.

Slatopolsky, E., Mercado, A., Morrison, A., Yates, J., and Klahr, S., 1976, Inhibitory effects of hypermagnesemia on the renal action of parathyroid hormone, *J. Clin. Invest.* **58**:1273.

Smith, R., Henderson, R. G., and Russell, R. G., 1975, The use of metabolically-active derivatives of vitamin D in rickets and osteomalacia due to renal glomerular failure, *J. Bone Joint Surg. Br.* **57**:247.

Spanos, E., Colston, K. W., and Evans, I. M. S., 1976, Effect of prolactin on vitamin D metabolism, *Mol. Cell. Endocrinol.* **5**:163.

Spencer, R., Charman, M., Emtage, J. S., and Lawson, D. E. M., 1976a, Production and properties of vitamin-D-induced mRNA for chick calcium-binding protein, *Eur. J. Biochem.* **71**:399.

Spencer, R., Charman, M., Wilson, P., and Lawson, E., 1976b, Vitamin D-stimulated intestinal calcium absorption may not involve calcium binding protein directly, *Nature (London)* **263**:161.

Stamp, T. C., 1975, Factors in human vitamin D nutrition and in the production and cure of classical rickets, *Proc. Nutr. Soc.* **34**:119.

Stanbury, S. W., Torkington, P., Lumb, G. A., Adams, P. H., de Silva, P., and Taylor, C. M., 1975, Asian rickets and osteomalacia: Patterns of parathyroid response in vitamin D deficiency, *Proc. Nutr. Soc.* **34**:111.

Steele, T. H., 1976, Selective lithium inhibition of hormonal phosphaturic responses, *J. Pharmacol. Exp. Ther.* **197**:206.

Steele, T. H., and DeLuca, H. F., 1976, Influence of dietary phosphorus on renal phosphate reabsorption in the parathyroidectomized rat, *J. Clin. Invest.* **57**:867.

Steele, T. H., Engle, J. E., Tanaka, Y., Lorenc, R. S., Dudgeon, K. L., and DeLuca, H. F., 1975, Phosphatemic action of 1,25-dihydroxyvitamin D_3, *Am. J. Physiol.* **229**:489.

Tanaka, Y., DeLuca, H. F., Ikekawa, N., Morisaki, M., and Koizumi, N., 1975, Determination of stereochemical configuration of the 24-hydroxyl group of 24,25-dihydroxyvitamin D_3 and its biological imporatnce, *Arch. Biochem. Biophys.* **170**:620.

Taylor, C. M., Mawer, E. B., and Reeve, A., 1975, The effects of a diphosphonate and dietary calcium on the metabolism of vitamin D_3 (cholecalciferol) in the chick, *Clin. Sci. Mol. Med.* **49**:391.

Taylor, C. M., Hughes, S. E., and DeSilva, P., 1976, Competitive protein binding assay for 24,25-dihydroxycholecalciferol, *Biochem. Biophys. Res. Commun.* **70**:1243.

Teitelbaum, S. L., Bone, J. M., Stein, P. M., Gilden, J. J., Bates, M., Boisseau, V. C., and Avioli, L. V., 1976, Calcifediol in chronic renal insufficiency: Skeletal response, *J. Am. Med. Assoc.* **235**:164.

Theiler, A., 1931, The pathological aspects of phosphorus and calcium deficiency in cattle, *Vet. Rec.* **11**:1143.

Theiler, A., and Green, H. H., 1932, Aphosphorosis in ruminants, *Nutr. Abstr. Rev.* **1**:359.

Theiler, A., Green, H. H., and DuTolt, P. J., 1927, Minimum mineral requirements of cattle, *J. Agric. Sci.* **17**:291.

Tougaard, L., Sorensen, E., Brochner-Mortensen, J., Christensen, M. S., Rodbro, P., and Sorensen, A. W., 1976, Controlled trial of 1-alpha-hydroxycholecalciferol in chronic renal failure, *Lancet* **1**:1044.

Trohler, U., Bonjour, J. P., and Fleisch, H., 1976, Renal tubular adaptation to dietary phosphorus, *Nature (London)* **261**:145.

Turton, C. W. B., Stanley, P., Stamp, T. C. B., and Maxwell, J. D., 1977, Altered vitamin-D metabolism in pregnancy, *Lancet* **1**:222.

Vergne-Marini, P., Parker, T. F., Pak, C. Y. C., Hull, A. R., DeLuca, H. F., and Fordtran, J. S., 1976, Jejunal and ileal calcium absorption in patients with chronic renal disease, *J. Clin. Invest.* **57**:861.

Wagonfeld, J. B., Nemchausky, B. A., Bolt, M., Vander Horst, J., Boyer, J. L., and Rosenberg, I. H., 1976 Comparison of vitamin D and 25-hydroxy-vitamin D in the therapy of primary biliary cirrhosis, *Lancet* **2**:391.

Walling, M. W., and Kimberg, D. V., 1975, Effects of 1-alpha,25-dihydroxyvitamin D_3 and *Solanum glaucophyllum* on intestinal calcium and phosphate transport and on plasma Ca, Mg and P levels in the rat, *Endocrinology* **97**:1567.

Walling, M. W., Kimberg. D. V., Wasserman, R. H., and Feinberg, R. R., 1976, Duodenal active transport of calcium and phosphate in vitamin D-deficient rats: Effects of nephrectomy, *Cestrum diurnum,* and 1-α-25-dihydroxyvitamin D_3, *Endocrinology* **98**:1130.

Wasserman, R. H., Corradino, R. A., Krook, L., Hughes, M. R., and Haussler, M. R., 1976, Studies on the 1-α, 25-dihydroxycholecalciferol-like activity in a calcinogenic plant. Cestrum diurnum, in the chick, *J. Nutr.* **106**:457.

Wezeman, F. H., 1976, 25-hydroxyvitamin D_3: Autoradiographic evidence of sites of action in epiphyseal cartilage and bone, *Science* **194**:1069.

Whedon, G. D., Lutwak, L., Rambaut, P. C., Whittle, M. W., Reid, J., Smith, M. C., Leach, C., Stadler, C. R., and Stanford, D. D., 1976, Mineral and nitrogen balance study observations: The second manned Skylab mission, *Aviat. Space Environ. Med.* **47**:391.

Wills, M. R., and Jenkins, M. V., 1976, The effect of uraemic metabolites on parathyroid extract-induced bone resorption *in vitro, Clin. Chim. Acta* **73**:121.

Yawata, Y., Craddock, P., Hebbel, R., Howe, R., Silvis, S., and Jacob, H., 1973, Hyperalimentation hypophosphatemia: hematologic, neurologic dysfunction due to ATP depletion, *Clin. Res.* **21**:729.

Zerwekh, J. E., Lindell, T. J., and Haussler, M. R., 1976. Increased intestinal chromatin template activity. Influence of 1-α,25-dihydroxyvitamin D_3 and hormone-receptor complexes, *J. Biol. Chem.* **251**:2388.

10

Nutrition, Growth, and Development

Myron Winick

10.1. Introduction

During 1976, there was considerable progress in investigating a number of areas concerned with nutrition and health. Three of these areas will be reviewed in detail:

1. Malnutrition and the mechanisms of cellular growth
2. Genetic obesity
3. Nutrition and pregnancy

10.2. Malnutrition and the Mechanisms of Cellular Growth

During the past two decades, numerous studies from a variety of sources have demonstrated that most organs undergo hyperplasia during early growth, whereas later growth is characterized by cellular hypertro-

MYRON WINICK • Institute of Human Nutrition, College of Physicians and Surgeons, Columbia University, New York, New York 10032.

phy. Malnutrition imposed during the hyperplastic phase retards the rate of cell division and results in an organ with fewer cells. This change is permanent. By contrast, malnutrition during hypertrophic growth prevents the enlargement of cells, but with rehabilitation, they fill up with protein and reach their expected size. Recently, a number of studies have been undertaken that have attempted to elucidate some of the mechanisms by which malnutrition produces these effects on cellular growth.

Since it has long been known that various hormones, particularly growth hormone and thyroid hormone, are very important in the control of normal growth, there has been a good deal of speculation that malnutrition exerts its effects on growth indirectly by reducing the amount or availability of one or both of these hormones. Some data have supported this concept of an indirect effect of malnutrition exerted primarily through the endocrine system, while other data have failed to support it. For example, certain workers have observed increased growth in malnourished animals injected with growth hormone (Zamenhof *et al.,* 1971). Others have not. In neonatally undernourished rats, reduced thyroid hormone in the circulation has been reported, as well as a reduced oxygen consumption in brain, a known consequence of thyroid deficiency (Muzzo *et al.*, 1973). Circulating growth hormone has been reported to be reduced in human infants with marasmus and their growth rate to be increased if they are treated with growth hormone (Monckeberg *et al.*, 1963). In the case of kwashiorkor, by contrast, growth hormone levels are elevated, and yet growth failure is prominent (Pimstone *et al.*, 1973). Recent data have begun to shed some light on the role of hormones in the growth retardation produced by early malnutrition.

In rats, hypothyroidism reduces the rate of cell division in brain, but extends the time during which cells divide from 21 days to about 35 days. The ultimate number of cells achieved is actually greater than in normal animals. In contrast, hyperthyroidism produces the reverse. The rate of cell division is increased, but the time is shortened and the ultimate number of cells is fewer (Muzzo and Brasel, 1973).

The effects of a change in nutritional status during early life, on the other hand, are always on the rate of cell division; the time during which cells divide is never altered. In rat brain, cell division ceases at 21 days, regardless of how the animal is fed.

We can see, therefore, that there is a fundamental difference between the action or lack of action of thyroid hormone and that of malnutrition. This difference is highlighted if one examines the activity of DNA polymerase (an enzyme involved in DNA synthesis) in hypothyroidism and in malnutrition. Hypothyroid animals show lower activity during the early hyperplastic phase of brain growth. However, activity remains elevated beyond the period of time when it drops to low levels in normal brain. In contrast, in malnourished animals, activity drops to these low (adult) levels at the normal time (Muzzo and Brasel, 1973).

These data clearly demonstrate that the effects of early malnutrition are not manifesting themselves, at a cellular level, by reducing either the secretion or the availability of thyroid hormone.

The role of pituitary growth hormone in producing the effect of malnutrition is less clearly defined. Growth-hormone deficiency reduces the rate of cell division without altering the time that cells divide. In this respect, then, its effect is similar to that of undernutrition. In growth-hormone deficiency, however, this reduction in the rate of cell division in all organs does not take place until the middle part of neonatal life. For example, in mice genetically devoid of growth hormone, organ growth and the rate of cell division in the various organs are normal during the first 10 days of life (Winick and Grant, 1968). Thus, early hyperplastic growth both prenatally and during early neonatal life is not under the control of growth hormone, yet undernutrition will reduce the rate of cell division during this period of life. These data suggest that at least during gestation and early lactation, the period when brain changes are most marked, malnutrition exerts its effects independent of growth hormone. The possibility still exists, however, that one of the effects of malnutrition is to inhibit the secretion of growth hormone and therefore to limit its availability when it is needed. Assuming that this were so, it would seem most logical that this effect is in addition to the primary effect of malnutrition on cellular growth, which continues to be the same both before and after growth hormone becomes important. Other data would support this interpretation. "Overnutrition" increases the rate of protein synthesis in pituitary dwarf mice during the time that cell division has stopped (Winick, 1968). Malnutrition reduces the activity of the enzyme serine dehyrogenase in growing liver. Hypophysectomy has no effect. When treated with growth hormone, malnourished animals show little or no increase in DNA synthesis (Jasper and Brasel, 1973). Finally, animals re-fed after malnutrition show a return to normal in cellular growth much more rapidly than do hypophysectomized rats treated with growth hormone. Thus, the data at present would indicate that malnutrition does not act solely through this mechanism. What then is the primary mechanism by which undernutrition affects cellular growth?

Amino acids from the general body pool are supplied directly for protein synthesis and for the synthesis of nucleotides, which then enter the general body nucleotide pool. The nucleotides are then utilized for either DNA or RNA synthesis. Newly formed DNA is quite stable, whereas the newly formed RNA turns over, and the rate of snythesis is in equilibrium with the rate of degradation. A number of enzymes are involved in all these processes; their activity depends, in part at least, on the quantitative and qualitative nature of protein synthesis. Thus, the availability of amino acids will affect both nucleic acid and protein synthesis, and the amount and quality of the protein synthesized will in turn affect the synthesis of nucleic acids. To complete the cycle, since RNA is an essential element in protein synthesis, changes in the quantity and quality of RNA will also affect the quantity and quality of the protein synthesized.

Where in this cycle does protein–calorie malnutrition exert its effect? Although the data are not complete, they certainly point to the fact that limitation of protein in the diet will decrease the availability of amino acids for protein synthesis. The work of Munro (1970) and that of Miller (1969) has demonstrated reduced protein synthesis both *in vivo* and *in vitro* when either protein or amino acids in the diet are limited. Further, Munro (1970) suggested that although any amino acid may be limiting under experimental conditions, tryptophan appears to be the limiting amino acid in most physiological situations.

More recently, it was shown that during protein restriction, muscle weight loss is due both to decreased protein synthesis and to increased protein catabolism (Li and Goldberg, 1976). These two mechanisms are under separate control and occur at different times, synthesis decreasing within 24 hr and catabolism increasing after 48 hr. Infusion with glucose alone appears to allow synthesis to proceed at relatively normal rates, at least in the neonatal guinea pig, whereas catabolism remains increased (Ogata and Holliday, 1976). In contrast, limitation of carbohydrate results in very low synthesis rates, which have been explained by the fact that the ability to recycle amino acids from muscle breakdown is an energy-dependent phenomenon (Stein *et al.*, 1976). Other studies have stressed the importance of reduced protein synthesis in the lack of growth during malnutrition, and have ascribed these reduced rates of synthesis to decreased ribosomal content and activity (Millward *et al.*, 1975; Nnanyelugo, 1976). Finally, it has been shown that early severe malnutrition will affect the activity of certain enzymes involved in protein metabolism. Heart lactic dehydrogenase activity is lowered after 13 weeks of malnutrition (Penney *et al.*, 1976). In contrast, muscle enzymatic activity involved in the α-decarboxylation of leucine was markedly elevated by 5 days of starvation (Harbhajan and Siamak, 1976).

Thus, at present, available data suggest that both synthesis and degradation of protein are affected by malnutrition. The quality of the diet, i.e., carbohydrate vs. protein content, may be very important in determining whether the major changes will be in synthesis or catabolism.

Measurements of amino acid pool size using ^{15}N nitrogen suggest an overall decrease in the pool or a compartmentalization of amino acids during malnutrition (Stein *et al.*, 1976). In contrast, there is some evidence that suggests that amino acids are preferentially converted to nucleotides. For example, total nucleotide pool size in brains of neonatally malnourished animals is unaffected. Incorporation of labeled orotic acid into the nucleotide pool is significantly increased, however, and preliminary data suggest that incorporation of labeled amino acids into the nucleotide pool is also increased. We may postulate, then, that the synthesis of nucleotides is increased in brains of neonatally malnourished rats. If the nucleotide pool size does not change in brain or actually decreases in liver, where are these nucleotides being distributed? Incorporation of labeled nucleotides into DNA is markedly reduced in the organs of malnourished animals, demonstrating that there is a decreased distribution into DNA synthesis (Dallman, 1971; Dallman and Maimes, 1973; Goldberg and Goldspink, 1975). In contrast, incorporation of labeled precursor into RNA is markedly increased in liver and brain of neonatally malnourished animals. Thus, the rate of DNA synthesis is reduced, whereas the rate of RNA synthesis is increased in neonatal protein–calorie restriction.

Recent experiments have demonstrated that nucleolar synthesis of 45 S rRNA is increased in rat liver during protein restriction for 1 week. Moreover, the rate of synthesis of other species of rRNA is increased. Transport to cytoplasm of 28 S and 18 S rRNA is normal (Lewis and Winick, 1977).

One effect of early malnutrition, then, is a redistribution of available nucleotides. How is this redistribution controlled? What are the mechanisms involved in the decreased DNA synthesis, and how can we explain an increase in RNA synthesis in the face of descriptive data that conclusively demonstrate a reduced RNA content per cell?

We can answer the second question by examining the rate of RNA degradation after early malnutrition. There is a marked increase in the rate of decay of previously labeled RNA in liver of malnourished rats, and in brain there is a drop in the RNA/DNA ratio at a time when RNA synthesis is increased (Quirin-Stricker and Mandel, 1968). Thus, although the rate of RNA synthesis is increased, the rate of degradation must also be increased. This latter increase is presumably greater than the former, resulting in a net loss of RNA that explains the drop in the RNA/DNA ratio or RNA content per cell.

During the past year, data have been collected that indicate not only that the rate of degradation of cytoplasmic rRNA is increased, but also that degradation of 28 S rRNA is increased more than that of 18 S rRNA. Hence, the cytoplasmic ratio of 18 S rRNA to 28 S rRNA is reversed (Lewis *et al.*, 1976).

In an attempt to explore some of the mechanisms by which these dynamic changes occur, the activity of certain of the enzymes involved in the regulation of the steps just described has been measured. DNA polymerase is an enzyme involved in the terminal phase of DNA synthesis. In a number of nonphysiological situations, the activity of this enzyme was shown to increase under conditions that stimulate DNA synthesis (Brasel *et al.*, 1969; Brasel, 1972). Moreover, the increase was shown to precede the increase in DNA synthesis (Brasel, 1972).

Activity of this enzyme in liver of growing rats is in part under the control of pituitary growth hormone. Hypophysectomy reduces enzyme activity and growth hormone replacement elevates the activity before any increase in DNA synthesis can be demonstrated (Jasper and Brasel, 1973).

In brain, the activity of DNA polymerase parallels the rate of cell division during normal growth (Brasel *et al.*, 1970), and this parallel relationship holds when various brain regions are studied. These data demonstrate that the activity of this enzyme is an excellent indicator of the rate of cell division, and suggest that during normal growth, DNA polymerase may play a role in regulating the rate of DNA synthesis. Neonatal malnutrition will reduce the activity of this enzyme in rat liver. Jasper and Brasel (1974) demonstrated that when malnourished animals are re-fed during the hyperplastic phase of growth, the activity of DNA polymerase returns to normal levels within 12 hr. By 24 hr, activity is 150% of normal. DNA synthesis, as measured either by [^{14}C]thymidine incorporation into DNA or by increases in total DNA content, does not increase for at least 48 hr. These data clearly demonstrate an increase in activity of DNA polymerase *before* any demonstrable increase in DNA synthesis, and suggest that increased levels in the activity of this enzyme stimulate DNA synthesis, rather than the reverse. These findings reinforce the other data in suggesting that DNA polymerase activity during both normal and abnormal growth plays a role in regulating the rate of cell division.

Other data suggest that thymidine kinase activity may be reduced when animals are malnourished during the proliferative period of growth (Tagliamante *et al.*, 1972).

Thus, the evidence at this stage suggests that one way by which early malnutrition may curtail the rate of DNA synthesis and perhaps indirectly regulate the distribution of available nucleotides is by reducing the activity of DNA polymerase or thymidine kinase.

Metcoff (1974) investigated the enzymes involved in RNA synthesis. He has demonstrated an increase in RNA polymerase activity in leukocytes of undernourished children and in placentas from mothers who were malnourished and whose infants demonstrated intrauterine growth failure. Suggestive as these data may be, experiments demonstrating an elevation in the activity of RNA polymerase in tissues exposed to neonatal malnutrition, and correlating this increased activity with an increase in the rate of RNA synthesis, are lacking.

The degradative phase of RNA metabolism is of particular interest, since it is the increased rate of degradation that accounts for the net loss of RNA per cell. The enzyme alkaline RNase has been shown to be involved in RNA catabolism (Kraft and Shortman, 1970, Rosso *et al.*, 1973; Rosso and Raguso, 1972).

Since, as previously pointed out, RNA catabolism is increased in brains of animals exposed to early malnutrition the effect of such malnutrition on the activity of alkaline RNase has been studied. Malnutrition imposed at birth will elevate the activity of this enzyme in rat brain (Rosso and Winick, 1975). This elevation increases progressively as the duration of malnutrition increases, so that increased activity is present regardless whether the data are expressed per milligram of DNA, per milligram of protein, or per milligram of RNA. Thus, neonatal malnutrition selectively elevates the activity of this enzyme in the face of a decrease in overall protein synthesis and a fall in tissue RNA content.

During the past year, two cytoplasmic RNAs have been described in liver and brain of immature animals. Both are heavier than 28 S, and both disappear around the time that cell division stops in these tissues (28 days in liver, 21 days in cerebrum, and 17 days in cerebellum). Malnutrition reduces the concentration of these species of RNA more than the concentration of 18 or 28 S rRNA. If these RNA species are somehow involved in the control of cell division, the data suggest that their preferential decrease might be, in part, responsible for the reduced rate of cell division (Lewis *et al.*, 1976).

Data collected during the past two years also suggest that RNA metabolism and hence protein synthesis may "adapt" to prolonged protein restriction. Synthesis of the polyamines putrecine and spermidine increases early in malnutrition, reaches a plateau, and returns to normal by 5 weeks. Activities of ornithine decarboxylase (ODC) and *S*-adenosylmethionine decarboxylase (SAMD) follow the same pattern as does the rate of synthesis of nuclear RNA. Refeeding produces similar changes—a marked increase in all these parameters during the first 48 hr and a return to normal shortly thereafter (Rozovski *et al.*, 1976).

Thus, during the past year, there has been considerable progress in elucidating some of the mechanisms by which malnutrition affects cellular growth. RNA synthesis increases, as does degradation. RNA content drops, and during proliferative growth, the heavier RNAs are affected more. DNA synthesis decreases, perhaps as a consequence of lowered activities of certain enzymes involved in its synthesis or because of a lowered concentration of specific RNA species involved in the synthesis of proteins necessary for cell replication. Protein synthesis decreases, and protein catabolism increases. These changes may represent the early phase of an adaptive response during which the organism preserves certain essential functions while disposing of other less essential functions, i.e., growth or cell division. A great deal more must be done to substantiate some of these hypotheses, but the experiments performed during the last few years have opened the way to our understanding of some of these mechanisms.

10.3. Genetic Obesity

10.3.1. Changes in Adipose Tissue during Normal Growth

Data during the past several decades have suggested that at least two types of obesity can be described. These types are classified by the number and size of adipocytes into hyperplastic and hypertrophic obesity (Björntorp and Sjöström, 1971; Hirsch and Knittle, 1970). Both animal data and human observations have suggested that the hyperplastic form of obesity is induced early in life, and that once an increased number of cells is present, weight reduction will not result in their decrease (Hirsch and Knittle, 1970; Hirsch and Han, 1969). In contrast, hypertrophic obesity begins later in life, and weight reduction results in a return to a normal cell size (Hirsch and Han, 1969). Thus, in terms of severity and prognosis, the childhood form of obesity presents a more difficult problem. An important question that these studies raise is: when do adipocytes stop dividing normally? Difficulty in answering this question has stemmed from the fact that the methods used for "counting" the number of fat cells all depended on the presence of fat within the cell. However, fat cells no longer divide once they have fat within them. Thus, although we could pinpoint the time when the number of fat cells reach their maximum, whether this is due to a cessation of cell division at that time or to an ending of lipid filling into cells that had previously divided was unknown. Greenwood and Hirsch (1974) approached this problem by studying the incorporation of [H^3]thymidine into DNA in the "stromovascular" and "adipocyte" fraction of various fat pads. They concluded that cell division occurred almost exclusively in the stromovascular compartment, and that in the rat, cells destined to become lipid-filled fat cells, preadipocytes, were synthesized by 35 days of age. However, not all these predestined cells were immediately detected in the fat-cell fraction. Some preadipocytes took as long as 50 days (animals 84–98 days of age) to fill with lipid and thus become detectable by the electronic cell-counting method.

In an attempt to develop a nonradioactive procedure for monitoring the rate of cell division of preadipocytes, the activities of thymidine kinase and DNA polymerase in various adipose depots during development were recently measured (Cleary *et al.*, 1975, 1976; Cleary, 1976). The data indicate that adult levels of these two enzymes are reached at some point between the fourth and fifth postnatal weeks and correlate well with the previous thymidine-uptake studies (Greenwood and Hirsch, 1974). To monitor lipid filling, the activity of lipoprotein lipase was measured during development. Activity of this enzyme increases fourfold between 17 and 35 days of age preceding the increase in fat-cell size (Hietanen and Greenwood, 1976). Thus, the possibility now exists that the actual sequence of hyperplastic and hypertrophic growth in young infants and children can be determined using safe and acceptable procedures. The signal(s) or feedback mechanism(s) controlling adipose tissue mass, or responsible for the switch in mechanisms controlling hyperplastic growth, or both, are unknown. However, recent assessment of several studies of rats and mice in which adipose tissue was removed surgically failed to show any lasting compensatory increase in adipose mass or fat-cell size (Faust *et al.*, 1976; Kral, 1976). These studies suggested that during normal adipose tissue growth, fat-cell size rather than total adipose mass or fat cell number is important in regulation of adipose mass.

10.3.2. Animal Models of Genetic Obesity

There is evidence both in animals and in humans that there is a genetic component in obesity. Whether this component is a contributing factor to the hyperplastic or hypertrophic type of obesity is unknown. A particular species of rat, the Zucker rat, shows a recessive pattern of genetic obesity. Affected animals become obese shortly after weaning. This obesity is primarily hyperplastic in nature. At present, studies using this animal model are seeking to determine the timing of the hyperplasia and the factors that control it. Bell and Stern (1976) confirmed the finding by Zucker and Antoniades (1972) that increased total body fat could be measured in a population of young (presumably homozygous for obesity; fafa) suckling Zucker rats preceding hyperinsulinemia as a characteristic of the obesity. Hyperphagia is a characteristic of the dynamic stage of the obesity (Zucker and Zucker, 1961; Bray and York, 1972; Greenwood *et al.*, 1974), and a recent paper on adult female Zucker rats showed some alterations of norepinephrine levels in obese animals as compared with lean (Cruce *et al.*, 1976). Significantly increased levels were found in the median eminence of fafa's, while significantly decreased levels were found in the paraventricular nucleus. The authors indicate no direct evidence that these results could account for either hyperphagia or the obesity, but mention that norepinephrine has been shown to be related to feeding behavior. It has also been shown that hypophysectomy of adult, 150-day-old, Zucker fatties does not reverse the obesity, but does prevent further weight gain (Powley and Morton, 1976). Thus, the pituitary and the endocrine pathways it controls are not the primary lesion of this obesity. A further attempt at restricting food intake and assessing the effect on body composition showed that lean and obese male animals respond differently to such treatment (Deb *et al.*, 1976). Lean Zucker rats the diets of which were restricted by 50% of *ad libitum* from 6 to 10 weeks of age decreased their body fat 50%, from 10 to 5%, while fatties restricted by the same amount decreased body fat 25%, from 44 to 33%. It would thus appear that the mechanism(s) responsible for controlling fat deposition are altered in the fatty rat.

It has previously been suggested that the defect in the fatty rat is an inability to shut off fat-cell proliferation at the appropriate time (Johnson *et al.*, 1973). Recent work showed that this may in fact be the case. Two proliferative enzymes, thymidine kinase and DNA polymerase, were shown to have elevated activities in adipose tissue of obese animals at 14 weeks of age (Cleary *et al.*, 1976).

Thus, this animal model is providing useful information about at least one type of genetic hyperplastic obesity. Cell division, as measured by activity of thymidine kinase and DNA polymerase, continues long beyond the normal period. In addition, the abnormal feeding behavior is not mediated through any known endocrine mechanism, but may involve a defect in one area of the hypothalamus. Whether these increased norepinephrine levels are a primary genetic defect or secondary to the increased number of fat cells is unknown.

Concomitant with these studies of genetic obesity in rats, a number of investigations have examined the problem in humans.

10.3.3. Human Studies

As previously mentioned, obesity that dates from early childhood may be the most severe form of the disease, and is usually accompanied by hyperplasia and hypertrophy of fat depots (Salans *et al.*, 1973; Brook *et al.*, 1972). Early-onset obesity has been attributed both to genetic factors and to early overnutrition. Overnutrition was studied indirectly by retrospective studies that assessed weight gain (Dörner *et al.*, 1976) or weight attained (Charney *et at.*, 1976) in early postnatal life. The data obtained were correlated with adult weight for height. These studies (in agreement with previous studies) indicated that infants who gained more weight or attained a higher body weight were more likely to be overweight adults. These authors do not discuss, however, the fact that the majority of these infants *do not* become overweight or obese. In contrast, some infants in the other groups who were average or low gainers or weight-attainers did become obese. In addition, economic data and their association with overweight indicate that poor female children tend to be lean but grow up to be fatter as adults (Garn, 1976). Thus, the nature of the association between obesity in early childhood and later adult obesity is still not totally clear.

More conclusive data have been reported in the area of genetic or familial association with the development of obesity in children. A study of 101 twin pairs that compared skinfold thickness of monozygous and like-sexed dizygotic twins showed excellent correlations of measurements between identical twins (Börjeson, 1976). It was concluded that early nutrition and environment were probably quite similar in both types of twin pairs. The differences were therefore attributed to genetic factors. Even when the monozygous twins had varied greatly in birth weight, their later skinfold thicknesses were quite similar. Analyses of the Ten-State Nutrition Survey to assess body fatness, also using skinfold thickness, indicated that there was a significant familial relationship of body fatness (Garn and Clark, 1976). Children whose parents had been identified as lean were the leanest, and children whose parents had been identified as obese were the fattest. By 17 years of age, children of obese parents were three times fatter (by skinfold determination) than children of lean parents.

Thus, although the evidence is far from conclusive, the data seem to be leading to the conclusion that certain forms of obesity in the human may be genetically determined.

10.4. Nutrition and Pregnancy

Informed opinion is divided as to the degree to which undernutrition influences the outcome of pregnancy. Some maintain that birth weight is readily affected by maternal diet. Others maintain that normal fetal growth will be continued at the expense of the mother's tissues in all but the most extreme nutritional circumstances. Information pertaining to the effects of undernutrition during gestation on the growth of the fetus in humans is difficult to collate, but what there is tends to suggest that severe malnutrition will result in fetal growth retardation, whereas milder forms of malnutrition will still yield a normal-sized fetus (Lechtig *et al.*, 1975; Blackwell *et al.*, 1973). Recent studies in primates lend further support to this view (Kohrs *et al.*, 1976; Riopelle *et al.*, 1976).

From these observations, it is obvious that some adjustment, biochemical or physiological or both, to pregnancy exists that safeguards both mother and fetus against deprivation.

The use of protein stored in early pregnancy to subsidize the rising cost of protein synthesis in late pregnancy could play a major part in reducing the influence of protein restriction on fetal growth. To test this hypothesis, Naismith and Morgan (1976) fed rats either a low-protein diet throughout pregnancy or the same diet supplemented with protein from days 6–10 inclusive. The supplement was therefore withdrawn before significant growth of the fetus had taken place. Analysis of the fetus at parturition showed that feeding extra protein in early pregnancy had promoted substantial increases in the protein content and cellularity of the tissues (this was undoubtedly caused in part through the influence on placental growth).

A number of enzymes involved in amino acid catabolism, including alanine aminotransferase (EC 2.6.1.2.), show greatly reduced activity in the latter half of pregnancy (Naismith and Fears, 1971). However, the activity of the enzyme tryptophan pyrrolase (EC 1.13.1.12), which initiates the degradation of tryptophan to nicotinic acid, was reported to rise in late pregnancy (Harding, *et al.*, 1961). A comparison of the activities of tryptophan pyrrolase and alanine aminotransferase measured in the livers of rats at different stages of gestation (Naismith and Morgan, 1975) shows that after an initial small rise, the activity of alanine aminotransferase fell to one-third the value for nonpregnant controls. In contrast, tryptophan pyrrolase activity was reduced in early pregnancy, then rose to a value three times that of the controls.

The rising tryptophan pyrrolase activity would cause a withdrawal of tryptophan from the amino acid pool, which would initiate and maintain the catabolism of muscle protein (Munro, 1970). Thus, the differing responses of these two inducible enzymes to the changing pattern of hormone secretions during pregnancy could provide a mechanism whereby amino acids released from the tissue proteins could be conserved for fetal tissue anabolism. There is some evidence to support this hypothesis, in that Naismith and Morgan (1975) found that the rise in tryptophan pyrrolase activity in the liver of pregnant rats was accompanied by a fall in the concentration of free tryptophan in their muscles. Furthermore, when an excess of nicotinic acid was fed to pregnant rats fed a low protein diet during the last week of pregnancy, the normal increase in tryptophan pyrrolase was suppressed by feedback inhibition, and a significant reduction in the weight, protein content, and cellularity of the offspring occurred.

It is of interest to recall the earlier work of Calloway (1974), since her measurements of nitrogen balance in pregnant women lend support to the existence of a biphasic cycle of events in women. She observed little difference in the retention of nitrogen between early and late pregnancy, even though the rate of protein accretion by the products of conception exhibits an eightfold increase between the second and last quarter of pregnancy (Hytten and Thomson, 1970).

Further evidence of other metabolic adaptations to pregnancy, to ensure a normal rate of accretion of nitrogen by the conceptus in times of maternal nutritional deprivation, have come to light from the endeavors of Freinkel and his colleagues. They observed, in both animals and humans, that during late gestation, overnight fasting gives rise to a more rapid mobilization and oxidation of fat and urinary loss of nitrogen than occur in the nonpregnant state (Herrera *et al.*, 1969; Freinkel *et al.*, 1974; Freinkel and Metzger, 1975). This "accelerated starvation" (Freinkel, 1965) cannot be accounted for by either basal hyperglucagonemia (Daniel *et al.*, 1974) or elevated glucagon insulin ratios (Nitzan *et al.*, 1975). In fact, the suppression of glucagon release in response to oral glucose is greater during gestation than postpartum (Daniel *et al.*, 1974).

Following mixed meals, these authors found that hyperglycemia was exaggerated and the insulin glucagon ratio was increased, but that there were smaller rises in total plasma amino acids compared with subjects receiving just oral glucose (Metzger *et al.*, 1977). Increments in plasma glucagon were, however, the same for the first 60 min antepartum as postpartum. This suggested that while α-cell suppressibility by glucose or insulin or both may be enhanced during pregnancy, α-cell stimulatory response to amino acids is essentially the same or even enhanced. The increased insulin glucagon ratio would tend to minimize intrahepatic losses and increase anabolism in the peripheral tissues from circulating dietary amino acids directly after a meal. Preserving and increasing the α-cell secretory response to aminogenic stimulation could then be a means of protecting the mother from the occurrence of hypoglycemia caused by high insulin release instigated by amino acids (Metzger *et al.*, 1977).

It has also been shown that while the fetal liver has a limited capacity to divert to fat metabolism during maternal nutritional deprivation, the maternal liver can increase its traffic in fat. The placenta and fetal brain would seem to be able to use lipid products as oxidative fuels during maternal starvation (Herrera and Freinkel, 1975). This may provide a mechanism for preferentially sparing amino acids and glucose for biosynthetic events in these tissues.

Recent evidence has contributed to the idea that severe protein restriction during gestation impairs the proper development of the fetal endocrine system, which is instrumental in producing permanent effects on development. Circulatory levels of triiodothyronine, thyroxine (Shrader *et al.*, 1977a, b), and insulin (Antinmo *et al.*, 1976a) are significantly reduced in the progeny of protein-deprived pregnant females. Furthermore, the metabolism of growth hormone is also seriously affected either by an impairment of the production, release, or breakdown of growth hormone or of its releasing factor (Antinmo *et al.*, 1976b).

The importance of deficiencies of trace elements in fetal development has long been recognized, but this area has seen an upsurge of interest in recent times with respect to zinc. Zinc deficiency in pregnant rats quickly produces anorexia and, in the fetus, impaired synthesis of nucleic acids, leading to decreased brain DNA and intrauterine growth retardation (McKenzie *et al.*, 1975), as well as chromosomal aberrations (Hurley, 1976). A recent study in Scandinavia showed that women who gave birth to immature or dysmature infants showed lower serum zinc concentrations during early pregnancy than women with normal deliveries and normal infants. It is becoming apparent that low serum zinc concentrations during human pregnancy may be a sign of zinc deficiency implying risks to mother and infant (Jameson, 1976).

There is still no good method of recognizing fetal malnutrition *in utero,* but much research is progressing to develop prenatal markers of fetal growth. Amniotic fluid tests in intrauterine growth retardation reveal that the lecithin/sphingomyelin ratios and creatinine levels are depressed (Doran *et al.,* 1976). Leukocyte alkaline phosphatase level in conjunction with urinary estriol excretion is another experimental marker. Low levels are seen in preeclampsia and seem to provide a good indication of fetal well-being and placental function (Leventhal *et al.*, 1976).

References

Antinmo, T., Baldijão, C., Pond, W. G., and Barnes, R. H., 1976a, Decreased dietary protein or energy intake and plasma growth hormone levels of the pregnant pig, its fetuses and developing progeny, *J. Nutr.* **106**:940.

Antinmo, T., Baldijão, C., Pond, W. G. and Barnes, R. H., 1976b, Maternal protein malnutrition during gestation alone and its effects on plasma insulin levels of the pregnant pig, its fetuses and the developing offspring, *J. Nutr.* **106**:1647.

Bell, G. E., and Stern, J. S., 1976, Development of obesity and hyperinsulinemia in the Zucker obese rat (fa/fa), *Fed. Proc. Fed. Amer. Soc. Exp. Biol.* **35**:657 (abstract).

Björntorp, P., and Sjöström, L., 1971, Number and size of adipose tissue fat cells in relation to metabolism in human obesity, *Metabolism* **20**:703.

Blackwell, R. Q., Chow, B. F., Chin, K. S., Blackwell, B., and Hsu, S. C., 1973, Prospective maternal nutrition study in Taiwan: Rationale, study design, feasibility, and preliminary findings, *Nutr. Rep. Int.* **7**:517.

Börjeson, M., 1976, The aetiology of obesity in children, *Acta Paediatr. Scand.* **65**:279.

Brasel, J. A., 1972, Age dependent differences in DNA polymerase activity following uninephrectomy in rats, *Growth* **36**:45.

Brasel, J. A., Coffey, D. S., and Williams-Ashman, H. G., 1968, Androgen induced changes in DNA polymerase activity of coagulating glands of castrated rats, *Med. Exp.* **18**:321.

Brasel, J. A., Ehrenkranz, R. A., and Winick, M., 1973, Patterns of DNA polymerase activity in normal rat forebrain and cerebellum in the suckling period, *Growth* **37**:301.

Bray, G. A., and York, D. A., 1972, Studies on food intake of genetically obese rats, *Amer. J. Physiol.* **223**:176.

Brook, C. G. D., Lloyd, J. K., and Wolff, O. H., 1972, Relation between age of onset of obesity and size and number of adipose cells, *Br. Med. J.* **2**:25.

Calloway, D. H., 1972, Nitrogen balance during pregnancy, in: *Current Concepts in Nutrition,* Vol. 2, *Nutrition and Fetal Development* (M. Winick, ed.), pp. 79–94, John Wiley & Sons, New York.

Charney, E., Goodman, H. C., McBride, M., Lyon, B., and Pratt, R., 1976, Childhood antecedents of adult obesity: Do chubby infants become obese adults?, *N. Engl. J. Med.* **295**:6.

Cleary, M. P., 1976, Postnatal growth and thymidine kinase activity in adipose tissue of normal, genetically obese, and overfed rats, Doctoral dissertation, Columbia University, New York.

Cleary, M. P., Greenwood, M. R. C., and Brasel, J. A., 1975, Thymidine kinase as a measure of adipocyte proliferation in normal and obese rats, *Fed. Proc. Fed. Amer. Soc. Exp. Biol.* **34**:908 (abstract).

Cleary, M. P., Klein, B. E., Greenwood, M. R. C., and Brasel, J. A., 1976, Proliferative enzymes in adipose tissue of normal and obese rats, *Fed. Proc. Fed. Amer. Soc. Exp. Biol.* **35**:502 (abstract).

Cruce, J. A., Thoa, N. B., and Jacobowitz, D. M., 1976, Catecholamines in the brains of genetically obese rats, *Brain Res.* **101**:165.

Dallman, P. R., 1971, Malnutrition: Incorporation of thymidine-^{3}H into nuclear and mitochondrial DNA, *J. Cell Biol.* **51**:549.

Dallman, P. R., and Maimes, E. C., 1973, Protein deficiency: Contrasting effects on DNA and RNA metabolism in rat liver, *J. Nutr.* **103**:1311.

Daniel, R. R., Metzger, B. E., Freinkel, N., Faloona, G., Unger, R. H., and Nitzan, M., 1974, Carbohydrate metabolism in pregnancy. XI. Response of plasma glucagon to overnight fast and oral glucose during normal pregnancy and in gestational diabetes, *Diabetes* **23**:771.

Deb, S., Martin, R. J., and Hirschberger, T. V., 1976, Maintenance requirement and energetic efficiency of lean and obese Zucker rats, *J. Nutr.* **106**:191.

Doran, T. A., Malone, R. M., Benzie, R. J., Jones O. V., Thompson, D. W., and New, M. L., 1976, Amniotic fluid tests for fetal maturity in normal and abnormal pregnancies, *Amer. J. Obstet. Gynecol.* **125**:586.

Dörner, G., Hagen, N., and Witthuhn, W., 1976, Die frühpostnatale Überernährung als ätiopathogenetischer Faktor der Erwachsenenfettsucht, *Acta Biol. Med. Ger.* **35**:799.

Faust, I. M., Johnson, P. R., and Hirsch, J., 1976, Noncompensation of adipose mass in partially lipectomized mice and rats, *Amer. J. Physiol.* **231**:538.

Freinkel, N., 1965, Effects of the conceptus on maternal metabolism during pregnancy, in: *On the Nature and Treatment of Diabetes* (B. S. Leibel and G. A. Wrenshall, eds.), pp. 679–691, Excerpta Medica, Amsterdam.

Freinkel, N., and Metzger, B. E., 1975, Some considerations of fuel economy in the fed state during late human pregnancy, in: *Early Diabetes in Early Life* (R. Camerini and H. Cole, eds.), pp. 289–301, Academic Press, New York.

Freinkel, N., Metzger, B. E., Nitzan, H., Daniel, R., Surmaczynska, B., and Nagel, T., 1974, Facilitated anabolism in late pregnancy: Some novel maternal compensations for accelerated starvation, in: *Proceedings of the VIIIth Congress of the International Diabetes Federation, Int. Cong. Ser. 312* (N.J. Malaise and J. Pirant, eds.), pp. 474–488, Excerpta Medica, Amsterdam.

Garn, S. M., 1976, The origins of obesity, *Amer. J. Dis. Child.* **130**:465.

Garn, S. M., and Clark, D. C., 1976, Trends in fatness and the origins of obesity, *Pediatrics* **57**:443.

Goldberg, A. L., and Goldspink, D. P., 1975, Influence of food deprivation and adrenal steroids on DNA synthesis in various mammalian tissues, *Amer. J. Physiol.* **228**:*310*.

Greenwood, M. R. C., and Hirsch, J., 1974, Postnatal development of adipocyte cellularity in the normal rat, *J. Lipid Res.* **15**:474.

Greenwood, M. R. C., Hirsch, J., Quartermain, D., Johnson, P., and Cruce, J. A. F., 1974, Food motivated behavior in the genetically obese and hypothalamic–hyperphagic rats and mice, *Physiol. Behav.* **13**:687.

Harbhajan, S. P., and Siamak, A. A., 1976, Assessment of effect of starvation, glucose, fatty acids and hormones on α-decarboxylation of leucine in skeletal muscle of rat, *J. Nutr.* **106**:1079.

Harding, H. R., Rosen, F., and Nichol, C. A., 1961, Influence of age, adrenolectomy and corticosteroids on hepatic transaminase activity, *Amer. J. Physiol.* **201**:271.

Herrera, E., and Freinkel, N., 1975, Metabolites in the liver, brain and placenta of fed or fasted mothers and fetal rats, *Horm. Metab. Res.* **7**:247.

Herrera, E., Knopp, R. H., and Freinkel, N., 1969, Carbohydrate metabolism in pregnancy. VI. Plasma fuels, insulin, liver composition, gluconeogenesis and nitrogen metabolism during late gestation in the fed and fasted rat, *J. Clin. Invest.* **48**:2260.

Hietanen, E., and Greenwood, M. R. C., 1976, Lipoprotein lipase activity in epididymal fat pads of growing rats, *Fed. Proc. Fed. Amer. Soc. Exp. Biol.* **35**:502 (abstract).

Hirsch, J., and Han, P. W., 1969, Cellularity of rat adipose tissue: Effects of growth, starvation, and obesity, *J. Lipid Res.* **10**:77.

Hirsch, J., and Knittle, J. L., 1970, Cellularity of obese and nonobese human adipose tissue, *Fed. Proc. Fed. Amer. Soc. Exp. Biol.* **29**:1516.

Hurley, L. S., 1976, Trace elements and teratogenesis, *Med. Clin. North Amer.* **60**:771.

Hytten, F. E., and Thomson, A. M., 1970, Maternal physiological adjustments, in: *Maternal Nutrition and the Course of Pregnancy,* pp. 41–73, National Academy of Sciences, Washington, D.C.

Jameson, S., 1976, Effects of zinc deficiency in human reproduction, *Acta Medica Scand., Suppl. 593,* p. 1.

Jasper, H. G., and Brasel, J. A., 1973, The effects of growth hormone on DNA polymerase activity in the liver of normal and hypophysectomized rats, *Endocrinology* **92**:194.

Jasper, H. G., and Brasel, J. A., 1974, Rat liver DNA synthesis in the "catch-up" growth of nutritional rehabilitation, *J. Nutr.* **104**:405.

Johnson, P. R., Stern, J. S., Greenwood, M. R. C., Zucker, L. M., and Hirsch, J., 1973, Effect of early nutrition on adipose cellularity and pancreatic insulin release in the Zucker rat, *J. Nutr.* **103**:738.

Kohrs, M. B., Harber, A. E., and Kerr, G. R., 1976, Effects of a low-protein diet during pregnancy of the rhesus monkey. 1. Reproductive efficiency, *Amer. J. Clin. Nutr.* **29**:136.

Kraft, N., and Shortman, K. A., 1970, A suggested control function for the animal tissue ribonuclease–ribonuclease inhibitor system, based on studies of isolated cells and phytohaemagglutinin-transformed lymphocytes, *Biochim. Biophys. Acta* **217**:164.

Kral, J. G., 1976, Surgical reduction of adipose tissue in male Sprague–Dawley rat, *Amer. J. Physiol.* **231**:1090.

Lechtig, A., Habicht, J.-P., Yarbrough, C., Delgado, H., Guzman, G., and Klein, R. E., 1975, Influence of food supplementation during pregnancy on birth weight in rural populations of Guatemala, in: *Nutrition, Proceedings of the IXth International Congress of Nutrition, Prognosis for the Undernourished Surviving Child,* Mexico, 1972, Vol. 2, (A. Chavez, H. Bourges, and S. Basta eds.), pp. 44–59, Karger, Basel.

Leventhal, H., Biale, Y., and Ben-Adert, N., 1976, Leukocyte alkaline phosphate determinations and urinary estriol excretion in normal and pathologic pregnancies, *J. Reprod. Med.* **16**:44.

Lewis, C. B., and Winick, M., 1977, Regulation of *in vivo* ribosomal RNA synthesis and ribosome formation in livers of protein-deficient rats, *Fed. Proc. Fed. Amer. Soc. Exp. Biol.* **36**:1155 (abstract).

Lewis, C. G., Rosso, P., and Winick, M., 1976, Demonstration of the existence of two "developmental" species of RNA in liver and brain cytoplasm, *Fed. Proc. Fed. Amer. Soc. Exp. Biol.* **35**:855 (abstract).

Li, J. B., and Goldberg, A. L., 1976, Effects of food deprivation on protein synthesis and degradation in rat skeletal muscles, *Amer. J. Physiol.* **231**:441.

McKenzie, J. M., Fosmire, G. J., and Sandstead, H. H., 1975, Zinc deficiency during the latter third of pregnancy: Effects on fetal rat brain, liver and placenta, *J. Nutr.* **105**:1466.

Metcoff, J., 1972, Biochemical markers of intrauterine malnutrition, in: *Current Concepts in Nutrition,* Vol. 2, *Nutrition and Fetal Development* (M. Winick, ed.), pp. 27–44, John Wiley & Sons, New York.

Metzger, B. E., Unger, R. H., and Freinkel, N., 1977, Carbohydrate metabolism in pregnancy. XIV. Relationships between circulating glucagon, insulin, glucose and amino acids in response to a "mixed meal" in late pregnancy, *Metabolism* **26**:151.

Miller, S. A., 1969, Protein metabolism during growth and development, in: *Mammalian Protein Metabolism,* Vol. 3 (H. N. Munro, ed.) pp. 183–233, Academic Press, New York.

Millward, D. J., Garlick, P. J., Stewart, R. J. C., Nnanyelugo, D. O., and Waterlow, J. C., 1975, Skeletal-muscle growth and protein turnover, *Biochem. J.* **150**:235.

Monckeberg, F., Donoso, G., Oxman, S., Pak, N., and Meneghello, J., 1963, Human growth hormone in infant malnutrition, *Pediatrics* **31**:58.

Munro, H. N., 1970, Free amino acid pools and their role in regulation, in: *Mammalian Protein Metabolism,* Vol. 4 (H. N. Munro, ed.), pp. 299–386, Academic Press, New York.

Muzzo, S., and Brasel, J. A., 1973, Neonatal hypothyroidism and DNA synthesis in rat cerebellum, presented at the 55th Annual Meeting of the Endocrine Society, June, 1973.

Muzzo, S., Gregory, T., and Gardner, L. I., 1973, Oxygen consumption by brain mitochondria of rats malnourished *in utero* in the metabolism, *J. Nutr.* **103**:314.

Naismith, D. J., and Fears, R. B., 1971, Adaptations of protein during pregnancy in the rat, *Proc. Nutr. Soc.* **31**:8A.

Naismith, D. J., and Morgan, B. L. G., 1975, The regulation of protein metabolism during pregnancy in the rat, *Proc. Nutr. Soc.* **34**:27A.

Naismith, D. J., and Morgan, B. L. G., 1976, The biphasic nature of protein metabolism during pregnancy in the rat, *Br. J. Nutr.* **36**:563.

Nitzan, M., Freinkel, N., Metzger, B. E., Unger, R. H., Faloona, G. R., and Daniel, R. R., 1975, The interrelations of glucose, insulin and glucagon after overnight fast and in response to oral glucose during late pregnancy, *Isr. J. Med. Sci.* **11**:617.

Nnanyelugo, D. O., 1976, Changes in RNA content during chronic protein deprivation in the hind limb muscles of rats, *Nutr. Rep. Int.* **14**:209.

Ogata, E. S., and Holliday, M. A., 1976, The effects of starvation glucose infusion and normal feeding on muscle protein synthesis and catabolism in the newborn guinea pig, *Biol. Neonate* **29**:247.

Penney, D., Anderson, D., and Dongas, J., 1976, Effects of early severe malnutrition on heart and skeletal muscle lactate dehydrogenase, *J. Nutr.* **106**:1235.

Pimstone, B. L., Beck, D. J., and Hansen, J. D. L., 1973, Human growth hormone and sulphation factor in protein–calorie malnutrition, in: *Endocrine Aspects of Malnutrition, Kroc Found. Symp., No. 1* (L. I. Gardner and P. Amacher, eds.), pp. 73–90, Kroc Foundation, Santa Ynez, California.

Powley, T. L., and Morton, S. A., 1976, Hypophysectomy and regulation of body weight in the genetically obese Zucker rat, *Amer. J. Physiol.* **230**:982.

Quirin-Stricker, C., and Mandel, P., 1968, Etude du renouvellement du RNA des polysomes, du RNA de transfert et du RNA "messager" dans le foie de rat soumis a un jeune proteique, *Bull. Soc. Chim. Biol.* **50**:31.

Riopelle, A. J., Hale, P. A., and Watts, E. S., 1976, Protein deprivation in primates. VII. Determinants of size and skeletal maturity at birth in Rhesus monkeys, *Hum. Biol.* **48**:203.

Rosso, P., and Raguso, L., 1972, RNase activity: Rate of RNA degradation and cellular RNA content, *Fed. Proc. Fed. Amer. Soc. Exp. Biol.* **31**:697.

Rosso, P., and Winick, M., 1975, Effects of early undernutrition and subsequent refeeding on alkaline ribonuclease activity of rat cerebrum and liver, *J. Nutr.* **105**:1104.

Rosso, P., Nelson, M., and Winick, M., 1973, Changes in cellular RNA content and alkaline ribonuclease activity in rat liver during development, *Growth* **37**:143.

Rozovski, J., Winick, M., and Rosso, P., 1976, Adaptive changes in polyamine metabolism during malnutrition and refeeding, *Fed. Proc. Fed. Amer. Soc. Exp. Biol.* **35**:341 (abstract).

Salans, L. B., Cushman, S. W., and Weismann, R. E., 1973, Studies of human adipose tissue—adipose cell size and number in nonobese and obese patients, *J. Clin. Invest.* **52**:929.

Shrader, R. E., Hastings-Roberts, M. M., Ferlatte, M. L., and Zeman, F. J., 1977a,

Effect of prenatal protein deprivation on fetal and neonatal thyroid morphology in the rat, *J. Nutr.* **107**;213.

Shrader, R. E., Ferlatte, M. I., Hastings-Roberts, M. M., Schoenborne, B. M., Hoernicke, C. A., and, Zeman, F. J., 1977b, Thyroid funcion in prenatally protein-deprived rats, *J. Nutr.* **107**:221.

Stein, T. P., Oram-Smith, J. C., Leskiw, M. J., Wallace, H. W., Long, L. C., and Leonard, J. M., 1976, Effect of nitrogen and calorie restriction on protein synthesis in the rat, *Amer. J. Physiol.* **230**:1321.

Tagliamonte, B., Benedetti, C., and Spadoni, M. A., 1972, Effect of refeeding on liver thymidine-kinase activity of food restricted suckling rats, *Nutr. Rep. Int.* **5**:305.

Winick, M., 1968, Cellular response with increased feeding in pituitary dwarf mice, *J. Nutr.* **94**:121.

Winick, M., and Grant, P., 1968, Cellular growth in the organs of the hypopituitary dwarf mouse, *Endocrinology* **83**:544.

Zamenhof, S., Van Marthens, E., and Grauel, L., 1971, Prenatal cerebral development: Effect of restricted diet, reversal by growth hormone, *Science* **174**:954.

Zucker, L. M., and Antoniades, H. N., 1972, Insulin and obesity in the Zucker genetically obese rat "fatty," *Endocrinology* **90**:1320.

Zucker, L. M., and Zucker T. F., 1961, Fatty, a new mutation in the rat, *J. Hered.* **52**:275.

11

Metabolic Aspects of Renal Stone Disease

Hibbard E. Williams

11.1. Introduction

The problems of diagnosis and treatment of renal stone disease remain much the same as they have for the past several years. The most important of these is the question of basic pathogenetic mechanisms in stone formation and growth, particularly in the so-called "idiopathic stone-formers." Solutions to this problem are slowly emerging and are essential for the development of rational and effective treatment programs. The causes of the common idiopathic hypercalciuria syndrome continue to be debated throughout the world, and some consensus is beginning to develop. The importance of urate in the nucleation of calcium oxalate stones and the role of relatively minor changes in urinary oxalate excretion in the development of these stones also remain as key issues in our understanding of recurrent nephrolithiasis.

Research in all these areas continues to be hampered by difficulties in the definition of clinical activity of stone disease and the necessity of

HIBBARD E. WILLIAMS • Medical Service, San Francisco General Hospital Medical Center; Department of Medicine, University of California, San Francisco, California.

following patients closely with adequate frequent urinary analyses for long periods of time. The latter is particularly important in evaluating the effectiveness of new treatment programs. Nevertheless, important improvements have occurred during the past year, and these will be focused on in this chapter.

11.2. Incidence of Renal Stone Disease

Renal stone disease continues to be an extremely common problem in clinical medicine, although no new figures of incidence or prevalence have appeared. It seems likely that older estimates of one episode of stone disease for every 1000 individuals per year is still accurate today. In other words, good preventive measures for recurrent stone disease have yet to be developed.

An international symposium on bladder stone disease in Southeast Asia (*Proceedings,* 1977) held this year in Washington, D.C. emphasized again the very high incidence of this problem in male children below the age of 10 in Southeast Asia and parts of the Middle East. These stones are composed largely of urates and calcium oxalate. The mechanism of stone formation remains elusive, although malnutrition and particularly phosphate depletion may play a major role (Van Reen, 1976). The high phytate content of the diet of afflicted children may lead to or aggravate the phosphate deficiency. Phosphate supplementation has reduced oxalate crystalluria in these patients and seems to diminish the incidence of stone episodes (Van Reen, 1976).

11.3. Classification of Renal Stone Disease

In this chapter, the author will continue to use the following classification scheme for stone disease:

1. Increased crystalloid excretion, particularly calcium, oxalate, uric acid, cystine, and xanthine
2. Physicochemical changes in urine that predispose to stone formation at normal crystalloid content, i.e., changes in pH and inhibitors of stone formation
3. Idiopathic stone disease in which the mechanism is not known or in which combinations of the preceding two mechanisms may play a role

Regardless of which mechanism is primary, the actual formation of a urinary stone may be looked on as a stepwise process involving four stages (Robertson, 1976): (1) In the first stage, nucleation of a crystal occurs. It may occur either by homogeneous nucleation (secondary to oversaturation) or by heterogeneous nucleation (precipitated by some nucleating factor such as another salt or crystal). (2) The second stage is that of crystal growth and aggregation. In this stage, the phenomenon of epitaxy may take place, in which one crystalline substance grows on the surface of a crystal of different composition (Nancollas, 1976). (3) In the third stage, one of the crystal aggregates may become lodged or trapped in some area of the urinary tract. (4) In the final stage, growth of the stone into a macroscopic clinically significant calculus occurs. Although disagreement exists as to the most important of these steps, in general, this dynamic process probably occurs in most types of renal calculus disease.

11.4. Renal Stone Disease Secondary to Increased Crystalloid Excretion

11.4.1. Hypercalciuria

This phenomenon remains an important one in the etiology of stone disease. Hyperparathyroidism and renal tubular acidosis, type I or distal type, both have an increased incidence of stone disease secondary to hypercalciuria. Other causes of hypercalciuria such as hyperthyroidism, multiple myeloma, and metastatic malignancy are rarely associated with an increased incidence of stone disease because the disease process is either rapidly diagnosed and corrected or the patients succumb before renal calculi have sufficient time to develop. The most common and most controversial hypercalciuric state associated with stone disease is the syndrome of idiopathic hypercalciuria. This syndrome occurs most commonly in adult men, often with a family history of stone disease, and is diagnosed by the finding of persistent elevation of urinary calcium excretion in the absence of hypercalcemia or other causes of hypercalciuria. Plasma phosphate concentration is usually low in these patients, although there is great variability (Nordin *et al.*, 1976). Ionized calcium in serum is found to be elevated in some of these patients (Muldowney *et al.*, 1973), and parathyroid hormone levels have been reported to be either low, normal, or high (Nordin *et al.*, 1976; Pak, 1976).

The mechanism for the hypercalciuria continues to be debated. A small number of these patients may have normocalcemic hyperparathyroidism although well-documented cases of this are rare. A primary renal leak of calcium was suggested by some studies (Coe *et al.*, 1973), but again, direct documentation of this mechanism has not been forthcoming.

The most consistent finding in most patients with idiopathic hypercalciuria is increased GI absorption of calcium (Nordin *et al.*, 1976). Is this a primary defect or is it secondary to some other abnormality? This important question is unsolved at present. The studies of Nordin *et al.* (1976) suggested that the hypercalciuria and increased absorption of calcium observed in patients with idiopathic hypercalciuria and stone disease may represent the upper end of the normal distribution of urine calcium absorption and urinary excretion of calcium. Coe and Kavalach (1974) suggested, however, that the primary abnormality in these patients is phosphate depletion, and that this leads secondarily to hypercalciuria, increased parathormone secretion, and increased 1,25-dihydroxy-vitamin D synthesis that in turn leads to increased calcium absorption. Several problems have been voiced in criticism of this theory, including lack of evidence for definite phosphate depletion in idiopathic hypercalciuria, lack of correlation between plasma phosphate and calcium absorption, and the tendency for phosphate depletion to raise serum calcium and decrease plasma parathormone (Nordin *et al.*, 1976). Despite this argument, raised 1,25-dihydroxy-vitamin D levels in these patients have been reported (Pak, 1976), suggesting that the calcium hyperabsorption is in some way secondary to abnormalities in this controlling factor.

11.4.2. Hyperoxaluria

The causes of hyperoxaluria were reviewed in detail in the first volume of this series (Williams, 1976a), and will not be covered again in this chapter. The most common form of hyperoxaluria in man remains the syndrome of enteric hyperoxaluria. This syndrome has now been reported to occur in a wide variety of GI disorders, including regional enteritis, granulomatous bowel disease, bowel resection, blind loop syndrome, bacterial overgrowth, chronic biliary tract disease, chronic pancreatitis, and jejunoileal bypass procedures (Williams, 1976b). Although hyperoxaluria has been demonstrated in most of the patients with jejunoileal bypass procedures, the incidence of stone disease has generally been less than 20%. Cases of acute renal failure secondary to renal oxalosis have been reported in this group, and in at least one patient, restoration of normal GI continuity reversed the renal failure (Cryer *et al.*, 1975; Earnest *et al.*, 1977).

The mechanism for the hyperoxaluria in this syndrome is hyperabsorption of dietary oxalate. Because certain substrates such as glycine may be converted to oxalate in the lumen of the GI tract in the presence of bacterial overgrowth, it has not always been possible to return oxalate excretion to normal with a "low oxalate" diet. The mechanism of the hyperoxaluria appears to be largely due to competition of intraluminal oxalate and fatty acids for the calcium ion. In the presence of large intraluminal fatty acid concentrations, calcium is no longer available to oxalate, and more oxalate is free to diffuse across the GI mucosa (Williams, 1976b). The effect of cholestyramine on lowering oxalate excretion in this group of patients has suggested a role for unabsorbed bile acids in increasing oxalate absorption, but no direct proof for this hypothesis exists. Cholestyramine may bind intraluminal oxalate directly, making it unavailable for absorption.

Perhaps a more important feature of oxalate lies not in its excessive excretion in the definite hyperoxaluric states, but in its variable excretion within the normal range in idiopathic stone-formers. Mean urinary oxalate excretion is significantly higher in groups of idiopathic stone-formers when compared with control subjects (Robertson *et al.*, 1976). Because studies by Robertson and co-workers emphasized the role of moderate changes in urinary oxalate in controlling calcium oxalate solubility (Robertson *et al.*, 1972), the slightly higher oxalate excretion in stone-formers may assume a much greater importance than other factors in the genesis of the stone disease. No studies have been reported explaining the mechanism for this increased oxalate excretion in idiopathic stone-formers, and the possibilities of either increased production of endogenous oxalate or increased intake or absorption of exogenous oxalate must be evaluated carefully in the future.

11.4.3. Hyperuricosuria

Hyperuricosuria leading to an increased concentration of uric acid in urine and supersaturation of the urine with respect to uric acid remains a major cause of uric acid nephrolithiasis. Most often, this hyperuricosuria is secondary to overproduction of uric acid, as in the genetic hyperuricemic syndrome or those myeloproliferative disorders associated with increased turnover of nucleoproteins (Seegmiller, 1976).

Recently, an increased incidence of hyperuricosuria was reported in patients with recurrent calcium oxalate calculi (Coe and Kavalach, 1974). This hyperuricosuria was due primarily to increased ingestion of dietary purines (Coe and Kavalach, 1974). These findings have led to speculations that urate may act as a heterogeneous nucleator of calcium oxalate. This seems unlikely in view of the difficulty in finding urates in most calcium oxalate stones and the fact that the urine of calcium oxalate stone-formers is never sufficiently supersaturated with sodium urate and rarely with sufficient uric acid to cause spontaneous precipitation. Nevertheless, success in the treatment of calcium oxalate stone-formers with allopurinol has been claimed (Coe and Raisen, 1973).

11.4.4. Cystine and Xanthine Stones

No new studies have appeared relative to the formation of cystine and xanthine stones. Cystine stones are found only in the genetic disease cystinuria, and form because of supersaturation of the urine with this amino acid. A new drug (α-mercaptopropionyl glycine) was reported to be effective in the treatment of cystine stones (Remien *et al.*, 1975). Xanthine stones have been found in three conditions: the rare hereditary xanthinuria syndrome, after allopurinol therapy in patients with the Lesch–Nyhan syndrome, and in patients given allopurinol for hyperuricemia secondary to chemotherapeutic treatment of myeloproliferative disorders.

An interesting new type of renal stone was recently described in patients with a hereditary deficiency of the enzyme adenine phosphoribosyl transferase, which catalyzes the conversion of adenine to adenosine monophosphate (Simmonds *et al.*, 1976; Cartier *et al.*, 1974). In this condition, stones composed of 2,8-dihydroxyadenine have been identified. This compound is produced under conditions of adenine accumulation by the action of xanthine oxidase.

11.5. Renal Stone Disease Secondary to Physicochemical Changes in Urine Composition

Examples of this mechanism of stone formation include the development of uric acid stones secondary to persistent acidification of the urine and the development of apatite–struvite stones in patients with chronic urinary tract infection and alkaline urine secondary to urea-splitting microorganisms (Griffith and Musher, 1976). In the latter condition, recent studies emphasized the importance of urease production by the microorganism in the genesis of the stone formation, and also suggested that urease inhibition may be useful in the treatment of these stones (Griffith *et al.*, 1976).

The most active research activities in this area have focused on the potential role of urinary inhibitors in renal stone formation. A number of naturally occurring inhibitors of stone growth have been identified in urine, including urea, citrate, amino acids, trace metals, acid mucopolysaccharides, pyrophosphate, and small polypeptides. The mechanisms whereby these inhibitors actually interrupt stone growth have been well studied (Nancollas, 1976). Four possible mechanisms exist: (1) complexing of calcium by the inhibitor, reducing the effective concentration of calcium ion; (2) absorption of the inhibitor at growth sites on the crystal surface, blocking further crystal growth; (3) interference with morphology of the growing crystal; and (4) a change in ionic strength of the urine, altering the effective solubility of the precipitating salt.

Studies of total inhibitory activity of urine in normal subjects and stone-formers were summarized recently (Robertson, 1976). *In vitro* measurement of total inhibitory activity of urine showed that idiopathic stone-formers have significantly less inhibitory activity than do normal subjects.

In addition, the size of crystals found in the urine of stone-formers is inversely related to the amount of inhibitory activity. Unfortunately, it has not been possible to identify the lack of a specific inhibitor to account for this diminished total inhibitory activity. In some patients with renal tubular acidosis, however, decreased citrate excretion may explain in part the propensity for stone formation.

The two most important inhibitors of stone formation found in urine are pyrophosphate, which accounts for about 10–15% of total inhibitory activity, and acid mucopolysaccharides, which may account for the largest percentage of total inhibitory activity (Robertson *et al.*, 1976). It has not been possible to correlate the decrease in total inhibitory activity of urine from stone-formers with their concentration of urinary acid mucopolysaccharide. It has been shown that the higher the concentration of urate in urine, the less effective are the acid mucopolysaccarides as inhibitors. On the basis of these data, it was speculated that the decrease in total inhibitory activity in stone-formers' urine may be a function of the relative concentrations of urate and acid mucopolysaccharides (Robertson *et al.*, 1976). Additional data in this fascinating area will be awaited with interest.

Changes in urinary organic matrix substance have not been correlated in the past with the activity of the stone disease, and the matrix nucleation theory of stone formation has not been a fashionable one. A recent study by Spector *et al.* (1976) rekindled an interest in this theory. These investigators studied the organic matrices of kidney stones composed of different mineral composition. The organic matrix of calcium oxalate stones was found to contain different patterns of acidic amino acids than those of the organic matrix of uric acid or apatite–struvite stones. This difference in amino acids composition of the organic matrices suggested that the organic matrix may play a role in certain types of stone disease.

11.6. Idiopathic Renal Stone Disease

Idiopathic renal stone disease, the most common type of recurrent nephrolithiasis, is generally defined as that form of stone disease in which no single abnormality discussed in Sections 11.4 and 11.5 is identified as the primary pathogenetic mechanism. Recently, a series of elegant studies by Robertson *et al.* (1976) shed some light on the basic mechanisms of stone formation in this group of patients. The findings of this group of investigators are summarized as follows:

1. The urine of idiopathic stone-formers (ISF) is more saturated with respect to calcium oxalate than that of normal subjects.

2. Urinary calcium and oxalate excretion in ISF is significantly higher than in normal subjects.
3. The size of calcium oxalate crystals in the urine of ISF is greater than that in normal subjects.
4. Total inhibitory activity of urine from ISF is significantly lower than that of normal subjects.
5. The ratio of saturation to total inhibitory activity (the saturation–inhibitor index) is greater in ISF than in normal subjects, and there is a positive correlation between the percentage of large calcium oxalate crystals and the saturation–inhibition index of urine samples of ISF.

From these important observations, a reasonable explanation for stone formation in ISF is beginning to emerge. Discordant changes in the degrees of saturation and inhibition of stone formation appear to combine to cause the eventual development of recurrent renal stones in this group of patients. The exact mechanism whereby these changes take place is not known at present. Alterations in both parameters can result from variations in dietary intake and intestinal absorption, diurnal and seasonal variations in the urinary excretion of urinary crystalloids, and variations in the excretion of urinary inhibitors, particularly the acid mucopolysaccharides. Continued research in the control of these variables should lead to valuable information in the future.

11.7. Treatment of Renal Stone Disease

The rational treatment of renal stone disease is dependent on the accurate identification of pathogenetic mechanisms. In those patients with stone disease secondary to increased crystalloid excretion, control of excessive urinary excretion of the particular crystalloid should decrease the activity of the stone disease. Many of the treatment modalities for patients in this category are discussed in the first volume of this series and in other reviews (Pak, 1976, 1977; Smith, 1976) and will not be repeated here. In patients who have stone disease on the basis of some abnormality in the physicochemical state of the urine, correction of the abnormality should improve the stone problem, i.e., urinary acidification and control of infection in the apatite–struvite stone-former and urinary alkalinization in patients with uric acid stones. One interesting new approach to therapy in patients with apatite–struvite stones is the use of acetohydroxamic acid, a urease inhibitor (Griffith *et al.*, 1976). This compound reduces urinary pH and ammonia, and has been proposed for the treatment of patients with this stone problem. No long-term clinical studies have yet been reported.

The most important clinical problem in recurrent stone disease is the treatment of those patients with idiopathic nephrolithiasis. Because many of these patients have slightly elevated urine calcium and oxalate excretion and decreased total inhibitory activity, treatment programs have been directed at the correction of these abnormalities. Several approaches have been used to treat patients with elevated or high normal urine calcium levels. A low calcium diet is certainly indicated in the patient with hyperabsorption of calcium. In patients who do not have increased GI absorption, however, a low calcium diet may increase urinary oxalate. This dietary program should therefore not be applied randomly to all patients with idiopathic stone disease. Cellulose phosphate does lower urinary calcium, but may also increase urinary oxalate (Pak, 1976). For this reason, this drug is most useful in hyperabsorbers of calcium, and probably should not be used in other patients with idiopathic stone disease. Thiazides lower urinary calcium excretion, and although urine oxalate may increase slightly, the saturation of urine with respect to calcium oxalate is lowered (Pak, 1976). Thiazides may also increase urinary pyrophosphate, an important inhibitor of stone formation (Pak, 1976). Another approach to therapy in these patients has been to increase urinary inhibitory activity. The most useful drug programs in this regard have been orthophosphate and diphosphonate therapy. Orthophosphate therapy decreases urinary calcium and increases urinary pyrophosphate, thereby decreasing the state of saturation of the urine with respect to calcium oxalate and retarding the spontaneous nucleation of calcium oxalate. The author has had particular success with this form of therapy in patients with primary hyperoxaluria, and similar results have been reported from other laboratories (Smith, 1976). The diphosphonates are potent inhibitors of calcium oxalate nucleation, crystal growth, and crystal aggregation of calcium oxalate (Pak, 1976). Unfortunately, urinary oxalate and urine saturation with respect to calcium oxalate may increase with the use of these compounds, and osteomalacia may occur as a side effect (Pak, 1976). For this reason, these compounds cannot be recommended at this time in the treatment of idiopathic stone disease.

Finally, because hyperuricosuria is sometimes found in patients with recurrent calcium oxalate nephrolithiasis and because urates could theoretically cause heterogeneous nucleation of calcium oxalate, allopurinol has been recommended in the treatment of idiopathic calcium oxalate stone disease (see Section 11.1.4.3). In view of the significant toxicity of allopurinol, the author believes that this drug should be reserved for treatment of stone patients who have been shown to have persistent hyperuricosuria.

References

Cartier, P., Hamet, M., and Hamburger, J., 1974, Une nouvelle maladie métabolique: Le défecit complete en adénine-phosphoribosyl-transférase avec lithiases de 2,8-dihydroxyadénine, *C. R. Acad. Sci.* **279**:883.

Coe, F. L. Canterbury, J. M., Firpo, J. O., and Reiss, E., 1973, Evidence for secondary hyperparathyroidism in idiopathic hypercalciuria, *J. Clin. Invest.* **52**:134.

Coe, F. L., and Kavalach, A. G., 1974, Hypercalciuria and hyperuricosuria in patients with calcium nephrolithiasis, *N. Engl. J. Med.* **291**:1344.

Coe, F. L., and Raisen, L., 1973, Allopurinol treatment of uric-acid disorders in calcium-stone formers, *Lancet* **1**:129.

Cryer, P. E., Garber, A. J., Hoffstein, P., Lucas, B., and Wise, L., 1975, Renal failure after small intestinal bypass for obesity, *Arch. Intern. Med.* **135**:1610.

Earnest, D., Campbell, J., Hunt, T. K., and Naughton, J., 1977, Progressive renal failure with hyperoxaluria: a new complication of jejunoileal bypass, *Gastroenterology* **72**:1054.

Griffith, D. P., Gibson, J. R., Clinton, C. W., and Musher, D. M., 1976, Acetohydroxamic acid: Initial investigations in man, in: *Urolithiasis Research* (H. Fleisch, W. G. Robertson, L. H. Smith, and W. Vahlensieck, eds.), pp. 545–548, Plenum Press, New York.

Griffith, D. P., and Musher, D. M., 1976, Urease: Principal cause of infection stones, in *Urolithiasis Research* (H. Fleisch, W. G. Robertson, L. H. Smith, and W. Vahlensieck, eds.), pp. 451–454, Plenum Press, New York.

Muldowney, F. P., Freaney, R., Spillane, E. A., and O'Donoghue, P., 1973, Ionised calcium levels in "Normocalcaemic" hyperparathyroidism, *Ir. J. Med. Sci.* **14**:223.

Nancollas, G. H., 1976, The kinetics of crystal growth and renal stone formation, in: *Urolithiasis Research* (H. Fleisch, W. G. Robertson, L. H. Smith, and W. Vahlensieck, eds.), pp. 5–23, Plenum Press, New York.

Nordin, B. E. C., Peacock, M., and Marchall, D. H., 1976, Calcium excretion and hypercalciuria, in: *Urolithiasis Research* (H. Fleisch, W. G. Robertson, L. H. Smith, and W. Vahlensieck, eds.), pp. 101–116, Plenum Press, New York.

Pak, C. Y. C., 1976, Idiopathic renal lithiasis: New developments in evaluation and treatment, in: *Urolithiasis Research* (H. Fleisch, W. G. Robertson, L. H. Smith, and W. Vahlensieck, eds.), pp. 213–224, Plenum Press, New York.

Pak, C. Y. C., 1977, Physicochemical and clinical aspects of nephrolithiasis, in: *International Colloquium on Renal Lithiasis* Gainesville, Florida, January 1976 (in press).

Proceedings of the International Symposium on Bladder Stone Disease in Southeast Asia, 1977, Washington, D.C., April 1976 (in press).

Remien, A., Kallistratos, G., and Burchardt, P., 1975, Treatment of cystinuria with Thiola (α-mercaptopropionyl glycine), *Eur. Urol.* **1**:227.

Robertson, W. G., 1976, Physical chemical aspects of calcium stone-formation in the urinary tract, in: *Urolithiasis Research* (H. Fleisch, W. G. Robertson, L. H. Smith, and W. Vahlensieck, eds.), pp. 25–39, Plenum Press, New York.

Robertson, W. G., Peacock, M., and Nordin, B. E. C., 1972, Measurement of activity products in urine from stone-formers and normal subjects, in: *Urolithiasis—Physical Aspects* (B. Finlayson, L. L. Hench, and L. H. Smith, eds.), pp. 79–95, National Academy of Sciences, Washington, D.C.

Robertson, W. G., Knowles, F., and Peacock, M., 1976, Urinary acid mucopolysaccharide inhibitors of calcium oxalate crstallization, in: *Urolithiasis Research* (H. Fleisch, W. G. Robertson, L. H. Smith, and W. Vahlensieck, eds.), pp. 331–334, Plenum Press, New York.

Seegmiller, J. E., 1976, Genetic defects in human purine metabolism leading to urolithiasis, in: *Urolithiasis Research* (H. Fleisch, W. G. Robertson, L. H. Smith, and W. Vahlensieck, eds.), pp. 147–154, Plenum Press, New York.

Simmonds, H. A., Van Acker, K. J., Cameron, J. S., and Snedden, W., 1976, A new cause of urinary calculi: 2,8-Dihydroxyadenine stones in supposed "uric acid" crystalluria, in: *Urolithiasis Research* (H. Fleisch, W. G. Robertson, L. H. Smith, and W. Vahlensieck, eds.), pp. 517–521, Plenum Press, New York.

Smith, L. H., 1976, Application of physical, chemical, and metabolic factors to the management of urolithiasis, in: *Urolithiasis Research* (H. Fleisch, W. G. Robertson, L. H. Smith, and W. Vahlensieck, eds.), pp. 199–211, Plenum Press, New York.

Spector, A. R., Gray, A., and Prien, E. L., Jr., 1976, Kidney stone matrix: Difference in acidic protein composition, *Invest. Urol.* **13**:387.

Van Reen, R., 1976, Idiopathic urinary bladder stone disease, in: *Urolithiasis Research* (H. Fleisch, W. G. Robertson, L. H. Smith, and W. Vahlensieck, eds.), pp. 569–572, Plenum Press, New York.

Williams, H. E., 1976a, Metabolic aspects of renal stone disease, in: *The Year in Metabolism 1975–1976* (N. Freinkel, ed.), pp. 299–316, Plenum Press, New York.

Williams, H. E., 1976b, Oxalic acid: Absorption, excretion and metabolism, in: *Urolithiasis Research* (H. Fleisch, W. G. Robertson, L. H. Smith, and W. Vahlensieck, eds.), pp. 181–188, Plenum Press, New York.

12

Metabolism and Metabolic Actions of Ethanol

Charles S. Lieber

12.1. Metabolism of Ethanol

12.1.1. Role of Alcohol Dehydrogenase and Interaction of Dietary Factors with Ethanol and Acetaldehyde Metabolism

According to prevailing concepts, the rate-limiting factor in the metabolism of ethanol by the alcohol dehydrogenase (ADH) pathway is the capacity of the liver to reoxidize the NADH produced from the reduction of NAD by the hydrogen from the ethanol rather than the activity of ADH itself. It appears now, however, that ADH is not necessarily present in excess, and that under a variety of circumstances, it is the level of the enzyme itself that actually becomes rate-limiting (Crow *et al.*, 1977). The concept that rates of ethanol metabolism may be determined by the level of ADH activity has been the subject of controversy for many years and

CHARLES S. LIEBER • Section and Laboratory of Liver Disease, Nutrition and Alcoholism, Veterans Administration Hospital, Bronx, New York 10468; Mount Sinai School of Medicine (CUNY), New York, New York 10029.

has attracted more recent attention because ADH was found to be heterogeneous, and several isoenzymes have been described in human liver (Schenker *et al.*, 1971; Pietruszko *et al.*, 1972; Smith *et al.*, 1971, 1972; Li and Magnes, 1975). In addition, an atypical ADH was isolated (von Wartburg *et al.*, 1965) that, *in vitro,* has a much higher activity at physiologic pH than does the normal variety. Although those individuals with "atypical" ADH have enzyme activities several times higher than normal *in vitro,* this is not accompanied by an acceleration of the metabolism of ethanol *in vivo* (Edwards and Price Evans, 1967). This discrepancy supported the view that in the process of ADH-mediated ethanol oxidation, ADH itself is not rate-limiting provided that an at least normal amount of enzyme is present. Under these conditions, velocities may depend on availability of the cofactor NAD, especially the speed of the reoxidation of the ADH–NADH complex.

The studies of Crow *et al.* (1977) confirmed that the levels of cytosolic NAD^+ and NADH may be important factors in regulation of ethanol oxidation when rates are lower than those set by the V_{max} of ADH. They also show, however, that ADH is not present in the liver in as great an excess as was believed, and in some cases, the rate of ethanol oxidation is limited principally by the V_{max} of liver ADH. If ADH is not present in the liver in much excess, one expects that circumstances that might reduce ADH activity, if only modestly, would also diminish rates of ethanol oxidation. This is indeed what was found. An experimental example of the role of the decreased ADH level on the rate of ethanol metabolism can be furnished by the effect of low-protein diets, which have been shown to reduce hepatic ADH levels in rats (Horn and Manthei, 1965; Bode, C., *et al.*, 1970) and to considerably slow the metabolism of ethanol both in rats (Bode, C., *et al.*, 1970) and in man (Bode, C., *et al.*, 1971). It was also confirmed recently (Bode, J. C., and Thiele, 1975) that prolonged fasting markedly slows the metabolism of ethanol. Thus, in malnourished alcoholics, the pharmacologic effects of ethanol (including those on the brain) may be greater, due to slower ethanol metabolism causing higher and more sustained blood ethanol levels; in contrast, effects of ethanol secondary to its metabolism may be less striking.

Dietary factors may not only alter ethanol metabolism, but may also change the rate of the oxidation of its product, namely, acetaldehyde. Indeed, it had been noted that in some groups of rats, alcohol resulted in much higher acetaldehyde levels than ordinarily observed (Lindros *et al.*, 1975; Marchner and Tottmar, 1976a). This puzzling finding has now been explained. The acetaldehyde produced by the oxidation of ethanol is in turn oxidized to acetate by a mitochondrial acetaldehyde dehydrogenase of the liver. It was found that the activity of the mitochondrial enzyme was 2–3 times lower in rats fed the commercial diet in question. This explains why the acetaldehyde blood levels were 2–4 times higher in rats fed this diet. The unknown dietary factor was shown to be located in the calcinated bonemeal fraction of the diet, and was identified as cyanamide (Marchner and Tottmar, 1976b).

12.1.2. Role, Nature, and Metabolic Consequences of Non-ADH Pathways for Ethanol Oxidation

It is now well recognized that in addition to ADH, other hepatic enzyme systems can oxidize ethanol, namely, catalase and the microsomal ethanol-oxidizing system (MEOS). Catalase is located primarily in peroxisomes, with some activity found in microsomal fractions, probably as a contaminant rather than a component of the microsomal membranes (Redman *et al.*, 1972). It was shown by Keilin and Hartree (1945) that catalase is capable of oxidizing ethanol *in vitro* in the presence of H_2O_2-generating systems. It is generally accepted that the rate of H_2O_2-mediated peroxidation of ethanol by catalase is limited by the rate of H_2O_2 generation, rather than by the activity of catalase itself. The rate of H_2O_2 generation in the liver, however, has been reported to be very low: 3.6 μmol/hr per g liver under physiologic conditions (Boveris *et al.*, 1972). This rate represents only 2% of the rate of ethanol oxidation *in vivo* (178 μmol/hr per g liver) (Lieber and DeCarli, 1972). In perfused liver experiments, a similar low rate of H_2O_2 generation (3–5 μmol/hr/g of liver) was reported by Oshino *et al.* (1973). Furthermore, recent studies showed that not all the H_2O_2 generated in the liver could be utilized for the peroxidation of ethanol by catalase (Oshino *et al.*, 1975). Ethanol peroxidation by catalase can therefore theoretically account for only an insignificant fraction of ethanol oxidation under normal conditions.

The other non-ADH alcohol-oxidizing system of the liver is the MEOS. This system was previously differentiated from alcohol dehydrogenase by its subcellular localization (microsomes vs. cytosol), pH optimum (7.4 vs. 9–11), cofactor requirements (NADPH vs. NAD), and relative lack of sensitivity to pyrazole (Teschke *et al.*, 1974, 1976; Lieber and DeCarli, 1970; Lieber, 1977). The activity of the MEOS was also differentiated from catalase by its relative insensitivity to catalase inhibitors such as azide and cyanide, and by the inability of a H_2O_2-generating system (glucose–glucose oxidase) to sustain ethanol oxidation both in microsomes (Teschke *et al.*, 1974) and in liver slices (Teschke *et al.*, 1976).

Recently, the reconstitution of the ethanol-oxidizing activity with the three microsomal components cytochrome *P*-450, NADPH cytochrome *c* reductase, and lecithin was achieved by Ohnishi and Lieber (1976, 1977). In these experiments, cytochrome *P*-450 was partially purified by protease treatment and subsequently by column chromatography on DEAE–cellulose using a stepwise KCl gradient (Comai and Gaylor, 1973). NADPH cytochrome *c* reductase was partially purified essentially by the method of

Levin *et al.* (1974). The activity of the reconstituted microsomal ethanol-oxidizing system (reconstituted MEOS) was dependent on cytochrome *P*-450 and the reductase and required synthetic phospholipids (such as lecithin) for its maximal activity. The K_m of the reconstituted MEOS for ethanol was 10 mM, which is similar to the K_m measured in crude microsomes and the MEOS fraction isolated by column chromatography (Lieber and DeCarli, 1968, 1970; Teschke *et al.*, 1974). This reconstituted system required NADPH as a cofactor, but did not react to a H_2O_2-generating system, and was insensitive to the catalase inhibitor azide. These characteristics were also similar to those observed in crude microsomes.

Thus, despite the considerable controversy that has surrounded this issue, it is now agreed by the principal contenders involved that catalase cannot account for microsomal ethanol oxidation (Thurman and Brentzel, 1977; Teschke *et al.*, 1977). There is still disagreement, however, on the relative importance of the ADH and non-ADH pathways for the metabolism of ethanol in the liver.

That ethanol metabolism can persist even in the presence of pyrazole (a potent ADH inhibitor) was shown before both *in vivo* (Lieber and DeCarli, 1972) and *in vitro* in isolated perfused liver (Papenberg *et al.*, 1970), liver slices (Lieber and DeCarli, 1970), and isolated liver cells (Thieden, 1971; Grunnet *et al.*, 1973; Matsuzaki and Lieber, 1975). Furthermore, in the presence of pyrazole, glucose labeling from [1R-^{3}H] ethanol was nearly abolished, while [H^3]HO production was inhibited less than 50%. In view of the stereospecificity of ADH for [1R-^{3}H]ethanol, these findings again suggested "the presence of a significant pathway not mediated by cytosolic ADH" (Rognstad and Clark, 1974). Additional evidence that this pyrazole-insensitive residual ethanol metabolism is not ADH-mediated was derived from the fact that the cytosolic redox state was unaffected (Grunnet and Thieden, 1972). The rate of this non-ADH-mediated oxidation varied depending on the concentrations of ethanol used, from 20 to 25% (Lieber and DeCarli, 1970, 1972; Papenberg *et al.*, 1970) to half or more (Thieden, 1971; Grunnet *et al.*, 1973; Matsuzaki and Lieber, 1975) of the total ethanol metabolism. However, estimates of the magnitude of the non-ADH pathway obtained by measurements of residual ethanol metabolism after inhibition with the ADH inhibitors pyrazole or 4-methyl-pyrazole are actually underestimations, in view of the recently recognized fact that these inhibitors also reduce the activity of the microsomal alcohol-oxidizing system (Teschke *et al.*, 1977). This is also illustrated by the fact that when Rognstad (1974) used isotopic probes to assess rates of ethanol metabolism, he found the contribution of the non-ADH pathway to be 35% under conditions that yielded somewhat lower results in the presence of pyrazole. In comparing the rate of utilization of deuterated and nondeuterated ethanol by liver cells, Rognstad concluded not only that a significant non-ADH pathway exists, but also that it is unlikely that catalase contributes to its operation.

This increasing ethanol metabolism with rising ethanol concentration was not only found in the presence of an ADH inhibitor, but also could be observed in its absence, in isolated hepatocytes (Grunet *et al.*, 1973; Matsuzaki and Lieber, 1975), and in isolated perfused livers (Gordon, E. R., 1968).

That ethanol metabolism increases with rising ethanol concentrations well above the level needed to fully saturate ADH clearly indicates the involvement of an non-ADH pathway. Moreover, the acceleration of ethanol metabolism at higher ethanol concentrations explains sporadic observations, which were recently confirmed (Lereboullet *et al.,* 1976; Feinman *et al.,* 1977), that ethanol disappearance from the blood is not linear at high ethanol concentrations that fully saturate the ADH pathway. In addition to its scientific interest, the observation of nonlinearity of ethanol disappearance in the blood at high ethanol concentration is of particular significance for the medicolegal application of blood ethanol measurements. Heretofore, a common procedure to determine retrospectively the blood ethanol concentrations at a given time was to extrapolate linearly from a subsequent determination with the additional assumption of a standard rate of metabolism. In view of the recent findings corroborating the nonlinear disappearance of ethanol, and the adaptive increase after chronic consumption (discussed in the next section), conventional calculations should be interpreted with caution. Indeed, another important aspect of the non-ADH pathway is its selective involvement in the process of the adaptive increase in ethanol metabolism secondary to chronic ethanol consumption.

12.1.3. Effects of Chronic Ethanol Consumption on Ethanol Metabolism

Regular drinkers tolerate large amounts of alcoholic beverages, mainly because of CNS adaptation. In addition, alcoholics also develop increased rates of blood ethanol clearance, so-called "metabolic tolerance" (Kater *et al.*, 1969; Ugarte *et al.*, 1972). Experimental ethanol administration also results in an increased rate of ethanol metabolism (Lieber and DeCarli, 1970; Tobon and Mezey, 1971; Misra *et al.,* 1971). The mechanism of this acceleration has been the subject of debate. In *The Year in Metabolism 1975–1976* (Lieber, 1976), I discussed in detail how the theory that increased mitochondrial reoxidation of the NADH (possibly as a consequence of a "hypermetabolic state" in the liver) has been invoked to explain accelerated ethanol metabolism after chronic ethanol consumption. In addition to NADH reoxidation and acceleration of ethanol metabolism via the ADH pathway, it appeared that the MEOS is also involved. This view was supported by the observation that unlike ADH, the MEOS actually increases in activity after chronic ethanol consumption.

That chronic ethanol feeding results in an increased activity in liver tissue of a non-ADH and noncatalase pathway has now been shown in isolated hepatocytes. Liver cells were obtained from rats pair-fed with ethanol (36% of total calories) in a nutritionally adequate liquid diet for 4–6 weeks; the diet of the corresponding littermates contained additional carbohydrates instead of ethanol. With the use of this experimental model, ethanol oxidation was enhanced in isolated parenchymal liver cells by increasing the ethanol concentration employed *in vitro* from 10 to 30 mM. Of particular interest was the observation that this phenomenon was more pronounced in ethanol-fed rats than in their pair-fed controls (Teschke *et al.*, 1977). To test whether or not the MEOS is involved in this adaptive increase, ADH and catalase activities were inhibited by pyrazole and sodium azide, respectively. The activity of the non-ADH and noncatalase pathway (which is most likely due to the MEOS) was significantly higher in ethanol-fed rats than in controls. In addition, the difference between the two groups was more striking at 30 than at 10 mM. These data indicate that the MEOS represents a major mechanism for the acceleration of ethanol metabolism at high ethanol concentrations. The role of the increased activity of a non-ADH pathway to explain the accelerated ethanol metabolism in alcoholics was also shown by Salaspuro *et al.* (1975), who found that alcoholics (particularly those with poor nutrition), when given 4-methyl pyrazole (a potent ADH inhibitor), had a high residual rate of ethanol metabolism.

The MEOS pathway could contribute to the acceleration of ethanol metabolism after chronic ethanol consumption both directly and indirectly. The direct effect may be mediated by the induction of MEOS activity itself, which is known to occur after chronic ethanol feeding (Lieber and DeCarli, 1970). Indirectly increased MEOS activity might accelerate oxidation by the ADH pathway. Indeed, MEOS activity is associated with enhanced NADPH utilization, and the NADPH:NADP and NADH:NAD systems are linked (Veech *et al.*, 1969). For instance, NADH could reduce oxaloacetate to malate, which could be oxidized to pyruvate with generation of NADPH (Fig. 1). Pyruvate could regenerate the oxaloacetate in an ATP-requiring reaction. The hypothesis of the link of the oxidation of ethanol with the reduction of oxaloacetate was already proposed before (Lieber, 1968). Experimental evidence that tends to support this concept was provided more recently by Damgaard *et al.*(1972) and Grunnet and Thieden (1972), who showed the expected changes in hepatic malate and pyruvate in the presence of high concentrations of ethanol and pyrazole.

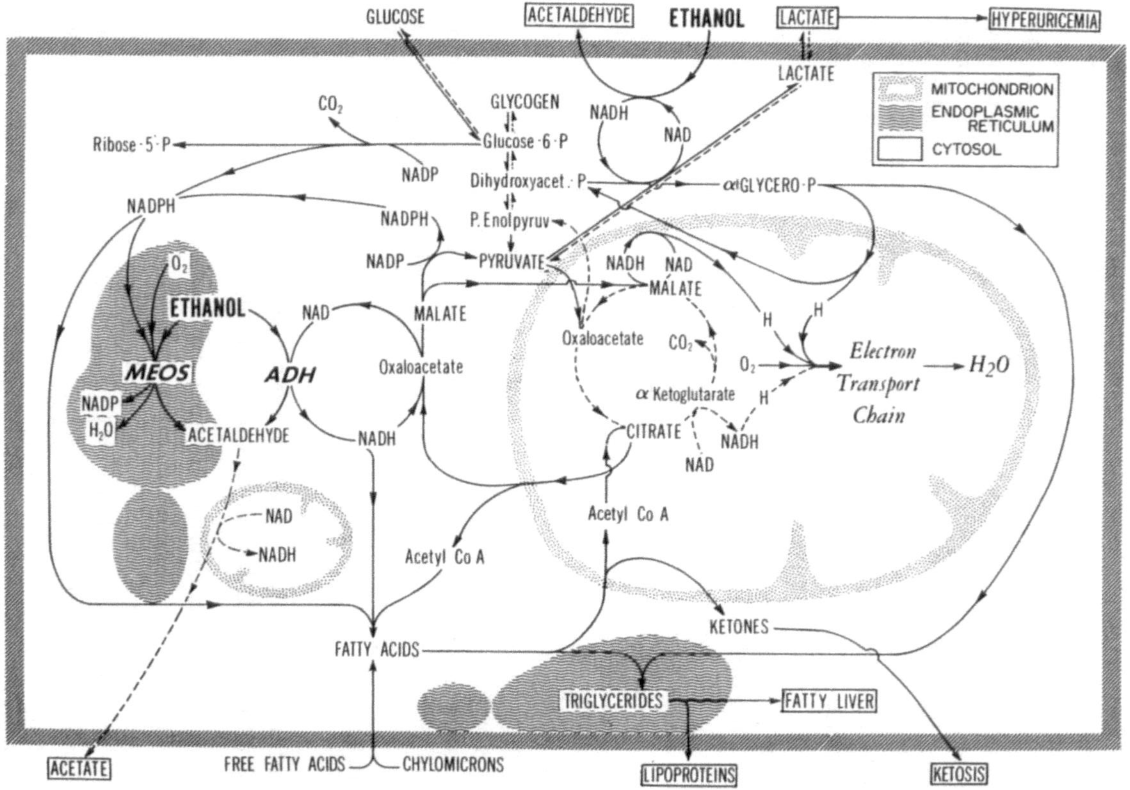

Fig. 1. Metabolism of ethanol in the hepatocyte. (---) Pathways that are decreased after ethanol abuse. (ADH) alcohol dehydrogenase; (MEOS) microsomal ethanol-oxidizing system; (NAD) nicotinamide adenine dinucleotide; (NADH) nicotinamide adenine dinucleotide, reduced form; (NADP) nicotinamide adenine dinucleotide phosphate; (NADPH) nicotinamide adenine dinucleotide phosphate, reduced form. From Lieber (1977).

It is now recognized that after chronic alcohol consumption, not only is there a quantitative increase of the activity of MEOS, but also the MEOS undergoes a qualitative change. Indeed, it was recently suggested by different groups that ethanol feeding results in the appearance of a form of cytochrome *P*-450 different by its catalytic activity. Ullrich *et al.* (1975) reported that tetrahydrofuran specifically inhibited 7-ethoxycoumarin *O*-dealkylation by microsomes of ethanol-treated rats, but not of controls. In addition, a cytochrome *P*-450 species showing high affinity for cyanide was reported as preferentially induced by ethanol (Joly *et al.*, 1972; Comai and Gaylor, 1973; Hasumura *et al.*, 1975). Moreover, SDS–polyacrylamide gel electrophoresis showed an induction of microsomal protein of 53,400 molecular weight, presumably an apoprotein of cytochrome *P*-450. The activity of azide-insensitive microsomal alcohol- (ethanol-, propanol-, butanol-) oxidizing system (MEOS) strikingly increased in ethanol-fed rats whether expressed as specific activity (nmol aldehyde/min per mg protein) or turnover number (nmol aldehyde/min per nmol cytochrome *P*-450). The partially purified cytochrome *P*-450 from ethanol-fed rats was more active for alcohol oxidation than the control preparation in the presence of an excess of NADPH-cytochrome *c* reductase and L-α-dioleoyl lecithin. There was no significant difference in the capacity of partially purified NADPH-cytochrome *c* reductase from either ethanol-fed rats or controls to promote ethanol oxidation in the presence of cytochrome *P*-450 and L-α-dioleoyl lecithin (Ohnishi and Lieber, 1977).

Studies by Joly *et al.* (1977) also showed that chronic ethanol administration to rats is associated with the appearance of a form of cytochrome *P*-450 with spectral and catalytic properties different from those of cytochrome *P*-450 of control, phenobarbital-treated, and methylcholanthrene-treated rats.

12.1.4. Influence of Liver Disease, Ethnic Background, Circadian Rhythm, and Other Factors on Ethanol Metabolism

As discussed before, chronic ethanol consumption is associated with an increase in rate of ethanol disappearance from the blood. When alcohol abuse results in severe liver disease, however, this acceleration disappears, and on occasion, there may be an actual reduction in blood alcohol clearance. This occurs, however, only with very severe liver disease shown to be associated with reduced liver ADH (Dow *et al.*, 1975). In patients with moderate cirrhosis, the rate of alcohol metabolism can be normal (Dacruz *et al.*, 1975). In general, understanding of the mechanisms responsible for changes of the rate of alcohol metabolism *in vivo* is often difficult because of the multiplicity of the factors involved. In addition to the activity of the enzymes of the pathways discussed before, total hepatic mass and blood flow through the liver are important parameters not often measureable. Availability of cofactors and the capacity of the liver to dispose of the products (NADH and acetaldehyde) also play a key role. Most studies also fail to mention the time of day they were done. Such information would be useful, however, in view of the circadian variation of ethanol metabolism (Wilson *et al.*, 1956; Sturtevant *et al.*, 1976), which is particularly manifest and perhaps even altered in the alcoholic (Jones and Paredes, 1974).

Individual differences in rates of ethanol metabolism also appear, in part, genetically controlled (Vessell *et al.*, 1971), and the possible role of heredity for the development of alcoholism in man was emphasized by Goodwin (1971). Differences in rates of ethanol metabolism (Fenna *et al.*, 1971) and sensitivity to alcohol (Wolff, 1972) according to racial background were reported. Fenna *et al.* (1971) found that blood ethanol clearance is significantly faster in Caucasians than in Eskimos and Indians, whereas Indians had a greater capacity for acceleration of blood ethanol clearance after chronic ethanol consumption. The differences could not be correlated with previous ethanol intake or dietary habits, suggesting that a genetic mechanism may be implicated, although the influence of environmental factors was not fully excluded. Moreover, the results cannot be generalized. Indeed, Ewing *et al.* (1974) found that Caucasians and Orientals did not differ significantly in their rate of ethanol metabolism, and Bennion and Li (1976) recently reported that American Indians from Arizona metabolized ethanol at the same rate as Caucasians, and that the activity of their liver ADH was the same. Specifically, no atypical form was found. In contrast, Fukui and Wakasugi (1972) observed a strikingly increased incidence of atypical ADH in the Japanese population, compared with the reported results in Caucasians (von Wartburg and Schürch, 1968; Smith *et al.*, 1971). Furthermore, recent studies carried out by Reed *et al.* (1976) in Ojibwa Indians revealed a high rate of alcohol metabolism. The same study also showed that Chinese subjects metabolize ethanol more rapidly than Caucasians. The apparent acceleration in Chinese could possibly be explained on the basis of their relative leanness compared with the Caucasians under investigation. Indeed, a difference in adipose tissue may strikingly affect calculations of ethanol metabolism as carried out by the Widmark technique. The variable results among American Indians may be understood on the basis of the considerable difference in ethnic background of the various tribes studied. On the other hand, interpretation of the results is complicated by a variable and not well defined degree of alcoholism in the assessed populations. As discussed before, chronic alcohol consumption is known to affect rates of alcohol metabolism. Moreover, the techniques used are not uniform (oral vs. intravenous alcohol administration) and do not carefully distinguish rates of ethanol metabolism at high and low blood levels. Some studies also used breath alcohol measurements, the accuracy and reproducibility of which have been seriously questioned recently (Alobaidi *et al.*, 1976). In any event, although it is likely that ethnic differences exist not only in terms of ethanol metabolism, but also with respect to physiologic responses to ethanol, additional studies are needed to define respective roles of racial background, habitual alcohol consumption, and associated nutritional factors.

12.2. Interaction of Ethanol with Androgen Metabolism

Male alcoholics with overt liver disease are known to exhibit certain hypogonadal features, such as testicular atrophy; gynecomastia is also commonly associated with alcoholic cirrhosis (Lloyd and Williams, 1948). The underlying endocrine abnormalities are complex, and result in part from increased plasma sex hormone binding protein (Galvao-Teles *et al.*, 1973), enhanced conversion of androgenic precursors to estrogens *in vivo* (Gordon, G. G., *et al.*, 1975; Baker *et al.*, 1976), and decreased catabolism of the latter (Breuer and Breuer, 1973). Recent studies have indicated that in addition to abnormalities of androgen and estrogen metabolism associated with liver disease, alcohol itself may affect androgen metabolism even prior to the development of chronic liver injury. Indeed, after feeding rats ethanol as part of a liquid diet, according to a modification of the technique described by DeCarli and Lieber (1967), Van Thiel *et al.* (1975) found atrophy of the testes and accessory sex glands (prostate and seminal vesicles) in the alcohol-treated animals. The testicular weight of isocalorically fed controls was twice that of the alcohol-treated group. The loss of testicular weight was related to reduction of mean seminiferous tubular diameter and to a decrease in the amount of germinal epithelium within the tubules. The pituitary glands did not show any histological changes in this study. Furthermore, vitamin A, which is essential for spermatogenesis (Howell *et al.*, 1967), is absorbed and transported in plasma as retinol, but peripheral oxidation to retinal is essential for activation (Olson, 1967). As in the liver and in the retina (Mezey and Holt, 1971), testicular retinal formation is dependent on ADH activity which was found to be indeed present in testes (Van Thiel *et al.*, 1974). Ethanol competitively inhibits testicular retinal formation *in vitro.* Testicular deficiency of activated vitamin A could result in the aspermatogenesis and the gonadal atrophy observed by Van Thiel *et al.* (1975). In addition, because of the ADH activity of the testicles, it is probable that ethanol ingestion is associated with high testicular concentrations of NADH, which could also alter testicular sex steroidogenesis. Specifically, the conversion of pregnenolone to progesterone, a rate-controlling step in testosterone formation, is NAD-dependent and might be inhibited by the excessive accumulation of NADH. Similarly, the 3- and 17β-OH-steroid reductases are NAD-dependent and important in androgen biosynthesis. Thus, alcohol ingestion may directly decrease testosterone biosynthesis. In addition to decreased production, enhanced testosterone degradation might also occur secondary to the "induced" activity of hepatic microsomal testosterone reductase (Rubin *et al.*, 1976). Because of decreased production and enhanced degradation, one could expect decreased plasma testosterone levels. Indeed, feeding of alcohol to mice (Badr and Bartke, 1974) and rats (Van Thiel *et al.*, 1975) resulted in decreased plasma testosterone concentration. Studies in chronic alcoholics (Mendelson and Mello, 1974) also suggested that alcohol ingestion may lower plasma testosterone. The effect of alcohol in normal nonalcoholic males was less clear, since one group showed no effect in acute studies (Toro *et al.*, 1973), while another group reported decreases in plasma levels of testosterone during the "hangover" period following the experimental administration of alcohol (Ylikahari *et al.*, 1974). A recent study by G. G. Gordon *et al.* (1976) clearly showed, however, that in normal males, relatively short-term alcohol ingestion can result in significant alterations in testosterone metabolism and blood levels. There was a decrease in the mean plasma concentration and production rate of the androgen. During the first 5 days of alcohol administration, there was initially a dampening of the episodic bursts of testosterone secretion followed by a fall in the plasma levels of the hormone. More prolonged administration of alcohol resulted in further decreases in the mean plasma level of the steroid (Fig. 2). The volunteers were maintained on adequate nutritional regimen, and none lost weight during the study, which tended to exclude a nutritional disturbance as the cause of the decreased testosterone levels. The changes in plasma luteinizing hormone suggested both a central (hypothalamus–pituitary) and gonadal effect of alcohol. In addition, alcohol consumption altered the peripheral metabolism of testosterone, as manifested by an increase in the metabolic clearance rate of testosterone in most of the subjects studied. The increased plasma clearance of testosterone may have been secondary to the combined effects of decreased plasma binding capacity for the androgen and increased hepatic testosterone A-ring reductase activity (Fig. 3), both of which were demonstrated in this study. In contrast to alcoholic cirrhosis, there were no significant changes in circulating estradiol or androstenedione or the conversion ratios of testosterone to these product steroids. Thus, the results of this study established that alcohol, *per se,* has significant effects on testosterone metabolism independent of cirrhosis or nutritional factors.

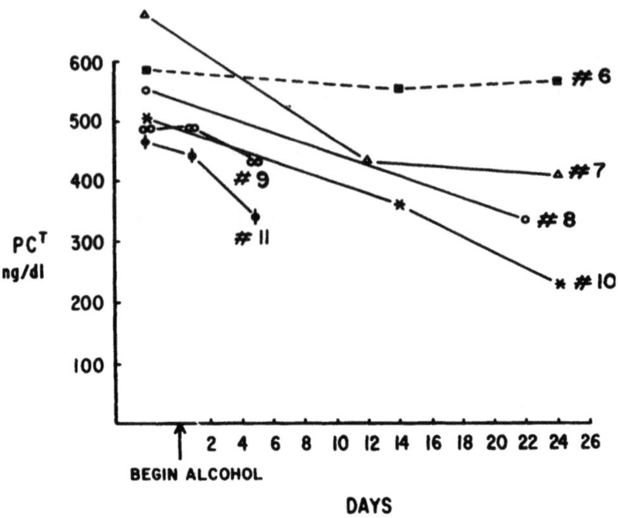

Fig. 2. Effect of 3–4 weeks of alcohol consumption on the mean plasma concentration of testosterone (PCT) in 6 normal male volunteers. Subject 6 developed gastric discomfort after 12 days on alcohol, and the dose was reduced by two-thirds. (From G. G. Gordon *et al.*, (1976).

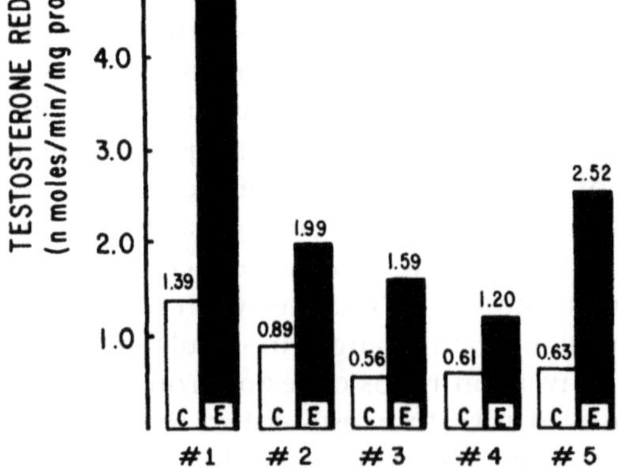

Fig. 3. Effect of alcohol (ethanol) on the activity of testosterone A-ring reductase in male volunteers measured in liver biopsy specimens. Subjects 2 and 3 are abstinent alcoholics; the other subjects are nonalcoholics. (C) Control value; (E) after ethanol administration. From G. G. Gordon *et al.* (1976).

12.3. Interaction of Ethanol with Amino Acid Metabolism

Unlike the wealth of information available concerning the interaction of ethanol with lipid and carbohydrate metabolism, its effects on amino acids are relatively uncharted. What little information is available concerns primarily the action of ethanol on brain amino acid metabolism (Noble and Tewari, 1977). However, recent investigations in the baboon fed alcohol as 50% of total calories along with an adequate diet (Lieber and DeCarli, 1974) led to the discovery of characteristic abnormalities of plasma amino acids produced by chronic but not acute ethanol consumption consisting of a six- to sevenfold increase in plasma α-amino-n-butyric acid (AANB) (Shaw and Lieber, 1975). This increase did not depend on the presence of ethanol in the blood, and was of equal magnitude in baboons that had developed steatosis and those that had developed in addition varying degrees of alcoholic hepatitis and fibrosis. Furthermore, the increase developed gradually over a period of weeks to months, thus reflecting chronic rather than acute ethanol consumption. The changes also occurred independent of the degree of liver injury.

Investigations in humans also revealed that AANB was increased by chronic but not acute alcohol consumption (Shaw and Lieber, 1976). However, the level in the plasma was also decreased by dietary protein deficiency. Indeed, clinical protein malnutrition is associated with characteristic plasma amino acid abnormalities, including a depression of branched-chain amino acids (BCAA) (Holt *et al.*, 1968). Thus, in chronic alcoholic patients, plasma amino acid abnormalities may reflect a complex interaction of many factors: nutrition, alcoholic liver disease, alcohol-induced injury in other organs, and associated disease states. The frequent concurrence of chronic alcoholism and nutritional deficiency makes the separation of these variables especially difficult. However, whereas AANB was found to be markedly increased (compared with BCAA) in the plasma of baboons fed alcohol as 50% of total calories (Shaw and Lieber, 1975), both AANB and BCAA are all depressed (and to a similar degree) when measured in protein deficiency. Therefore, as a means to correct for nutritional factors, the level of AANB was expressed relative to BCAA, used as a marker of dietary protein intake. For convenience, leucine was selected, but similar results were obtained with valine and isoleucine. In man, the plasma AANB level relative to leucine was found to be increased in the majority of alcoholics regardless of nutritional status or degree of liver injury (Shaw *et al.*, 1976, 1978). This increase persisted for days to weeks, but eventually was reversible following cessation of drinking. It did not require the presence of alcohol and was not present in nonalcoholics with liver disease of viral etiology. Furthermore, the plasma AANB level was increased in a majority of both ambulatory and hospitalized alcoholics, and there was a statistically significant positive correlation between the corrected plasma level of AANB and the amount of ethanol consumed in the recent past. Thus, the plasma AANB level (expressed relative to leucine to correct for nutritional status) provides an objective biochemical test of recent heavy drinking. Its reversibility following cessation of drinking may make it especially valuable in the monitoring and evaluation of treatment modalities for alcoholism.

It is particularly noteworthy that in baboons fed alcohol and that developed liver lesions (including steatosis, inflammation, and fibrosis) (Lieber *et al.*, 1975), the characteristic amino acid changes (especially the elevation of BCAA) differed strikingly from those observed in malnutrition; these findings indirectly support the concept that liver disease in the alcoholic can develop under metabolic conditions different from those that prevail in malnutrition. The mechanism of the amino acid changes induced by alcohol has not been fully elucidated yet. Preliminary research was conducted in the rat during chronic alcohol feeding. A threefold increase in free AANB in plasma was accompanied by a sixfold increase in the liver. Furthermore, a two- to threefold increase in hepatic production of AANB was observed in liver slices of alcohol-fed animals fasted overnight to eliminate acute effects of ethanol. These results support the thesis that chronic alcohol consumption results in increased release of AANB from the liver (Shaw and Lieber, 1977).

12.4. Effects of Ethanol on the Gastrointestinal Tract

12.4.1. Metabolic Consequences of Gastric Alterations Induced by Alcohol

It is well recognized that gastritis is commonly associated with alcoholism, and changes produced in the stomach by chronic alcohol consumption were reviewed in detail by Chey, (1972). Metabolic consequences of these changes, however, have been appreciated only recently. As a follow-up to initial studies that revealed significant blood loss associated with atrophic gastritis (Dinoso *et al.*, 1976), these investigators have now assessed the impact of alcoholic gastritis on plasma protein loss during ethanol ingestion (Chowdhury *et al.*, 1977). Albumin loss in the feces was quantitated before and during ingestion of 40% ethanol using ^{51}Cr-labeled albumin. The study included 5 subjects in each of three classifications: normal gastric mucosa, superficial gastritis, and chronic atrophic gastritis. During the control period, plasma albumin loss was minimal and similar in all three groups. Exposure to ethanol resulted in a greater output of plasma albumin in the feces of all subjects. This loss was statistically significant in subjects with superficial gastritis ($p < 0.01$) and chronic atrophic gastritis ($p < 0.005$). In each group, 2 subjects underwent gastric clearance studies of ^{51}Cr-labeled albumin. Increased GI clearance of plasma albumin was observed in all 6 subjects during ethanol ingestion; the increase was highly significant in subjects with atrophic gastritis ($p < 0.001$). The augmented loss observed in subjects with chronic atrophic gastritis is in keeping with a previous study in which greater loss of fecal red blood cells occurred in subjects with atrophic gastritis after exposure to ethanol in comparison with subjects with normal mucosa or with chronic superficial gastritis (Dinoso *et al.*, 1973). In this study, however, loss of plasma protein in the feces was considerably greater than the loss of red blood cells, and was observed to be significant also in subjects with superficial gastritis.

There are several possibilities that may account for the greater loss of plasma in subjects with chronic atrophic gastritis after ingestion of alcohol. One dose of alcohol in an amount comparable to that commonly taken by alcoholics is capable of producing hemorrhagic and exudative lesions both in the stomach and in the duodenum (Gottfried *et al.,* 1976). In subjects with previous gastritis, such a response to alcohol may be enhanced, in view of the increased susceptibility of these subjects to develop erosions in the gastric mucosa when given alcohol (Dinoso *et al.,* 1973). In any event, the study of Chowdhury *et al.* (1977) showed that ethanol ingestion can cause an increased loss of plasma proteins in the feces that may become of clinical significance in subjects with atrophic gastritis. The mechanism underlying the gastric effects of alcohol has not been elucidated as yet. It is possible that the ethanol-induced damage of gastric mucosa is at least partly due to the decreased mucosal content of cyclic AMP (cAMP). Indeed, in a study by Puurunen and Karppanen (1975), 5 and 25 min after the administration of 10% ethanol into the stomach, the gastric mucosal content of cAMP was decreased by approximately 50%. Also, *in vitro,* the mucosal content of cAMP was decreased by ethanol within 5 min. The decrease was about 30% with 2.5% ethanol and approximately 60% with 10% ethanol. Ethanol caused a concentration-dependent inhibition of the activity of the gastric mucosal adenyl cyclase. With 0.166 M (9.4%) alcohol, the inhibition was nearly 100%.

12.4.2. Metabolic Consequences of Intestinal Changes Produced by Alcohol

Alcoholics frequently experience diarrhea and abdominal colics suggestive of malabsorptive disorders. An absorption defect was documented in 10 chronic alcoholic patients within a few days of admission after an acute alcoholic episode (Krasner *et al.,* 1976). Impaired absorption of D-xylose was noted in 3 patients and low leukocyte ascorbic acid and serum folate levels in 5. No abnormality in jejunal histology was detected. The absorption of water and electrolytes from the jejunum was studied in these patients using a triple-lumen tube perfusion system. The mean rate of absorption of water in the alcoholic subjects (50.0 ± 2.3 ml/hr) was significantly lower ($p < 0.001$) than the mean value in 14 healthy control subjects 205 ± 15.9 ml/hr). Significant reduction in Na^+ and Cl^- absorption was also demonstrated in the alcoholic subjects. These results indicate that alcoholics, after acute alcohol abuse, may have a functional impairment of water and electrolyte absorption from the jejunum. This may account in part for symptoms such as diarrhea that may be present (Krasner *et al.,* 1976). Generally, however, the biochemical evidence of malabsorption correlates poorly with intestinal symptoms in the alcoholic (Lindenbaum and Lieber, 1975). Food intolerance, particularly of lactose, secondary to defective intestinal digestion could contribute to the production of these symptoms. Low lactase activity in adulthood exists in a majority of the world's population (Bayless *et al.*, 1971). Furthermore, location of lactase on the villus (Nordström *et al.*, 1968) makes it vulnerable to the corrosive effects of luminal toxins such as alcohol (Baraona *et al.*, 1974, 1975). Indeed, disaccharidase activities often decrease with intestinal injury (Herbst *et al.*, 1970; Berchtold *et al.*, 1971; Giannella *et al.*, 1971). To ascertain whether alcohol ingestion affects intestinal disaccharidase activities and influences the incidence of symptomatic lactose intolerance, lactase activity and lactose tolerance were studied in alcoholics and nonalcoholics of two human population groups with genetically determined low and high intestinal lactase levels, namely, blacks and whites (of Northern European origin) (Perlow *et al.*, 1977). After an overnight fast, biopsies of the jejunum were obtained with a Quinton Multipurpose Suction Biopsy Tube positioned fluoroscopically at the level of the ligament of Treitz. When measured within 10 days of alcohol withdrawal, sucrase activity was decreased by 33% in the alcoholics. Lactase activity was less than 1 U/g in 100% of the black and 20% of the white alcoholics as compared with 50% of the black and none of the white controls (Fig. 4). Lactase activity was virtually absent in 45% of the black alcoholics. A second jejunal biopsy following an additional 2-week period of alcohol abstinence exhibited significant secondary increases in the activities of both disaccharidases. Oral administration of lactose (1 g/kg body wt.) resulted in significantly lower blood glucose concentration and higher incidence of adverse effects in alcoholics, mainly among the blacks.

The mechanism for the disaccharidase depression in alcoholics has not been fully elucidated. Since these effects were observed in alcoholics without nutritional deficiencies, the reduction in disaccharidase activity

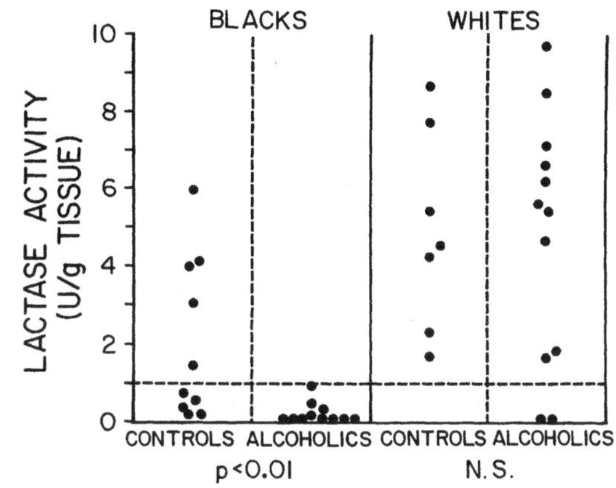

Fig. 4. Comparison of jejunal lactase activity in per oral biopsies between 21 black and 19 white males of similar nutritional status with and without a history of recent alcoholism. While 100% of black alcoholics had lactase activity lower than 1 U/g, only 50% of nonalcoholic blacks were deficient ($p<0.01$). The difference among whites was not significant. From Perlow *et al.*, (1977).

appears to be an effect of chronic alcohol ingestion *per se*. Ethanol administration to human volunteers for 3–6 days was reported to inhibit glycolytic and gluconeogenic intestinal enzyme activities (Greene *et al.*, 1974). Similar depressions of intestinal disaccharidase as well as alkaline phosphatase activities were produced in rats ingesting alcohol either acutely or chronically with nutritionally adequate diets (Baraona *et al.*, 1974). The dose of ethanol given to these rats resulted in ethanol concentrations within the intestinal lumen comparable to those found in human subjects after drinking (Halsted *et al.*, 1973). Evidence of gut injury and subsequent regeneration of intestinal epithelium was found in rats fed ethanol-containing diets (Baraona *et al.*, 1974), and in humans endoscoped after controlled alcohol administration (Gottfried *et al.*, 1976). The concomitant improvement in disaccharidase activities and increase in mitotic activity after alcohol abstinence (Perlow *et al.*, 1977) are consistent with the possibility of regeneration. It is intriguing, however, that the time required for the disaccharidase activities to improve was considerably longer than that expected for the epithelium to regenerate. This suggests that these effects of alcohol may not merely reflect villus cell desquamation, but may also alter cell renewal or maturation. The low values of lactase activity in the jejunal biopsies of alcoholics were also accompanied by poor lactose absorption, as measured by the rise in blood glucose concentration after an oral load. This indicates that the alteration produced by alcohol was not restricted to the upper segment of the jejunum, but was sufficiently extensive to impair total lactose absorption. This effect was again more apparent in the black alcoholics. Lactose malabsorption was associated with increased incidence of colic, diarrhea, and a dumping-like syndrome severe enough to require medical attention. Thus, not only may disaccharidase deficiency in alcoholics be an indication of the damaging effect of alcohol on the intestinal epithelium, but also this association may lead to increasing morbidity from primary lactase deficiency, a rather common disorder. As little as 3 g lactose was shown to produce symptoms in individuals with low intestinal lactase activity (Bedine and Bayless, 1973). Thus, milk intolerance may be unmasked or exaggerated in those populations in which both alcoholism and genetically determined low lactase levels are common. In view of the likelihood of significant milk intolerance in alcoholics, the common practice of liberal milk supplementation for "nutritional restoration" or the treatment of gastritis- or ulcer-associated symptoms should be reconsidered, particularly in ethnic groups (such as blacks) with preexisting low lactase activities.

References

Alobaidi, T. A. A., Hill, D. W., and Payne, J. P., 1976, Significance of variations in blood breath partition coefficient of alcohol, *Br. Med. J.* **2**:1479–1481.

Badr, F. M., and Bartke, A., 1974, Effect of ethyl alcohol on plasma testosterone level in mice, *Steroids* **23**:921–928.

Baker, H. W. G., Burger, H. G., DeKretser, D. M., Dulmanis, A., Hudson, B., O'Connor, S., Paulsen, C. A., Purcell, N., Rennie, G. C., Seah, C. S., Taft, H. P., and Wang, C., 1976, A study of the endocrine manifestations of hepatic cirrhosis, *Q. J. Med.* **45**:145–178.

Baraona, E., Pirola, R. C., and Lieber, C. S., 1974, Small intestinal damage and changes in cell population produced by ethanol ingestion in the rat, *Gastroenterology* **66**:226–234.

Baraona, E., Pirola, R. C., and Lieber, C. S., 1975, Acute and chronic effects of ethanol on intestinal lipid metabolism, *Biochim. Biophys. Acta.* **388**:19–28.

Bayless, T. M., Paige, D. M., and Ferry, G. D., 1971, Lactose intolerance and milk drinking habits, *Gastroenterology* **60**:605–608.

Bedine, M. S., and Bayless, T. M., 1973, Intolerance of small amounts of lactose by individuals with low lactase levels, *Gastroenterology* **65**:735–743.

Bennion, L. J., and Li, T. K., 1976, Alcohol metabolism in American Indians and whites, *New Eng. J. Med.* **294**:9–13.

Berchtold, P., Dahlqvist, A., Gustafson, A., and Asp, N.-G., 1971, Effects of a biguanide (metformin) on vitamin B_{12} and folic acid absorption and intestinal enzyme activities, *Scand. J. Gastroenterol.* **6**:751–754.

Bode, C., Goebell, H., and Stahler, M., 1970, Änderungen der Alkoholdelhydrogenase-Aktivität in der Rattenleber durch Eiweissmangel und Äthanol, *Z. Gesamte Exp. Med.* **152**:111–124.

Bode, C., Buckwald, B., and Goebell, H., 1971, Inhibition of ethanol breakdown due to protein deficiency in man, *Ger. Med.* **1**:149–150.

Bode, J. C., and Thiele, D., 1975, Hemmung des Äthanolabbaus beim Menschen durch Fasten: Reversibilität durch Fructose-Infusion, *Dtsch. Med. Wochenschr.* **100**:1849–1851.

Boveris, A., Oshino, N., and Chance, B., 1972, The cellular production of hydrogen peroxide, *Biochem. J.* **128**:617–630.

Breuer, V. J., and Breuer, H., 1973, Halbwertszeit von [4-^{14}C] Östradiol-17β *in vivo* sowie Stoffwechsel von [4-^{14}C] Östron und [4-^{14}C] Östriol *in vitro* bei Lebergesunden und bei Patienten mit Lebercirrhose, *Z. Klin. Chem. Klin. Biochem.* **11**:263–269.

Chey, W. Y., 1972, Alcohol and gastric mucosa, *Digestion* **7**:239–251.

Chowdhury, A. R., Malmud, L. S., and Dinoso, V. P., Jr., 1977, Gastrointestinal plasma protein loss during ethanol ingestion, *Gastroenterology* **72**:37–40.

Comai, K., and Gaylor, J. L., 1973, Existence and separation of three forms of cytochrome P-450 from rat liver microsomes, *J. Biol. Chem.* **248**:4947–4955.

Crow, K. E., Cornell, N. W., and Veech, R. L., 1977, The rate of ethanol metabolism in isolated rat hepatocytes, *Alcoholism: Clin. Exp. Res.* **1**:43–47.

Dacruz, A. G., Correia, J. P., and Menezes, L., 1975, Ethanol metabolism in liver cirrhosis and chronic alcoholism, *Acta Hepato-Gastroenterol.* **22**:369–374.

Damgaard, S. E., Sestoft, L., Lundquist, F., and Tygstrup, N., 1972, The interrelationship between fructose and ethanol metabolism in the isolated perfused pig liver, *Acta Med. Scand. Suppl. 542,* pp. 131–140.

DeCarli, L. M., and Lieber, C. S., 1967, Fatty liver in the rat after prolonged intake of ethanol with a nutritionally adequate new liquid diet, *J. Nutr.* **91**:331–336.

Dinoso, V. P., Jr., Meshkinpour, H., and Lorber, S. H., 1973, Gastric mucosal morphology and faecal blood loss during ethanol ingestion, *Gut* **14**:289–292.

Dinoso, V. P., Jr., Chuang, J., and Murthy, S. N. S., 1976, Changes in mucosal and venous histamine concentrations during instillation of ethanol in the canine stomach, *Dig. Dis.* **21**:93–97.

Dow, J., Krasner, N., and Goldberg, A., 1975, Relation between hepatic alcohol dehydrogenase activity and the ascorbic acid in leucocytes of patients with liver disease, *Clin, Sci. Mol. Med.* **49**:603–608.

Edwards, J. A., and Price Evans, D. A., 1967, Ethanol metabolism in subjects possessing typical and atypical liver alcohol dehydrogenase, *Clin. Pharmacol. Ther.* **8**:824–829.

Ewing, J. A., Rouse, B. A., and Pellizzari, E. D., 1974, Alcohol sensitivity and ethnic background, *Amer. J. Psychiatry* **131**:206–210.

Feinman, L., Baraona, E., Matsuzaki, S., Korsten, M., and Lieber, C. S., 1977, Concentration dependence of ethanol metabolism *in vivo* in rats and man, *Clin. Res.* **25**:269.

Fenna, D., Mix, L., Schaefer, O., and Gilbert, J. A. L., 1971, Ethanol metabolism in various racial groups, *Can. Med. Assoc. J.* **105**:472–475.

Fukui, M., and Wakasugi, C., 1972, Liver alcohol dehydrogenase in a Japanese population, *Jpn. J. Legal Med.* **26**:46–51.

Galvao-Teles, A., Anderson, D. C., Curke, C. W., and Marshall, J. S., 1973, Biologically active androgens and estradiol in men with chronic liver disease, *Lancet* **1**:173–177.

Giannella, R. A., Routh, W. R., and Toskes, P. P., 1971, Jejunal brush border injury and impaired sugar and amino acid uptake in the blind loop syndrome, *Gastroenterology* **67**:965–974.

Goodwin, D. W., 1971, Is alcoholism hereditary?, *Arch. Gen. Psychiatry* **25**:545–549.

Gordon, E. R., 1968, The utilization of ethanol by the isolated perfused rat liver, *Can. J. Physiol. Pharmacol.* **46**:609–616.

Gordon, G. G., Olivo, J., Rafii, F., and Southren, A. L., 1975, Conversion of androgen to estrogens in cirrhosis of the liver, *J. Clin. Endocrinol. Metab.* **40**:1018–1026.

Gordon, G. G., Altman, K., Southren, A. L., Rubin, E., and Lieber, C. S., 1976, Effect of alcohol (ethanol) administration on sex-hormone metabolism in normal men, *New Engl. J. Med.* **295**:793–797.

Gottfried, E. B., Korsten, M. A., and Lieber, C. S., 1976, Gastritis and duodenitis induced by alcohol: An endoscopic and histologic assessment, *Gastroenterology* **70**:890.

Greene, H. L., Stifel, F. B., Herman, R. H., Herman, Y. F., and Rosensweig, N. S., 1974, Ethanol-induced inhibition of human intestinal enzyme activities: Reversal by folic acid, *Gastroenterology* **67**:434–440.

Grunnet, N., and Thieden, H. I. D., 1972, The effect of ethanol concentration upon *in vivo* metabolic levels of rat liver, *Life Sci. (Part II)* **11**:983.

Grunnet, N., Quistorff, B., and Thieden, H. I. D., 1973, Rate-limiting factors in ethanol oxidation by isolated rat-liver parenchymal cells, *Eur. J. Biochem.* **40**:275–282.

Halsted, C. H., Robles, E. A., and Mezey, E., 1973, Distribution of ethanol in the human gastrointestinal tract, *Amer. J. Clin. Nutr.* **26**:831–834.

Hasumura, Y., Teschke, R., and Lieber, C. S., 1975, Hepatic microsomal ethanol-oxidizing system (MEOS): Dissociation from reduced nicotinamide adenine dinucleotide phosphate oxidase and possible role of Form I of cytochrome P-450, *J. Pharmacol. Exp. Ther.* **194**:469–474.

Herbst, J. J., Hurwitz, R., Sunshine, P., and Kretchmer, N., 1970, Effect of colchicine on intestinal disaccharidases: Correlation with biochemical aspects of cellular renewal, *J. Clin. Invest.* **49**:530–536.

Holt, L. E., Jr., Snyderman, S. E., Norton, P. M., and Roitman, E., 1968, The plasma aminogram as affected by protein intake, in: *Protein Nutrition and Free Amino Acid Patterns* (J. H. Leathem, ed.), pp. 32–39, Rutgers University Press, New Brunswick, New Jersey.

Horn, R. S., and Manthei, R. W., 1965, Ethanol metabolism in chronic protein deficiency, *J. Pharmacol. Exp. Ther.* **147**:385–390.

Howell, J. McC., Thompson, J. N., and Pitt, G. A. J., 1967, Changes in the tissues of guinea-pigs fed on a diet free from vitamin A but containing methyl retinoate, *Br. J. Nutr.* **21**:37–44.

Joly, J.-G., Ishii, H., and Lieber, C. S., 1972, Microsomal cyanide-binding cytochrome: Its role in hepatic ethanol oxidation, *Gastroenterology* **62**:174.

Joly, J.-G., Villeneuve, J.-P., and Mavier, P., 1977, Chronic ethanol administration induces a form of cytochrome P-450 with specific spectral and catalytic properties, *Alcoholism: Clin. Exp. Res.* **1**:17–20.

Jones, B. M., and Paredes, A., 1974, Circadian variation of ethanol metabolism in alcoholics, *Br. J. Addict.* **69**:3–10.

Kater, R. M. H., Carulli, N., and Iber, F. L., 1969, Differences in the rate of ethanol metabolism in recently drinking alcoholic and non-drinking subjects, *Amer. J. Clin. Nutr.* **22**:1608–1617.

Keilin, D., and Hartree, E. F., 1945, Properties of catalase. Catalysis of coupled oxidation of alcohols, *Biochem. J.* **39**:293–301.

Krasner, N., Cochran, K. M., Russell, R. I., Carmichael, H. A., and Thompson, G. G., 1976, Alcohol and absorption from the small intestine. I. Impairment of absorption from the small intestine in alcoholics, *Gut* **17**:245–248.

Lereboullet, J., Barres, G., and Briard, J.-P., 1976, La courbe d'alcoolemie de Widmark est-elle toujours fiable?, *Bull. Acad. Nat. Med. Paris* **160:**312–315.

Levin, W., Ryan, D., West, S., and Lu, A. Y. H., 1974, Preparation of partially purified lipid-depleted cytochrome P-450 and reduced nicotinamide adenine dinucleotide phosphate-cytochrome *c* reductase from rat liver microsomes, *J. Biol. Chem.* **249**:1747–1754.

Li, T. K., and Magnes, L. J., 1975, Identification of a distinctive molecular form of alcohol dehydrogenase in human livers with high activity, *Biochem. Biophys. Res. Commun.* **63**:202–208.

Lieber, C. S., 1968, Metabolic effects produced by alcohol in the liver and other tissues, *Adv. Intern. Med.* **14**:151–199.

Lieber, C. S., 1976, Metabolism and metabolic aspects of ethanol, in: *The Year in Metabolism 1975–1976* (N. Freinkel, ed.), pp. 317–342, Plenum Press, New York.

Lieber, C. S., 1977, *Metabolic Aspects of Alcoholism,* University Park Press, Baltimore.

Lieber, C. S., and DeCarli, L. M., 1968, Ethanol oxidation by hepatic microsomes: Adaptive increase after ethanol feeding, *Science* **162**:917–918.

Lieber, C. S., and DeCarli, L. M., 1970, Hepatic microsomal ethanol oxidizing system: *In vitro* characteristics and adaptive properties *in vivo, J. Biol. Chem.* **245**:2505–2512.

Lieber, C. S., and DeCarli, L. M., 1972, The role of the hepatic microsomal ethanol oxidizing system (MEOS) for ethanol metabolism *in vivo, J. Pharmacol. Exp. Ther.* **181**:279–288.

Lieber C. S., and DeCarli, L. M., 1974, An experimental model of alcohol feeding and liver injury in the baboon, *J. Med. Primatol.* **3**:153–163.

Lieber, C. S., DeCarli, L. M., and Rubin, E., 1975, Sequential production of fatty liver, hepatitis and cirrhosis in sub-human primates fed ethanol with adequate diets, *Proc. Natl. Acad. Sci. U.S.A.* **72**:437–441.

Lindenbaum, J., and Lieber, C. S., 1975, Effects of chronic ethanol administration on intestinal absorption in man in the absence of nutritional deficiency, *Ann. N. Y. Acad. Sci.* **252**:228–234.

Lindros, K. O., Koivula, T., and Eriksson, C. J. P., 1975, Acetaldehyde levels during ethanol oxidation: A diet-induced change and its relation to liver aldehyde dehydrogenases and redox states, *Life Sci.* **17**:1589–1598.

Lloyd, C. W., and Williams, R. H., 1948, Endocrine changes associated with Laennec's cirrhosis of the liver, *Amer. J. Med.* **4**:315–330.

Marchner, H., and Tottmar, O., 1976a, Influence of the diet on the metabolism of acetaldehyde in rats, *Acta Pharmacol. Toxicol.* **38**:59–71.

Marchner, H., and Tottmar, O., 1976b, Inhibition of the acetaldehyde dehydrogenases in rat liver by a cyanamide derivative present in a commercial standard diet for small animals, *Acta Pharmacol. Toxicol.* **39**:331–343.

Matsuzaki, S., and Lieber, C. S., 1975, ADH-independent ethanol oxidation in the liver and its increase by chronic ethanol consumption, *Gastroenterology* **69**:845.

Mendelson, J. H., and Mello, N. K., 1974, Alcohol, aggression and androgens, *Aggression* **52**:225–247.

Mezey, E., and Holt, P. R., 1971, The inhibitory effect of ethanol on retinol oxidation by human liver and cattle retina, *Exp. Mol. Pathol.* **15**:148–156.

Misra, P. S., Lefevre, A., Ishii, H., Rubin, E., and Lieber, C. S., 1971, Increase of ethanol, meprobamate and pentobarbital metabolism after chronic ethanol administration in man and in rats, *Amer. J. Med.* **51**:346–351.

Noble, E. P., and Tewari, S., 1977, Metabolic aspects of alcoholism in the brain, in: *Metabolic Aspects of Alcoholism* (C. S. Lieber, ed.), pp. 149–186, University Park Press, Baltimore.

Nordström, C., Dahlqvist, A., and Josefsson, L., 1967, Quantitative determination of enzymes in different parts of the villi and crypts of rat small intestine. Comparisons of alkaline phosphatase, disaccharidases and dipeptidases, *J. Histochem. Cytochem.* **15**:713–721.

Ohnishi, K., and Lieber, C. S., 1976, Reconstitution of the hepatic microsomal ethanol oxidizing system, *Fed. Proc. Fed. Amer. Soc. Exp. Biol.* **35**:706.

Ohnishi, K., and Lieber, C. S., 1977, Reconstitution of the microsomal ethanol-oxidizing system: qualitative and quantitative changes of cytochrome *P*-450 after chronic ethanol consumption, *J. Biol. Chem.* **252**:(in press).

Olson, J. A., 1967, The metabolism of vitamin A., *Pharmacol. Rev.* **19**:559–596.

Oshino, N., Chance, B., Sies, H., and Bücher, T., 1973, The role of H_2O_2 generation in perfused rat liver and the reaction of catalase compound I and hydrogen donors, *Arch. Biochem. Biophys.* **154**:117–131.

Oshino, N., Jamieson, D., and Chance, B., 1975, The properties of hydrogen peroxide production under hyperoxic and hypoxic conditions of perfused rat liver, *Biochem. J.* **146**:53–65.

Papenberg, J., von Wartburg, J. P., and Aebi, H., 1970, Metabolism of ethanol and fructose in the perfused rat liver, *Enzymol. Biol. Clin.* **11**:237–250.

Perlow, W., Baraona, E., and Lieber, C. S., 1977, Symptomatic intestinal disaccharidase deficiency in alcoholics, *Gastroenterology,* **72**:680–684.

Pietruszko, R., Theorell, H., and de Zalenski, C., 1972, Heterogeneity of alcohol dehydrogenase from human liver, *Arch. Biochem. Biophys.* **153**:279–293.

Puurunen, J., and Karppanen, H., 1975, Effects of ethanol on gastric acid secretion and gastric mucosal cyclic AMP in the rat, *Life Sci.* **16**:1513–1520.

Redman, C. M., Grab, D. J., and Irukulla, R., 1972, The intracellular pathway of newly formed rat liver catalase, *Arch. Biochem. Biophys.* **152**:496–501.

Reed, T. E., Kalant, H., Gibbins, R. J., Kapur, B. M., and Rankin, G., 1976, Alcohol and acetaldehyde metabolism in Caucasians, Chinese and Amerinds, *Can. Med. Assoc. J.* **115**:851–854.

Rognstad, R., 1974, Isotopic probes into pathways of ethanol metabolism, *Arch. Biochem. Biophys.* **163**:544–551.

Rognstad, R., and Clark, D. G., 1974, Tritium as a tracer for reducing equivalents in isolated liver cells, *Eur. J. Biochem.* **42**:51–60.

Rubin, E., Lieber, C. S., Altman, K., Gordon, G. G., and Southren, A. L., 1976,

Prolonged ethanol consumption increases testosterone metabolism in the liver, *Science* **191**:563–564.

Salaspuro, M. P., Lindros, K. O., and Pikkarainen, P., 1975, Ethanol and galactose metabolism as influenced by 4-methylpyrazole in alcoholics with and without nutritional deficiencies, *Ann. Clin. Res.* **7**:269–272.

Schenker, T. M., Teeple, L. J., and von Wartburg, J. P., 1971, Heterogeneity and polymorphism of human-liver alcohol dehydrogenase, *Eur. J. Biochem.* **24**:271–279.

Shaw, S., and Lieber, C. S., 1975, Plasma amino acids in alcoholic liver injury: Contrast with protein malnutrition, *Clin. Res.* **23**:459A.

Shaw, S., and Lieber, C. S., 1976, Characteristic plasma amino acid abnormalities in the alcoholic: Respective role of alcoholism, nutrition and liver injury, *Clin. Res.* **24**:291A.

Shaw, S., and Lieber, C. S., 1977, Increased plasma α-amino-n-butyric acid (AANB) due to excess hepatic production: A biochemical marker of alcoholism, *Clin. Res.* **25**:499.

Shaw, S., Stimmel, B., and Lieber, C. S., 1976, Plasma alpha-amino-n-butyric acid to leucine ratio: An empirical biochemical marker of alcoholism, *Science* **194**:1057–1058.

Shaw, S., Lue, S.-L., and Lieber, C. S., 1978, Biochemical tests for the detection of alcoholism: comparison of plasma alpha amino-n-butyric acid with other available tests, *Alcoholism: Clin. Exp. Res.* **2**:(in press).

Smith, M., Hopkinson, D. A., and Harris, H., 1971, Developmental changes and polymorphism in human alcohol dehydrogenase, *Ann. Hum. Genet. London* **34**:251–271.

Smith, M., Hopkinson, D. A., and Harris, H., 1972, Alcohol dehydrogenase isozymes in adult human stomach and liver: Evidence for activity of the ADH_3 locus, *Ann. Hum. Genet. London* **35**:243–253.

Sturtevant, F. M., Sturtevant, R. P., Scheving, L. E., and Pauly, J. E., 1976, Chronopharmacokinetics of ethanol. II. Circadian rhythm in rate of blood level decline in a single subject, *Naunyn-Schmiedeberg's Arch. Pharmakol.* **293**:203–208.

Teschke, R., Hasumura, Y., and Lieber, C. S., 1974, Hepatic microsomal ethanol oxidizing system: Solubilization, isolation and characterization, *Arch. Biochem. Biophys.* **163**:404–415.

Teschke, R., Hasumura, Y., and Lieber, C. S., 1976, Hepatic ethanol metabolism: Respective role of alcohol dehydrogenase, the microsomal ethanol oxidizing system and catalase, *Arch. Biochem. Biophys.* **175**:635–643.

Teschke, R., Matsuzaki, S., Ohnishi, K., DeCarli, L. M., and Lieber, C. S., 1977, Microsomal ethanol oxidizing system (MEOS): Current status of its characterization and its role, *Alcoholism: Clin. Exp. Res.* **1**:7–15.

Thieden, H. I. D., 1971, The effect of ethanol concentration on ethanol oxidation rate in rat liver slices, *Acta Chem. Scand.* **25**:3421–3427.

Thurman, R. G., and Brentzel, H. J., 1977, The role of alcohol dehydrogenase in microsomal ethanol oxidation and the adaptive increase in ethanol metabolism due to chronic treatment with ethanol, *Alcoholism: Clin. Exp. Res.* **1**:33–38.

Tobon, F., and Mezey, E., 1971, Effect of ethanol administration on hepatic ethanol and drug-metabolizing enzymes and on rates of ethanol degradation, *J. Lab. Clin. Med.* **77**:110–121.

Toro, G., Kolodny, R. C., Jacobs, L. S., Masters, W. H., and Daughaday, W. H., 1973, Failure of alcohol to alter pituitary and target organ hormone levels, *Clin. Res.* **21**:505.

Ugarte, G., Pereda, T., Pino, M. E., and Iturriaga, H., 1972, Influence of alcohol intake, length of abstinence and meprobamate on the rate of ethanol metabolism in man, *Q. J. Stud. Alcohol* **33**:698–705.

Ullrich, V., Weber, P., and Wollenberg, P., 1975, Tetrahydrofurane—an inhibitor for ethanol-induced liver microsomal cytochrome P-450, *Biochem. Biophys. Res. Commun.* **64**:808–813.

Van Thiel, D. H., Gavaler, J., and Lester, R., 1974, Ethanol inhibition of vitamin A metabolism in the testes: Possible mechanism for sterility in alcoholics, *Science* **186**:941–942.

Van Thiel, D. H., Gavaler, J. S., Lester, R., and Goodman, M. D., 1975, Alcohol-induced testicular atrophy. An experimental model for hypogonadism occurring in chronic alcoholic men, *Gastroenterology* **69**:326–332.

Veech, R. L., Eggleston, L. V., and Krebs, H. A., 1969, The redox state of free nicotinamide-adenine dinucleotide phosphate in the cytoplasm of rat liver, *Biochem. J.* **115**:609-619.

Vesell, E. S., Page, J. G., and Passananti, G. T., 1971, Genetic and environmental factors affecting ethanol metabolism in man, *Clin. Pharmacol. Ther.* **12**:192–201.

von Wartburg, J. P., and Schürch, P. M., 1968, Atypical human liver alcohol dehydrogenase, *Ann. N. Y. Acad. Sci.* **151**:936–946.

von Wartburg, J. P., Papenberg, J., and Aebi, H., 1965, An atypical human alcohol dehydrogenase, *Can. J. Biochem.* **43**:889–898.

Wilson, R. H. L., Newman, E. J., and Newman, H. W., 1956, Diurnal variation in rate of alcohol metabolism, *J. Appl. Physiol.* **8**:556–558.

Wolff, P. H., 1972, Ethnic differences in alcohol sensitivity, *Science* **175**:449–450.

Ylikahari, R., Huttumen, M., Harkonen, M., and Adlercrentz, H., 1974, Letter to the editor: Hangover and testosterone, *Br. Med. J.* **2**:445.

Index

AANB, *see* α-amino-*n* butyric acid
ABMT, *see* Average basement membrane thickness
A-cell glucoreceptor, 112
Acetaldehyde metabolism, alcohol dehydrogenase and, 411-413
Acetazolamide, 349
Acetohydroxamic acid, in renal stone disease, 406
Acetylcholine, cGMP and, 12
Acidosis, electrolyte loss in, 175
Acyl-CoA dehydrogenases, inhibition of by methylenecyclopropylacetic acid, 241-244
ADA (adenosine deaminase)
  cofomycin and, 265
  in drug action and metabolism, 268-269
  immunodeficiency disease and, 265
  in monocyte maturation, 264
  tissue distribution and, 274
  tissue forms of, 274-275
ADA activity
  genetic heterogeneity of, 275
ADA activity (*cont'd*)
  in hereditary hemolytic anemia, 277-278
  inhibition of, 266
  residual, 275
ADA deficiency, 255-256
  frequency of, 270
  metabolic consequences of, 272-274
  metabolic studies of, 270-271
  pathological mechanism of, 275-277
  purine metabolism and, 273
  SCID and, 269-277
  treatment of, 271-272
Adenine arabinoside, 268, 306
Adenine metabolism, 273
Adenine phosphoribosyltransferase deficiency, 254-256, 295-298
  in cell culture, 298
  clinical presentation of, 295-298
  in erythrocytes, 297
  genetics of, 298
  purine metabolites in, 297-298
  therapy in, 297
  urinary calculi in, 296-297

Adenosine
in adenine nucleotide synthesis, 276-277
toxicity of, 273
Adenosine deaminase, *see* ADA
Adenosine metabolism, mitogenic stimulation of, 266
Adenosine kinase, in gouty arthritis, 300
Adenosine toxicity, 268
Adenosine triphosphate
in ADA deficiency, 270-271
conversion of to cAMP, 8, 330
guanylate cyclase and, 6
intracellular compartmentalization of, 263
Adenylate cyclase activity, increase in, 4
Adenylic acid cycle, in ammonia production, 258-260
ADH, *see* Alcohol dehydrogenase
Adipose mass, obesity and, 173
Adrenalectomy, cGMP and, 11-12, 22
α-adrenergic agonists, cGMP and, 13
Alanine aminotransferase, 390
Alanine synthesis, in muscle, 153-156
Alcohol, *see also* Ethanol
intestinal changes produced by, 425-428
Alcohol consumption, *see also* Ethanol metabolism
alcohol metabolism and, 415-418
liver and, 416
Alcohol dehydrogenase, in ethanol metabolism, 411-413
Alcoholic cirrhosis, vitamin D and, 347-348
Alcoholic gastritis, 424
Alcoholics
jejenum of, 426-427
lactase activity in, 427-428
sucrase activity in, 426
water and electrolyte absorption in, 426
Alcoholics Anonymous, 178
Alcoholism, α-amino-*n*-butyric acid level in, 423
Allopurinol
orotic aciduria and, 305-306
in oxypurine excretion, 289
Alloxan diabetes, insulin secretion in, 45
American Heart Association, 209
American Indians, diabetes in, 55
American Journal of Clinical Nutrition, 179
American Medical News, 174
Amino acid metabolism, 153-157
ethanol and, 423-424
glucagon and, 110
Amino acids
branched-chain, 156-157, 423
in glucagon secretion, 113
malnutrition and, 381-382
metabolism of, 219-238
transport of in γ-glutamyl cycle, 235-238
α-Amino-*n*-butyric acid, 423
Ammonia
adenylic acid cycle and, 260
purines in production of, 258-260
Amylase secretion, cGMP and, 18
Androgen metabolism, ethanol and, 420-422
Anemia, hereditary hemolytic, 277-278
Angiotensin, cGMP and, 17
Anticonvulsants, vitamin D and, 348
Antipancreatic autoimmunity, 39
Antiviral drugs, 306
APRT, *see* Adenine phosphoribosyltransferase deficiency
Ara-A (adenine arabinoside), 268, 306
Arabian horses, immunodeficiency disease in, 274
9-β-D-arabinofuranosyl-adenine, 268
Ara-C (cytosine arabinoside), 306
Arachidonic acid, 14
Arginine deficiency, pyridine metabolism and, 305
Arthritis, gouty, *see* Gouty arthritis
Aspartate transcarbamylase, 304
Aspermatogenesis, ethanol and, 420
ATP, *see* Adenosine triphosphate
ATP/ADP ratio, in cytosol, 263
Autonomic neuropathy, diabetes and, 75-76
Average basement membrane thickness, in diabetes, 65
Azaserine, 262
Azide, cGMP and, 15-16

Basement membrane lesions, of diabetes, 64
Basement membrane thickening, in diabetes, 64-66
Behavior modification, in obesity treatment, 176-178
Beta-adrenergic receptors, isoprotenol and, 261

Beta-cell secretory products, measurement of, 48-49
Big plasma glucagon, 104
Bihormonal abnormality hypothesis, 123-126
Bihormonal unit, concept of, 110-111
Biliary cirrhosis, vitamin D and, 347
Birmingham Diabetes Survey (1961), 56
Blindness, in diabetes mellitus, 66-68
Body fuel metabolism, 143-163
  amino acid metabolism and, 153-157
  in exercise, 160-163
  fatty acid metabolism and, 157-159
  glucose metabolism and, 143-153
  ketone metabolism and, 157-159
Bone, calcium and phosphate in, 328
Bone cells, vitamin D and, 340
BPG, *see* Big plasma glucagon
Brain, ammonia production and, 258
Branched-chain amino acids, 156-157, 423
Broad-beta disease, 193
8-bromo cGMP, 19
Butyrylglycine, 243

Calcitonin, 327
Calcium
  in bone, 328
  cGMP levels and, 14
  in glucagon secretion, 113-114
  renal handling of, 331
  vitamin D and, 333, 339
Calcium absorption
  in uremia, 352
  vitamin D and, 337
Calcium-binding protein, 337-338
Calcium diet, in renal stone disease, 407
Calcium homeostasis, regulation of, 327-356
Calcium oxalate stones, 399
cAMP (adenosine 3′-5′-cyclic phosphate)
  ATP conversion to, 8, 330
  beta-adrenergic receptors and, 261
  binding proteins for, 268
  in cell growth and proliferation, 19
  in cystic fibrosis, 22
  free, 8
  in glucagon secretion, 114
  guanylate cyclases and, 3-8
  in immunosuppression, 267-268
  mRNA and, 10-11
  in parathyroid disorders, 21
cAMP (*cont'd*)
  parathyroid hormone and, 17, 366
  propranolol and, 262
  tissue content reduction in, 8
  tumors and, 20-21
cAMP concentrations, refractoriness of, 9
cAMP hydrolysis, 9
cAMP level
  guanylate cyclase and, 5
  variation in, 1-2
cAMP metabolism, compared with cGMP, 3
cAMP synthesis, prostaglandins and, 13-14
Canine tissues, IRG moieties of, 104
Capping of receptors, 266
Carbachol, cGMP and, 12-13
Carbamylphosphate synthetase, 304
Carbohydrate, in diabetes, 81-82
Carnitine, 243
Catecholamines, cGMP and, 17
Cell growth
  cGMP and, 19
  malnutrition and, 379-386
Cerebral edema, ketoacidosis and, 84
Cerebrotendinous xanthomatosis, 203-204
cGMP (cyclic guanosine monophosphate)
  adrenalectomy and, 11-12, 22
  α-adrenergic agonists and, 13
  amylase secretion and, 18
  angiotensin and, 17
  azide and, 15-16
  biogenic amines and other agents in relation to, 1-22
  calcium and, 14-15
  carbachol and, 12-13
  in cell growth and proliferation, 19
  catecholamines and, 17
  choline esters and, 12-13
  in Cushing's disease, 22
  in cystic fibrosis, 22
  different pools of, 7
  discovery of, 2
  in extracellular fluids, 8-9
  formation and degradation of, 3-11
  heart and, 18
  histamine and, 16-19
  hydroxylamine and, 15-16
  hypophysectomy and, 11-12, 22
  insulin and, 20
  in intestinal mucosa, 18
  metabolism and, 1-22

cGMP (*cont'd*)
nitrosamines and, 16
in parathyroid disorders, 21
parathyroid hormone and, 16
in PHA stimulation, 267
phosphodiesterase inhibitors and, 17
physiologic effects and, 17-20
prostaglandins and, 13-14
regulation of in tissues, 11-17
serotonin and, 14-15
smooth-muscle contraction and, 17-18
thymidine and, 263
tumors and, 20-21
in urine, 2, 11
cGMP levels, acetylcholine and, 12
cGMP metabolism, compared with cAMP, 3
Chemical diabetes, 56-58, *see also* Diabetes mellitus
Chenodeoxycholic acid, 204
Children
Lesch-Nyhan syndrome,in, 254
purine overproduction in, 253-254
Cholestanol, 204
Cholesterol level
in Pima Indians, 73-74
probucol and, 210-211
Cholesterol metabolism, 194-198
in cultured cells, 196-199
in intact humans, 194-196
LDL receptors in, 196-198
production rate for, 195
Cholestyramine, 210
oxalate excretion and, 402-403
Cholinesterase-resistant analogue, cGMP and, 12
Choline esters, cGMP and, 12-13
Choreoathetosis, 291
Ciba Foundation Symposium, 256-257
Circadian rhythm, ethanol metabolism and, 418
Cirrhosis, vitamin D and, 347-348
Coformycin
adenosine deaminase and, 265
toxic effects of, 276
Colestipol hydrochloride, 210
Collagen, vitamin D and, 340
Connecting peptide, beta-cell secretory products and, 48-49
Coronary Drug Project, 210
Coronary heart disease, *see also* Heart disease
Coronary heart disease (*cont'd*)
high-density-lipoprotein levels and, 189-193
hypertryglyceridemia and, 206-207
C-peptide, *see* Connecting peptide
CTX, *see* Cerebrotendinous xanthomatosis
Cushing's disease, cGMP and, 22
Cyclic AMP, *see* cAMP
Cyclic GMP, *see* cGMP
Cyclic nucleotide phosphodiesterases, 8-10
forms of, 9
Cyclic nucleotide protein kinases, 10-11
Cyclic nucleotides, *see also* cAMP; cGMP
clinical studies with, 20-22
enzymatic degradation of, 8-9
in extracellular fluids, 21-22
in parathyroid disorders, 21
psoriasis and, 20
in tissues, 20
in tumors, 20-21
Cystic fibrosis, cyclic nucleotides and, 22
Cytosine arabinoside, 306

Diabetes mellitus, 33-88
A-cell function in, 123
adrenergic activity in, 46
aging in, 77-78
alloxan diabetes and, 45
in American Indians, 54-55
autoimmunity in, 38-42
autonomic neuropathy and, 75-76
basement membrane lesions of, 64
basement membrane thickening in, 64-66
biochemical studies in, 64
blindness in, 66-68
blood glucose control in, 59
carbohydrates in, 81-82
cell-mediated immunity in, 41-42
chemical, *see* Chemical diabetes
chemical agents in, 42-43
chronic therapy in, 85
control of, 59-62
diabetic microangiopathy and, 62
diabetic retinopathy in, 66-69
diet in, 79-82
environmental factors in, 42-43
epidemiological findings in, 54-59
exercise and, 161-163
genetic heterogeneity of, 33-43
genetic susceptibility to, 34-36
glucagon and, 53, 123-129
glycosylated hemoglobin and, 60-62

Diabetes mellitus (*cont'd*)
growth disturbances in, 77-78
heart rate and, 76
heterogeneity of, 33-54
HLA system and, 34-36, 40-42
hyperaldosteronism and, 72-73
hyperglycemia and, 33, 59
hyperketonemia in, 158-159
insulin deficiency in, 124
insulin receptors in, 52-53
insulin release to glucose in, 45-46
insulin-requiring, 43
insulin resistance in, 49-54
insulin response heterogeneity in, 43-44
insulin secretion in, 43-48
insulin treatment in, 82-86
juvenile onset type, *see* Juvenile-onset-type diabetes
ketoacidosis and, 82-85
kidney damage in, 69-74
lipoatrophy and, 85
long-term complications in, 62-78
microvascular permeability changes in, 63-64
oral glucose tolerance test-sugar area in, 80
oral hypoglycemia treatment and, 86-88
phenformin in, 87-88
plasma glucose levels in, 45-46
plasma protein changes in, 62-63
plasma renin activity in, 72
post-glucose plasma level in, 54-56
in pregnancy, 78-79
renal failure in, 70-71
somatostatin and, 54
sulfonylureas in, 86-87
susceptibility to, 34-36
treatment of, 79-88
type A and type B patients in, 53
virus-induced, 36-38, 423
vitamin D and, 354
Diabetic ketoacidosis, 73
Diabetic macroangiopathy, 73-75
Diabetic microangiopathy, 62
Diabetic nephropathy, 69-73
clinical course in, 71
lesions in, 69-70
treatment in, 71-72
Diabetic neuropathy, 75-78
postural hypotension and, 75
prevention and treatment of, 78
Diabetic retinopathy, 66-69
Diadenosine tetraphosphate, 262
Dihydrobiopterin, 221
Dihydrofolate reductase, 222
Dihydropteridine reductase deficiency, 224-226
Diphenolhydantoin, osteomalacia and, 351
Divalent ion metabolism, 327-367
see also Calcium metabolism; Magnesium metabolism; phosphate metabolism; Vitamin D
DNA, cyclic nucleotides and, 20
DNA polymerase
in adipose tissue, 386-388
cell growth and, 384
DNA synthesis
in malnutrition, 383-385
nucleotide pool and, 381
DOPA, tyrosine hydroxylation to, 225
Dysbetalipoproteinemia, 193

EHNA, *see* Erythro-9-(2-hydroxy-3-nonyl) adenine
Electron-transferring flavoprotein, 244, 246
Encephalomyocarditis virus, 37, *see also* EMC diabetes
Endocrine pancreas, morphofunctional interrelationships of, 120
Epinephrine-induced hyperglucagonemia, 114
Erythrocyte metabolism, in PNP deficiency, 283-284
Erythro-9-(2-hydroxy-3-nonyl) adenine, 264-268
ADA activity and, 266
cell line killing by, 268
toxic effects and, 276
Escherichia coli, 5
ETF, *see* Electron-transferring flavoprotein
Ethanol, *see also* Alcohol; Alcoholism
amino acid metabolism in, 423-424
gastrointestinal tract and, 424-428
intestinal changes produced by, 425-428
Ethanol consumption, metabolism and, 411-420
Ethanol metabolism
androgen metabolism and, 420-422
ethnic background and, 418-420
liver disease and, 418
testosterone and, 421
Ethanol oxidation, non-ADH pathways for, 413-415, *see also* Ethanol metabolism

Ethnic background, in ethanol metabolism, 418-420
Euglycemia, glucose infusion and, 151
Exercise
 fuel metabolism in, 160-163
 insulin and, 161-163
Extracellular fluids, cyclic nucleotides and, 21-22

Familial hypercholesterolemia, 195, 199-203
 genetics of, 199
 therapy for, 201-202
 pathogenesis of, 199-201
Fat metabolism, in fetal liver, 391
Fatty acid metabolism, 157-159
Fatty acid oxidation, hypoglycin and, 240
Fatty acids, glucose-sparing effect and, 160-161
Fetal malnutrition, 389-392
FH, *see* Familial hypercholesterolemia
Fibroblasts
 in purine nucleoside phosphorylase deficiency, 283-284
 cholesterol metabolism in, 196
Flavoprotein, electron-transferring, 244, 246
Fuel, body, *see* Body fuel

Gastric inhibitory polypeptide, 47-48
Gastrointestinal D cells, role of, 120
Gastrointestinal tract, ethanol and, 424-428
GCTP, *see* γ-glutamyltranspeptidase
Genetic obesity, 386-389, *see also* Obesity
 animal models of, 387-388
GIP, *see* Gastric inhibitory polypeptide
GLI, *see* Glucagonlike immunoreactivity
Glomerulosclerosis, nodular intercapillary, 71
Glucagon, *see also* Hyperglucagonemia
 amino acids and, 113
 β-adrenergic mechanism and, 114
 bihormonal abnormality hypothesis in, 124-126
 calcium and, 113-114
 cAMP and, 114
 clearance and degradation of, 106-107
 in clinical medicine, 123-129
 defined, 101
 effects on lipids and ketones, 110
 extrapancreatic, 116-117
 in fuel homeostasis, 109
Glucagon (*cont'd*)
 gastrointestinal hormones and, 114-115
 in gluconeogenic pathway, 108
 growth hormone and, 115
 in hepatic ketogenesis, 109
 immunoreactive, *see* Immunoreactive glucagon
 physiologic actions of, 107-109
 prostaglandins and, 115
 immunologic relationships in, 105
 immunoreactive, 101-104
 neurotensin and, 115
 structure of, 101-102
 structure-function relationships in, 104-106
 transitory nature of, 148
Glucagon actions, molecular basis for, 106
Glucagon biosynthesis, 102-103
"Glucagonlike immunoreactivity," 102
Glucagon metabolism, 106-107
Glucagonoma syndrome, 104, 112, 127-129
Glucagon secretion
 control of, 111-113
 glucose and, 112
Glucocorticoids, glucagon and, 115
Gluconeogenesis, 108-109
 glutaryl CoA in, 244
 insulin/glucagon ratio in, 111
 in starvation, 147
Glucose
 as fuel, 111-112
 in glucagon secretion, 112
Glucose absorption, somatostatin and, 143-145
Glucose-fatty acid cycle, 160-161
Glucose ingestion, exercise and, 160-161
Glucose intolerance, as insulin-receptor disorder, 53
Glucose metabolism, body fuel and, 143-146
Glucose production, 145-151
 during protein meals, 109-110
 maintenance of, 109
 protein ingestion and, 145-146
 starvation and, 146-148
Glucose-tolerance tests, 38
 blood glucose level and, 56
 diabetes control and, 61
 insulin levels in, 49-50
 in pregnancy, 79
Glucose uptake, insulin and, 51-52

γ-Glutamyl cycle, 219, 229, 231-232
in amino acid transport, 235-238
γ-Glutamyl cyclotransferase, 232-233
γ-Glutamyltranspeptidase, 231
Glutaric aciduria, 219
type II, 238-246
Glutathione, 231
Glycerol, circulating, 158
Glycogen, carcass, 147
Glycogenolysis
hepatic, 107-108
in starvation, 147
Glycogen storage disease, uric acid in, 300
Glycosylated hemoglobin, diabetic control and, 60-62
Gout, metabolic abnormalities in, 299-301, *see also* Gouty arthritis
Gouty arthritis, 299-304
clinical features of, 301
kidney and, 303
monosodium urate crystal in, 302-303
treatment of, 303-304
urate deposition in, 301-302
Growth, nutrition and, 379-392
Growth hormone
in DNA synthesis, 381
metabolism of, 391
role of, 380
GSH concentration, in sheep and rabbit erythrocytes, 236-237, *see also* Glutathione
GTP, *see* Guanosine triphosphate
GTT, *see* Glucose tolerance tests; *see also* Chemical diabetes
Guanase deficiency, in lymphoblast lines, 284
Guanylate cyclase
arachidonic acid and, 14
ATP and, 6
detergents and, 4-6
in formation and degradation of cGMP, 3-8
GTP and, 6-7
multiple forms of, 6
particulate nature of, 4
Guthrie test, in phenylketonuria, 225

HDL, *see* High-density lipoprotein levels
Heart, cGMP and, 18
Heart disease, hyperlipidemia and, 211-212, *see also* Coronary heart disease
Hemodialysis, hyperlipidemia in, 208
Hemoglobin A_{1C}, in diabetes control, 61
Hemolytic anemia, ADA activity in, 277-278
Hepatic glucose production
exercise and, 110
increase in, 51-52
maintenance of, 109-110
Hereditary hemolytic anemia, ADA activity in, 277-278
Herpes hominis, 306
HGP, *see* Hepatic glucose production
High-density lipoprotein, possible mechanisms of, 192-193
Histamine release, cGMP and, 16-19
Histocompatibility system, 34-36, *see also* HLA antigens
HLA antigens
diabetes and, 34-36
pancreatic islet cell antibodies and, 40
and virus-induced diabetes, 36-38
HLA-B8 antigens, 35
HLA-BW15 antigens, 35
HLA-CW3 antigens, 35
HLA-DW3 antigens, 35
HLA-DW4 antigens, 35
HMG CoA reductase activity, 197
Hormones, glucagon and, 114-115, *see also* Growth hormones
HPRT, *see* Hypoxanthine-guanine phosphoribosyltransferase
Hunger, starvation and, 176
Hydrochloric acid, somatostatin and, 119
β-hydroxybutyrate/acetoacetate ratio, 159
Hydroxylamine, cGMP and, 15-16
Hydroxylation system, phenylalanine and, 221-222
5-Hydroxytryptophan, HPRT deficiency and, 291
25-Hydroxyvitamin D_3, 333-343, *see also* Vitamin D
alcoholism and, 348
defective production of, 347
in renal failure, 353
Hyperalpha lipoproteinemia, 191-192
Hyperammonemia, with orotic aciduria, 305
Hypercalciuria, 361
renal stone disease and, 401-402
Hypercholesterolemia, 195
colestipol hydrochloride in, 210
familial, 199-203
Hyperglucagonemia
in accelerated starvation, 391

Hyperglucagonemia (*cont'd*)
arginine and, 123-124
of cirrhosis, 115
evanescent effects of, 148-151
Hyperglycemia
diabetes mellitus and, 33-34, 59
endogenous, 125
exogenous, 125
postprandial, 126
Hyperketonemia, ketone disposal in, 158-159
Hyperlipidemias, 187-189, 195
definition and classification of, 187-188
diet in, 208-209
drugs used in, 210-211
epidemiology of, 188-189
ischemic heart disease and, 211-212
partial ileal bypass surgery in, 211
renal failure and, 207-208
treatment of, 208-212
Hyperlipoproteinemia, type III, 193-194
Hyperparathyroidism, 350, 360
renal stone disease and, 401
Hyperphagia
defense of, 173
as learned behavior, 177
Hyperphenylalaninemia, benign, 223-224
Hypertriglyceridemia, 204-207
coronary heart disease and, 206-207
insulin in, 205
Hyperuricemia, 291
in gouty arthritis, 299
Hyperuricosuria, renal stone disease and, 403, 407
Hypervitaminosis D, phosphate depletion in, 361
Hypoaldosteronism, diabetes mellitus and, 72-73
Hypocalcemia
hypomagnesia and, 366
in jejunoileal shunt, 179
Hypocalcemic phase, of PTH action, 331
Hypogammaglobulinemia
clinical presentation of, 287-288
purine nucleotidase deficiency in, 286-287
Hypoglucagonemia, somatostatin and, 149-150
Hypoglycemia
insulin, 152-153
neonatal, 153
sulfonylureas in, 86-87
Hypoglycin
fatty acid oxidation and, 240
metabolic effects of, 239-241
structure of, 239
Hypomagnesia, hypocalcemia and, 365-366
Hypophosphatemia, phosphate depletion and, 360-361
Hypophosphaturia, phosphate depletion and, 361
Hypophysectomy, cGMP and, 11-12, 22
Hypothyroidism, cell division and, 380
Hypotonia, 255
Hypoxanthine
differentiation and, 264
in HPRT-deficient cells, 261
in Lesch-Nyhan syndrome, 285
in purine metabolism, 258
Hypoxanthine-guanine phosphoribosyltransferase deficiency, 256, 289-294
chemical correlations with, 290-291
enzyme abnormality in, 292
erythrocyte differentiation and, 264
genetics of, 293-294
other conditions associated with, 294
purine overproduction in, 293

ICA, *see* Pancreatic-islet-cell antibodies
"Idiopathic stone-formers," 399, 403, *see also* Renal stone disease
Ileal bypass surgery, in hyperlipidemia, 211
Immunoreactive glucagon, 103-104, 106, 108, 112-116
calcium and, 120
glucagonoma and, 127-129
radioimmunoassay for, 116
somatostatin and, 120
Indian Health Service, 56
Inosine triphosphate, in NTPH deficiency, 298-299
Insulin
cGMP and, 20
in diabetic retinopathy, 68
in diabetes treatment, 82-86
in endogenous hypertriglyceridemia, 205
exercise and, 161-163
hepatic glucose output and, 151
hypoglycemia effects of, 152
ketoacidosis and, 82-85
in ketone utilization, 159
Insulin binding, in type A and type B patients, 53

Insulin hypoglycemia, counterregulation during, 152-153
Insulin-induced lipoatrophy, 86
Insulin-receptors
disorders of, 53-54
insulin binding to, 52-54
Insulin release, inhibition and stimulation of in diabetes, 46
Insulin resistance
in diabetes, 49-54
evidence for, 49-50
mechanism of, 52-54
Insulin secretion
in diabetes mellitus, 43
mechanism of, 44-48
Insulin standard groups, 86
Insulin-variable groups, 86
Interfering factor, glucagon and, 104
Intestinal mucosa, cGMP and, 18
IPTH, *see* Parathyroid hormone immunoassay
IQ scores, in phenylketonuria, 227
IRG, *see* Immunoreactive glucagon
Ischemic heart disease, primary prevention of, 211-212
ISF, *see* Stone-formers, idiopathic
Islet cell antibodies, 38-40, *see also* Pancreatic-islet-cell antibodies, ICA
Islets of Langerhans
somatostatin and, 120
subcellular specialization in, 121
transplantation of, 78
Isoleucine, oxidation of, 242
Isovalerylglycine, 242-243

Jamaican vomiting sickness, 219, 238-239
recent studies in, 244-245
Jejunoileal shunt, in obesity treatment, 179-180
Jejunum, in alcoholics, 426-427
JOD, *see* Juvenile-onset-type diabetes
Juvenile-onset-type diabetes, 34-36
carbohydrate intolerance in, 43
glucagon suppression in, 126-127
growth disturbances in, 77-78
pancreatic-islet-cell antibodies in, 38-39

Ketoacidosis, 125
cerebral tumor and, 84-85
in diabetes mellitus, 82-85
lactic acidosis and, 88
Ketogenesis
hormonal regulation of, 157-158
glucagon and, 109
substrate regulation of, 158
Ketone disosal, in hyperketonemia, 158-159
Ketosis, as counterforce to hunger, 175
Kidney
calcium handling by, 355-356
extracellular volume expansion in, 359
in magnesium homeostasis, 364-365
parathyroid hormone and, 331-332
phosphate metabolism and, 356-359
uric acid and, 303
vitamin D metabolism in, 334-336
Kidney transplants, in diabetic patients, 70-71

Lactic acidosis, ketoacidosis and, 88
Last Chance Diet, The, 174
LDL, *see* Low-density lipoproteins
LDL receptor, 196
bypassing of, 198
in familial hypercholesterolemia, 200
Lecithin/sphingomyelin ratios, 392
Lesch/Nyhan syndrome, 254, 256, 285
HPRT deficiency and, 261
PNP deficiency and, 285
Lipid metabolism, *see* Lipoprotein metabolism
Lipids, glucagon and, 110
Lipoatrophy, in diabetes mellitus, 85
Lipoprotein Lp(a), 185-186
Lipoproteinemia, familial hyperalpha and familial hyperbeta, 191-192
Lipoprotein levels
coronary heart disease and, 189-193
high-density, 189-191
low-density, *see* Low-density lipoproteins
Lipoprotein metabolism, 184-185
Lipoprotein metabolism disorders, therapy for, 201-202
Lipoprotein structure, 184-187
Lipoprotein-X, liver disease and, 187
Liver
ketone formation in, 159
in purine processing, 257-258
Liver cells, in ethanol consumption, 416
Liver disease
ethanol metabolism and, 418-420
lipoprotein-X and, 187
Low-density lipoproteins, 189-190
apoprotein and, 201

Low-density lipoproteins (*cont'd*)
cholesterol metabolism and, 195-196
in familial hypercholesterolemia, 201-202
ferritin-labeled, 198
possible mechanisms of, 192-193
Lp(a), *see* Lipoprotein Lp(a)
LP-X, *see* Lipoprotein-X
Lubrol PX detergent, 4
Lymphocytes, mitogen-stimulated, 284

Magnesium depletion, 365-366
Magnesium homeostasis, kidney in, 364-365
Magnesium metabolism, 364-366
Malnutrition
cellular growth and, 379-386
DNA synthesis in, 385
pituitary growth hormone and, 381
protein synthesis and, 381-382
RNA catabolism and, 385
thyroid hormone and, 380-381
Maturity-onset-type diabetes
carbohydrate intolerance in, 43
diabetic retinopathy and, 67
gastric inhibitory polypeptide in, 48
glucose tolerance test and, 57
growth disturbances in, 77-78
islet-cell antibodies in, 40
insulin secretion in, 45-47
MBMT, *see* Minimum basement membrane thickness
MCPA, *see* Methylenecyclopropylacetic acid
MEOS, *see* Microsomal ethanol-oxidizing system
Messenger RNA, *see* mRNA
Metabolic acidosis, 229-230
Methylenecyclopropylacetic acid, 239-241
Acyl-CoA dehydrogenases and, 241-244
Microsomal ethanol oxidizing system, 413, 416, 418
Microvascular permeability, changes in, 63-64
Milk, in alcoholic gastritis, 427-428
Minimum basement membrane thickness, in diabetes, 65
Mitogenic stimulation, in adenosine metabolism, 266-267
MOD, *see* Maturity-onset-type diabetes
Monoamine oxidase, in HPRT deficiency, 291
mRNA
cAMP and, 10-11
vitamin D and, 337
Multiple Risk Factor Intervention Trial, 212
Muscle, alanine synthesis in, 153-156
Muscle metabolism, of branched-chain amino acids, 156-157
Mystromys albicaudatus, 65

NADH (reduced nicotinamide adenine dinucleotide), 235
in ethanol metabolism, 411-412
NADP (nicotinamide adenine dinucleotide phosphate), 221
NADPH (reduced nicotinamide adenine dinucleotide phosphate), 221-222
in ethanol oxidation, 413-414
NADPH: NADP system, in ethanol metabolism, 416-417
National Heart, Lung, and Blood Institute, 212
Nephrolithiasis, *see* Renal stone disease
Neurological defect, biochemical mechanism and, 291-292
Niacin, *see* Nicotinic acid
Nicotinamide adenine dinucleotide phosphate, *see* NADP
Nicotinic acid, in hyperlipidemia, 210
Nitro compounds, cGMP and, 15-16
Non-ADH pathways, in ethanol oxidation, 413-415
Norepinephrine, scorpion toxin and, 114
NTPH (nucleoside triphosphate pyrophosphohydrolase) deficiency, 298-299
Nucleotide pool, growth and, 381-382
Nutrition
genetic obesity and, 386-389
growth and, 379-392
pregnancy and, 389-392

Obesity, *see also* Hyperphagia
adipose mass and, 173
behavior modification and, 176-178
core problem in, 170
genetic, 386-389
hyperlipidemia and, 209
hyperphagia in, 170-171
hypothetical defended variables in, 170-173
insulin levels in, 175
jejunoileal shunt and, 179-180

Obesity (*cont'd*)
ketogenic diet in, 175
as life style, 172-173
protein-sparing modified fast in, 174-175
starvation in, 175-176
treatment of, 169-181
Oligophrenia, 291
Orotic acid, 273
Orotic aciduria
hyperammonemia and, 305
in other errors of metabolism, 306
in PNP deficiency, 285
Orthophosphate, inorganic, 263
Osteomalacia
of anticonvulsant therapy, 349
barbiturates and, 351
Overeaters Anonymous, 178
Overweight problem, *see* Obesity
5-Oxoproline, 230
5-Oxoprolinuria, 219, 229-230
biochemical basis of, 232-235
γ-glutamyl cycle and, 232
GSH and, 237
Oxypurine excretion, allopurinol in, 289

Pancreas, transplantation of, 78
Pancreatic D cells, role of, 120
Pancreatic exocrine function, somatostatin and, 119
Pancreatic islet cell antibodies, 38-40
Pancreozymin, 14, 16
Parathyroid action, hypocalcemic phase of, 331
Parathyroid disorders, cyclic nucleotides and, 21
Parathyroidectomy, low calcium diet and, 330
Parathyroid glands, vitamin D and, 340
Parathyroid hormone, 328-330
bone and, 330-331
calcium regulation, 327
cAMP and, 366
cGMP and, 16
divalent ion control of, 328-330
immunoassay for, 332-333
kidney and, 331-332
in phosphate metabolism, 356-357
Patching, of receptors, 266
Pentanoic acids, branched-chain, 243
Pentolamine, 114
Phenformin, in hypoglycemic therapy, 87-88
Phenoxybenzine, 114
Phenylalanine
hydroxylation system and, 221-222
tyrosine and, 220
Phenylalanine hydroxylation, 221-229
Phenylalanine-restricted diet, 227
Phenylketonuria, 219-221
as balanced polymorphism, 226-227
clinical, 226-229
cross-reacting material in, 222
defect in, 222-223
dietary treatment of, 227-228
IQ and, 227-228
maternal, 229
Phosphate
in bone, 328
renal handling of, 331
Phosphate absorption, in uremia, 352
Phosphate depletion, 359-364
bone cells and, 363-364
soft tissue and, 363
Phosphate level, vitamin D and, 337
Phosphate metabolism, 356-364
parathyroid hormone in, 357
serum calcium level in, 358
vitamin D and, 358-359
Phosphatė restriction, sex difference in, 363
Phosphodiesterase inhibitors, 14
cGMP and, 17
Phosphodiesterase-resistant cGMP analogue, 19
Phosphoribosylpyrophosphate synthetase
APRT and, 260
increased activity of, 294-295
inheritance of, 295
kinase and, 273
PHA addition and, 266
PNP deficiency and, 285
Phosphorus, dietary intake of, 356-357
Phosphorus regulation, kidney and, 331-332
Phenylketonuria, in children, 227-228
PICA, *see* Pancreatic-islet-cell antibodies
Pima Indians
blood glucose levels in, 54
cholesterol levels in, 73-74
diabetic retinopathy in, 66
hyperglucagonemia in, 123-124
Pitressin, 359
Pituitary growth hormone, in malnutrition, 381, 391

PKU, *see* Phenylketonuria
Plasma IRG, hyperglycemia and, 123
Plasma proteins, changes in, 62-63
Platelet aggregation, cGMP and, 19-20
PN, *see* Pyrimidine-5′-nucleotidase
PNP (purine nucleoside phosphorylase) deficiency, 278-286
  blood and serum metabolites in, 282-283
  clinical presentation of, 278-280
  erythrocyte metabolism and, 283-284
  immunodeficiency disease and, 265
  Lesch-Nyhan syndrome and, 285
  possible mechanisms of, 284-285
  PP-ribose-P deficiency and, 285
  urine metabolites in, 280-282
PNP enzyme activity, erythrocyte metabolism and, 283-284
Postglucose plasma level, in diabetes mellitus, 54-56
Postheparin plasma, lipoprotein lipase activity of, 205
Postprandial plasma glucose response, 81
PP-ribose-P, *see* Phosphoribosylpyrophosphate synthetase
PP-ribose-P-glutamine amidotransferase, 261
Pregnancy
  alanine aminotransferase in, 390
  nutrition and, 389-392
  protein restriction in, 391
  vitamin D and, 341-342
Primary hypogammaglobulinemia, 287-288
Probucol, in hyperlipidemia, 210-211
Proglucagon, 102, 104
Proinsulin, transformation to insulin, 48
Propranolol, glucagon and, 114
Prostaglandin endoperoxide, 19
Prostaglandins
  cAMP synthesis and, 13-14
  cGMP and, 13-14
  glucagon and, 115
Protein kinases, activation of with cAMP or cGMP, 10-11
Protein-sparing modified fast, in obesity treatment, 80, 174-176
Protein storage, in pregnancy, 389-390
Protein synthesis
  RNA and, 382
  in malnutrition, 381-382
Pseudohypoparathyroidism, vitamin D and, 354
PSMF, *see* Protein-sparing modified fast
PTH, *see* Parathyroid hormone
PTX, *see* Parathyroidectomy
Purine metabolism
  disorders of, 253-307
  liver and, 257-258
  role of, 257-269
Purine nucleoside phosphorylase deficiency, 253, 278-286
Purine 5′-nucleotidase deficiency, in primary hypogammaglobulinemia, 286-287
Purine overproduction
  in children, 253-254
  in cultured fibroblasts, 284
  in HPRT deficiency, 292
Purines
  in ammonia production, 258-260
  immune system and, 263-266
  in malignant cells, 306
Purine synthesis, regulation of, 260-263
Pyrimidine metabolism
  abnormalities of, 304-306
  disorders of, 253-307
  drug and nutritional factors in, 305
Pyrimidine-5′-nucleotidase deficiency, 304-305
Pyrimidine nucleotide, ADA deficiency and, 270
Pyrimidines, in malignant cells, 306-307
Pyroglutamic acid, 230, *see also* 5-Oxoproline
Pyroglutamic aciduria, 229, *see also* 5-Oxoprolinuria

Renal failure
  hyperlipidemia and, 207-208
  vitamin D and, 350, 353
Renal stone disease
  classification of, 400-401
  crystalloid excretion and, 401-404
  cystine and xanthine stones in, 403-404
Renal stone disease
  diagnosis of, 399
  hypercalciuria and, 401-403
  hyperoxaluria and, 402-403
  hyperuricosuria and, 403, 407
  idiopathic, 405-406
  incidence of, 400
  low calcium diet in, 407
  metabolic aspects of, 399-407
  and physicochemical urine changes, 404-405
  treatment in, 406-407

Renal transplantation, hyperlipidemia in, 207-208
Retinopathy, diabetic, *see* Diabetic retinopathy
Reye's syndrome, Jamaican vomiting sickness and, 245
Ribavirin, 306
Rickets, vitamin D and, 344-346, 350, 360
RNA
in malnutrition, 383, 385
messenger, *see* mRNA
in protein synthesis, 382
RNA synthesis, nucleotides and, 381
RNA virus infections, in animals, 306

Salivary glands, phosphate regulation and, 332
SCID, *see* Severe combined immunodeficiency disease
Scorpion toxin, norepinephrine and, 114
Secretin, cGMP and, 16
Serine dehydrogenase, malnutrition and, 381
Serotonin, cGMP and, 14
Severe combined immunodeficiency disease, 269-277
β-sitosterolemia, 203-204
Smooth-muscle contraction, cGMP and, 17-18
Sodium azide, guanylate cyclase and, 7
Sodium oxonate, urate and, 303
Solanum glaucophyllum, 337
Solanum malacoxylon, 354
Somatostatin, 54, 117-128
blood xylose and, 144
endocrine actions of, 118-120
gastrointestinal function and, 144
gastrointestinal tract and, 119
glucose and, 113, 143-146
hypoglucagonemia and, 149-150
IRG and, 120
norepinephrine and, 114
pancreatic, 118-120
paracrine actions of, 118
prolonged infusion of, 149-150
splanchnic blood flow and, 145
as tetradecapeptide, 144
SSPI, *see* Steady state plasma insulin
Starvation
carcass glycogen and, 147
glucose levels and, 146-147
hypoglucagonemia in, 391
obesity and, 176
Steady-state plasma insulin, 50
Stone-formers
apatite-struvite, 406, *see also* Renal stone disease
idiopathic, 399, 403
Substance P, glucagon and, 115
Sulfonylureas, in hypoglycemia therapy, 86-87

Take Off Pounds Sensibly, 178
T-cell dysfunction, in immunodeficiency disease, 253
Testosterone metabolism, "hangover" and, 421
Tetrahydrobiopterin, 221-222
6-Thioguanine, as differentiation inducer, 264
Thymidine
in ADA deficiency, 271-272
cGMP and, 267
in human lymphocytes, 263
Thymidine kinase
in adipose tissue, 386-388
malnutrition and, 384
Thyroid hormone, growth and, 380
Tolbutamide, 86-87
Triiodothyronine, in pregnancy, 391
Triton X-100 detergent, 4
Tryptophan pyrrolase, 390
Tumors, cyclic nucleotides and, 20-21
Tyrosine, phenylalanine and, 220

University Group Diabetes Program, 86, 88
Uremia, calcium and phosphate absorption in, 352
Uric acid
kidneys and, 303
overproduction of, 299
Urinary tract calculi, xanthine and, 288
Urine composition, renal stone disease and, 404-405

Vasopressin, 359
Vitamin D
actions of, 337-342
alcoholism and, 347-348
assays for, 342-343
biliary cirrhosis and, 347
bone cells, and, 340
in calcium homeostasis, 333
chemistry and metabolism of, 334-337
cholecalciferol-25-hydroxylase and, 334
collagen and, 340

Vitamin D (*cont'd*)
in diabetes, 354
25-hydroxy-vitamin D_3 and, 333-343
international unit of, 333
malabsorption of, 346-347
muscle and, 341
neonatal-maternal relationships and, 341
parathyroid glands and, 340-341
phosphate depletion and, 361
in phosphate metabolism, 358-359
in plants, 337
plasma calcium levels and, 339
plasma transport of, 342
in pregnancy, 341-342
in renal failure, 350-351
rickets and, 344-346, 350
sterols of, 334-337, 342-343
toxicity of, 343-344
Vitamin D action, absence of, 344-355
Vitamin D deficiency, 344-347
parathyroid hormone and, 331
Vitamin-D-dependent rickets, 344-346, 350
Vitamin D_3, intestinal absorption of, 349
VLDL (very low density lipoproteins), 193-194
Vomiting, 230, 238-239

Weight Watchers, 178
World Health Organization, 212

Xanthine
in ureteral calculi, 254
in urinary tract calculi, 288
Xanthine oxidase activity, 289
Xanthinuria, 254
hereditary, 288
Xanthomatosis, cerebrotendinous, 203-204
Xyl-A (9-β-D-xylofuranosyl-adenine), 268
Xylose absorption, somatostatin and, 119-120

MIX
Papier aus verantwortungsvollen Quellen
Paper from responsible sources
FSC® C105338
FSC
www.fsc.org

If you have any concerns about our products,
you can contact us on
ProductSafety@springernature.com

In case Publisher is established outside the EU,
the EU authorized representative is:
Springer Nature Customer Service Center GmbH
Europaplatz 3, 69115 Heidelberg, Germany

Printed by Libri Plureos GmbH
in Hamburg, Germany